SECOND EDITION

KAPLAN & SADOCK'S

CONCISE TEXTBOOK OF CHILD AND ADOLESCENT PSYCHIATRY

SECOND EDITION

KAPLAN & SADOCK'S

CONCISE TEXTBOOK OF CHILD AND ADOLESCENT PSYCHIATRY

EDITORS

Caroly S. Pataki, M.D.
Health Sciences Clinical Professor
Department of Psychiatry and Biobehavioral Sciences
David Geffen School of Medicine at UCLA
Los Angeles, California

Robert J. Boland, M.D.
Senior Vice President and Chief of Staff
The Menninger Clinic
Professor and Vice Chair
Menninger Department of Psychiatry and Behavioral Sciences
The Brown Foundation Endowed Chair in Psychiatry
Baylor College of Medicine
Houston, Texas

Marcia L. Verduin, M.D.
Associate Dean for Students
Professor of Psychiatry
University of Central Florida College of Medicine
Orlando, Florida

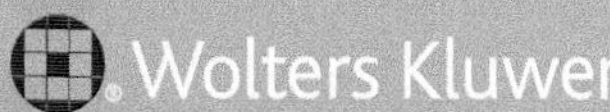

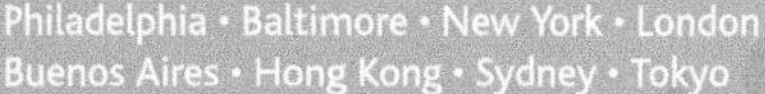

Acquisitions Editor: James Sherman
Development Editor: Ariel S. Winter
Senior Editorial Coordinator: Sean Hanrahan
Marketing Manager: Kristen Watrud
Production Project Manager: Matthew West
Manager, Graphic Arts & Design: Stephen Druding
Manufacturing Coordinator: Lisa Bowling
Prepress Vendor: Aptara, Inc.

2nd edition

9 8 7 6 5 4 3 2 1

Printed in the United States of America

Library of Congress Cataloging-in-Publication Data

Names: Sadock, Benjamin J., 1933- Kaplan & Sadock's concise textbook of child and adolescent psychiatry. | Pataki, Caroly S., editor. | Boland, Robert Joseph, editor. | Verduin, Marcia L., editor.
Title: Kaplan and Sadock's concise textbook of child and adolescent psychiatry / [edited by] Caroly S. Pataki, Robert J. Boland, Marcia L. Verduin.
Other titles: Concise textbook of child and adolescent psychiatry | Kaplan & Sadock's synopsis of psychiatry.
Description: Second edition. | Philadelphia : Wolters Kluwer, [2026] | Condensed version of the child and adolescent sections of Kaplan & Sadock's Synopsis of Psychiatry, twelfth edition, 2022. | Includes bibliographical references and index. | Summary: "This derivative text presents updated clinical material on child and adolescent psychiatry from the best-selling Kaplan and Sadock's Synopsis of Psychiatry. Coverage includes clinically relevant information on normal and abnormal development; examination; neuroimaging; learning, communication and behavioral disorders; adolescent substance use disorder; forensic issues; and the spectrum of psychiatric problems such as depression and bipolar disorders. Treatment chapters include a broad range of psychopharmacologic and psychotherapeutic techniques, as well as the many controversies related to appropriate use of medication in children. The proposed 2nd Edition will be derived from the 12th Edition of Kaplan & Sadock's Synopsis of Psychiatry with Dr. Pataki providing updates and additions as necessary. Some additional topics including Racism and Diversity, LGBTQ topics, internet gaming, and the impact of social media on children and adolescents will also be added"– Provided by publisher.
Identifiers: LCCN 2025004537 (print) | LCCN 2025004538 (ebook) | ISBN 9781975222925 (paperback) | ISBN 9781975222932 (epub)
Subjects: MESH: Mental Disorders–diagnosis | Mental Disorders–therapy | Child | Adolescent
Classification: LCC RC454 (print) | LCC RC454 (ebook) | NLM WS 350 | DDC 616.89–dc23/eng/20250515
LC record available at https://lccn.loc.gov/2025004537
LC ebook record available at https://lccn.loc.gov/2025004538

shop.lww.com

MPP0625

To my family and readers of this book who make my work in this field meaningful.

—Caroly S. Pataki

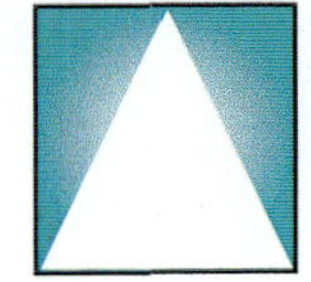

Preface

The Kaplan and Sadock series comes in a myriad of sizes. The *Concise Textbook of Child and Adolescent Psychiatry* is one of the briefest books in the series. It is a condensed version of the child and adolescent sections of *Kaplan & Sadock's Synopsis of Psychiatry*, twelfth edition, which is a reduced version of the child and adolescent chapters within the *Comprehensive Textbook of Psychiatry*. The *Synopsis* covers both the behavioral sciences and the diagnosis and treatment of psychiatric disorders.

The *Concise Textbook of Child and Adolescent Psychiatry* focuses on the most clinically relevant chapters. It is designed for readers who need a compact but thorough clinical child and adolescent psychiatry book.

The *Concise Textbook of Child and Adolescent Psychiatry* is intended for psychiatrists and nonpsychiatric physicians, medical students, psychologists, social workers, psychiatric nurses, and other mental health professionals, such as occupational and art therapists, among others.

The organization here follows the organization used in the *Synopsis*. Whenever possible, disorders are grouped syndromally. For example, various depressive disorders' phenomenology is presented before discussing diagnosis and then treatment. This approach was a strategic choice, as much modern research no longer groups patients by clinical diagnoses, and many incorporate larger groupings, such as patients with depression or patients with psychosis.

The overarching philosophy in this work is that mental health is a part of physical health, and one needs to discuss psychiatric disease within the context of all medicine. Even the term "mind–body" seems obsolete, implying a divide that does not exist.

COMPREHENSIVE TEACHING SYSTEM

The *Concise Textbook of Child and Adolescent Psychiatry* is one part of a comprehensive system developed to facilitate the teaching of psychiatry and the behavioral sciences. At the head of the system is the *Comprehensive Textbook of Psychiatry*, which is global in depth and scope; it is designed for and used by psychiatrists, behavioral scientists, and all mental health professionals. The *Synopsis of Psychiatry* is a briefer, highly modified, and current version suitable for medical students, psychiatric residents, practicing psychiatrists, and mental health professionals. The *Concise Textbook of Child and Adolescent Psychiatry* describes all psychiatric disorders, including their diagnosis and treatment in adolescents and children.

Another part of the system, *Study Guide and Self-Examination Review of Psychiatry*, consists of multiple-choice questions and answers; it is designed for students of psychiatry and for clinical psychiatrists who require a review of the behavioral sciences and general psychiatry in preparation for a variety of examinations. The questions are consistent with the format used by most standardized examinations. Other parts of the system include the *Pocket Handbook of Clinical Psychiatry,* and the *Pocket Handbook of Psychiatric Drug Treatment*. They are designed and written to be carried by clinical trainees and practicing physicians, whatever their specialty, as a practical reference. Together, these books create multiple approaches to the teaching, study, and learning of psychiatry.

CLASSIFICATION OF DISORDERS DSM-5-TR

The *Diagnostic and Statistical Manual of Mental Disorders, Fifth Edition, Text Revision (DSM-5-TR)* was published by the American Psychiatric Association in 2022.

DSM-5-TR contains the official nomenclature used by psychiatrists and other mental health professionals in the United States, and in many other countries. It involved more than 200 experts in the field, many of whom contributed to DSM-5. The psychiatric disorders discussed in the textbook are consistent with and follow that nosology. Four new review groups (Culture, Sex and Gender, Suicide, and Forensic) participated in developing DSM-5-TR.

DSM-5-TR is not directly reproduced in prose or table form in the *Concise Textbook of Child and Adolescent Psychiatry*. It is expected that most child and adolescent psychiatrists and trainees will already have access to the DSM-5-TR; if not, it is highly recommended. Some tables outline the primary symptoms, time courses, and other criteria associated with the significant diagnoses to aid the reader with diagnostic reasoning.

ICD-11

Readers should be aware of the classification system developed by the World Health Organization (WHO), the *International Statistical Classification of Diseases and Related Health Problems* (ICD-11). ICD-11 was adopted by the World Health Assembly in 2019 and came into effect globally on January 1, 2022.

ICD-11, which is fully electronic, is the international standard for up-to-date systematic coding of all medical diagnoses and all psychiatric disorders.

Although many diagnostic categories overlap within DSM-5-TR and ICD-11, certain disorders may differ in specific criteria. Additionally, differences in the number of symptoms and the severity criteria can vary for some disorders according to DSM-5-TR and ICD-11.

There are textual differences between DSM and ICD, but according to treaties between the United States and the WHO, the diagnostic code numbers are identical to ensure uniform national and international psychiatric statistics. ICD diagnoses and numerical codes are accepted by Medicare, Medicaid, and private insurance companies for reimbursement purposes.

CASE HISTORIES

Case histories are an integral part of the *Concise Textbook of Child and Adolescent Psychiatry*. They are used extensively throughout the text to add clarity and bring to life the clinical disorders described. Cases come from various sources. Many case studies have been preserved from past editions of various textbooks within the series since they expertly illustrate the concepts described. We thank the many contributors for allowing the *Concise Textbook of Child and Adolescent Psychiatry* to use these cases in the current editions.

ACKNOWLEDGMENTS

A special thanks to the editorial team at Wolters Kluwer, particular thanks go to our Acquisitions Editors, Chris Teja, and James Sherman, Senior Editorial Coordinator Sean Hanrahan, and Ariel S. Winter, our Senior Development Editor.

Our deepest thanks go to Benjamin and Virginia Sadock, who created an immensely valuable series of references. It is our honor to help continue their tradition of scholarship, scientific pursuit, and humanism.

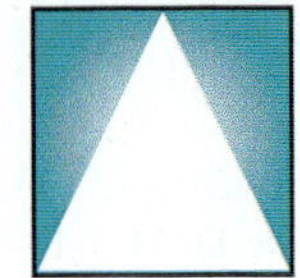

Acknowledgments

We deeply appreciate the work of our colleagues whose contributions to the eleventh edition of *Kaplan & Sadock's Comprehensive Textbook of Psychiatry* have been incorporated into this book.

Child Maltreatment—*Heather Williams, M.D. and Bradley Freeman, M.D.*

School Consultation and Collaborating with the Educational System—*Sheryl Kataoka, M.D., M.S.H.S., Ilaina Blum, M.A., M.F.T., Edward Castelo, M.D., and Roya Ijadi-Maghsoodi, M.D., M.S.H.P.M.*

Pediatric Sleep Disorders—*Jess P. Shatkin, M.D., M.P.H., and Anna Ivanenko, M.D., Ph.D.*

Internet Gaming Disorder in Youth—*Michael Feldmeier, M.D., Michael Ogata, M.D., Caroly Pataki, M.D., and Roxy Szeftel, M.D.*

Gay, Bisexual, Transgender, Queer/Questioning, Intersex, and Asexual (LGBTQIA) Youth—*Natalia Ramos, M.D., M.P.H., Serena Chang, M.D., B.A., Mikko Thelwell, M.D., M.P.H.*

Racism and Discrimination's Impact on the Health and Well-Being of Developing Children and Adolescents—*Wanjiku F.M. Njoroge, M.D., Ewurama Sackey, M.D., Nana Asabere, M.D., and Eraka Bath, M.D.*

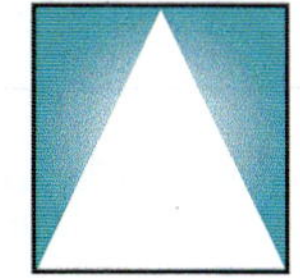

About the Editors

Caroly S. Pataki, M.D.

Dr. Pataki is Health Sciences Clinical Professor of Psychiatry & Biobehavioral Sciences at the University of California, David Geffen School of Medicine at UCLA.

Dr. Pataki has devoted most of her career to being an educator, curriculum developer, mentor, and writer/editor of educational materials for child and adolescent psychiatry trainees and junior faculty in the child and adolescent psychiatry field. Dr. Pataki served as the Associate Director of Training and Education for the University of California, Los Angeles Child and Adolescent Psychiatry Fellowship program for 11 years.

Following that, Dr. Pataki became the Director of Training and Education and the Chief of Child and Adolescent Psychiatry at the University of Southern California's Division of Child and Adolescent Psychiatry during her tenure on the faculty for 6 years.

Dr. Pataki has held clinical leadership positions in the five medical centers where she has worked. Dr. Pataki was the first Medical Director of a Children's Psychiatry Inpatient unit at the State University of New York at Stony Brook Medical Center. Following that position, Dr. Pataki became the Medical Director of the Adolescent Psychiatry Partial Hospital program at the NYU/Bellevue Medical Center. While a faculty member at NYU Medical Center, Dr. Pataki also served as the Division Chief of Child and Adolescent Psychiatry at Lenox Hill Hospital, an affiliate of NYU. Dr. Pataki was then recruited to UCLA Medical Center where she served as the Medical Director of the Adolescent Psychiatry Partial Hospital program.

Dr. Pataki is currently a consultant to the Los Angeles County Edelman Children's Dependency Court as a member of the Juvenile Court Mental Health Service. In that role, she provides consultations to attorneys and judicial officers regarding optimal psychiatric treatment of children and adolescents in the child welfare system.

Dr. Pataki first worked with Dr. Benjamin Sadock in the early 1990s as a lecturer on child and adolescent psychiatry topics in the annual Bellevue/NYU Medical School Comprehensive Psychiatry Review course, which Dr. Sadock led. She then lectured on child and adolescent psychiatry topics in the Bellevue/NYU Medical School Postgraduate Medical School Faculty Psychiatry Oral Board Review course, led by Dr. Sadock.

Dr. Pataki was recruited by Dr. Sadock to write and edit for the Kaplan & Sadock series, starting with the *Study Guide and Self-examination Review for Kaplan and Sadock's Synopsis of Psychiatry* (fifth edition), and *Kaplan & Sadock's Synopsis of Psychiatry* (seventh edition) in 1994. Dr. Pataki remains a writer and editor for the Kaplan & Sadock book series. Dr. Pataki became the section editor for the Child and Adolescent Psychiatry chapters in *Kaplan & Sadock's Comprehensive Textbook of Psychiatry* in 1998. She has remained in that role until the present.

Dr. Pataki's collaboration with Kaplan & Sadock's textbook series has enabled her to make a significant contribution to the training and education of child and adolescent psychiatrists over the years. Dr. Pataki's longstanding collaboration with Kaplan & Sadock's textbook series has been a meaningful and fulfilling educational activity for her.

Robert J. Boland, M.D.

Dr. Boland is the chief of staff and senior vice president at The Menninger Clinic in Houston, Texas. He is also a vice-chair of the Menninger Department of Psychiatry and Behavioral Sciences at Baylor College of Medicine (BCM) and the Brown Foundation Endowed Chair in Psychiatry at BCM.

Before coming to Houston, he served as vice-chair of education and director of the psychiatry residency program at Brigham and Women's Hospital in Boston, Massachusetts, and as an associate professor of psychiatry at Harvard Medical School. He is board-certified in psychiatry with expertise in medical education, consultation-liaison, and geriatric psychiatry. He is an alumnus of Georgetown University, where he earned his undergraduate and medical degrees. Before joining Brigham and Women's Hospital, Dr. Boland had an 18-year tenure at the Alpert School of Medicine at Brown University, Providence, Rhode Island. For more than 30 years, he has been an active member of the American Psychiatric Association. Dr. Boland is the former president of the American Association of Directors of Psychiatric Residency Training, the Academy of Consultation-Liaison Psychiatry, and the Association for Academic Psychiatry. He is currently a Director of the American Board of Psychiatry and Neurology.

Dr. Boland has authored or co-authored over 100 publications and is a frequent speaker at grand rounds and national meetings. In addition, he is the coeditor of the Kaplan and Sadock series of textbooks, which are the most popular texts in psychiatry. Dr. Boland is also the co-host of the Menninger Clinic's Mind Dive Podcast.

Marcia L. Verduin, M.D.

Dr. Verduin is the Associate Dean for Students and a Professor of Psychiatry at the University of Central Florida College of Medicine in Orlando, Florida. She graduated from the University of Florida College of Medicine and completed her residency training and addiction psychiatry fellowship at the Medical University of South Carolina. She is a Fellow of the American College of Psychiatrists and a Distinguished Fellow of both the American Psychiatric Association and the Association for Academic Psychiatry. In 2007, Dr. Verduin became the first psychiatry faculty member at UCF's new medical school, where she played an integral role in developing the overarching undergraduate medical education curriculum and securing LCME accreditation.

In addition to her roles at the University of Central Florida College of Medicine, Dr. Verduin currently serves as the President of the American College of Psychiatrists. She is a Past President for the Association for Academic Psychiatry, Immediate Past Chair of the Association of American Medical College's (AAMC) Group on Student Affairs, prior Associate Editor of the Psychiatry Residency In-Training Examination, and has served as an examiner for the American Board of Psychiatry and Neurology.

Dr. Verduin has a special interest in combatting the burden of stigma associated with mental health disorders, particularly in faith-based communities. She has been invited to speak around the world, including in Australia, New Zealand, Fiji, the Philippines, Southeast Asia, and Nigeria. Her contributions to advancing mental health care in those areas of the world have been covered in various U.S. and international media.

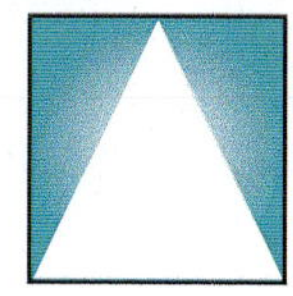

Contents

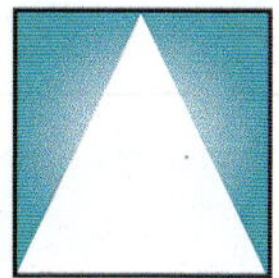

1 Infant, Child, and Adolescent Development

Development throughout infancy, childhood, and adolescence consists of a continuous interplay between biologic predisposition and environmental experiences, forming the basis of current conceptualizations of development. There is much evidence that observed developmental outcomes evolve from interactions between particular genetic substrates and specific environmental events. For example, the serotonin transporter gene sensitizes a child with early adverse experiences of abuse or neglect to increased risk for later development of a depressive disorder. Also, the degree of resilience and adaptation, that is, the ability to withstand adversity without damaging effects, is likely to be mediated by endogenous glucocorticoids, cytokines, and neurotrophins. Thus, allostasis, the process of achieving stability in the face of adverse environmental events, results from interactions between specific environmental challenges and particular genetic backgrounds that combine to result in a response. Adverse childhood experiences (ACEs) are likely to alter the trajectory of development in a given individual, and during early development, the brain is especially vulnerable to injury. Acquiring subtle social skills, for example, relates to changes in the adolescent brain. Adolescents' keen abilities, competencies, and interests in a host of technologic advances—including the Internet and ever-changing social media, for example—shed some light on their potential to adapt to new and challenging demands.

PRENATAL, INFANT, AND CHILD

The phases of development described in this section include the following: prenatal is defined as the time frame from conception to 8 weeks; the fetus, from 8 weeks to birth; infancy, from birth to 15 months; the toddler period, from 15 months to 2½ years; the preschool period, from 2½ years to 6 years; and the middle years, from 6 to 12 years.

PRENATAL

Historically, the analysis of human development began with birth. The influence of endogenous and exogenous in utero factors, however, now requires that developmental schemes consider intrauterine events. The infant is not a tabula rasa, a smooth slate upon which outside influences etch patterns. On the contrary, myriad factors within the womb have already influenced the newborn. For example, the studies of Stella Chess and Alexander Thomas (described later) have demonstrated a wide range of temperamental differences among newborns. Maternal stress, through the production of adrenal hormones, also influences the behavioral characteristics of newborns.

The time frame in which the development of the embryo and fetus occurs is known as the prenatal period. After implantation, the egg begins to divide and is known as an embryo. Growth and development occur at a rapid pace; by the end of 8 weeks, the shape is recognizably human, and the embryo has become a fetus. Figure 1-1 illustrates a sonogram of a 9-week and 15-week fetus in utero.

The fetus maintains an internal equilibrium that, with variable effects, interacts continuously with the intrauterine environment. In general, most disorders that occur are multifactorial—the result of a combination of effects, some of which can be cumulative. Damage at the fetal stage usually has a more global impact than damage after birth, because rapidly growing organs are the most vulnerable. Boys are more vulnerable to developmental damage than girls are; geneticists recognize that in humans and animals, female fetuses show a propensity for greater biologic vigor than male fetuses, possibly because of the second X chromosome in the female.

Prenatal Life

Much biologic activity occurs in utero. A fetus is involved in a variety of behaviors that are necessary for adaptation outside the womb. For example, a fetus sucks on thumb and fingers; folds and unfolds its body, and eventually assumes a position in which its occiput is in an anterior vertex position, which is the position in which fetuses usually exit the uterus.

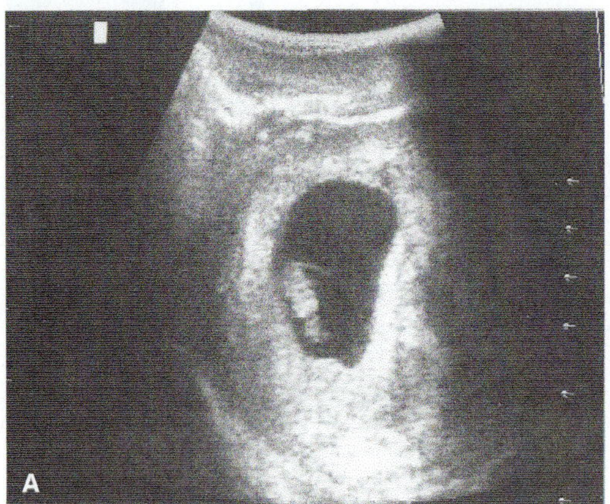

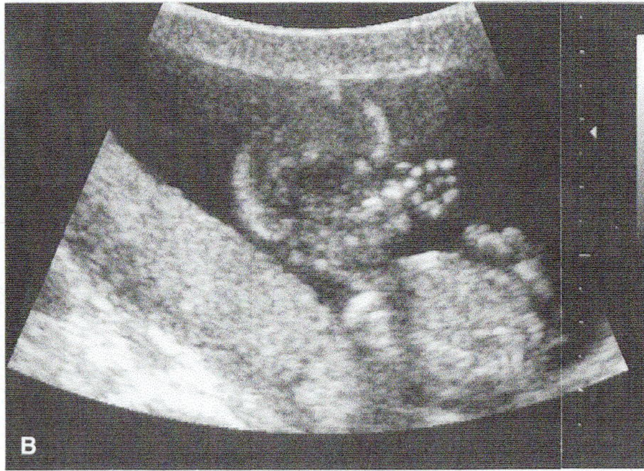

FIGURE 1-1. **A**: Sonogram of fetus at 9 weeks. **B**: Same fetus at 15 weeks. (Courtesy K.C. Attwell, M.D.)

Behavior. Pregnant women are extraordinarily sensitive to fetal movements. They describe their unborn babies as active or passive, as kicking vigorously or rolling around, as quiet when the mothers are active, but as kicking as soon as the mothers try to rest.

Women usually detect fetal movements 16 to 20 weeks into the pregnancy; the fetus can be artificially set into total body motion by in utero stimulation of its ventral skin surfaces by the 14th week. The fetus may be able to hear by the 18th week, and it responds to loud noises with muscle contractions, movements, and an increased heart rate. A bright light flashed on the abdominal wall of the 20-week pregnant woman causes changes in fetal heart rate and position. The retinal structures begin to function at that time. Eyelids open at 7 months. Smell and taste develop then, and the fetus can respond to substances injected into the amniotic sac, such as contrast medium. Some reflexes present at birth exist in utero: the grasp reflex, which appears at 17 weeks; the Moro (startle) reflex, which appears at 25 weeks; and the sucking reflex, which appears at about 28 weeks.

Nervous System. The nervous system arises from the neural plate, which is a dorsal ectodermal thickening that appears on about day 16 of gestation. By the sixth week, part of the neural tube becomes the cerebral vesicle, which later becomes the cerebral hemispheres (Fig. 1-2).

The cerebral cortex begins to develop by the 10th week, but layers do not appear until the sixth month of pregnancy; the sensory cortex and the motor cortex form before the association cortex. Some brain function has been detected in utero by fetal encephalographic responses to sound. The human brain weighs about 350 g at birth and 1,450 g at full adult development, a fourfold increase, mainly in the neocortex. This increase is almost entirely because of the growth in the number and branching of dendrites establishing new connections. After birth, the number of new neurons is negligible. Uterine contractions can contribute to fetal neural development by causing the developing neural network to receive and transmit sensory impulses.

Pruning. Pruning refers to the programmed elimination during the development of neurons, synapses, axons, and other brain structures from the original number, present at birth, to a lesser number. Thus, the developing brain contains structures and cellular elements that are absent in the older brain. The fetal brain generates more neurons than it will need for adult life. For example, in the visual cortex, neurons increase in number from birth to 3 years of age, at which point they diminish in number. The adult brain contains fewer neural connections than were present during the early and middle years of childhood. About twice as many synapses are present in certain parts of the cerebral cortex during early postnatal life than during adulthood.

Pruning occurs to rid the nervous system of cells that have served their function in the development of the brain. Some neurons, for example, exist to produce neurotrophic or growth factors and are programmed to die once they complete their task, a process called *apoptosis*.

These observations imply that the immature brain can be vulnerable in locations that lack sensitivity to injury later on. The developing white matter of the human brain before 32 weeks of gestation is especially sensitive to damage from hypoxic and ischemic injury and metabolic insults. Neurotransmitter receptors located on synaptic terminals are subject to injury from excessive stimulation by excitatory amino acids, (e.g., glutamate, aspartate), a process referred to as excitotoxicity. This process may be relevant to the etiology of disorders such as schizophrenia.

Maternal Stress

Maternal stress correlates with high levels of stress hormones (epinephrine, norepinephrine, and adrenocor-

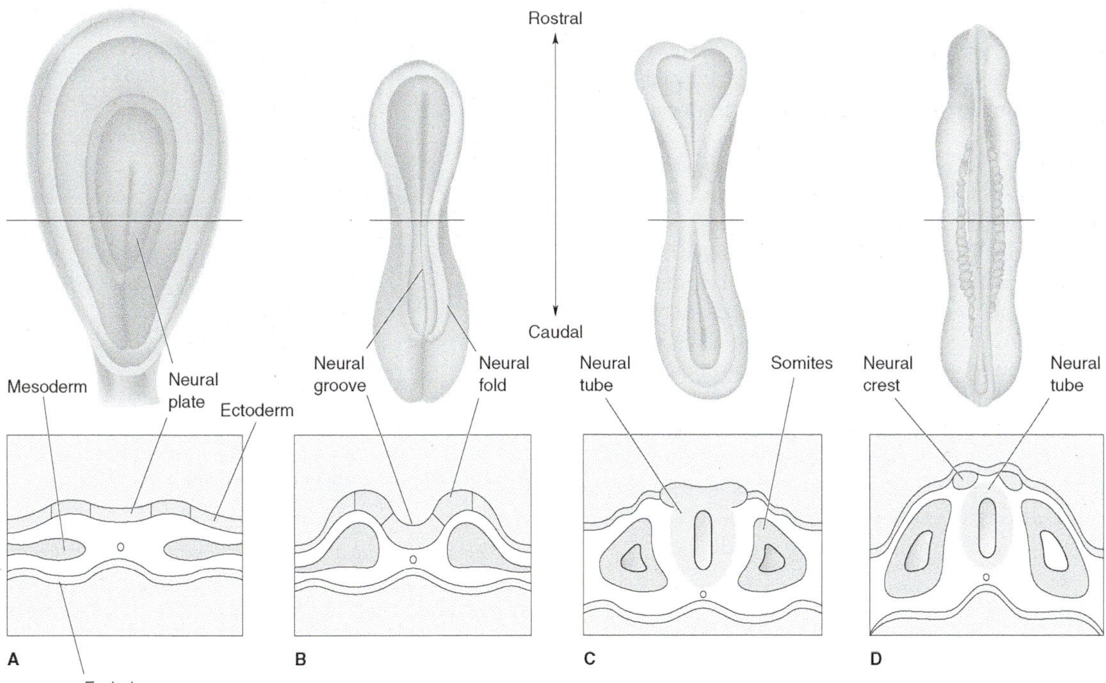

FIGURE 1-2. Formation of the neural tube and neural crest. These schematic illustrations follow the early development of the nervous system in the embryo. The drawings above are dorsal views of the embryo; those below are cross sections. **A**: The primitive embryonic central nervous system (CNS) begins as a thin sheet of ectoderm. **B**: The first important step in the development of the nervous system is the formation of the neural groove. **C**: The walls of the groove, called neural folds, come together and fuse, forming the neural tube. **D**: The bits of neural ectoderm that are pinched off when the tube rolls up are called the neural crest, from which the peripheral nervous system (PNS) will develop. The somites are mesoderm that will give rise to much of the skeletal system and the muscles. (Reprinted from Bear MF, Conners BW, Paradiso MA, eds. *Neuroscience: Exploring the Brain*. 2nd ed. Lippincott Williams & Wilkins; 2001:179, with permission.)

ticotropic hormone) in the fetal bloodstream, which act directly on the fetal neuronal network to increase blood pressure, heart rate, and activity level. Mothers with high levels of anxiety are more likely to have babies who are hyperactive, irritable, and of low birth weight, and who have problems feeding and sleeping than are mothers with low anxiety levels. Fever in the mother causes the fetus's temperature to rise.

Maternal Drug Use

Alcohol. Alcohol use in pregnancy is a significant cause of severe physical and mental congenital disabilities in children. Each year, up to 40,000 babies are born with some degree of alcohol-related damage. The National Institute on Drug Abuse (NIDA) reports that 19% of pregnant women used alcohol during their pregnancy, the highest rate being among white women.

Fetal alcohol syndrome affects about one-third of all infants born to alcoholic women. Table 1-1 lists the characteristics of the disorder. The incidence of infants born with fetal alcohol syndrome is about 0.5 per 1,000 live births.

Some studies suggest that alcohol use during pregnancy may also contribute to attention-deficit/hyperactivity disorder (ADHD).

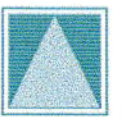

Table 1-1. Characteristics of Fetal Alcohol Syndrome

Growth retardation of prenatal origin (height, weight)
Facial dysmorphism
Microcephaly (head circumference below the third percentile)
Hypertelorism (large distance between eyes)
Microphthalmia (small eyeballs)
Short palpebral fissures
Inner epicanthal folds
Midface hypoplasia (underdevelopment)
Smooth or short philtrum
Thin upper lip
Short, turned up nose
Cardiac defects
Central nervous system (CNS) manifestations
Delayed development
Hyperactivity
Attention deficits
Learning disabilities
Intellectual deficits
Seizures

Smoking. Smoking during pregnancy may cause both premature births and below-average infant birth weight. Some reports have associated sudden infant death syndrome (SIDS) with mothers who smoke.

Other Substances. Chronic marijuana use is associated with low infant birth weight, prematurity, and withdrawal-like symptoms, including excessive crying, tremors, and hyperemesis (severe and chronic vomiting). Crack cocaine use by women during pregnancy may cause behavioral abnormalities such as increased irritability and crying and decreased desire for human contact. Infants born to mothers dependent on narcotics go through a withdrawal syndrome at birth.

Prenatal exposure to various prescribed medications can also result in abnormalities. Common drugs with teratogenic effects include antibiotics (tetracyclines), anticonvulsants (valproate, carbamazepine, phenytoin), progesterone-estrogens, lithium, and warfarin.

INFANCY

The average newborn weighs about 3,400 g (7.5 lb). Small fetuses (birth weight below the 10th percentile for their gestational age) occur in about 7% of all pregnancies. From the 26th to the 28th week of gestation, the prematurely born fetus has a good chance of survival. Arnold Gesell described developmental landmarks that are widely used in both pediatrics and child psychiatry. These landmarks outline the sequence of children's motor, adaptive, and personal–social behavior from birth to 6 years (Table 1-2).

Premature infants are born before 34 weeks or weigh less than 2,500 g (5.5 lb). Such infants are at increased risk for learning disabilities, such as dyslexia, emotional and behavioral problems, mental retardation, and child abuse. With each 100 g increment of weight, beginning at about 1,000 g (2.2 lb), infants have a progressively better chance of survival.

Developmental Milestones in Infants

Reflexes and Survival Systems at Birth. Primitive reflexes are present at birth. They include the rooting reflex (puckering of the lips in response to perioral stimulation), the grasp reflex, the plantar (Babinski) reflex, the knee reflex, the abdominal reflexes, the startle (Moro) reflex (Fig. 1-3), and the tonic neck reflex. In healthy children, the grasp reflex, the startle reflex, and the tonic neck reflex disappear by the fourth month. The Babinski reflex usually disappears by the 12th month.

Survival systems—breathing, sucking, swallowing, and circulatory and temperature homeostasis—are relatively functional at birth, but the sensory organs are still developing. Further differentiation of neurophysiologic functions depends on an active process of stimulatory reinforcement from the external environment, such as persons touching and stroking the infant. The newborn infant is awake for only a short period each day; rapid eye movement (REM) and non-REM sleep are present at birth. Other spontaneous behaviors include crying, smiling, and penile erection in males. Infants 1 day old can detect the smell of their mother's milk, and those 3 days old distinguish their mother's voice.

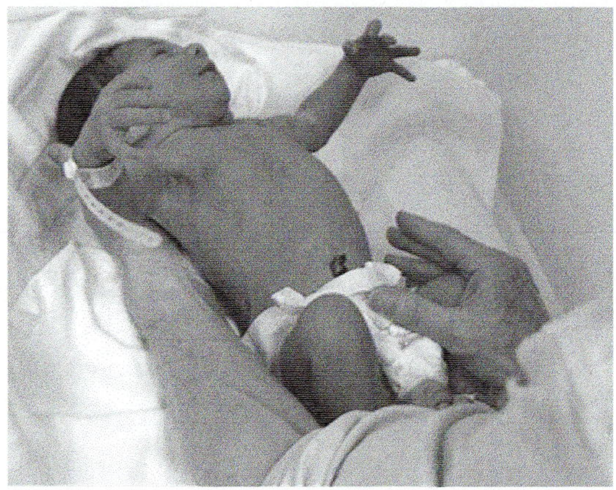

FIGURE 1-3. The Moro reflex. The head is allowed to fall backward. The arms abduct and extend.

Language and Cognitive Development. At birth, infants can make noises, such as crying, but they do not vocalize until about 8 weeks. At that time, guttural or babbling sounds occur spontaneously, especially in response to the mother. The persistence and further evolution of children's vocalizations depend on parental reinforcement. Language development occurs in well-delineated stages, as outlined in Table 1-3.

By the end of infancy (about 2 years), infants have transformed reflexes into voluntary actions that are the building blocks of cognition. They begin to interact with the environment, to experience feedback from their bodies, and to become intentional in their actions. By the end of the second year of life, children begin to use symbolic play and language.

Jean Piaget (1896–1980), a Swiss psychologist, observed the growing capacity of young children (including his own) to think and to reason. Table 1-4 outlines Piaget's stages of cognitive development.

Emotional and Social Development. By the age of 3 weeks, infants imitate the facial movements of adult caregivers. They open their mouths and thrust out their tongues in response to adults who do the same. By the third and fourth months of life, we can easily elicit these behaviors. These imitative behaviors are likely the precursors of the infant's emotional life. The smiling response occurs in two phases: the first phase is

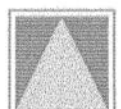

Table 1-2.
Common Malformations and Congenital Disorders in Humans

Genetic (20–25%)	**Condition**
Trisomy 21	Down syndrome
Mutation in *CFTR* gene	Cystic fibrosis
Mutation in *HEXA* gene	Tay–Sachs disease
Mutation in *HBB* gene (Beta-thalassemia) or *HBA1/HBA2* genes (Alpha-thalassemia)	Thalassemia
Mutation in *HBB* gene	Sickle cell anemia
FMR1 gene CGG repeat expansion	Fragile X syndrome
Deletion or uniparental disomy affecting paternal chromosome 15q11.2–q13	Prader–Willi syndrome
Trisomy 18	Edwards syndrome
Mutation in *NF1* gene	Neurofibromatosis type 1 (NF1)
Mutation in *FBN1* gene	Marfan syndrome
Mutation in *FGFR3* gene	Achondroplasia
Monosomy X	Turner syndrome (45, X)
Extra X chromosome	Klinefelter syndrome (47, XXY)
Environmental (4–5%)	
Maternal methamphetamine, opioid, and other substance use during pregnancy	Can cause neurodevelopmental disorders, neonatal abstinence syndrome
Maternal alcohol use during pregnancy	Can cause fetal alcohol syndrome
Folate deficiency	Neural tube defects
Lead exposure	Neurodevelopmental impairment and neurobehavioral problems
Mercury (in utero methylmercury exposure)	Can cause neurologic, visual, and hearing defects
Maternal diabetes (pregestational diabetes)	Increased risk of neural tube defects, caudal regression syndrome, congenital heart defects
Ionizing radiation	Can cause microcephaly, intellectual disability if exposed early in pregnancy
Valproic acid	Teratogenic—neural tube defects, facial anomalies, neurodevelopmental disorders
Retinoic acid (Accutane)	Severe birth defects (craniofacial, cardiac, thymic, CNS anomalies)
Maternal infection during pregnancy (3–4%)	
Toxoplasmosis	Hydrocephalus, intracranial calcifications, chorioretinitis, seizure
Syphilis	Can cause congenital disorders, congenital syphilis, preterm
Rubella	Congenital rubella syndrome—can cause deafness, vision problems, heart defects, intellectual disability
Cytomegalovirus (CMV)	Can cause congenital CMV, microcephaly, enlarged liver and spleen
HSV (herpes simplex virus)	Skin, eye, and mouth lesions; encephalitis; microcephaly; seizures
Zika virus	Can cause microcephaly, congenital Zika syndrome, and brain damage
Unknown cause (50–70%)	Congenital disorders and infant malformations

endogenous smiling, which occurs spontaneously within the first 2 months and is unrelated to external stimulation; the second phase is exogenous smiling, usually stimulated by the mother, and occurs by the 16th week.

The stages of emotional development parallel those of cognitive development. The caregiving person provides the primary stimulus for both aspects of mental growth. Human infants depend totally on adults for survival. Through warm and predictable interactions, an infant's social and emotional repertoire expands with the interplay of caregivers' social responses (Table 1-5).

In the first year, infants' moods are highly variable and intimately related to internal states such as hunger. Toward the second two-thirds of the first year, infants' moods grow increasingly related to external social cues; a parent can get even a hungry infant to smile. When the infant is internally comfortable, a sense of interest and pleasure in the world and its primary caregivers should prevail. Prolonged separation from the mother (or other primary caregivers) during the second 6 months of life can lead to depression that may persist into adulthood as part of an individual's character.

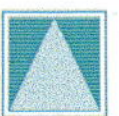

Table 1-3.
Language Development

Age	Typical Comprehension	Typical Expression	Intelligibility	Articulation
12–18 mo	Understands names of common objects and can identify them from a group; may know up to 150 words by 18 mo	Uses single words; often speaks using a combination of babbling and real words	25%	Articulates vowels correctly, but may omit first and final consonants
18–24 mo	Responds to simple directions or action commands (e.g., "sit down"); begins to understand complex sentences; understands pronouns	Uses two-word phrases; uses language to meet their needs; begins to use three-word telegraphic phrases	25–50%	
24–36 mo	Understands names of objects and family members (e.g., mom, grandpa); understands bigger and smaller; understands hunger and thirst	Babbling becomes less common; uses full sentences; announces intentions; vocabulary may grow from 270 words at 2 y to 895 words at 3 y	50–80%	*p*, *b*, and *m* clearly articulated; rhythmic disturbances such as stuttering may be present
36–54 mo	Understands prepositions (e.g., under, before), cause and effect, may know 3,500 words at 3 y and 5,500 at 4 y	Uses language to describe past events; likes rhymes or exaggerations; can define some words	90%	Correct articulation of *n*, *w*, *ng*, *h*, *t*, *d*, *k*, *g*
55+ mo	Understands concepts like speed, time, and numbers; understands left and right; understands abstract terms	Can tell stories; grammar is varied; self-correction of grammatical errors	100%	Improved articulation of *f*, *v*, *s*, *z*, *l*, *r*, *th*, and consonant blends

Temperamental Differences

Infants vary in their autonomic reactivity and temperament. Chess and Thomas identified nine behavioral dimensions in which reliable differences among infants can be observed (Table 1-6).

In studies of temperament, most temperamental dimensions of individual children remain stable through adulthood, but some do not persist. This is likely due to genetic and environmental effects on personality. A complex interplay exists among the initial characteristics of infants, the mode of parental interactions, and children's subsequent behavior. Observations of the stability and plasticity of certain temperamental traits support the importance of interactions between genetic endowment (nature) and environmental experience (nurture) in behavior.

Attachment

Bonding is the term used to describe the intense emotional and psychological relationship a mother develops for her baby. Attachment is the relationship the baby develops with its caregivers. Infants in the first months after birth become attuned to social and interpersonal interaction. They show a rapidly increasing responsivity to the external environment and an ability to form a special relationship with significant primary caregivers—that is, to form an attachment. Table 1-7 lists the commonly observed attachment styles.

Harry Harlow. Harry Harlow studied social learning and the effects of social isolation on monkeys. Harlow placed newborn rhesus monkeys with two types of surrogate mothers—one a wire-mesh surrogate with a feeding bottle and the other a wire-mesh surrogate covered with terry cloth. The monkeys preferred the terry-cloth surrogates, which provided contact and comfort, to the feeding surrogate. (When hungry, the infant monkeys would go to the feeding bottle but then would quickly return to the terry-cloth surrogate.) When frightened, monkeys raised with terry-cloth surrogates showed intense clinging behavior and appeared to be comforted, whereas those raised with wire-mesh surrogates gained no comfort and appeared to be disorganized. The results of Harlow's experiments suggest that infant attachment is not merely the result of feeding.

Both types of surrogate-reared monkeys were subsequently unable to adjust to life in a monkey colony and had extraordinary difficulty learning to mate. When impregnated, the female monkeys failed to mother their young.

John Bowlby. John Bowlby studied the attachment of infants to mothers and concluded that early separation of infants from their mothers had severe adverse effects on children's emotional and intellectual

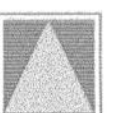

Table 1-4.
Piaget's Stages of Cognitive Development

Period of Development	Cognitive Spatial Stages and Associated Concepts	Cognitive Achievements
Gestational		Fetus can "learn" sounds and respond differentially to them after birth
Infancy: Birth–2 yr	Sensorimotor	Infants "think" with their eyes, ears, and senses
Birth–1 mo	Reflective; egocentric (newer research refutes this)	Newborns can learn to associate stroking with sucking
4–8 mo	Secondary circular: looks for objects partially hidden	Newborns can learn to suck to produce certain visual displays or music
8–12 mo	Secondary circulation coordinated: peek-a-boo, finds hidden objects	Can remember for 1-mo periods Can play with parent by looking for partially hidden objects
12–18 mo	Tertiary circular: explores properties and drops objects	Memory improves
18 mo–2 yr	Mental representation, make-believe play; memory of objects	Body parts used as objects Can stack one object within another Remembers hidden objects Drops objects over crib Knows animal sounds; names objects Knows body parts and familiar pictures Can understand causes not visible
Early Childhood: 2–7 yr	Preoperational	
2–7 yr	Egocentrism: "I want you to eat this too." Animistic: "I'm afraid of the moon." Lack of hierarchy: "Where do these blocks go?" Centration: "I want it now, not after dinner." Irreversibility: "I don't know how to go back to that room."	Preschoolers use symbols Development of language and make-believe No sign of logic 3-yr-olds can count 2–3 objects; know colors and age 4-yr-olds can fantasize without concrete props
2–5 yr	Transductive reasoning: "We have to go this way because that's the way Daddy goes."	5–6-yr-olds get humor; understand good and bad; can do some chores 7–11-yr-olds have good memory; recall; can solve problems
Middle Childhood: 7–11 yr	Concrete operational Hierarchical classification—arranges cars by types Reversibility—can play games backward and forward (e.g., checkers, triple kings) Conservation—lose two dimes and look for same Decentration—worry about small details, obsessive Spatial operations—likes models for directions Horizontal decalage—conservation of weight, logic Transitive inference—syllogisms; compare everything, brand names important	Children begin to think logically Understand conservation of matter Frozen milk same amount as melted Can organize objects into hierarchies Children seem rational and organized
Adolescence: 11–19 yr	Formal operational	
11 yr onward	Hypothetical-deductive reasoning; adolescent quick thinking or excuses Imaginary audience—everyone is looking at them Personal fable—inflated opinion of themselves Propositional thinking—logic	Abstraction and reason Can think of all possibilities

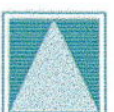

Table 1-5.
Emotional Development

Stages First Seen	Emotional Skills	Emotional Behavior
Gestational–Infancy: 0–2 yr		
0–2 mo onward	Love, evoked by touching Fear, evoked by loud noise Rage, evoked by body restrictions Brain pathways for emotion forming	Social smile and joy shown Responds to emotions of others All emotions there
3–4 mo onward	Self-regulation of emotions starts; brain pathways of emotion growing	Laughter possible and more control over smiles Anger shown
7–12 mo	Self-regulation of emotion grows Increased intensity of basic three	Able to elicit more responsiveness Denies to cope with stress
1–2 yr	Shame and pride appear; envy, embarrassment appear Displaces onto other children	Some indications of empathy starting Expressions of feeling: "I like you, Daddy", "I'm sorry" Likes attention and approval. Enjoys play alone or next to peers
Early Childhood: 2–5 yr		
3–6 yr	Can understand causes of many emotions Can begin to find ways for regulating emotions and for expressing them Identifies with adult to cope	Empathy increases with understanding More response and less reaction; self-regulation: "Use your words to say that you are angry with him" Aggression becomes competition By age 5, shows sensitivity to criticism and cares about feelings of others
Middle Childhood: 5–11 yr		Ego rules until age 6
7–11 yr	Can react to the feelings of others More aware of other's feelings	Empathy becomes altruism: "I feel so bad about their fire, I'm going to give them some of my things" Superego dominates

development. He described attachment behavior, which develops during the first year of life, as the maintenance of physical contact between the mother and child when the child is hungry, frightened, or in distress.

Mary Ainsworth. Mary Ainsworth expanded on Bowlby's observations and found that the interaction between mother and baby during the attachment period influences the baby's current and future behavior significantly. Many observers believe that patterns of infant attachment affect future adult emotional relationships. Patterns of attachment vary among babies; for example, some babies signal or cry less than others. Sensitive responsiveness to infant signals, such as cuddling the baby when it cries, causes infants to cry less in later months. Close bodily contact with the mother when the baby signals for her fosters self-reliance, rather than clinging dependence. Unresponsive mothers produce anxious babies.

Ainsworth also confirmed that attachment serves to reduce anxiety. What she called the secured base effect enables a child to move away from the attachment figure and explore the environment. Inanimate objects, such as a teddy bear or a blanket (called the transitional object by Donald Winnicott), also serve as a secure base, one that often accompanies children as they investigate the world. A growing body of literature derived from direct observation of mother–infant interactions and longitudinal studies has expanded on and refined Ainsworth's original descriptions. Maternal sensitivity and responsiveness are the main determinants of secure attachment. However, when the attachment is insecure, the type of insecurity (avoidant, anxious, or ambivalent) is determined by infant temperament. Overall, male infants are less likely to have secure attachments and are more vulnerable to changes in maternal sensitivity than are female infants.

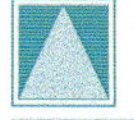

Table 1-6.
Temperament—Newborn to 6 Years

Dimension	Description
Activity level	Percent of time spent in activities
Distractibility	Degree to which stimuli are allowed to alter behavior
Adaptability	Ease moving into change
Attention span	Amount of time spent on attending
Intensity	Energy level
Threshold of responsiveness	Intensity required for response
Quality of mood	Amount positive compared to amount negative behavior
Rhythmicity	Regulation of functions
Approach/withdrawal	Response to new situations

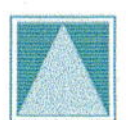

Table 1-7. Types of Attachment

Secure Attachment	Children show fewer adjustment problems; however, these children have typically received more consistent and developmentally appropriate parenting for most of their life. The parents of securely attached children are likely better able to maintain these aspects of parenting through a divorce. Given that the family factors that lead to divorce also impact the children, there could be fewer securely attached children in divorcing families.
Insecure/Avoidant Attachment	Children become anxious, clinging, and angry with the parent. These children typically come from families with adults who were also insecurely attached to their families and, thus, were unable to provide the kind of consistency, emotional responsiveness, and care that securely attached parents could offer. Such parents have a more difficult time with divorce and are more likely to become rejecting.
Insecure/Ambivalent Attachment	Children generally are raised with disorganized, neglecting, and inattentive parenting. The parents are even less able to provide stability and psychological strength for them after a divorce and, as a result, the children are even more likely to become clinging but inconsolable in their distress, as well as to act out, suffer mood swings, and become oversensitive to stress.

The birth of a second child decreases the attachment of the firstborn child. This decrease is most notable when the firstborn is 2 to 5 years of age as opposed to younger. Not surprisingly, the extent of the decrease also depends on the mother's sense of security, confidence, and mental health.

Social Deprivation Syndromes and Maternal Neglect. Investigators, especially René Spitz, have long documented the severe developmental retardation that accompanies maternal rejection and neglect. Infants in institutions characterized by low staff-to-infant ratios and frequent turnover of personnel tend to display marked developmental retardation, even with adequate physical care and freedom from infection. The same infants, placed in adequate foster or adoptive care, exhibit marked acceleration in development.

Primary Attachment Figures. Babies become most attached to the primary caregiver that takes care of them. Babies raised in extended families or with multiple caregivers can establish many attachments.

Stranger Anxiety. A developmentally expected fear of strangers typically appears in infants at about 26 weeks of age and is more fully developed by 32 weeks. At the approach of a stranger, infants may cry or cling to their primary attachment figure. Babies exposed to only one caregiver are more likely to have stranger anxiety than babies exposed to a variety of caregivers. Stranger anxiety likely results from a baby's growing ability to distinguish caregivers from all other persons.

Separation anxiety, which occurs between 10 and 18 months of age, is related to stranger anxiety but is not identical to it. Separation from the person to whom the infant is attached precipitates separation anxiety. Stranger anxiety, however, occurs even when the infant is in the mother's arms. The infant learns to separate as it starts to crawl and move away from the mother, but the infant continually looks back and frequently returns to the mother for reassurance.

Margaret Mahler (1897–1985) proposed a theory to describe how young children acquire a sense of identity separate from that of their mothers'. Her observations of children and their mothers lead to her theory of separation-individuation. Table 1-8 lists Mahler's stages of separation-individuation.

Infant Care

Infants' behavior influences caregivers' behavior, just as mothers' behavior modulates infants' behavior. A calm,

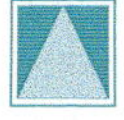

Table 1-8. Stages of Separation-Individuation Proposed by Mahler

1. Normal autism (birth–2 mo)
   Periods of sleep outweigh periods of arousal in a state reminiscent of intrauterine life.
2. Symbiosis (2–5 mo)
   Developing perceptual abilities gradually enable infants to distinguish the inner from the outer world; mother–infant is perceived as a single fused entity.
3. Differentiation (5–10 mo)
   Progressive neurologic development and increased alertness draw infants' attention away from self to the outer world. Physical and psychological distinctiveness from the mother is gradually appreciated.
4. Practicing (10–18 mo)
   The ability to move autonomously increases children's exploration of the outer world.
5. Rapprochement (18–24 mo)
   As children slowly realize their helplessness and dependence, the need for independence alternates with the need for closeness. Children move away from their mothers and come back for reassurance.
6. Object constancy (2–5 yr)
   Children gradually comprehend and are reassured by the permanence of mother and other important people, even when not in their presence.

smiling, predictable infant is a powerful reward for tender caregiver response. A jittery, irregular, irritable infant may cause stress in the primary caregiver. When a primary caregiver has limited capacity for dealing with a given infant's needs, the caregiver may withdraw from the child and thus not meet the child's needs.

Goodness of Caregiver Fit

Goodness of fit describes how well the primary caregivers relate to the newborn or developing infant; the concept takes into account the temperamental characteristics of both parent and child. Each newborn has innate psychophysiologic characteristics, which are known collectively as temperament. Chess and Thomas identified a range of standard temperamental patterns, from the difficult child at one end of the spectrum to the easy child at the other end.

Children who fit the definition of displaying a difficult temperament make up about 10% of all children and may exhibit hyperalert physiologic reactions. Compared to children who fit the definition of having an easy temperament, those with difficult temperaments typically overreact to stimuli (cry easily at loud noises), sleep poorly, eat at unpredictable times, and are difficult to comfort. Children who fit the definition of having an easy temperament make up 40% of all children and tend to be more regular in eating, eliminating, and sleeping; more flexible, and better at adapting to change and new stimuli with minimal distress, and are more easily comforted when they cry. The other 50% of children are mixtures of these two types. A child with a difficult temperament is harder to raise and places higher demands on the caregivers than the easy child. Chess and Thomas used the term *goodness of fit* to characterize the harmonious and consonant interaction between a primary caregiver and a child in their motivations, capacities, and styles of behavior. Poor fit is likely to lead to distorted development and maladaptive functioning. A difficult child must be recognized because parents of such infants often have feelings of inadequacy and believe that they are doing something wrong to account for the child's difficulty in sleeping and eating and their problems comforting the child.

Good-Enough Mothering. Winnicott believed that infants begin life in a state of nonintegration, with unconnected and diffuse experiences, and that mothers provide the relationship that enables infants' incipient selves to emerge. Primary caregivers supply a holding environment in which infants are contained and experienced. During the last trimester of pregnancy and for the first few months of a baby's life, the mother is in a state of primary maternal preoccupation, absorbed in fantasies about, and experiences with, her baby. The mother need not be perfect, but she must provide good-enough mothering. The primary caregiver plays a vital role in bringing the world to the child and offering empathic anticipation of the infant's needs. If the primary caregiving parent can resonate with the infant's needs, the baby can become attuned to its bodily functions and drives that are the basis for the gradually evolving sense of self.

TODDLER PERIOD

Accelerated motor and intellectual development occur in the second year. The ability to walk gives toddlers some control over their actions; this mobility enables children to determine when to approach and when to withdraw. The acquisition of speech profoundly extends their horizons. Typically, children learn to say "no" before they learn to say "yes." Toddlers' negativism (i.e., saying "no") is vital to the development of independence, but if it persists and becomes predominant, oppositional behavior becomes problematic.

Learning language is a crucial task in the toddler period. Vocalizations become distinct, and toddlers can name a few objects and make needs known in one or two words. Near the end of the second year and into the third year, toddlers sometimes use short sentences. The pace of language development varies considerably from child to child, and although a small number of children are genuinely late developers, most child experts recommend a hearing test if the child is not making two-word sentences by age 2.

Developmental Milestones in Toddlers

Language and Cognitive Development. Toddlers begin to listen to explanations that can help them tolerate delay. They create new behaviors from old ones (originality) and engage in symbolic activities, for instance, using words and playing with dolls when the dolls represent something, such as a feeding sequence. Toddlers have varied capacities for concentration and self-regulation.

Emotional and Social Development. In the second year, pleasure and displeasure become further differentiated. Social referencing is often apparent at this age; the child looks to parents and others for emotional cues about how to respond to novel events. Toddlers show exploratory excitement, assertive pleasure, and pleasure in discovery and in developing new behavior (e.g., new games), including teasing and surprising or fooling the parent (e.g., hiding). The toddler has capacities for an organized demonstration of love, as when the toddler runs up and hugs, smiles, and kisses the parent at the same time, and of protest when the toddler turns away, cries, bangs, bites, hits, yells, and kicks. Comfort with family and apprehension with strangers may increase. Anxiety appears to be related to disapproval and the loss of a loved caregiver and can be disorganizing.

Sexual Development. Sexual differentiation is evident from birth when parents start dressing and treating infants differently because of the expectations evoked by sex typing. Through imitation, reward, and coercion, children assume the behaviors that their cultures define as appropriate for their sexual roles. Children exhibit curiosity about anatomical sex. When their curiosity is recognized as healthy and elicits age-appropriate replies, children acquire a sense of the wonder of life and are comfortable with their roles. If the subject of sex is taboo and parents rebuff children's questions, shame, and discomfort may result.

Gender identity, the conviction of being male or female, begins to manifest at 18 months of age and is often fixed by 24 to 30 months. It was once widely believed that gender identity was primarily a function of social learning. John Money reported on children with ambiguous or damaged external genitalia who were raised as the sex opposite to their chromosomal sex. Long-term follow-up of those individuals suggests that a major part of gender identity is innate and that rearing may not affect the genetic diathesis.

Gender role describes the behavior that society deems appropriate for one sex or another. There may be different expectations for boys and girls in what and with whom they play, their tone of voice, the expression of emotions, and how they dress. Boys are often more likely than girls to engage in rough-and-tumble play. Female primary caregivers often talk more to girls than to boys, and by the time the child is 2 years of age, male caregivers may pay more attention to male children.

Toilet Training. The second year of life is a period of increasing social demands on children. Toilet training serves as a paradigm of the family's general training practices; that is, the parent who is overly severe in the area of toilet training is likely to be punitive and restrictive in other areas also. Control of daytime urination is usually complete by the age of 2½, and control of nighttime urination is usually complete by the age of 4 years. Since 1900, the pendulum has swung between extremes of permissiveness and control in toilet training. The trend in the United States has been toward delayed training, but in the last few years, this trend appears to be shifting back to early training.

Toddlers may have sleep difficulties related to fear of the dark, which may be helped with a nightlight. Most toddlers generally sleep about 12 hours a day, including a 2-hour nap. Parents must be aware that children of this age may need reassurance before going to bed and that the average 2-year-old takes about 30 minutes to fall asleep.

Parenting Challenges. In infancy, the primary responsibility for parents is to meet the infant's needs sensitively and consistently. The parental task in the toddler stage requires firmness about the boundaries of acceptable behavior and encouragement of the child's progressive emancipation. Parents must be careful not to be too authoritarian at this stage; children must be allowed to operate for themselves and to learn from their mistakes and must be protected and assisted when challenges are beyond their abilities.

During the toddler period, children are likely to struggle for the exclusive affection and attention of their parents. They may compete with siblings or one or another parent for the starring role in the family. Although children are beginning to be able to share, they do so reluctantly. When the demands for exclusive possession are not resolved effectively, the result is likely to be jealous competitiveness in relationships with peers and lovers. The fantasies aroused by the struggle lead to fear of retaliation and displacement of fear onto external objects. In an equitable, loving family, a child elaborates on a moral system of ethical rights. Parents need to balance between punishment and permissiveness and set realistic limits on a toddler's behavior.

PRESCHOOL PERIOD

Marked physical and emotional growth occurs during the preschool period. Generally, between 2 and 3 years of age, children reach half their adult height. The 20 baby teeth are in place at the beginning of the stage, and by the end, they begin to fall out. Children are ready to enter school by the time the stage ends at age 5 or 6. They have mastered the tasks of primary socialization—to control their bowels and urine, to dress and feed themselves, and to control their tears and temper outbursts, at least most of the time.

The term preschool for the age group of 2½ to 6 years may be a misnomer; many children are already in school-like settings, such as preschool nurseries and daycare centers, where working mothers must often place their children. Preschool education can be valuable, but stressing academic advancement too far beyond a child's capabilities can be counterproductive.

Developmental Milestones in Preschoolers

Language and Cognitive Development. In the preschool period, children's use of language expands, and they use sentences. Individual words have regular and consistent meanings at the beginning of the period, and children begin to think symbolically. In general, however, their thinking is egocentric; they cannot place themselves in the position of another child and are incapable of empathy. Children think intuitively and prelogically and do not understand causal relations.

Emotional and Social Behavior. At the start of the preschool period, children can express such complex emotions as love, unhappiness, jealousy, and envy, both preverbally and verbally. Their emotions are still easily influenced by somatic events, such as tiredness and hunger. Although they still think mostly egocentrically, children's capacity for cooperation and sharing is emerging.

Various losses, such as of a loved person or approval, may cause anxiety. Although still potentially disorganizing, preschool children can tolerate anxiety better than when they were younger. Four-year-olds are learning to share and to have concern for others and may express feelings of tenderness.

By the end of the preschool period, children have many relatively stable emotions. The child balances expansiveness, curiosity, pride, and gleeful excitement related to the self and the family with coyness, shyness, fearfulness, jealousy, and envy. Shame and humiliation are evident. Capacities for empathy and love are developed but are fragile and quickly lost if competitive or jealous strivings intervene. Anxiety and fears are related to bodily injury and loss of respect, love, and emerging self-esteem. Guilt feelings are possible.

Children between the ages of 3 and 6 years are aware of their bodies and differences between the sexes. Their physical awareness extends beyond genitalia. Children may be preoccupied with illness or injury, and some call this "the Band-Aid phase." Every injury must be examined and taken care of by a parent.

Children develop a division between what they want and what others tell them to do. The division increases until a gap grows between their set of expanded desires, their exuberance at unlimited growth, and their parents' restrictions; they gradually turn parental values into self-obedience, self-guidance, and self-punishment.

At the end of the preschool stage, the child's conscience is evolving. The development of a conscience sets the tone for the moral sense of "right and wrong." Until about 7 years of age, children typically experience rules as "absolute" and as existing for their own sake. They do not understand that more than one point of view on a moral issue may exist; a violation of the rules calls for absolute retribution—that is, children have the notion of immanent justice.

SIBLING RIVALRY. In the preschool period, children relate to others in new ways. The birth of a sibling (a common occurrence during this time) tests a preschool child's capacity for further cooperation and sharing but may also evoke sibling rivalry, which is most likely to occur at this time. Sibling rivalry depends on child-rearing practice. Favoritism, for any reason, commonly aggravates such rivalry. Children who get special treatment because they are gifted, are defective in some way, or have a preferred gender are likely to receive angry feelings from their siblings. Experiences with siblings can influence growing children's relationships with peers and authority; for example, a problem may result if the needs of a new baby prevent the mother from attending to a firstborn child's needs. If not handled properly, the displacement of the firstborn can be a traumatic event.

PLAY. In the preschool years, children begin to distinguish reality from fantasy, and play reflects this growing awareness. Pretend games are popular and playfully help test real-life situations. Dramatic play in which children act out a role is typical. One-to-one play relationships advance to complicated patterns with rivalries, secrets, and two-against-one intrigues. Children's play behavior reflects their level of social development.

Between 2½ and 3 years, children commonly engage in parallel play, solitary play alongside another child with no interaction between them. By age 3, play is often associative, that is, playing with the same toys in pairs or small groups, but still with no real interaction among them. By age 4, children are usually able to share and engage in cooperative play. Real interactions and taking turns become possible.

Between 3 and 6 years of age, drawings may trace growth. A child's first drawing of a human being is a circular line with marks for the mouth, nose, and eyes; they add ears and hair later; arms and stick-like fingers appear next, and then legs appear. Last to appear is a torso in proportion to the rest of the body. Intelligent children can deal with details in their art. Drawings express creativity throughout a child's development: They are representational and formal in early childhood, make use of perspective in middle childhood, and become abstract and affect-laden in adolescence. Drawings also reflect children's body image concepts and sexual and aggressive impulses.

IMAGINARY COMPANIONS. Imaginary companions most often appear during preschool years, usually in children and usually in the form of persons. Imaginary companions may also be things, such as anthropomorphized toys. Some studies suggest that up to 50% of children between the ages of 3 and 10 years have imaginary companions at one time or another. Their significance is not clear, but these figures are usually friendly, relieve loneliness, and reduce anxiety. In most instances, imaginary companions disappear by age 12, but they can occasionally persist into adulthood.

MIDDLE YEARS

The period between age 6 and puberty is the middle years. During this time, children enter elementary school. The formal demands for academic learning and accomplishment become significant determinants of further personality development.

Developmental Milestones in School-Age Children

Language and Cognitive Development. In the middle years, language expresses complex ideas with relations among several elements. Logical exploration tends to dominate fantasy, and children show an increased interest in rules and orderliness and an increased capacity for self-regulation. During this period, children's conceptual skills develop, and thinking becomes organized and logical. The ability to concentrate is well established by age 9 or 10, and by the end of the period, children begin to think in abstract terms. Improved gross motor coordination and muscle strength enable children to write fluently and draw artistically. They are also capable of complex motor tasks and activities, such as tennis, gymnastics, golf, baseball, and skateboarding.

Recent evidence has shown that changes in thinking and reasoning during the middle years result from maturational changes in the brain. Children are now capable of increased independence, learning, and socialization. Theorists consider moral development a gradual, stepwise process spanning childhood, adolescence, and young adulthood.

In the middle years, both girls and boys make new identifications with other adults, such as teachers and counselors. These identifications may so influence both girls and boys to emulate them that they may develop goals of wanting to emulate their same-sex major attachment figures or to pursue goals that are quite different.

The school-age period is a time when peer interaction assumes significant importance. Interest in relationships outside the family takes precedence over those within the family. Nevertheless, a special relationship exists with the same-sex parent, with whom children identify and who is now an ideal and a role model.

Empathy and concern for others begin to emerge early in the middle years; by the time children are 9 or 10, they have well-developed capacities for love, compassion, and sharing. They have a capacity for long-term, stable relationships with family, peers, and friends, including best friends. Emotions about sexual differences begin to emerge as either excitement or shyness with the opposite sex. School-age children prefer to interact with children of the same sex. Although the middle years have sometimes been referred to as a latency period—a moratorium on psychosexual exploration and play until the eruption of sexual impulses with puberty—it is now recognized that a considerable amount of sexual interest continues through these years. Sex play and curiosity are typical, especially among boys, but also among girls. Boys compare genitals and may engage in peer masturbation. Interest in anal humor and toilet jokes is also typical. Children this age often start using sexual and excretory words as expletives.

BEST FRIEND. Harry Stack Sullivan postulated that a buddy, or best friend, is an influential phenomenon during the school years. By about 10 years of age, children tend to develop close same-sex relationships, which Sullivan believed is necessary for further healthy psychological growth.

SCHOOL REFUSAL. School refusal may emerge at this time in some children, generally because of separation anxiety. An anxious mother may transmit her own separation anxiety to a child, or a child who is prone to anxiety as well. School refusal in a child may not be an isolated problem since it is often a symptom of separation anxiety disorder. Children with separation anxiety disorder are at higher risk for other anxiety disorders such as generalized anxiety disorder and social anxiety disorder.

Sex Role Development

Persons' sex roles are related to their sense of gender identity; persons may see themselves as predominantly male or female, or gender fluid Sex roles also involve identification with culturally acceptable masculine, feminine, or more gender fluid ways of behaving; in current times, changing societal expectations of what constitutes masculine, feminine, and more gender fluid behaviors has modernized a previously narrow view of masculine and feminine.

Parents often react differently to their male and female children, sometimes without realizing it. Independence, physical play, and aggressiveness are generally more encouraged in boys, and prosocial behavior and verbal communication may be more encouraged in girls. Nowadays, boys are encouraged to verbalize their feelings and girls are encouraged to pursue careers traditionally dominated by males and to participate in competitive sports. As society becomes more accepting and less rigid in its expectations of sex roles, opportunities for boys and girls enlarge and broaden.

Biologically, boys are more physically aggressive than girls; and parental expectations have traditionally reinforced this trait. Differences also exist between boys and girls in the influence of persons outside the family. As school-age children, girls tend to respond to the expectations and opinions of girls and teachers. Boys, on the other hand, tend to respond to other boys when they are of school age.

Dreams and Sleep

Children's dreams can have a profound effect on behavior. During the first year of life, when reality and fantasy are not yet fully differentiated, dreams may be experienced as if they were, or could be, real. At age 3, many children believe dreams are shared directly by more than one person, but most 4-year-olds understand that dreams are unique to each person. Children view dreams either with pleasure or, as is most often reported, with fear. The dream content depends on the children's life experience, developmental stage, mechanisms used during dreaming, and sex.

Disturbing dreams are most common when children are 3, 6, and 10 years of age. Two-year-old children may dream about being bitten or chased; at the age of 4, they may have many animal dreams and also dream of persons who either protect or destroy. At age 5 or 6, dreams of being killed or injured, of flying and being in cars, and of ghosts become prominent; the role of conscience, moral values, and increasing conflicts are concerned with these themes. In early childhood, aggressive dreams rarely seem to occur; instead, dreamers are in danger, a state that perhaps reflects children's dependent position. By about the age of 5, children realize that their dreams are not real; before then, they believed them to be real events. By age 7, children know that they create their dreams themselves.

Between the ages of 3 and 6 years, children usually want to keep their bedroom door open or to have a night-light, so that they can either maintain contact with their parents or view the room in a realistic, nonfearful way. At times, children resist going to sleep to avoid dreaming. Disorders associated with falling asleep, therefore, are often connected with dreaming. Children often create rituals to protect themselves in the withdrawal from the world of reality into the world of sleep. Parasomnias, such as sleepwalking, sleep talking, enuresis (bed-wetting), and night terrors, are common at this age. They usually occur during stage 4 sleep when dreaming is minimal, and they do not indicate emotional trouble or underlying psychopathology. Most children grow out of parasomnias by adolescence.

Periods of REM occur about 60% of the time during the first few weeks of life, a period when infants sleep two-thirds of the time. Premature babies sleep even longer than full-term babies, and a higher proportion of their sleep is REM sleep. The sleep-wake cycle of newborns is about 3 hours long. Adults spend about 20% of sleep dreaming. Even newborns have brain activity similar to that of the dreaming state.

Birth Order

The effects of birth order vary. Firstborn children may be more highly valued or given more attention than subsequent children. Firstborn children appear to be more achievement oriented and motivated to please their parents than subsequent children born to the same parents. Some studies show that people in certain competitive occupational areas, such as architecture, accounting, and engineering, tend to be firstborn children.

Second and third children have the advantage of their parents' previous experience. Younger children also learn from their older siblings. For example, they may show a more sophisticated use of pronouns at an earlier age than firstborns did. When spacing children too tightly, however, there may not be enough time for each child. The arrival of new children in the family affects not only the parents but also the siblings. Firstborn children may resent the birth of a new sibling, who threatens their sole claim on parental attention. In some cases, regressive behavior, such as enuresis or thumb sucking, occurs.

Some researchers have suggested that there is a relationship between birth order and personality. However, extensive multicohort analyses have not supported this.

Children and Divorce

Many children live in homes in which divorce has occurred. Approximately 30% to 50% of all children in the United States live in homes in which one parent (usually the mother) is the sole head of the household, and 61% of all children born in any given year can expect to live with only one parent before they reach the age of 18 years. A child's age at the time of the parents' divorce affects the child's reaction to the divorce. Immediately after a divorce, an increase in behavioral and emotional disorders appears in all age groups. Infants do not understand anything about separation or divorce; however, they do notice changes in their parents' responses to them and may experience changes in their eating or sleeping patterns; have bowel problems; and seem more fretful, fearful, or anxious. Children 3 to 6 years of age may not understand what is happening, and those who do understand often assume that they are somehow responsible for the divorce. Older children, especially adolescents, comprehend the situation and may believe that they could have prevented the divorce had they intervened in some way, but they are still hurt, angry, and critical of their parents' behavior.

Some children harbor the fantasy that their parents will reunite. Such children may show animosity toward a parent's real or potential new mate. Adaptation to the effects of divorce in children typically takes several years; however, up to about one-third of children from divorced homes may have lasting psychological trauma. Among boys, physical aggression is a common sign of distress. Adolescents tend to spend more time away from the parental home after the divorce. Children who adapt best to divorce are typically in a situation in which both parents make genuine efforts to spend time and relate to the child despite the child's potential anger about the divorce. The predivorce stability of the household is another influence, as are economic factors. To facilitate adaptation in children, a divorced couple who are amicable and avoid arguing with one another is most likely to succeed.

Family Factors in Child Development

Family Stability. Parents and children living under the same roof in harmonious interaction is the idealized cultural norm in Western society. Within this framework, childhood development presumably proceeds most optimally. Children of divorced parents who are in perpetual conflict are at higher risk of a range of psychological and psychiatric problems including low self-esteem, depressive disorders, and anxiety disorders. Some children from unstable or highly conflictual homes are more resilient than others due to a variety of genetic and environmental factors.

Adverse Events. It is now well known that childhood adverse events, especially multiple events and in early childhood, have long-term negative effects on emotional and physical well-being. Sexual and physical abuse, neglect, or loss of a parent interact with genetic background in a given child and influence the trajectory of development. For example, as mentioned earlier, early severe maltreatment such as sexual abuse increases the risk of multiple psychosocial difficulties and the emergence of many psychiatric disorders. Among young, maltreated children, those with particular genetics, that is, who have the "short" variant of the serotonin transporter gene (short 5-HTTLPR polymorphism), may be more vulnerable to chronic depression in adulthood. This example of specific gene–environment interaction plays a vital role in a child's development as well as in the risk for future psychopathology. Current investigations are also seeking insight into what factors lead to resilience in youth exposed to adverse events, yet maintain allostasis, that is, stability in the face of stressful events. Hormones of the adrenal glands, thyroid, gonads, as well as metabolic hormones, play a role in the brain's ability to maintain stability upon exposure to stress, and the prefrontal cortex, hippocampus, and amygdala play critical roles in regulating emotionality, aggression, and resilience.

Daycare Centers. The role and impact of daycare centers on children's development has been studied with varying results. The National Institute of Child Health and Human Development reported that 4½-year-olds who had spent more than 30 hours a week in childcare were more demanding, more aggressive, and more noncompliant than those raised only in their home, and showed higher cognitive skills, particularly in math and reading. These same children continued to score higher in math and reading skills but had more poor work habits and social skills in third grade. The researchers were careful to note that this behavior was within the normal range, however.

All studies of daycare must take into account the quality of both the daycare center and the homes from which children come. For example, a child from a disadvantaged home may be better off at a daycare center than a child from an advantaged home. Similarly, a woman who wishes to leave home to work for financial or other reasons and cannot do so may resent remaining in the home in a child-rearing role, which may adversely affect the child.

Parenting Styles. How children are raised varies considerably between families in the same environment and within different cultures. Rutter has clustered this diversity into four general styles. Subsequent research has confirmed that certain styles tend to correlate with particular behavior in children, although the outcomes are by no means absolute. The authoritarian style, characterized by strict, inflexible rules, can lead to low self-esteem, unhappiness, and social withdrawal. The indulgent-permissive style, which includes little or no limit setting coupled with unpredictable parental harshness, can lead to low self-reliance, poor impulse control, and aggression. The indulgent-neglectful style, one of noninvolvement in the child's life and rearing, puts the child at risk for low self-esteem, impaired self-control, and increased aggression. The authoritative-reciprocal style, marked by firm rules and shared decision-making in a warm, loving environment, is believed to be the style most likely to result in self-reliance, self-esteem, and a sense of social responsibility.

Developmental Trajectories

Children who don't meet expected developmental milestones may be impacted by environmental and genetic influences. Specific developmental disorders, particularly developmental language disorders, often are diagnosed in the preschool years. Delayed development of language is a common parental concern. Children who do not use words by 18 months or phrases by 2½ to 3 years may need assessment, particularly if they do not appear to understand typical verbal cues or much language at all. Mild intellectual disability or specific learning problems often are not diagnosed until after the child begins elementary school. Disruptive behavior disorder will become more apparent at that time, as the child begins to interact with peers. Similarly, attention-deficit disorders may only be apparent in school with its need for sustained attention.

ADOLESCENCE

Adolescence, marked by the physiologic signs and surging sexual hormones of puberty, is the period of maturation between childhood and adulthood. Adolescence is a transitional period in which peer relationships deepen, autonomy in decision-making grows, and they seek intellectual pursuits and social belonging. Adolescence is mostly a time of exploration and making choices, a gradual process of working toward an integrated concept of self. Adolescents are "works in progress," characterized by increasing ability for mastery over complex challenges of academic, interpersonal, and emotional tasks while searching for new interests, talents, and social identities. A body of growing literature of the specific mechanisms of brain development in adolescence has increased our understanding of broadening social skills in adolescents, in addition to the three expected developmental changes in adolescence: increased risk-taking, increased sexual behavior, and a move toward peer affiliation rather than a primary family attachment. The total cortical gray matter is at its peak at about age 11 years in girls and 13 years in boys, which enhances the ability to understand subtle social situations, control impulses, make long-range plans, and think ahead. White matter volume increases throughout childhood and adolescence, which may allow for increased "connectivity," thereby enhancing the abilities of adolescents to acquire new competencies, such as those needed to master today's technology.

What Is Typical Adolescence?

The concept of typical in adolescent development refers to the degree of psychological adaptation displayed by an adolescent while navigating the hurdles and meeting the milestones characteristic of this period. For up to approximately 75% of youth, adolescence is a period of successful adaptation to physical, cognitive, and emotional changes, mostly continuous with their previous functioning. Psychological maladjustment, self-loathing, disturbance of conduct, substance abuse, affective disorders, and other impairing psychiatric disorders emerge in approximately 20% of the adolescent population.

Adolescent adjustment is continuous with previous psychological function; thus, psychologically disturbed children are at higher risk for psychiatric disorders during adolescence. Adolescents with psychiatric disorders are at increased risk for more significant conflicts with families and for feeling alienated from their families. Although up to 60% of adolescents endorse occasional distress or a psychiatric symptom, this group of adolescents functions well academically and with peers and describes themselves as generally satisfied with their lives.

The developmentalist Erik Erikson characterizes the normative task of adolescence as identity versus role confusion. The integration of past experiences with current changes takes place in what Erikson calls *ego identity*. Adolescents explore various aspects of their psychological selves by becoming fans of heroes or other well-known musical or political idols. Some adolescents appear consumed by their identification with a particular idol, whereas others are more moderate in their expression. Adolescents who feel accepted by a peer group and are involved in a variety of activities are less likely to become consumed by adoration of an idol. Socially isolated adolescents feel socially rejected and become overly identified with an idol to the exclusion of all other activities, are at higher risk for serious emotional problems, and require psychiatric intervention.

Erickson uses the term moratorium to describe the interim period between the concrete thinking of childhood and a more evolved complex ethical development. Erikson defines identity crisis as a normative part of adolescence in which adolescents pursue alternative behaviors and styles and then successfully mold these different experiences into a stable identity. A failure to do so would result in identity diffusion, or role confusion, in which the adolescent lacks a cohesive or confident sense of identity. Adolescence is the time to bond with peers, experiment with new beliefs and styles, fall in love for the first time, and explore creative ideas for future endeavors.

Most adolescents go through this developmental process with optimism, develop good self-esteem, maintain good peer relationships, and sustain harmonious relationships with their families.

Stages of Adolescence

Early Adolescence. Early adolescence, from 12 to 14 years of age, is the period in which the most striking initial changes occur—physically, attitudinally, and behaviorally. Growth spurts often begin in these years for boys, whereas girls may have already had rapid growth for 1 to 2 years. At this stage, boys and girls begin to criticize usual family habits, insist on spending time with peers with less supervision, have a greater awareness of style and appearance, and may question previously accepted family values. A new awareness of sexuality may be displayed by increased modesty and embarrassment with their current physical development or may exhibit itself in an increased interest in the opposite sex.

Early adolescents engage in subtle or overt displays of their growing desire for autonomy, sometimes with challenging behaviors toward authority figures, including teachers and school administrators, and exhibit disdain for rules themselves. At this age, some adolescents begin to experiment with cigarettes, alcohol, and marijuana.

During early adolescence, there is a normal variation in when new defining behaviors are acquired. Overall, although many early adolescents make new friends and modify their public image, most maintain positive connections to family members, old friends, and their family's values. However, for some, early adolescence can a time of overwhelming turmoil, during which there is a dramatic rejection of family, friends, and lifestyle, resulting in an alienation of the adolescent from their family.

Jenna, a 13-year-old adolescent, entered the 8th grade with high hopes of having a good year and making some new friends. She has been an easy going, fun-loving, and cooperative student, but this year she found the school rules increasingly irritating and felt that her teachers were too strict. She has always been able to get good enough grades putting in a minimum of work. Her older sister Sienna, now in 11th grade, had established herself as serious, compliant, well liked by students and teachers, and a well-behaved student who always puts maximum effort into homework and school projects. Jenna has always been compared to her older sister, never quite measuring up, and Jenna resented these comparisons because she didn't want to be a "nerd, like her sister." Jenna was more rebellious, took more risks, and made friends with more popular peers. To distinguish herself from her older sister in school, Jenna began to challenge the rules, stating that they were "stupid" and "meaningless." Jenna began to skip classes, to stay out late, and to experiment with alcohol and marijuana. Jenna rejected her best friends from sixth and seventh grade and began to hang out with more daring peers. When Jenna was at home, she was able to relate to her older sister only when they listened to music or watched Netflix.

Jenna's grades began to drop only slightly, but her parents noted that on her report cards, her teachers rated her effort and behavior as unsatisfactory. During the second month of school, Jenna's parents received a phone call that she was being suspended for a week due to skipping. During a subsequent meeting with the assistant principal and school counselor, Jenna argued that the suspension was unfair because her grades were still pretty good, and she did not understand why skipping class had triggered a suspension when she was getting passing grades. When her school would not back down, Jenna became angry and continued to insist that they were mistreating her. She blurted out that all of her teachers and her parents favored her older sister Sienna and treated her like a second-class citizen. The school suspended Jenna for 5 days and suggested that she seek counseling.

Jenna begrudgingly began psychotherapy and entered a weekly therapy group specializing in teens. Jenna's parents also sought therapy to work on becoming more unified in their parenting. Jenna remained in psychotherapy for the next 1½ years, during which time her attitude and reasoning style changed and evolved considerably. At age 15, Jenna understood why her school had suspended her. Jenna became more open to making friends with a variety of peers, and she disclosed that she liked herself better now than when she was 13. She became closer with her older sister, and she felt that her parents appreciated her for "who she was." (Courtesy of Caroly S. Pataki, M.D.)

Middle Adolescence. During the middle phase of adolescence (roughly between the ages of 14 and 16), adolescents' lifestyles may reflect their efforts to pursue their own stated goals of being independent. Their abilities to combine abstract reasoning with realistic decision-making and judgment are put to the test. In this phase, sexual behavior intensifies, making romantic relationships more complicated, and self-esteem becomes a pivotal influence on positive and negative risk-taking behaviors.

In this phase of development, adolescents tend to identify with a group of peers who become highly influential in their choices of activities, styles, music, idols, and role models. Adolescents' underestimation of the risks associated with a variety of recreational behaviors and their sense of "omnipotence," mixed with their drive to be autonomous, frequently cause some conflict with parental requests and expectations. Most teens can achieve the challenge of defining themselves as unique and different from their families while still connected with family members.

Lucas, a 16-year-old junior in high school, had just gotten his driver's license. He realized that he was lucky to have a brand-new car at 16, since most of his friends did not have cars. Lucas was upset that his parents strongly disapproved of his willingness to drive all his friends to places that he did not even want to go. Lucas was a well-liked teen who had always been an "A" and "B" student, and never had conflicts in school with peers. He played the trumpet in the school band and was on the track team. After he got his new car, Lucas started "going out" with a girl in his grade, Nina, who was also 16 years old. Lucas felt that they had a close relationship. Since she did not yet have a car, he was the "identified driver" whenever they went out or to parties. Lucas was glad about this because he didn't like alcohol and was relieved that Nina would not be driving, given that she drank quite a bit at parties. Nina seemed to be more advanced socially than Lucas, who was somewhat socially immature, and Nina was more risk-taking than Lucas. Lucas had always gotten along reasonably well with his parents, who were considered "easy-going" by his friends and seemed to be pleased that Lucas had a girlfriend.

Things were going well until it became clear that Nina was ready to go further in their sexual relationship. When Lucas realized that Nina was waiting for him to initiate a more intimate sexual relationship with her, he became ashamed of himself for being uncomfortable. Nina began to pressure him about it. When the subject of sex had come up with his parents "hypothetically" in the past, they had dismissed the subject, indicating that when it was the right time for him, Lucas would know. Lucas knew that many of his classmates were sexually active, but Lucas was not an impulsive person and liked to plan things carefully so that they would feel right to him. Lucas and Nina felt strongly for each other and had a great time together, except for the sexual issue. Lucas carefully told Nina that he loved her, but she decided to break up with him anyway to pursue a more intimate relationship. Lucas was miserable for the next few months, while Nina seemed to have forgotten all about him. After a few months had passed, Lucas found that he was enjoying talking to Jessica, a girl who sat next to him in his math class. They continued to be friendly in school over the next few months, and one day, Jessica invited Lucas to a family outing celebrating her birthday. Lucas accepted and they had an enjoyable day together. Jessica was much more like Lucas socially, and they became extremely comfortable with each other and without any pressure. Lucas and Jessica continued their relationship into their senior year of high school, and decided to apply to the same colleges so they could remain together. (Courtesy of Caroly S. Pataki, M.D.)

Late Adolescence. Late adolescence (between the ages of 17 and 19) is a time when continued exploration of academic pursuits, musical and artistic tastes, athletic participation, and social bonds lead a teen toward a greater definition of self and a sense of belonging to specific groups or subcultures within mainstream society. Well-adjusted adolescents can be comfortable with current choices of activities, tastes, hobbies, and friendships, yet remain aware that they will continue to refine their "identities" during young adulthood.

Lisa was a second-semester freshman in college, living on campus, and had just turned 18 years of age. She reflected happily that she was no longer a "minor" and could make almost any decision for herself without involving her parents.

Lisa had always been close to her family, especially her father, but wanted to enjoy her newfound freedom.

Lisa felt liberated and happy with her peers and classes at college, yet during the second semester of college, she became confused and less sure of the life plan she had when she entered college. Since 10th grade, Lisa had planned to pursue a career in medicine like her father, who had strongly encouraged her to become a doctor. So, in the first semester of college she had taken a heavy load of premed science courses, which to her surprise, she strongly disliked. For the second semester, Lisa signed up for liberal arts classes, and no science or math classes. Lisa did not mention this to her father, who she knew would be very disappointed and try to convince her to change her mind. Lisa picked classes for the second semester that ranged from art history to architectural drafting to sociology, philosophy, and music. When her father learned this, he decided that she had been influenced by her roommate, Joanne, who was thinking about majoring in studio art, but had not decided yet, and by her boyfriend Tom, who was in the architecture program.

As the semester progressed, Lisa found that her favorite courses were architectural drafting and the art history class, and Lisa wondered whether she liked the art history class and drafting so much because of how much she liked her roommate, Joanne, or because she just enjoyed the class. Lisa talked this over many times with Joanne, who suggested that she should focus on enjoying her current classes, and not feel pressured to figure out the rest of her life during freshman year. Joanne suggested, and Lisa agreed, that she should take the next year to explore a variety of subjects, including more classes in architecture and art history before making a final decision about a career. Lisa realized that Joanne's approach to college and life was so much more open, the opposite of her own approach, following her parents' pressure to plan and make a commitment to a career before entering college. Joanne's approach left more room for exploring her experiences with a variety of subjects and making a choice of a major when she felt ready to make a commitment, rather than jumping into what she was "supposed" to do according to her parents, especially her father. Lisa took Joanne's advice and allowed herself another year to try out many subjects and then decide on a career. After experiencing courses in many varied subjects, Lisa decided that she did truly enjoy the architecture classes, and she successfully switched her major from premed to architecture. (Courtesy of Caroly S. Pataki, M.D.)

Components of Adolescence

Physical Development. Puberty is the process by which adolescents develop physical and sexual maturity, along with reproductive ability. The first signs of the pubertal process are an increased rate of growth in both height and weight. This process begins in girls by approximately 10 years of age. By the age of 11 or 12, many girls noticeably tower over their male classmates, who do not experience a growth spurt, on average, until they reach 13 years of age. By age 13, many girls have experienced menarche, and most have developed breasts and pubic hair.

Wide variation exists in the normal range of onset and timing of pubertal development and its components. A set sequence occurs, however, in the order in which pubertal development proceeds. Thus, secondary sexual characteristics in boys, such as increased length and width of the penis, for example, will occur after the release of androgens from developed enlarged testes.

Sexual maturity ratings (SMRs), also referred to as Tanner Stages, range from SMR 1 (prepuberty) to SMR 5 (adult). The SMR ratings include stages of genital maturity in boys and breast development in girls, as well as pubic hair development. Table 1-9 outlines SMRs for boys and girls.

The primary female sex characteristic is ovulation, the release of eggs from ovarian follicles, approximately once every 28 days. When adolescent girls reach SMR 3 to 4, ovarian follicles are producing enough estrogen to result in menarche, the onset of menstruation. When adolescent girls reach SMR 4 to 5, an ovarian follicle matures monthly, and ovulation occurs. Estrogen and progesterone promote sexual maturation, including further development of fallopian tubes and breasts.

For adolescent boys, the primary sex characteristic is the development of sperm by the testes. In boys, sperm development occurs in response to follicle-stimulating hormone acting on the seminiferous tubules within the testes. The pubertal process in boys consists of the growth of the testes stimulated by luteinizing hormone. An adolescent boy's ability to ejaculate generally emerges within 1 year of reaching SMR 2. Secondary sexual characteristics in boys include thickening of the skin, broadening of the shoulders, and the development of facial hair.

Cognitive Maturation. Cognitive maturation in adolescence encompasses a wide range of expanded abilities that fall within the global category of executive functions of the brain. These include the transition from concrete thinking to more abstract thinking; an increased ability to draw logical conclusions in scientific pursuits, with peer interactions, and in social situations; and new abilities for self-observation and self-regulation. Adolescents acquire increased awareness of their intellectual, artistic, and athletic gifts and talents, yet it often takes many more years into young adulthood to establish a practical application for these abilities.

The central cognitive change that occurs gradually during adolescence is the shift from concrete thinking (concrete operational thinking, according to Jean Piaget) to the ability to think abstractly (formal operational thinking, in Piaget's terminology). This evolution occurs as an adaptation to stimuli that demand an adolescent to produce hypothetical responses, as well as in response to the adolescent's expanded abilities to provide generalizations from specific situations. The development of abstract thinking is not a sudden epiphany but,

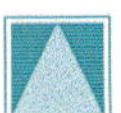

Table 1-9.
Sexual Maturity Ratings for Male and Female Adolescents

Sexual Maturity Rating	Girls	Boys
Stage 1	Preadolescent, papilla elevated No pubic hair	Penis, testes, scrotum preadolescent No pubic hair
Stage 2	Breast bud, small mound; areola diameter increased Sparse long pubic hair, mainly along labia	Penis size same, testes and scrotum enlarged, with scrotal skin reddened Sparse long pubic hair, mainly at the base of penis
Stage 3	Breast and areola larger; no separation of contours Pubic hair darker and coarser; spread over pubic area	Penis elongated, with increased size of testes and scrotum Pubic hair darker and coarser; spread over pubic area
Stage 4	Breast size increased Areola and papilla raised Pubic hair coarse and thickened; covers less area than in adults, does not extend to thighs	Penis increased in length and width Testes and scrotum larger Pubic hair coarse and thickened; covers less area than in adults, does not extend to thighs
Stage 5	Breasts resemble adult female breast; areola has recessed to breast contour Pubic hair increased in density; area extends to thighs	Penis, testes, scrotum appear mature Pubic hair increased in density; area extends to thighs

rather, a gradual process of expanding logical deductions beyond concrete experiences and achieving the capacity for idealistic and hypothetical thinking based on everyday life.

Adolescents often use an omnipotent belief system that reinforces their sense of immunity from danger, even when confronted with logical risks. Some degree of child-like magical thinking continues to coexist with more mature abstract thinking in many adolescents. Despite the persistence of magical thinking into adolescence, adolescent cognition departs from that of younger children insofar as the increased ability for self-observation and development of strategies to promote strengths and compensate for weaknesses.

One of the essential cognitive tasks in adolescence is to identify and gravitate toward those pursuits that seem to match the adolescent's cognitive strengths in academic courses and in thinking about future aspirations. Piaget believed that cognitive adaptation in adolescence is profoundly influenced by social relationships and the dialogue between adolescents and peers, making social cognition an integral part of cognitive development in adolescence.

Socialization. Socialization in adolescence encompasses the ability to find acceptance in peer relationships, as well as the development of more mature social cognition. The skills to develop a sense of belonging to a peer group are of central importance to a sense of well-being. Being viewed as socially competent by peers is a critical component in building good self-esteem for most early adolescents. Peer influences are powerful and can foster positive social interactions, as well as apply pressure in less socially accepted behaviors or even high-risk behavior. Belonging to a peer group is, in general, a sign of adaptation and a developmentally appropriate step in separating from parents and turning the focus of loyalty toward friends. Children between the ages of 6 and 12 can engage in exchanges of ideas and opinions and acknowledge feelings of peers, but the relationships often wax and wane in a discontinuous way based on altercations and good times. Friendships deepen with repeated good times, but, for some school-aged children, a variety of peers are often interchangeable—that is, a child may seek a companion when that child has free time, rather than out of a desire to spend time with a specific friend. As adolescence ensues, friendships become more individualized, and adolescents may share personal secrets with a friend rather than a family member. The adolescent may achieve a comfort level with one or several early adolescent peers, and the group may "stick together," spending most of their free time together. In early adolescence, a blend of the above two social modes may emerge, small "cliques" arise, and, even within the cliques, competition and jealousies regarding which dyads are "preferred" or higher ranked within the clique may result in some discontinuities in the relationships. In later adolescence, the peer group solidifies, leading to increased stability in the friendships and a greater mutuality in the quality of the interactions.

Moral Development. Morality is a set of values and beliefs about codes of behavior that conform to those shared by others in society. Adolescents, as do younger children, tend to develop patterns of behaviors characteristic of their family and educational environments and by imitation of specific peers and adults whom they admire. Moral development does not strictly follow chronologic age but, instead, is an outgrowth from cognitive development.

Piaget described moral development as a gradual process parallel to cognitive development, with expanded abilities in differentiating the best interests for society from those of individuals occurring during late adolescence. Preschool children simply follow the rules set forth by the parents; in the middle years, children accept rules but show an inability to allow for exceptions; and during adolescence, young persons recognize rules in terms of what is good for the society at large.

Lawrence Kohlberg integrated Piaget's concepts and described multiple stages of moral development within three significant levels of morality. The first level is preconventional morality, in which punishment and obedience to the parent are the determining factors. The second level is the morality of conventional role conformity, in which children try to conform to gain approval and to maintain good relationships with others. The third and highest level is the morality of self-accepted moral principles, in which children voluntarily comply with rules based on a concept of ethical principles and make exceptions to rules in certain circumstances.

Although Kohlberg's and Piaget's notions of moral development focus on a unified theory of cognitive maturation for both sexes, Carol Gilligan emphasizes the social context of moral development leading to divergent patterns in moral development. Gilligan points out that, in women, compassion and the ethics of caring are dominant features of moral decision-making, whereas, for men, predominant features of moral judgments are related more to a perception of justice, rationality, and a sense of fairness. Although influential, many psychologists and scholars criticize Gilligan's work as primarily observational and lacking scientific rigor. Feminist scholars note that Gilligan rarely considers the role of societal expectations in influencing gender-based behavior.

Developmental psychologists have incorporated insights from cognitive psychology and suggest that moral development goes beyond the rationality of Piaget and Kolberg. Psychologists such as Jonathan Haidt emphasize the role of intuition and preconceived beliefs based on the fundamental moral foundations found in a society. He suggests that the logical explanations one gives to justify one's actions are post hoc rationalizations meant to justify one's emotional (i.e., irrational) reactions to the moral dilemmas we face in society.

Self-Esteem. Self-esteem is a measure of one's sense of self-worth based on perceived success and achievements, as well as a perception of how much one is valued by peers, family members, teachers, and society in general. The most important correlates of good self-esteem are one's perception of attractive physical appearance and high value to peers and family. Secondary features of self-esteem relate to academic achievement, athletic abilities, and unique talents. Adolescent self-esteem is mediated, to a significant degree, by the positive feedback received from a peer group and family members, and adolescents often seek out a peer group that offers acceptance, regardless of negative behaviors associated with that group.

Current Environmental Influences and Adolescence

Adolescent Sexual Behavior. Sexual experimentation in adolescents often begins with fantasy and masturbation in early adolescence, followed by noncoital genital touching with the opposite sex or, in some cases, same-sex partners, oral sex with partners, and initiation of sexual intercourse at a later point in development. By high school, most male adolescents report experience with masturbation, and more than half of adolescent girls report masturbation. The balance between healthy adolescent sexual experimentation and emotionally and physically safe sexual practices remains a challenge for society.

Estimates vary, but about 50% of 9th- to 12th-grade students reported having had sexual intercourse. The median age at first intercourse is about 16 years for boys and 17 years for girls. Boys often have more sexual partners than do girls.

FACTORS INFLUENCING ADOLESCENT SEXUAL BEHAVIOR. Factors that affect sexual behavior in adolescents include personality traits, gender, cultural and religious background, racial factors, family attitudes, and sexual education and prevention programs.

Personality factors are associated with sexual behavior, as well as sexual risk-taking. Higher levels of impulsivity are associated with a younger age at the first experience of sexual intercourse; a higher number of sexual partners; sexual intercourse without the use of contraception, including condoms; and a history of a sexually transmitted disease (STD, chlamydia).

Historically, male adolescents have initiated sexual intercourse at a younger age than female adolescents. The younger a teenage girl is when she has sex for the first time, the more risk she has of having been pressured or acquiesced to an unwanted experience. Close to 4 of 10 girls who had first intercourse at 13 or 14 years of age report it was either not voluntary or unwanted. Three of four girls and over half of boys report that girls who have sex do so because their boyfriends pressure them to. In general, adolescents who initiate sexual intercourse at younger ages are also more likely to have a higher number of sexual partners.

The additive effects of a stable home and access to school-based educational programs can decrease high-risk sexual behavior among adolescents. Female empowerment strategies can play an essential role in decreasing unwanted sexual behavior and teenage pregnancies.

CONTRACEPTIVES. The majority of teenagers aged 15 to 19 years are aware of at least one method of birth control. The two most common methods are condoms and birth control pills. STDs, despite the use of condoms, are still at high levels in teens—approximately one in four sexually active teens contracts an STD every year.

PREGNANCY. Teenage pregnancy creates a plethora of health risks for both mother and child. Children born to teenage mothers have a higher chance of dying before the age of 5 years. Those who survive are more likely to perform poorly in school and are at higher risk of abuse and neglect. Teenage mothers are less likely to gain adequate weight during pregnancy, increasing the risk of premature births and low–birth-weight infants. Low–birth-weight babies are more likely to have organs that are not fully developed, resulting in bleeding in the brain, respiratory distress syndrome, and intestinal problems. Teenage mothers are also less likely to seek regular prenatal care and to take recommended daily multivitamins, and they are more likely to smoke, drink, or use drugs during pregnancy. Only about one-third of teenage mothers obtain high school diplomas, and only 1.5% have a college degree by the age of 30.

ABORTION. The abortion rate in many European countries tends to be far lower than that in the United States. The Centers for Disease Control and Prevention (CDC) reports that the abortion rate in the United States for girls between the ages of 15 and 19 is about 30 per 1,000. In France, about 10.5 of every 1,000 girls under the age of 20 had an abortion, according to World Health Organization statistics. The rate of abortion in Germany was 6.8; in Italy, 6.3; and in Spain, 4.5. Britain has a higher rate, 18.5. Family planning experts believe that more sex education and the availability of contraceptive devices help keep the number of abortions down. In Holland, where contraceptives are freely available in schools, the teenage pregnancy rate is among the lowest in the world.

Risk-Taking Behavior. Reasonable risk-taking is a necessary endeavor in adolescence, leading to confidence both in forming new relationships and in sports and social situations. High-risk behaviors among adolescents are associated with severe negative consequences, however, and can take many forms, including drug and alcohol use, unsafe sexual practices, self-injurious behaviors, and reckless driving.

Drug Use

ALCOHOL. About 30% of 12th graders report having five or more drinks in a row within 2 weeks. The average age when youths first try alcohol is 11 years for boys and 13 years for girls. The national average age at which Americans begin regular drinking is 15.9 years of age. People ages 18 to 25 show the highest prevalence of binge and heavy drinking. Drunk driving has declined since 2002. Alcohol dependence, along with other drugs, is associated with depression, anxiety, oppositional defiant disorder, antisocial personality disorder, and an increased rate of suicide.

NICOTINE. The number of young American smokers has declined since 1990. However, the rate of smoking among teenagers is still as high as or higher than that of adults. According to the American Cancer Society, on average more than one of five students have smoked cigarettes. Each day, more than 4,000 teenagers try their first cigarette, and another 2,000 become regular, daily smokers. Cigarette smokers are more likely to get into fights, carry weapons, attempt suicide, suffer from mental health problems such as depression, and engage in high-risk sexual behaviors. One of three will eventually die from smoking-related diseases. Cigarettes are the most common type of tobacco used among middle-school students, followed by cigars, smokeless tobacco, and pipes.

CANNABIS. Marijuana is the most popular drug, with 14.6 million people using it (6.2% of the population), two-thirds being under the age of 18. Its use, however, is slowly declining. About 6% of 12th graders report daily use of marijuana.

One of the primary reasons for such prevalence of marijuana use among teenagers is because many find that marijuana is easier to get than alcohol or cigarettes. This belief has declined in recent years. Once teenagers are dependent on marijuana, they often tumble into truancy, crime, and depression.

COCAINE AND METHAMPHETAMINE. About 13% of high school seniors have used cocaine, exceeding the national average of 3.6%. Crystal methamphetamine (ice) has an annual prevalence in 12th graders of about 2%.

OPIOIDS. In recent years, the number of teens using prescription pain relievers for nonmedical reasons has increased. Prescription drug abuse by people ages 18 to 25 has increased by 15%. Drugs of specific concern are the pain relievers oxycodone and hydrocodone. Oxycodone has gained ground among high school students since its emergence in 2001, with 5% of 12th graders, 3.5% of 10th graders, and 1.7% of 8th graders reporting use. About 9% of 12th graders use hydrocodone, 6% of 10th graders, and 2.5% of 8th graders.

Heroin use is prevalent among adolescents, although less so than cocaine. The average age of use is 19, but almost 2% of 12th graders use it. The nasal route (snorting) is the most common method of use.

Violence. Although rates of violent crime have decreased throughout the United States in recent years, violent crimes by young offenders are on the increase. Homicides are the second leading cause of death among people aged 15 to 25. (Accidents are first; suicides are third.) Black male teenagers are far more likely to be murder victims than are boys from any other racial or ethnic group or girls of any race. The factor most strongly associated with violence among adolescent boys is growing up in a household without a father or father surrogate; this factor aside, race, socioeconomic status, and education show no effect on the propensity toward violence.

BULLYING. *Bullying* is the use of one's strength or status to intimidate, injure, or humiliate another person of lesser strength or status. It can be physical, verbal, or social. Physical bullying involves physical injury or threat of injury to someone. Verbal bullying refers to teasing or insulting someone. Social bullying refers to the use of peer rejection or exclusion to humiliate or isolate a victim.

About 30% of 6th- through 10th-grade students experience moderate-to-frequent bullying, as a bully, a target, or both. Approximately 1.7 million children within this age group bully other children. Boys are more likely to be involved in bullying and violent behavior than girls. Girls tend to use verbal bullying rather than physical.

An estimated 160,000 students miss school each day because of fear of attack or intimidation from peers; some may drop out. Stresses of "victimization" can interfere with student's engagement and learning in school. Children who bully other children are at risk for engaging in more violent severe behaviors, such as frequent fighting and carrying a weapon.

Cyberbullying. During the last decade, electronic or internet bullying has become of great concern to adolescents. Cyberbullying is defined broadly to convey the use of electronic means to intimidate or harm someone intentionally. The reported prevalence of cyberbullying is variable, reports ranging from 1% to 62% of youth reporting that they were victims of cyber victimization. A study of about 700 Australian students, recruited at age 10 years, and followed until ages 14 to 15 years, found that 15% had engaged in cyberbullying, 21% had engaged in traditional bullying, and 7% had engaged in both. Another study of self-reported information collected from 399 teens in the 8th to 10th grades found that involvement in cyberbullying, either as a victim or a bully, specifically contributed to the prediction of depressive symptoms and suicidal ideation. This correlation between cyberbullying and depressive symptomatology is more reliable than the association of traditional bullying and affective disorder.

Gangs. Gang violence is a problem throughout the United States. There are 2,000 different youth gangs around the country, with more than 200,000 teens and young adults as members. Most members are between the ages of 12 and 24 years, with an average of 17 to 18 years. Gang membership is a brief phase for many teenagers; one-half to two-thirds leave the gang by the 1-year mark. Boys are more likely to join gangs than girls; however, female gang membership may be underrepresented. Female gang members are more likely to be found in small cities and rural areas and tend to be younger than male gang members. Female gang members are also involved in less delinquent or criminal activity than males and commit fewer violent crimes.

WEAPONS. Homicide is the third leading cause of death for people ages 10 to 24 years of age. Each day, on average, nearly 10 American children younger than the age of 18 years are killed in handgun suicides, homicides, and accidents. Many more are wounded. One in five youths in grades 9 to 12 carries a weapon: knife, gun, or club.

By law, anyone younger than 18 years cannot purchase a firearm. Two-thirds of students in grades 6 to 12 say that they can get a firearm within 24 hours, however. More than 22 million children live in a home with a firearm. In 40% of these homes, at least one gun is not locked, and 13% are unlocked and loaded. Two of three students involved in school shootings acquired their guns from their own home or that of a relative. At least 60% of suicide deaths in teens involve the use of a handgun.

SCHOOL VIOLENCE. According to the CDC, less than 2.6% of youth homicide occurred in schools over the last decade. Approximately 7% of teachers report they have been threatened with injury or physically attacked by a student from their school. Also, among students in grades 9 through 12, about 6% reported carrying a weapon on school property on one or more days in the 30 days before the survey.

Many factors can lead to violent acts in teenagers. Some inherited traits include impulsivity, learning difficulties, low IQ, or fearlessness. A correlation also exists between witnessing violent acts and involvement in violence. Children who witness violent acts are more aggressive and grow up more likely to become involved in violence—either as a victimizer or as a victim. Table 1-10

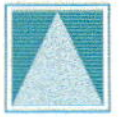

Table 1-10.
Warning Signs of School Violence

Early Warning Signs
Social withdrawal
Excessive feelings of isolation and being alone
Excessive feelings of rejection
Being a victim of violence
Feelings of being picked on and persecuted
Expression of violence in writings and drawings
Uncontrolled anger
Patterns of impulsive and chronic hitting, intimidating, and bullying behaviors
History of discipline problems
History of violent and aggressive behavior
Intolerance for differences and prejudicial attitudes
Drug and alcohol use
Affiliation with gangs
Inappropriate access to, possession of, and use of firearms
Serious threats of violence

Imminent Warning Signs
Serious physical fighting with peers or family members
Severe destruction of property
Severe rage for seemingly minor reasons
Detailed threats of lethal violence
Possession and/or use of firearms and other weapons
Other self-injurious behaviors or threats of suicide

lists some of the early and imminent warning signs of school violence.

On April 20, 1999, two teenage boys, ages 17 and 18 years, went on a shooting rampage through Columbine High School of Littleton, Colorado. Armed with shotguns, a semiautomatic rifle, and a pistol, they laughed and shouted as they shot classmates and teachers at point-blank range while hurling homemade explosives. Fifteen were killed, including the 2 gunmen, who also injured 25 people. This historical incident has become an unfortunate prototype for school shootings.

The gunmen were members of the "trench coat mafia" at the high school, a clique of social misfits who stood out at the school for their gothic style of dress and nihilistic attitude. The two gunmen were obsessed with violent video games and intrigued with Nazi culture, even though one was part Jewish. They chose the date of the attack to coincide with Adolf Hitler's birthday.

On the morning of December 14th, 2012, in Newtown, Connecticut, a 20-year-old young man drove his mother's car and entered Sandy Hook elementary school armed with an AR-15 rifle and two semiautomatic pistols purchased by his mother, and went on a shooting rampage, moving from classroom to classroom shooting children, teachers, and school administrators. Firing 154 rounds of ammunition, the gunman murdered a total of 20 children and 6 adults. Before driving to Sandy Hook Elementary school, the young man is believed to be the perpetrator of the shooting and killing of his mother in the home they shared. After the shootings, the gunman turned a shotgun on himself and took his own life. The Sandy Hook shootings were among the deadliest school attacks in the history of our country.

The gunman was a shy and awkward boy who was described as isolated, fidgety, and deeply troubled. He appeared to be obsessed with violence and mass killings. Numerous weapons, books, and articles describing other mass killings were found among his possessions. The gunman's mother was a gun enthusiast who purchased and kept multiple firearms in the home. Unlike him, the gunman's mother was outgoing and social. The gunman had been diagnosed with autism spectrum disorder. During investigation of his home, the gunman was found to have hundreds of pages of his writings and charts detailing incidents of mass killings that spanned several centuries. The gunman had become isolated and rejected by peers starting as a child, reportedly due to poor social skills, developmental speech delay, sensory sensitivities, anxiety, and obsessive-compulsive disorder. The gunman was home schooled by the 10th grade, where he spent most of his time playing violent video games and surrounding himself with his mother's weapons. The gunman became more and more reclusive during his high school years, losing touch with the activities of social engagement typical of his peers. The gunman was, reportedly, seething with anger internally and had serious contempt for people and his inability to develop positive relationships with peers or relatives. The gunman died a recluse who was deeply psychiatrically troubled.

SEXUAL OFFENSE. Adolescents younger than age 18 years account for about 20% of arrests for all sexual offenses (excluding prostitution), 20% to 30% of rape cases, 14% of aggravated sexual assault offenses, and 27% of child sexual homicides. These adolescent offenders account for the victimization of approximately one-half of boys and one-fourth of girls who are molested or sexually abused. Most instances have involved adolescent male perpetrators.

There appear to be two types of juvenile sex offenders: those who target children and those who offend against peers or adults. The age difference between the victim and the offender is the main difference between the two groups. Table 1-11 lists the differences and similarities between these two groups.

Etiologic factors of juvenile sex offending include significant maltreatment experiences and exposure to pornography, substance abuse, and exposure to aggressive role models. A significant number of offending adolescents have a childhood history of physical abuse (25% to 50%) or sexual abuse (10% to 80%). Half of the adolescent offenders lived with both parents and one other juvenile at the time of their offending. Evidence also suggests that most juvenile sex offenders are likely to become adult sex offenders. The most common psychosocial deficits of adolescent sexual offenders include low self-esteem, few social skills, minimal assertive skills, and poor academic performance. The most common psychiatric diagnoses are conduct disorder, substance use disorder, adjustment disorder, ADHD, specific phobia, and mood disorders.

Teen Prostitution.

Teenagers constitute a large portion of sexually trafficked victims of prostitution, with estimates ranging up to 1 million teenagers involved in prostitution. The average age of a recruit is 13 years; however, some are young as 9 years of age. A majority of adolescent prostitutes are vulnerable teens who are sexually trafficked by men who are abusive to the girls, and boys may become sexually trafficked same-sex victims of prostitution. Most teenagers who are sexually trafficked have a history of chaotic and unstable homes, sexual and/or physical abuse or neglect, and sometimes homelessness. Twenty-seven percent of teenage prostitution occurs in large cities, and incidents usually take place at an outside location, such as highways, roads, alleys, fields, woods, or parking lots. Teenage prostitutes are at high risk for acquired immunodeficiency syndrome (AIDS), and many (up to 70% in some studies) have HIV.

Tattoos and Body Piercing.

Body piercing and tattoos have been prevalent among adolescents since the 1980s. In the general population, approximately 10% to 13% of adolescents have tattoos. Of the more than 500 adolescents surveyed in a study, 13.2% report at least one

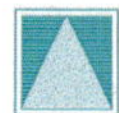

Table 1-11. Juvenile Sex Offender Subtypes

Juvenile Offenders Who Sexually Offend against Peers or Adults
Predominantly assault females and strangers or casual acquaintances
Sexual assaults occur in association with other types of criminal activity (e.g., burglary)
Have histories of nonsexual criminal offenses, and appear more generally delinquent and conduct disordered
Commit their offenses in public areas
Display higher levels of aggression and violence in the commission of their sexual crimes
More likely to use weapons and to cause injuries to their victims
Juvenile Offenders Who Sexually Offend against Children
Most victims are male and are related to them, either siblings or other relatives
Almost half of the offenders have had at least one male victim
The sexual crimes tend to reflect a greater reliance on opportunity and guile than injurious force. This appears to be particularly true when their victim is related to them. These youths may "trick" the child into complying with the molestation, use bribes, or threaten the child with loss of the relationship
Within the overall population of juveniles who sexually assault children are certain youths who display high levels of aggression and violence. Generally, these are youths who display more severe levels of personality and/or psychosexual disturbances, such as psychopathy, sexual sadism, and so on
Suffer from deficits in self-esteem and social competency
Many show evidence of depression
Characteristics Common to Both Groups
High rates of learning disabilities and academic dysfunction (30–60%)
The presence of other behavioral health problems, including substance abuse and disorders of conduct (up to 80% have some diagnosable psychiatric disorder)
Observed difficulties with impulse control and judgment

tattoo, and 26.9% report at least one body piercing, other than in their ear lobe, at some point in their lives. Both tattoos and body piercings are more common in girls than in boys. Adolescents who endorsed possession of at least one tattoo or body piercing are more likely to endorse the use of gateway drugs (cigarettes, alcohol, marijuana), as well as experience with hard drugs (cocaine, crystal methamphetamine, and ecstasy).

TRANSITION INTO ADULTHOOD: INTRODUCTION

Historically, in the field of developmental psychology, the predominant theory held that development ended with childhood and adolescence. Adults were considered to be finished products in whom the ultimate developmental states had been reached. Beyond adolescence, the developmental point of view was relevant only insofar as success or failure to reach adult levels or to maintain them determined the maturity or immaturity of the adult personality. Although the debate continues, the idea that development continues throughout life is increasingly accepted.

Development in adulthood, as in childhood, is always the result of the interaction among body, mind, and environment, never exclusively the result of any one of the three variables. Most adults are forced to confront and adapt to similar circumstances: establishing an independent identity, forming a marriage or other partnership, raising children, building and maintaining careers, and accepting the disability and death of one's parents.

In modern Western societies, adulthood is the most prolonged phase of human life. Although the exact age of consent varies from person to person, adulthood can be divided into three main parts: young or early adulthood (beginning at age 20), middle adulthood (beginning at age 40), and late adulthood or old age (age 65 and older).

YOUNG ADULTHOOD

Usually considered to begin at the end of adolescence (about age 20) and to end at age 40, early adulthood is characterized by peaking biologic development, the assumption of major social roles, and the evolution of an adult self and life structure. Successfully adapting to adulthood depends on the satisfactory resolution of childhood and adolescent crises and managing new adult challenges.

During late adolescence, young persons generally leave home and begin to function independently. Sexual relationships become serious, and the quest for intimacy begins. The 20s are spent, for the most part, exploring options for occupation and marriage or alternative relationships and making commitments in various areas.

Early adulthood requires choosing new roles (e.g., husband, father) and establishing an identity congruent with those new roles. It involves asking and answering the questions "Who am I?" and "Where am I going?" The choices made during this time may be tentative; young adults may make several false starts.

Transition from Adolescence to Young Adulthood

The transition from adolescence to young adulthood is characterized by real and intrapsychic separation from the family of origin and the engagement of new, phase-specific tasks (Table 1-12). It involves many important

Table 1-12.
Development Tasks of Young Adulthood

To develop a young-adult sense of self and other: the third individuation
To develop adult friendships
To develop the capacity for intimacy; to become a spouse
To become a biologic and psychological parent
To develop a relationship of mutuality and equality with parents while facilitating their midlife development
To establish an adult work identity
To develop adult forms of play
To integrate new attitudes toward time

events, such as graduating from high school, starting a job or entering college, and living independently. During these years, the individual resolves the issue of childhood dependency sufficiently to establish self-reliance and begins to formulate new, young-adult goals that eventually result in the creation of new life structures that promote stability and continuity.

Developmental Tasks

Establishing a self that is separate from parents is a significant task of young adulthood. For most individuals, the emotional detachment from parents that takes place in adolescence and young adulthood is followed by a new inner definition of themselves as comfortably alone and competent, able to care for themselves in the real world. This shift away from the parents continues long after marriage, and parenthood results in the formation of new relationships that replace the progenitors as the most influential individuals in the young adult's life.

Psychological separation from the parents is followed by the synthesis of mental representations from the childhood past and the young-adult present. The psychological separation from parents in adolescence has been called the *second individuation,* and the continued elaboration of these themes in young adulthood has been called the *third individuation.* The continuous process of elaboration of self and differentiation from others that occurs in the developmental phases of young and middle age continues to influence our meaningful adult relationships.

Further Readings

Alanko D. The health effects of video games in children and adolescents. *Pediatr Rev*. 2023;44(1):23–32.

Andrews JL, Ahmed SP, Blakemore SJ. Navigating the social environment in adolescence: the role of social brain development. *Biol Psychiatry*. 2021;89(2):109–118.

Blackmore SJ. Development of the social brain in adolescence. *J R Soc Med*. 2012;105(3):111–116.

Blair C, Raver CC. Child development in the context of adversity: experiential canalization of brain and behavior. *Am Psychol*. 2012;67(4):309–318.

Bonanno RA, Hymel S. Cyber bullying and internalizing difficulties: above and beyond the impact of traditional forms of bullying. *J Youth Adolesc*. 2013;42(5):685–697.

Braams BR, Krabbendam L. Adolescent development: from neurobiology to psychopathology. *Curr Opin Psychol*. 2022;48:101490.

Brown GW, Ban M, Craig TKJ, Harris TO, Herbert J, Uher R. Serotonin transporter length polymorphism, childhood maltreatment and chronic depression: a specific gene-environment interaction. *Depress Anxiety*. 2013;30(1):5–13.

Burgess AW, Garbarino C, Carlson MI. Pathological teasing and bullying turned deadly: shooters and suicide. *Victims & Offenders*. 2006;1(1): 1–14.

Burnett S, Sebastian C, Kadosh KC, Blakemore SJ. The social brain in adolescence: evidence from functional magnetic resonance imaging and behavioural studies. *Neurosci Biobehav Rev*. 2011;35(8): 1654–1664.

Busso DS, Pool AC, Kendall-Taylor N, Ginsburg KR. Reframing adolescent development: identifying communications challenges and opportunities. *J Res Adolesc*. 2022;32(4):1328–1340.

Cama SF, Sehgal P. Racial and ethnic considerations across child and adolescent development. *Acad Psychiatry*. 2021;45(1):106–109.

Casey BJ, Heller AS, Gee DG, Cohen AO. Development of the emotional brain. *Neurosci Lett*. 2019;693:29–34.

Franco P, Putois B, Guyon A, et al. Sleep during development: sex and gender differences. *Sleep Med Rev*. 2020;51:101276.

Giedd JN. Adolescent brain and the natural allure of digital media. *Dialogues Clin Neurosci*. 2020;22(2):127–133.

Giedd JN. The digital revolution and adolescent brain evolution. *J Adolesc Health*. 2012;51(2):101–105.

Hemphill SA, Kotevski A, Tollit M, et al. Longitudinal predictors of cyber and traditional bullying perpetration in Australian secondary school students. *J Adolesc Health*. 2012;51(1):59–65.

Henderson SW. Teleological perspectives in child and adolescent development. *J Am Acad Child Adolesc Psychiatry*. 2023;62(10): 1083–1085.

Karatoreos IN, McEwen BS. Annual research review: the neurobiology and physiology of resilience and adaptation across the life course. *J Child Psychol Psychiatry*. 2013;54(4):337–347.

Ladouceur CD, Peper JS, Crone EA, Dahl RE. White matter development in adolescence: the influence of puberty and implications for affective disorders. *Dev Cogn Neurosci*. 2012;2(1):36–54.

Maza MT, Fox KA, Kwon SJ, et al. Association of habitual checking behaviors on social media with longitudinal functional brain development. *JAMA Pediatr*. 2023;177(2):160–167.

Obradovic J. How can the study of physiological reactivity contribute to our understanding of adversity and resilience processes in development? *Dev Psychopathol*. 2013;24(2):371–387.

Pataki CS. Adolescent development In: Sadock BJ, Sadock VA, Ruiz P, eds. *Kaplan & Sadock's Comprehensive Textbook of Psychiatry*. 9th ed. Vol. 2. Lippincott Williams & Wilkins; 2009:3356.

Raffa BJ, Heerman WJ, Lampkin J, et al. Parental perspectives on the impact of the COVID-19 pandemic on infant, child, and adolescent development. *J Dev Behav Pediatr*. 2023;44(3):e204–e211.

Savopoulos P, Bryant C, Fogarty A, et al. Intimate partner violence and child and adolescent cognitive development: a systematic review. *Trauma Violence Abuse*. 2023;24(3):1882–1907.

Scott JC. Impact of adolescent cannabis use on neurocognitive and brain development. *Child Adolesc Psychiatr Clin N Am*. 2023;32(1):21–42.

Willoughby T, Good M, Adachi PJC, Hamza C, Tavernier R. Examining the link between adolescent brain development and risk taking form a social-developmental perspective. *Brain Cogn*. 2013;83(3):315–323.

Wright MF, Li Y. Kicking the digital dog: a longitudinal investigation of young adults' victimization and cyber-displaced aggression. *Cyberpsychol Behav Soc Netw*. 2012;15(9):448–454.

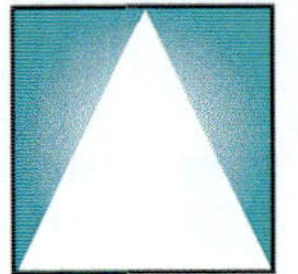

2 Examination and Diagnosis of Infants, Children, and Adolescents

A comprehensive evaluation of an infant, child, or adolescent is composed of interviews, observations of an infant, and observations as well as interviews with a child or adolescent. Parent or caregiver interviews are also an important component of a psychiatric evaluation. In addition, gathering of information from family members and current school or daycare programs are very helpful. If available, standardized assessments of the child's intellectual level and academic achievement are beneficial. When there are concerns about developmental milestones or trajectory, standardized measures of developmental level and neuropsychological assessments are useful. Children rarely request psychiatric evaluations, and youth often display varied emotional and behavioral responses at home and in school, so it is important to elicit information from a variety of sources. In some cases, the court or a child protective service agency may initiate a psychiatric evaluation. Children and adolescents can be excellent informants about symptoms related to mood and inner experiences, such as psychotic phenomena, sadness, fears, and anxiety. However, youth, especially younger children, have difficulty with remembering and reporting the chronology of symptoms and are sometimes reticent about reporting behaviors that have gotten them into trouble. Very young children often cannot articulate their experiences verbally and are more communicative about their feelings and preoccupations in a play or game situation. Assessment of an infant, child, or adolescent includes identifying the reasons for referral; assessing the nature and extent of the child's psychological and behavioral difficulties; and determining family, school, social, and developmental factors that are influencing the child's emotional well-being.

The first step in the comprehensive evaluation of a child or adolescent is to obtain a full description of the current concerns and a history of the child's previous psychiatric and medical problems. This interview is typically done first with the parents for young school-age children. In adolescents, it is important to understand the adolescent's perception of why they are being evaluated. A direct interview and observation of the child usually comes next, followed by psychological testing when indicated.

Clinical interviews offer the most flexibility in understanding the evolution of problems and in establishing the role of environmental factors and life events, but they may not systematically cover all psychiatric diagnostic categories. To increase the breadth of information generated, clinicians may use semi-structured interviews such as the *Kiddie Schedule for Affective Disorders and Schizophrenia for School-Age Children* (K-SADS); structured interviews such as the *National Institute for Mental Health Diagnostic Interview Schedule for Children Version IV* (NIMH DISC-IV); and rating scales, such as the *Child Behavior Checklist* and *Connors Parent or Teacher Rating Scale for ADHD*.

It is not uncommon for interviews from different sources, such as parents, teachers, and school counselors, to reflect different or even contradictory information about a given child. When faced with conflicting information, the clinician should determine whether apparent contradictions reflect an accurate picture of the child in different settings. Once obtaining a complete history from the parents, we should examine the child and assess the child's current functioning at home and school. Once a complete evaluation and psychological testing, if indicated, is completed, all the available information is considered to make a best-estimate diagnosis and followed by recommendations.

Once all of the necessary clinical information about a youth is obtained, before deciding on interventions, the clinician will make a determination of whether the youth meets criteria for one or more psychiatric disorders according to the Fifth Edition Text Revision of the *Diagnostic and Statistical Manual of Mental Disorders* (DSM-5-TR). Clinical interventions are often recommended to help ameliorate symptoms and situations even when a psychiatric disorder is not diagnosed.

CLINICAL INTERVIEWS

To conduct a useful child interview, a clinician must be familiar with typical development to place the child's responses in the proper perspective. For example, a young child's discomfort on separation from a parent and a school-age child's lack of clarity about the purpose of the interview are perfectly normal. Furthermore, behavior that is normal in a child at one age, such as temper tantrums in a 2-year-old, takes on a different meaning, for example, in a teenager.

The interviewer's first task is to engage the child and develop a rapport so that the child is comfortable. The interviewer should inquire about the child's concept of the purpose of the interview and should ask what the parents have told the child. If the child appears to be confused about the reason for the interview, the examiner may opt to summarize the parents' concerns in a developmentally appropriate and supportive manner. During the interview with the child, we seek to learn about the child's relationships with family members and peers, academic achievement, and peer relationships in school, and the child's pleasurable activities. An estimate of the child's cognitive functioning is a part of the mental status examination.

The extent of confidentiality in child assessment correlates with the age of the child. In most cases, almost all specific information can appropriately be shared with the parents of a very young child, whereas the privacy and permission of an older child or adolescent are necessary before we can share any information with parents. Clinicians should inform school-age and older children that if we become concerned that any child is dangerous to themselves or others, we must share this information with parents and, at times, additional adults. As part of all assessments, the clinician must determine whether that child is safe in their environment and must develop an index of suspicion about whether the child is a victim of abuse or neglect. Whenever there is a suspicion of child maltreatment, we are mandated by law to report it to the local child protective service agency.

Toward the end of the interview, the child may be asked in an open-ended manner whether they would like to bring up anything else. We should compliment each child for their cooperation and thank them for participating in the interview, and the interview should end on a positive note.

Infants and Young Children

Assessments of infants and very young children are done with the parents present, because very young children may be frightened by the interview situation. In addition, observation of the child with the parents present also allows clinicians to assess the parent–infant interaction. Infants may be referred for psychiatric evaluation for a variety of reasons, including high levels of irritability, difficulty being consoled, eating disturbances, poor weight gain, sleep disturbances, withdrawn behavior, lack of engagement in play, and developmental delay. Clinicians will assess areas of functioning that include motor development, activity level, verbal communication, ability to engage in play, problem-solving skills, adaptation to daily routines, relationships, and social responsiveness.

Clinical observations during the interview and standardized developmental measures will help determine a child's developmental level of functioning. Observations of play reveal a child's developmental level and reflect the child's emotional state and preoccupations. The examiner can interact with an infant aged 18 months or younger in a playful manner by using such games as peek-a-boo. We may observe children between the ages of 18 months and 3 years in a playroom. Children aged 2 years or older may exhibit symbolic play with toys, revealing more in this mode than through conversation. The use of puppets and dolls with children younger than 6 years of age is often an effective way to elicit information, particularly if questions are directed to the dolls, rather than to the child.

School-Age Children

Some school-age children are at ease when conversing with an adult; others may show fear, anxiety, poor verbal skills, or oppositional behavior. School-age children can usually tolerate a 45-minute session. The room should be sufficiently spacious for the child to move around, but not so large as to reduce intimate contact between the examiner and the child. We may reserve part of the interview for unstructured play, and various toys can be made available to capture the child's interest and to elicit themes and feelings. Children in lower grades may be more interested in the toys in the room, whereas by the sixth grade, children may be more comfortable with the interview process and less likely to show spontaneous play.

The first part of the interview explores the child's understanding of the reasons for the meeting. We should reassure the child that they are not here because they are "in trouble." Techniques that can facilitate disclosure of feelings include asking the child to draw peers, family members, a house, or anything else that comes to mind. We can then question the child about the drawings. We may ask children to reveal three wishes, to describe the best and worst events of their lives, and to name a favorite person to be stranded with on a desert island. Games such as Donald W. Winnicott's "squiggle," in which the examiner draws a curved line and then the child and the examiner take turns continuing the drawing, may facilitate conversation.

Questions that are partially open-ended with some multiple choices may elicit the best answers from school-age children. Simple, closed (yes or no) questions may not elicit sufficient information, and entirely open-ended questions can overwhelm a school-age child who cannot construct a chronologic narrative. These techniques often result in a shoulder shrug from the child. The use of indirect commentaries—such as, "I once knew a child who felt very sad when he moved away from all his friends"—is helpful, although we must be careful not to lead the child into confirming what the child thinks we want to hear. School-age children respond well to clinicians who help them compare moods or feelings by asking them to rate feelings on a scale of 1 to 10.

Adolescents

Adolescents usually have distinct ideas about why the evaluation was initiated and can usually give a chronologic account of the events leading to the evaluation, although some may disagree with the need for the evaluation. It is important for a clinician to communicate the value of hearing the story from an adolescent's point of view and essential for the clinician to reserve judgment and not assign blame. Adolescents may be concerned about confidentiality, and clinicians can assure them that permission will be requested from them before we share any specific information with parents, except in situations involving danger to the adolescent or others, in which case we must sacrifice confidentiality. Clinicians can approach adolescents in an open-ended manner; however, when silences occur during the interview, the interviewer should attempt to reengage the patient. We can explore what the adolescent believes the outcome of the evaluation will be (change of school, hospitalization, removal from the home, loss of privileges).

Some adolescents approach the interview with apprehension or hostility but open up when it becomes evident that we are neither punitive nor judgmental. We must be aware of our responses to adolescents' behavior (countertransference) and stay focused on the therapeutic process even in the face of defiant, angry, or difficult teenagers. Interviewers should set appropriate limits and should postpone or discontinue an interview if they feel threatened or if they become destructive or self-injurious. Every interview with an adolescent should include an exploration of suicidal thoughts, abuse, assaultive behavior, psychotic symptoms, substance use, and knowledge of safe sexual practices along with a sexual history. Once rapport is established, many adolescents appreciate the opportunity to tell their story and may reveal things that they have not disclosed to anyone else.

Family Interview

An interview with parents and the patient often takes place first with younger children, but with older children and adolescents, it often occurs later in the evaluation. Sometimes, an interview with the entire family, including siblings, can be informative. During an entire family meeting, a clinician can observe the interactions between the parents and children. Our clinical goal is to maintain a nonthreatening atmosphere in which each member of the family can speak freely without feeling that we are taking sides with any particular member. Although child psychiatrists generally function as advocates for their patients, in a family interview, we must validate each family member's feelings to enhance communication and elicit valuable information.

Parents

The interview with the patient's parents or caregivers is necessary to obtain a chronologic picture of the child's growth and development. A thorough developmental history is important as well as details of any stressors or significant events that have influenced the child's development. The clinician aims to elicit the parents' view of the family dynamics, as well as some details of their marital history and their own emotional adjustment. The family's psychiatric history and philosophy and style of their parenting are pertinent. Parents are usually the best informants about the child's early development and previous psychiatric and medical illnesses. They may be better able to provide an accurate chronology of past evaluations and treatment. In some cases, especially with older children and adolescents, the parents may be unaware of significant current symptoms or social difficulties of the child. Clinicians elicit the parents' formulation of the causes and nature of their child's problems and ask about their expectations for the current assessment.

DIAGNOSTIC INSTRUMENTS

The two main types of diagnostic instruments used by clinicians are diagnostic interviews and questionnaires. We administer diagnostic interviews to either children or their parents, which should elicit sufficient information on various aspects of functioning in order to determine whether the child meets DSM-5-TR criteria.

Semi-structured interviews, or "interviewer-based" interviews, such as K-SADS, the *Child and Adolescent Psychiatric Assessment* (CAPA), and the *Preschool Psychiatric Assessment* (PAPA), serve as guides. They help us clarify answers to questions about symptoms. Structured interviews, or "respondent-based" interviews, such as NIMH DISC-IV, the *Children's Interview for Psychiatric Syndromes* (ChIPS), and the *Diagnostic Interview for Children and Adolescents* (DICA), provide a script for the interviewer without interpretation of the patient responses during the interview process. Two other diagnostic instruments, the *Dominic-R* and the *Pictorial Instrument for Children and Adolescents* (PICA-III-R), use pictures as cues along with an accompanying question to elicit information about symptoms, which can be especially useful for young children as well as for adolescents.

Diagnostic instruments systematically aid the collection of information. Diagnostic instruments, even the most comprehensive, however, cannot replace clinical interviews, because clinical interviews are superior in understanding the chronology of symptoms, the interplay between environmental stressors and emotional responses, and developmental issues. Clinicians often find it helpful to combine data from diagnostic instruments with clinical material gathered in a comprehensive evaluation.

Questionnaires can cover a broad range of symptom areas, such as the *Achenbach Child Behavior Checklist (CBCL)*, or they can focus on a particular type of symptomatology, such as the *Connors Parent Rating Scale for ADHD*.

Semi-Structured Diagnostic Interviews

Kiddie Schedule for Affective Disorders and Schizophrenia for School-Age Children (K-SADS). The K-SADS is intended for children and adolescents from 6 to 18 years of age. It contains multiple items with some space for further clarification of symptoms. It elicits information on current diagnosis and symptoms present in the previous year. Another version can also ascertain lifetime diagnoses. This instrument has been used extensively, especially in the evaluation of mood disorders, and includes measures of impairment caused by symptoms. There is also a form for parents as well as the child. The schedule takes about 1 to 1.5 hours to administer. The interviewer should have some training in the field of child psychiatry but need not be a psychiatrist.

Child and Adolescent Psychiatric Assessment (CAPA). The CAPA is an "interviewer-based" instrument that can be used for children from 9 to 17 years of age. It comes in modular form so that we can focus on specific diagnostic entities without having to give the entire interview. It covers disruptive behavior disorders, mood disorders, anxiety disorders, eating disorders, sleep disorders, elimination disorders, substance use disorders, tic disorders, schizophrenia, PTSD, and somatization symptoms. It focuses on the 3 months before the interview, called the "primary period." In general, it takes about 1 hour to administer. It has a glossary to help clarify symptoms, and it provides separate ratings for the presence and severity of symptoms. The CAPA can be used to obtain information that applies to DSM-5-TR diagnoses. Training is necessary to administer this interview, and the interviewer must be prepared to use some clinical judgment in interpreting elicited symptoms.

Preschool Age Psychiatric Assessment (PAPA). The PAPA is a parent-report instrument based on the parent version of the CAPA for 9- to 18-year-olds. This assessment tool was created for 2-year-olds to 5-year-olds. The paper version of the PAPA and electronic version (ePAPA) are administered on a tablet device. The PAPA comes in 25 modules like the CAPA, so that specific diagnostic entities can be the focus of attention. There are a total of 25 modules; individual modules can be administered separately or in any combination. Like the CAPA, the PAPA includes the following modules: Modules Brief Developmental Assessment; Family Structure and Functioning; Parental Psychopathology; Childcare; Play and Peer Relationships; Depression; Mania; Conduct Problems; Attention-Deficit/Hyperactivity Disorder; Tics and Trichotillomania; Stereotypies and Unusual Speech (screening for Pervasive Developmental Disorders); Regulation/Habits; Eating and Food-Related Behaviors; Sleep; Somatization; Elimination; Separation Anxiety; Anxious Affect; Worries; Rituals and Repetitions; Psychosis; Reactive Attachment Disorder Symptoms; Life Events; Posttraumatic Stress Syndrome; Incapacity/Disability/Impairment; Socioeconomic Status and other demographic information.

Structured Diagnostic Interviews

National Institute of Mental Health Interview Schedule for Children Version IV (NIMH DISC-IV). The NIMH DISC-IV is a highly structured interview designed to assess more than 30 DSM-IV diagnostic entities administered by trained "laypersons." Although developed for DSM-IV, it can still be helpful diagnoses in DSM-5-TR. It is available in parallel child and parent forms. The parent form can be used for children from 6 to 17 years of age, and the direct child form of the instrument was designed for children from 9 to 17 years of age. A computer scoring algorithm is available. This instrument assesses for diagnoses present within the last 4 weeks, and also within the last year. Because it is a fully structured interview, the instructions serve as a complete guide for the questions, and the examiner need not have any knowledge of child psychiatry to administer the interview correctly.

Children's Interview for Psychiatric Syndromes (ChIPS). The ChIPS is a highly structured interview designed for use by trained interviewers with children from 6 to 18 years of age. It is composed of 15 sections, and it elicits information on psychiatric symptoms as well as psychosocial stressors targeting 20 psychiatric disorders, according to DSM-IV criteria; however, it also applies to diagnoses in DSM-5-TR. There are parent and child forms. It takes approximately 40 minutes to administer the ChIPS. Diagnoses covered include depression, mania, ADHD, separation disorder, OCD, conduct disorder, substance use disorder, anorexia, and bulimia. The ChIPS is a screening instrument for clinicians and a diagnostic instrument for clinical and epidemiologic research.

Diagnostic Interview for Children and Adolescents (DICA). The current version of the DICA was developed in 1997 to assess information resulting in diagnoses according to either DSM-IV or DSM-III-R. This instrument is relevant to DSM-5-TR as well.

Although designed as a highly structured interview, it can be used in a semi-structured format. This means that, although interviewers are allowed to use additional questions and probes to clarify elicited information, the method of probing is standardized so that all interviewers will follow a specific pattern. When using the interview with younger children, more flexibility is built-in, allowing interviewers to deviate from written questions to ensure that the child understands the question. Parent and child interviews are expected to be used. The DICA is designed for use with children 6 to 17 years of age and generally takes 1 to 2 hours to administer. It covers externalizing behavior disorders, anxiety disorders, depressive disorders, and substance use disorders, among others.

Pictorial Diagnostic Instruments

Dominic-R. Dominic-R is a pictorial, fully structured interview designed to elicit psychiatric symptoms from children 6 to 11 years of age. The pictures illustrate abstract emotional and behavioral content of diagnostic entities according to the DSM-III-R; however, information gleaned from this instrument also applies in conjunction with clinical information to the DSM-5-TR. The instrument uses a picture of a child called "Dominic," who is experiencing the symptoms in question. Some symptoms have more than one picture, with a brief story. Each picture includes a question about the situation depicted and whether the child has experienced something similar. Diagnostic entities covered by the Dominic-R include separation anxiety, generalized anxiety, depression and dysthymia, ADHD, oppositional defiant disorder, conduct disorder, and specific phobia. The symptom list is comprehensive; however, the interview does not explicitly ask about the frequency, duration, or age of onset of the symptom. The paper version of this interview takes about 20 minutes, and the computerized version of this instrument takes about 15 minutes. Trained lay interviewers can administer this interview. Computerized versions of this interview are available with pictures of a child who is White, Black, Latino, or Asian.

Pictorial Instrument for Children and Adolescents (PICA-III-R). PICA-III-R is composed of 137 pictures organized in modules and designed to cover five diagnostic categories, including disorders of anxiety, mood, psychosis, disruptive disorders, and substance use disorder. It is designed to be administered by clinicians and can be used for children and adolescents ranging from 6 to 16 years of age. The PICA-III-R provides a categorical (diagnosis present or absent) and a dimensional (range of severity) assessment. This instrument presents pictures of a child experiencing emotional, behavioral, and cognitive symptoms. The clinician asks the child, "How much are you like them?" and a five-point rating scale with pictures of a person with open arms in increasing degrees is shown to the child to help the child identify the severity of the symptoms. It takes about 40 minutes to 1 hour to administer the interview. This instrument was designed for DSM-III-R but is useful for DSM-5-TR diagnoses. This assessment can be used to aid in clinical interviews and research diagnostic protocols.

QUESTIONNAIRES AND RATING SCALES

Achenbach Child Behavior Checklist (CBCL)

The parent, teacher, and youth versions of the *Achenbach Child Behavior Checklist (CBCL)* cover a broad range of symptoms and several positive attributes related to academic and social competence. The parent version consists of 113 items to be rated 0 (not true), 1 (sometimes true), or 2 (very true). The teacher version is similar, but without the items that apply only to home life. The CBCL is completed by parents. The other companion versions are the Teacher's Report Form (TRF) (completed by teachers), and the Youth Self-Report (YSR) (completed by the child or adolescent).

In school-age groups, the CBCL includes items that pertain to mood, anxiety, and behavior with subscales for attention problems, aggressive behaviors, and delinquent behaviors. There are separate versions of the CBCL for preschool (CBCL/1.5 years to 5 years), and school-age (CBCL/6 years to 18 years). CBCL/1.5 to 5 years elicits caregivers' ratings of 99 problem areas, which are scored on the following syndrome scales: Emotionally Reactive, Anxious/Depressed, Somatic Complaints, Withdrawn, Attention Problems, Aggressive Behavior, and Sleep Problems.

This checklist identifies specific problem areas that we might otherwise overlook, and it may point out areas in which the child's behavior deviates from that of normal children of the same age group. The checklist does not make diagnoses.

The development and validation of a new subscale within the CBCL/6–18 for autism spectrum disorder was accomplished by Offermans and colleagues in 2023.

In a study of 152 preschoolers with a neurodevelopmental genetic disorder (neurogenetic syndromes), including fragile X, Prader–Willi, Angelman syndrome, and Williams syndrome, by Neo and colleagues (2021), the authors' findings suggest that the CBCL/1.5–5 appears to be a psychometrically sound narrowband and broadband measure of challenging behaviors in young children with neurogenetic syndromes.

Connors Abbreviated Parent–Teacher Rating Scale for ADHD

In its original form, the *Connors Abbreviated Parent–Teacher Rating Scale for ADHD* consisted of 93 items rated on a 0 to 3 scale, divided into 25 clusters, including problems with restlessness, temper, school, stealing, eating, and sleeping. Over the years, multiple versions of this scale were developed and used to aid in the systematic identification of children with ADHD. A highly abbreviated form of this rating scale, the *Connors Abbreviated Parent–Teacher Questionnaire,* was developed in 1973. It consists of 10 items that assess both hyperactivity and inattention.

Brief Impairment Scale

The *Brief Impairment Scale* (BIS) is a validated 23-item instrument suitable to obtain information on children ranging from 4 to 17 years of age that evaluates three domains of functioning: interpersonal relations, school/work functioning, and care/self-fulfillment. This scale is administered to an adult informant about their child, does not take long to administer, and provides a global measure of impairment along the above three dimensions. This scale does not make clinical decisions on individual patients, but it can provide information on the degree of impairment that a given child is experiencing in a particular area.

COMPONENTS OF THE CHILD PSYCHIATRIC EVALUATION

Psychiatric evaluation of a child includes a description of the reason for the referral, the child's past and present functioning, and any test results. Table 2-1 gives an outline of the evaluation.

Identifying Data

Identifying data for a child includes the child's gender, age, as well as the family constellation surrounding the child.

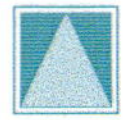

Table 2-1.
Child Psychiatric Evaluation

Identifying data
Identified patient and family members
Source of referral
Informants
History
Chief complaint
History of present illness
Developmental history and milestones
Psychiatric history
Medical history, including immunizations
Family social history and parents' marital status
Educational history and current school functioning
Peer relationship history
Current family functioning
Family psychiatric and medical histories
Current physical examination
Mental status examination
Neuropsychiatric examination (when applicable)
Developmental, psychological, and educational testing
Formulation and summary
DSM-5-TR diagnosis
Recommendations and treatment plan

History

A comprehensive history contains information about the child's current and past functioning from the child's report, from clinical and structured interviews with the parents, and information from teachers and previous treating clinicians. We usually obtain the chief complaint and the history of the present illness from both the child and the parents. Naturally, the child will articulate the situation according to their developmental level. The parents are usually the best source for determining the child's developmental history. Past clinicians can help augment psychiatric and medical histories. The child's report is critical for understanding the current situation regarding peer relationships and adjustment to school. Adolescents are the best informants regarding knowledge of safe sexual practices, drug or alcohol use, and suicidal ideation. The parents are usually the best source to understand the family's psychiatric and social histories and family functioning.

Mental Status Examination

We should obtain a detailed description of the child's current mental functioning through observation and specific questioning. Table 2-2 presents an outline of the mental status examination, and Table 2-3 lists components of a comprehensive neuropsychiatry mental status.

Physical Appearance. The examiner should document the child's size, grooming, nutritional state, head circumference, physical signs of anxiety, facial expressions, and mannerisms, as well as note any bruising.

Parent–Child Interaction. Before the interview, the examiner can observe the interactions between parents and the child in the waiting area. How the parents and child interact, both verbally and emotionally, is pertinent.

Separation and Reunion. The examiner should note how the child responds to separation from a parent, and how they react to the reunion. Either lack of affect at separation and reunion or severe distress on separation or

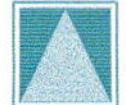

Table 2-2.
Mental Status Examination for Children

1. Physical appearance
2. Parent–child interaction
3. Separation and reunion
4. Orientation to time, place, and person
5. Speech and language
6. Mood
7. Affect
8. Thought process and content
9. Social relatedness
10. Motor behavior
11. Cognition
12. Memory
13. Judgment and insight

Table 2-3.
Neuropsychiatric Mental Status Examination[a]

A. General Description
1. General appearance and dress
2. Level of consciousness and arousal
3. Attention to environment
4. Posture (standing and seated)
5. Gait
6. Movements of limbs, trunk, and face (spontaneous, resting, and after instruction)
7. General demeanor (including evidence of responses to internal stimuli)
8. Response to examiner (eye contact, cooperation, ability to focus on interview process)
9. Native or primary language

B. Language and Speech
1. Comprehension (words, sentences, simple and complex commands, and concepts)
2. Output (spontaneity, rate, fluency, melody or prosody, volume, coherence, vocabulary, paraphasic errors, complexity of usage)
3. Repetition
4. Other aspects
   a. Object naming
   b. Color naming
   c. Body part identification
   d. Ideomotor praxis to command

C. Thought
1. Form (coherence and connectedness)
2. Content
   a. Ideational (preoccupations, overvalued ideas, delusions)
   b. Perceptual (hallucinations)

D. Mood and Affect
1. Internal mood state (spontaneous and elicited; sense of humor)
2. Future outlook
3. Suicidal ideas and plans
4. Demonstrated emotional status (congruence with mood)

E. Insight and Judgment
1. Insight
   a. Self-appraisal and self-esteem
   b. Understanding of current circumstances
   c. Ability to describe personal psychological and physical status
2. Judgment
   a. Appraisal of major social relationships
   b. Understanding of personal roles and responsibilities

F. Cognition
1. Memory
   a. Spontaneous (as evidenced during interview)
   b. Tested (incidental, immediate repetition, delayed recall, cued recall, recognition; verbal, nonverbal; explicit, implicit)
2. Visuospatial skills
3. Constructional ability
4. Mathematics
5. Reading
6. Writing
7. Fine sensory function (stereognosis, graphesthesia, two-point discrimination)
8. Finger gnosis
9. Right-left orientation
10. "Executive functions"
11. Abstraction

[a]Questions should be adapted to the age of the child.
Courtesy of Eric D. Caine, M.D. and Jeffrey M. Lyness, M.D.

reunion can indicate problems in the parent–child relationship or other psychiatric disturbances.

Orientation to Time, Place, and Person. Impairments in orientation can reflect neurologic damage, low intelligence, or a thought disorder. The age of the child must be kept in mind, however, because very young children may not know the date, other chronologic information, or the name of the interview site.

Speech and Language. The examiner should evaluate the child's speech and language acquisition. Is it appropriate for the child's age? A disparity between expressive language usage and receptive language is notable. The examiner should also note the child's rate of speech, rhythm, latency to answer, the spontaneity of speech, intonation, articulation of words, and prosody. Echolalia, repetitive stereotypical phrases, and unusual syntax are significant psychiatric findings. Children who do not use words by age 18 months or who do not use phrases by ages 2.5 to 3 years, but who have a history of typical babbling and responding appropriately to nonverbal cues, are probably developing typically. The examiner should consider the possibility that hearing loss is contributing to a speech and language deficit.

Mood. A child's sad expression, lack of appropriate smiling, tearfulness, anxiety, euphoria, and anger are valid indicators of mood, as are verbal admissions of feelings. Persistent themes in play and fantasy also reflect the child's mood.

Affect. The examiner should note the child's range of emotional expressivity, appropriateness of affect to thought content, ability to move smoothly from one affect to another, and sudden labile emotional shifts.

Thought Process and Content. In evaluating a thought disorder in a child, we must always consider what is typical for the child's age and what is deviant for any age group. The evaluation of thought-form considers loosening of associations, excessive magical thinking, perseveration, echolalia, the ability to distinguish fantasy from reality, sentence coherence, and the ability to reason logically. The evaluation of thought content considers delusions, obsessions, themes, fears, wishes, preoccupations, and interests.

Suicidal ideation is always a part of the mental status examination for children who are sufficiently verbal to understand the questions and old enough to understand the concept. Generally, children of average intelligence who are older than 4 years of age have some understanding of what is real and what is make-believe and may be asked about suicidal ideation, although a firm concept of the permanence of death may not be present until several years later.

We should also assess aggressive thoughts and homicidal ideation. Perceptual disturbances, such as hallucinations, are also evaluated. Very young children are expected to have short attention spans and may change the topic and conversation abruptly without exhibiting a symptomatic flight of ideas. Transient visual and auditory hallucinations in very young children do not necessarily represent major psychotic illnesses, but they do deserve further investigation.

Social Relatedness. The clinician should assess the child's social response to the interviewer, general level of social skills, eye contact, and degree of familiarity or withdrawal in the interview process. Overly friendly or familiar behavior may be as troublesome as extremely retiring and withdrawn responses. The examiner assesses the child's self-esteem, areas of confidence, and success with family and peer relationships.

Motor Behavior. The motor behavior part of the mental status examination includes observations of the child's coordination and activity level and ability to pay attention and carry out developmentally appropriate tasks. It also involves involuntary movements, tremors, motor hyperactivity, and any unusual focal asymmetries of muscle movement.

Cognition. We also should assess the child's intellectual functioning and problem-solving abilities. We can estimate the relative level of intelligence from a child's general information, vocabulary, and comprehension. For a specific assessment of the child's cognitive abilities, we can use a standardized test.

Memory. School-age children typically can remember three objects after 5 minutes and can repeat five digits forward and three digits backward. Anxiety can interfere with a child's performance, but an inability to repeat digits or to add simple numbers may reflect brain damage, intellectual disability, or learning disorders.

Judgment and Insight. The child's view of the problems, reactions to them, and suggested solutions may give us a good idea of the child's judgment and insight. Also, the child's understanding of what they can realistically do to help and what we can do adds to the assessment of the child's judgment.

Neuropsychiatric Assessment

A neuropsychiatric assessment is appropriate for children suspected of having a psychiatric disorder that coexists with neuropsychiatric impairment, or psychiatric symptoms that may be caused by neuropsychiatric dysfunction, or a neurologic disorder. Although a neuropsychiatric assessment is not sufficient in most cases to make a psychiatric diagnosis, neuropsychological profiles have been, in some cases, correlated with particular psychiatric symptoms and syndromes. For example, neuropsychological differences in executive function, language, and memory functions, as well as measures of mood and anxiety, have been found between youth with histories of childhood maltreatment and those without it. The neuropsychiatric evaluation combines information from neurologic, neuropsychological testing, and mental status examinations. The neurologic examination can identify asymmetrical abnormal signs (hard signs) that may indicate lesions in the brain. A physical examination can evaluate the presence of physical stigmata of specific syndromes in which neuropsychiatric symptoms or developmental aberrations play a role (e.g., fetal alcohol syndrome [FAS], Down syndrome).

A neuropsychiatric examination also includes neurologic soft signs and minor physical anomalies. Loretta Bender coined the term *neurological soft signs* in the 1940s to describe the nondiagnostic abnormalities in the neurologic examinations of children with schizophrenia. Soft signs do not indicate focal neurologic disorders, but they are associated with a wide variety of developmental disabilities and frequently occur in children with low intelligence, learning disabilities, and behavioral disturbances. Soft signs may refer to both behavioral symptoms (which are sometimes associated with brain damage, such as severe impulsivity and hyperactivity), physical findings (including contralateral overflow movements), and a variety of nonfocal signs (e.g., mild choreiform movements, poor balance, mild incoordination, asymmetry of gait, nystagmus, and the persistence of infantile reflexes). Soft signs include those that are normal in a young child but become abnormal when they persist in an older child and those that are abnormal at any age. The *Physical and Neurological Examination for Soft Signs* (PANESS) is an instrument used with children up to the age of 15 years. It consists of 15 questions about the general physical status and medical history and 43 physical tasks (e.g., touch your finger to your nose, hop on one foot to the end of the line, tap quickly with your finger). Neurologic soft signs are useful to note, but they are not useful in making a specific psychiatric diagnosis.

Minor physical anomalies or dysmorphic features occur with a higher than usual frequency in children with developmental disabilities, learning disabilities, speech and language disorders, and hyperactivity. As with soft signs, the documentation of minor physical anomalies is part of the neuropsychiatric assessment, but it is rarely helpful in the diagnostic process and does not imply a good or bad prognosis. Minor physical anomalies include a high-arched palate, epicanthal folds, hypertelorism, low-set ears, transverse palmar creases, multiple hair whorls, a large head, a furrowed tongue, and partial syndactyly of several toes.

When considering a seizure disorder in the differential diagnosis or a structural abnormality in the brain, electroencephalography (EEG), CT, or MRI may be indicated.

Developmental, Psychological, and Educational Testing

Psychological testing, structured developmental assessments, and achievement testing are valuable in evaluating a child's developmental level, intellectual functioning, and academic difficulties. A measure of adaptive functioning (including the child's competence in communication, daily living skills, socialization, and motor skills) is the most definitive way to determine the level of intellectual disability in a child. Table 2-4 outlines the general categories of psychological tests.

Development Tests for Infants and Preschoolers. The *Gesell Infant Scale,* the *Cattell Infant Intelligence Scale, Bayley Scales of Infant Development,* and

Table 2-4.
Commonly Used Child and Adolescent Psychological Assessment Instruments

	Name of Test	Age Range (yr)
Cognitive, Language, and Neuropsychological Assessments		
Tests of Intellectual Function	Wechsler Preschool and Primary Scale of Intelligence, 4th ed. (WPPSI-IV)	2½–7¾
	Wechsler Intelligence Scale for Children, 5th ed. (WISC-V)	6–16
	Wechsler Abbreviated Scale of Intelligence, 2nd ed. (WASI-II)	6–90
	Wechsler Intelligence Scale, 4th ed. (WAIS-IV)	16–90
	Stanford-Binet, 5th ed. (SB-5)	2–85+
	Kaufman Assessment Battery for Children, 2nd ed. (KABC-2)	3–19
	Differential Ability Scales, 2nd ed. (DAS-II)	2½–18
Achievement Tests	Woodcock-Johnson Tests of Achievement, 4th ed. (WJ-IV)	2–90+
	Kaufman Test of Educational Achievement, 3rd ed. (KTEA-3)	4–26
	Wechsler Individual Achievement Test, 3rd ed. (WIAT-III)	4–50
	Peabody Individual Achievement Test	5–19
	Wide Range Achievement Test, 4th ed. (WRAT-4)	5–95
Neuropsychological Tests	Halstead-Reitan Neuropsychological Test Batteries	5–15+
	Luria-Nebraska Neuropsychological Battery: Children's Revision	8–12
	Reitan-Indiana Neuropsychological Test Battery	5–8
	Comprehensive Test of Nonverbal Intelligence (CTONI-II)	6–90
	Leiter International Performance Scale (Leiter-3)	3–75+
	Test of Nonverbal Intelligence (TONI-4)	6–90
Language Tests	Clinical Evaluation of Language Fundamentals (CELF-5)	5–21
	Peabody Picture Vocabulary Test	2.6–90
	Expressive One-Word Picture Vocabulary Test	2–80
Memory Tests	Wide Range Assessment of Memory and Learning (WRAML-2)	5–90
	California Verbal Learning Test (CVLT-C, CVLT-II)	5–89
	Wechsler Memory Scale (WMS-IV)	16–90
Diagnostic, Behavioral, and Observational Assessments		
Diagnostic Interviews	Anxiety Disorders Interview Schedule for Children (ADIS-P/C)	8–17
	Kiddie Schedule for Affective Disorders and Schizophrenia (K-SADS)	6–17
	Mini International Neuropsychiatric Interview for Children and Adolescents (MINI-KID)	6–17
Behavioral Rating Scales	Achenbach Child Behavior Checklist	1.5–5
	Achenbach Youth Self Report	11–18
	Achenbach Teacher Report Form	6–18
	Strengths and Difficulties Questionnaire (SDQ)	2–17
	Early Childhood Inventory-5 (ECI-5)	3–6
	Child Autism Rating Scale (CARS-2)	2+
	SNAP-IV Teacher and Parent ADHD Rating Scale	6–18
	Conners ADHD Rating Scale 4th Edition (Conners 4™)	6–18
	Children's Depression Inventory (2nd Edition)	6–18
	Screen for Anxiety and Related Disorders (SCARED)	8–18
	Revised Children's Anxiety and Depression Scale (RCADS)	8–18
	Obsessive-Compulsive Inventory – Child & Parent version (OCI-PV)	7–17
Observational Assessments	Autism Diagnostic Observational Schedule (ADOS)	Various
	Disruptive Behavior-Diagnostic Observational Schedule (DB-DOS)	Preschool

the *Denver Developmental Screening Test* include developmental assessments of infants as young as 2 months of age. When used with very young infants, the tests focus on sensorimotor and social responses to a variety of objects and interactions. When using these instruments with older infants and preschoolers, the emphasis is on language acquisition. The *Gesell Infant Scale* measures development in four areas: motor, adaptive functioning, language, and social.

An infant's score on one of the above developmental assessments is not a reliable way to predict the child's future IQ in most cases. Infant assessments are valuable, however, in detecting developmental deviation and intellectual disability, and in raising suspicions of a developmental disorder. Whereas infant assessments rely heavily on sensorimotor functions, intelligence testing in older children and adolescents includes later-developing functions, including verbal, social, and abstract cognitive abilities.

Intelligence Tests for School-Age Children and Adolescents. The most widely used test of intelligence for school-age children and adolescents is the Fifth Edition of the *Wechsler Intelligence Scale for Children* (WISC-V). It can be given to children from 6 years to 16.11/12 years of age. The WISC-V yields an overall measure of intellectual function. It generates a verbal IQ, a performance IQ, and a combined full-scale IQ. The verbal subtests consist of vocabulary, information, arithmetic, similarities, comprehension, and digit span (supplemental) categories. The performance subtests include block design, picture completion, picture arrangement, object assembly, coding, mazes (supplemental), and symbol search (supplemental). The IQ computation does not include the scores of the supplemental subtests.

Each subcategory is scored from 1 to 19, with 10 being the average score. An average full-scale IQ is 100; 70 to 80 is very low average; 80 to 90 is in the low average range; 90 to 109 is average; 110 to 119 is a high average, and above 120 is in the superior or very superior range. The multiple breakdowns of the performance and verbal subscales allow great flexibility in identifying specific areas of deficit and scatter in intellectual abilities. Because a large part of intelligence testing measures abilities used in academic settings, the breakdown of the WISC-V can also point out skills in which a child is weak and may benefit from remedial education. According to the DSM-5-TR, an intellectual disability must include both intellectual and adaptive function deficits in social, conceptual, and/or practical domains, which emerge before 18 years of age. Deficits in intellectual functions include reasoning, problem solving, abstract thinking, judgment, and academic learning, confirmed by both clinical assessment and individual standardized intelligence testing such as the WISC-5. Deficits in adaptive function lead to failure to meet developmental and social/cultural standards for independence and social responsibility. The adaptive function deficits leading to limitations in communication, social functioning, or independent living require ongoing supports.

The *Stanford-Binet Intelligence Scale* covers an age range from 2 to 24 years. It relies on pictures, drawings, and objects for very young children and verbal performance for older children and adolescents. This intelligence scale, the earliest version of an intelligence test of its kind, leads to a mental age score as well as an IQ.

The *McCarthy Scales of Children's Abilities* and the *Kaufman Assessment Battery for Children* are two other intelligence tests that are available for preschool and school-age children. They do not cover adolescents.

LONG-TERM STABILITY OF INTELLIGENCE. Although a child's intelligence is relatively stable throughout the school-age years and adolescence, some factors can influence intelligence and a child's score on an intelligence test. The intellectual functions of children with severe mental illnesses and of those from deprived and neglectful environments may decrease over time, whereas the IQs of children with intensively enriched environments may increase over time. Factors that influence a child's score on a given test of intellectual functioning and, thus, affect the accuracy of the test are motivation, emotional state, anxiety, and cultural milieu. The interactions between cognitive ability and anxiety and depression, and psychosis are complex. One study of 4,405 youth from the Canadian National Longitudinal Study of Children and Youth (NLSCY), by Weeks and colleagues (2013), found that more exceptional cognitive ability was associated with less risk for anxiety and depressive symptoms in youth from 12 to 13 years of age; however, by ages 14 to 15 years, cognitive ability did not affect the odds of anxiety or depression.

Perceptual and Perceptual Motor Tests. The *Bender Visual-Motor Gestalt Test* can be given to children between the ages of 4 and 12 years. The test consists of a set of spatially related figures that the child copies. The number of errors determines the score. Although not a diagnostic test, it is useful in identifying developmentally age-inappropriate perceptual performances.

Personality Tests. Personality tests are not typically used to make diagnoses in youth, but they can help elicit themes and fantasies.

The Rorschach test is a projective technique in which ambiguous stimuli—a set of bilaterally symmetrical inkblots—are shown to a child, who then describes what they see in each. The hypothesis is that the child's interpretation of the vague stimuli reflects the basic characteristics of their personality. The examiner notes the themes and patterns.

A more structured projective test is the *Children's Apperception Test* (CAT), which is an adaptation of the *Thematic Apperception Test* (TAT). The CAT consists of cards with pictures of animals in scenes that are somewhat ambiguous but are related to parent–child and sibling issues, caretaking, and other relationships. The child describes what is happening and tells a story about the scene. The choice to use animals for the pictures is because some believe that children might respond more readily to animal images than to human figures.

Drawings, toys, and play are also applications of projective techniques used to evaluate children. Dollhouses, dolls, and puppets have been especially helpful in allowing a child who is reticent to engage in conversation a modality in which to express attitudes and feelings. Play materials that reflect household situations are likely to elicit a child's fears, hopes, and conflicts about the family.

Educational Tests. Achievement tests measure the attainment of knowledge and skills in a particular academic curriculum. The *Wide-Range Achievement Test*, Fifth Edition (WRAT-5), consists of tests of knowledge and skills and timed performances of reading, spelling, and mathematics. It is used with children from 5 years of age to adulthood. The test yields a score that we can compare to the average expected score for the child's chronologic age and grade level.

The *Peabody Individual Achievement Test* (PIAT) includes word identification, spelling, mathematics, and reading comprehension.

The *Kaufman Test of Educational Achievement*, the *Gray Oral Reading Test-Revised* (GORT-R), and the *Sequential Tests of Educational Progress* (STEP) are achievement tests that determine whether a child has achieved the educational level expected for their grade level. Often, children whose achievement is significantly lower than expected for their grade level in one or more subjects exhibit a specific learning disorder.

Biopsychosocial Formulation. The goal of the psychiatric examination in youth is to integrate all the information obtained into a formulation that takes into account the biologic predisposition, psychodynamic factors, environmental stressors, and life events that have led to the child's current level of functioning. We must consider psychiatric disorders and any specific physical, neuromotor, or developmental abnormalities in the formulation of etiologic factors for current impairment. Our conclusions are an integration of clinical information along with data from standardized psychological and developmental assessments. The psychiatric formulation includes an assessment of family function as well as the appropriateness of the child's educational setting. We should then determine the child's overall safety in their current situation and report any suspected maltreatment to the local child protective service agency. We then consider the child's overall well-being regarding growth, development, and academic and play activities.

Diagnosis

Structured and semi-structured (evidence-based) assessment tools often enhance a clinician's ability to make the most accurate diagnoses. These instruments described earlier include the K-SADS, the CAPA, and the NIMH DISC-IV interviews. The advantages of including a semi-structured or structured interview in the diagnostic process include decreasing clinician bias and systematically reviewing all the symptoms. Semi-structured and structured interviews can aid in increasing accuracy of DSM-5-TR diagnoses when there are overlapping symptoms.

Some clinical situations do not fulfill the criteria for DSM-5-TR diagnoses but cause impairment and require psychiatric attention and intervention. Clinicians who evaluate children are frequently in the position of determining the impact of the behavior of family members on the child's well-being. In many cases, a child's level of impairment is related to factors extending beyond a psychiatric diagnosis, such as the child's adjustment to their family life, peer relationships, and educational placement.

RECOMMENDATIONS AND TREATMENT PLAN

To recommend a treatment plan, we should use our formulation, integrating all of the data gained during our assessments. Optimal treatment often flows from this formulation. That is, identification of a biologic predisposition to a particular psychiatric disorder may be clinically relevant to inform a psychopharmacologic recommendation. An understanding of the psychodynamic interactions between family members may lead a clinician to recommend treatment that includes a family component. Educational and academic problems addressed in the formulation may lead to a recommendation to seek a more effective academic placement. We should also consider the overall social situation of the child or adolescent when recommending treatment. Most importantly in our treatment plan is to maintain the physical and emotional safety of a child or adolescent.

The child or adolescent's family, school life, peer interactions, and social activities often have a direct impact on the child's success in overcoming their difficulties. The psychological education and cooperation of a child or adolescent's family are essential ingredients in the successful application of treatment recommendations. Patients and families often see communications that balance the observed positive qualities of the child and family with the weak areas as more helpful than a focus only on the problem areas. Finally, the most successful treatment plans are those developed cooperatively between us, the child, and the family.

INTELLECTUAL DEVELOPMENTAL DISORDER (INTELLECTUAL DISABILITY) PSYCHIATRIC INTERVIEW AND TESTS

Psychiatric Interview

A psychiatric interview of a child or adolescent with intellectual developmental disorder (intellectual disability) requires clinical sensitivity in order to elicit information at the appropriate intellectual level while remaining respectful of the patient's age and emotional development. The patient's verbal abilities, including receptive and expressive language, can be initially noted by observing the communication between the caregivers and the patient. If the patient communicates mostly through gestures or sign language, the parents may serve as interpreters. Patients with milder forms of intellectual disability are often aware of their differences from others and their failures and may be anxious and ashamed during the interview. Approaching patients with a clear, supportive, concrete explanation of the diagnostic process, particularly patients with sufficiently receptive language ability, may allay anxiety and fears. Providing support and praise in language appropriate to the patient's age and understanding is beneficial. Subtle direction, structure, and reinforcement may be necessary to keep patients focused on the task or topic.

In general, the psychiatric examination of an intellectually disabled child or adolescent should reveal how the patient has coped with stages of development. Frustration tolerance, impulse control, and over-aggressive motor and sexual behavior are essential areas of attention in the interview. It is equally crucial to elicit the patient's self-image, areas of self-confidence, and an assessment of tenacity, persistence, curiosity, and willingness to explore the environment.

Structured Instruments, Rating Scales, and Psychological Assessment

In children and adolescents who have acquired language, we usually use one of several standardized instruments that include numerous domains of cognitive function. For children aged 6 to 16 years, the WISC-V is most common, and for children aged 3 to 6 years, the most commonly used is the Wechsler Preschool and Primary Scale of Intelligence-Revised. The Stanford-Binet Intelligence Scale, Fourth Edition, has the advantage that it can be administered to children even younger, starting at the age of 2 years. The Kaufman Assessment Battery for Children is appropriate for children ages 2½ to 12½ years, whereas the Kaufman Adolescent and Adult Intelligence Test apply to a wide range of ages, from 11 to 85 years. All of these standardized instruments evaluate cognitive abilities across multiple domains, including verbal, performance, memory, and problem-solving. Standardized instruments measuring adaptive function (functions of "everyday" life) assume that adaptive skills increase with age, and that adaptation may vary across different settings such as school, peer relationships, and family life. The Vineland Adaptive Behavior Scales can be used in infants through youth 18 years of age and includes four basic domains including *Communication* (Receptive, Expressive, and Written); *Daily Living Skills* (Personal, Domestic, and Community); *Socialization* (Interpersonal Relations, Play and Leisure, and Coping Skills); *Motor Skills* (Fine and Gross).

Several behavioral rating scales exist for the population with intellectual disabilities. General behavioral rating scales include the Aberrant Behavior Checklist (ABC) and the Developmental Behavior Checklist (DBC). The Behavior Problem Inventory (BPI) is a useful screening instrument for self-injurious, aggressive, and stereotyped behaviors. The Psychopathology Inventory for Mentally Retarded Adults (PIMRA) helps identify the presence of comorbid psychiatric symptoms and disorders.

Examining clinicians can use several screening instruments for developmental and intellectual delay or disability in infants and toddlers. However, the controversy over the predictive value of infant psychological tests is heated. Some report the correlation of abnormalities during infancy with later abnormal functioning as very low, and others report it to be very high. The correlation rises in direct proportion to the age of the child at the time of the developmental examination. Some exercises such as copying geometric figures, the *Goodenough Draw-a-Person Test,* the *Kohs Block Test,* and geometric puzzles all are useful quick screening tests of visual-motor coordination. For infants, the *Gesell* and *Bayley scales* and the *Cattell Infant Intelligence Scale* are useful.

The *Peabody Vocabulary Test* is the most widely used picture-based vocabulary test. Other tests often found useful in detecting intellectual disability are the *Bender Gestalt Test* and the *Benton Visual Retention Test.* The psychological evaluation should assess perceptual, motor, linguistic, and cognitive abilities.

Several comparisons between parent-report on behavior checklists and standard interviews in guiding psychiatric diagnoses were found to be equivalent in accuracy, according to Boyle and colleagues in 2023.

Furthermore, classifying children and adolescents based on a semi-structured diagnostic interview was not statistically different from making diagnoses based on a symptom checklist in terms of diagnostic accuracy and predictions of potential clinical outcomes, according to an 8-year follow-up study of children into adulthood in Brazil by Hoffman and colleagues (2024). The authors concluded that formulating diagnoses and estimating severity of outcome based on behavior and emotional checklists may be a valid alternative to the more time consuming and costly structured and semi-structured interviews to identify youth at risk for future psychiatric problems.

Physical Examination

A physical examination may demonstrate identifying characteristics of specific conditions associated with intellectual disabilities, and other genetic disorders that may require further investigation by a pediatrician or neurologist. For example, the configuration and the size of the head may offer clues to a variety of conditions, such as microcephaly, hydrocephalus, or Down syndrome. A patient's facial characteristics, for example, hypertelorism, a flat nasal bridge, prominent eyebrows, and epicanthal folds, may provide clues to a recognizable syndrome such as FAS. Facial characteristics including corneal opacities, retinal changes, low-set and small or misshapen ears, a protruding tongue, and disturbance in dentition may be stigmata of a variety of known syndromes. The facial expression, color, and texture of the skin and hair, a high-arched palate, the size of the thyroid gland, and the proportions of a child's trunk and extremities may offer clues for medical conditions. Dermatoglyphics (studying skin markings) may offer another diagnostic tool because unique ridge patterns and flexion creases on the hand occur in persons who are intellectually disabled, including chromosomal disorders and rubella. A pediatric examination is helpful in identifying potential medical diagnoses present along with psychiatric symptoms and disorders.

Further Readings

Achenbach TM, Dumenci L, Rescorla LA. *Ratings of Relations between DSM-IV Diagnostic Categories and Items of the CBCL/6–18, TRF, and YSR*. University of Vermont, Research Center for Children, Youth, & Families; 2001.

Allott K, Proffitt TM, McGorry PD, et al. Clinical neuropsychology within adolescent and young-adult psychiatry: conceptualizing theory and practice. *Appl Neuropsychol Child*. 2013;2(1):47–63.

Beck A, LeBlanc JC, Morissette K, et al. Screening for depression in children and adolescents: a protocol for a systematic review update. *Syst Rev*. 2021;10(1):24.

Bird HR, Canino GJ, Davies M, et al. The Brief Impairment Scale (BIS): a multidimensional scale of functional impairment for children and adolescents. *J Am Acad Child Adolesc Psychiatry*. 2005;44(7): 699–707.

Boyle MH, Duncan L, Wang L, Georgiades K. Problem checklists and standardized diagnostic interviews: evidence of psychometric equivalence for classifying psychiatric disorder among children and youth in epidemiological studies. *J Child Psychol Psychiatry*. 2023;64(5): 779–786.

Boyle MH, Duncan L, Wang L, Georgiades K. The 25-Item Ontario Child Health Study Emotional Behavioural Scales-Brief Version (OCHS-EBS-B): Test-retest reliability and construct validity when used as categorical measures. *Can J Psychiatry*. 2022;67(4):305–314.

Bryant-Waugh R, Micali N, Cooke L, Lawson EA, Eddy KT, Thomas JJ. Development of the Pica, ARFID, and Rumination Disorder Interview, a multi-informant, semi-structured interview of feeding disorders across the lifespan: a pilot study for ages 10–22. *Int J Eat Disord*. 2019;52(4):378–387.

Chambers WJ, Puig-Antich J, Hirsch M, et al. The assessment of affective disorders in children and adolescents by semistructured interview. Test-retest reliability of the schedule for affective disorders and schizophrenia for school-age children, present episode version. *Archives of General Psychiatry*. 1985;42(7):696–702.

Cleary MJ, Scott AJ. Developments in clinical neuropsychology: implications for school psychological services. *J School Health*. 2011;81(1):1–7.

Connors EH, Moffa K, Carter T, et al. Advancing mental health screening in schools: innovative, field-tested practices and observed trends during a 15-month learning collaborative. *Psychol Sch*. 2022;59(6): 1135–1157.

De Bellis MD, Woolley DP, Hooper SR. Neuropsychological findings in pediatric maltreatment: relationship of PTSD, dissociative symptoms and abuse/neglect indices to neurocognitive outcomes. *Child Maltreat*. 2013;18(3):171–183.

Egger HL, Erkanli A, Keeler G, Potts E, Walter BK, Angold A. Test-Retest Reliability of the Preschool Age Psychiatric Assessment (PAPA). *J Am Acad Child Adolesc Psychiatry*. 2006;45(5):538–549.

Faraone SV, Rostain AL, Blader J, et al. Practitioner review: emotional dysregulation in attention-deficit/hyperactivity disorder–implications for clinical recognition and intervention. *J Child Psychol Psychiatry*. 2019;60(2):133–150.

Hoffmann MS, Pine DS, Georgiades K, et al. Comparing mental health semi-structured diagnostic interviews and symptom checklists to predict poor life outcomes: an 8-year cohort study from childhood to young adulthood in Brazil. *Lancet Glob Health*. 2024;12(1):e79–e89.

Jeffrey J, Klomhaus A, Enenbach M, Lester P, Krishna R. Self-report rating scales to guide measurement-based care in child and adolescent psychiatry. *Child Adolesc Psychiatr Clin N Am*. 2020;29(4):601–629.

Kavanaugh B, Holler KI, Selke G. A neuropsychological profile of childhood maltreatment within an adolescent inpatient sample. *Appl Neuropsychol Child*. 2015;4(1):9–19.

Mattis S, Papolos D, Luck D, Cockerham M, Thode HC Jr. Neuropsychological factors differentiating treated children with pediatric bipolar disorder from those with attention-deficit/hyperactivity disorder. *J Clin Experi Neuropsychology*. 2011;33(1):74–84.

Neo WS, Suzuki T, Kelleher BL. Structural validity of the Child Behavior Checklist (CBCL) for preschoolers with neurogenetic syndromes. *Res Dev Disabil*. 2021;109:103834.

Offermans JE, de Bruin EI, Lange AMC, et al. The Development and Validation of a Subscale for the School-Age Child Behavior Check-List to Screen for Autism Spectrum Disorder. *J Autism Dev Disord*. 2023;53(3):1034–1052.

Posner K, Brown GK, Stanley B, et al. The Columbia–Suicide Severity Rating Scale: initial validity and internal consistency findings from three multisite studies with adolescents and adults. *Am J Psychiatry*. 2011;168(12):1266–1277.

Puig-Antich J, Orraschel H, Tabrizi MA, Chambers W. *Schedule for Affective Disorders and Schizophrenia for School-Age Children-Epidemiologic Version*. New York State Psychiatric Institute and Yale School of Medicine; 1980.

Recupero PR. The mental status examination in the age of the internet. *J Am Acad Psychiatry Law*. 2010;38(1):15–26.

Shaffer D, Fisher P, Lucas CP, Dulcan MK, Schwab-Stone ME. NIMH Diagnostic Interview Schedule for Children Version IV (NIMH DISC-IV): description, differences from previous versions, and reliability of some common diagnoses. *J Am Acad Child Adolesc Psychiatry*. 2000;39(1):28–38.

Schlechter AD, O'Brien KH, Stewart C. The positive assessment: a model for integrating well-being and strengths-based approaches into the child and adolescent psychiatry clinical evaluation. *Child Adolesc Psychiatr Clin N Am*. 2019;28(2):157–169.

Tsai AP, Smith RK, Gonzalez M, et al. Diagnostic accuracy of Achenbach scales in detecting youths' substance use disorders. *Psychol Assess*. 2022;34(6):570–582.

Vannest J, Szaflarski JP, Eaton KP, et al. Functional magnetic resonance imaging reveals changes in language localization in children with benign childhood epilepsy with centrotemporal spikes. *J Child Neurol*. 2013;28(4):435–445.

Weeks M, Wild TC, Poubidis GB, et al. Childhood cognitive ability and its relationship with anxiety and depression in adolescence. *J Affect Disord*. 2013.

Winters NC, Collett BR, Myers KM. Ten-year review of rating scales, VII: scales assessing functional impairment. *J Am Acad Child Adolesc Psychiatry*. 2005;44(4):309–338.

Wong MM, Brower KJ, Conroy DA, Craun EA. Convergence between the child behavior checklist sleep items, actigraphy and other sleep measures among children of parents with alcoholic disorders and controls. *Nat Sci Sleep*. 2022;14:2107–2121.

Youngstrom EA, Van Meter A, Frazier TW, Youngstrom JK, Findling RL. Developing and validating short forms of the parent general behavior inventory mania and depression scales for rating youth mood symptoms. *J Clin Child Adolesc Psychol*. 2020;49(2):162–177.

3 Intellectual Developmental Disorder (Intellectual Disability)

Intellectual Developmental Disorder (IDD; also referred to as Intellectual disability) can be caused by a range of environmental and genetic factors that lead to a combination of cognitive and social impairments. The American Association on Intellectual and Developmental Disabilities (AAIDD) defines intellectual disability as a disability characterized by significant limitations in both intellectual functioning (reasoning, learning, and problem solving) and in adaptive behavior (conceptual, social, and practical skills) that emerges before the age of 18 years. Approximately 1% to 3% of the global population has an intellectual disability.

The widespread acceptance of this definition has led to the international consensus that an assessment of both social adaptation and intelligence quotient (IQ) is the best way to determine the level of intellectual disability. Measures of adaptive function assess competency in social functioning, understanding of societal norms, and performance of everyday tasks, whereas measures of intellectual function focus on cognitive abilities. Individuals with a given intellectual level do not all have identical levels of adaptive function, however, epidemiologic data suggest that the combination of a person's intellectual level and level of adaptive function largely determine the prevalence of intellectual disability.

The *Diagnostic and Statistical Manual of Mental Disorders,* Fifth Edition Text Revision (DSM-5-TR), defines the levels of severity of IDD based on deficits in reasoning, judgment, and learning; and deficits in adaptive functioning causing failure to meet developmental milestones for independent living and social functioning. These deficits must begin in the developmental period. The change in emphasis from IQ scores in earlier diagnostic criteria to adaptive functioning criteria is because impairment in adaptive function determines the level of support that is required. The severity level of intellectual disability, according to DSM-5-TR, includes an assessment of functioning in a conceptual domain (e.g., academic skills), a social domain (e.g., relationships), and a practical domain (e.g., personal hygiene).

The International Classification of Diseases, 11th Edition (ICD-11) considers both the IQ as well as adaptive function to determine the level of IDDs.

A vital force in the current care of children with IDD is the philosophy of "normalization" in living situations, and "inclusion" in educational settings. Since the late 1960s, concepts of normalization and inclusion of children and adolescents with IDD remains prominent among advocacy groups and parents.

The passage of Public Law 94–142 (the Education for all Handicapped Children Act) in 1975 mandates that the public school system provides appropriate educational services to all children with disabilities. The Individuals with Disabilities Act (IDEA) in 1990 extended and modified the above legislation. Currently, the provision of public education for all children, including those with disabilities, "within the least restrictive environment" is mandated by law.

In addition to the educational system, advocacy groups, including the Council for Exceptional Children (CEC) and the Arc of the United States (The Arc), are well-known parental lobbying organizations for children with intellectual disability and were instrumental in advocating for Public Law 94–142. The AAIDD is the most prominent advocacy organization in this field. It has been very influential in educating the public about and supporting research and legislation relating to IDD.

The AAIDD promotes a view of IDD as a functional interaction between an individual and the environment, rather than a static designation of a person's limitations. Within this conceptual framework, a child or adolescent with an intellectual disability is determined to need intermittent, limited, extensive, or pervasive "environmental support" concerning a specific set of adaptive function domains. These include communication, self-care, home living, social or interpersonal skills, use of community resources, self-direction, functional academic skills, work, leisure, health, and safety.

The United Nations Convention on the Rights of Persons with Disabilities (2006) has created a forum to promote the full social inclusion of people with intellectual disabilities. Through its recognition and focus on social barriers, this international forum aims to provide protections for individuals with intellectual disabilities and to seek more inclusion of those with intellectual disabilities in social, civic, and educational activities.

NOMENCLATURE

An accurate definition of IDD has been a challenge for clinicians over the centuries. All current classification systems underscore that intellectual disability is more than a cognitive deficit. That is, it also includes impaired social adaptive function. According to DSM-5-TR, we should only make a diagnosis of IDD when there are deficits in intellectual functioning and deficits in adaptive functioning (see Table 3-1). Once intellectual deficits are recognized, the severity is determined by the level of deficits in intellectual functions, such as reasoning, problem solving, and judgment, and by the level of deficits in adaptive functioning, such as personal independence and social responsibility in home, school, and work. Deficits in intellectual functions are confirmed by both clinical assessment and standardized intelligence testing.

The diagnostic term intellectual developmental disorder (intellectual disability) is used in DSM-5-TR to match the diagnostic term in ICD-11, which is Disorders of Intellectual Development. The terms intellectual developmental disorder and intellectual disability are equivalent; however in educational settings and in advocacy settings, the term intellectual disability is more often used.

CLASSIFICATION

The DSM-5-TR diagnosis of IDD includes three criteria: (1) Deficits in intellectual functions such as reasoning, problem solving, academic learning, and learning from experience confirmed by both clinical evaluation and standard intelligence testing. (2) Deficits in adaptive functioning resulting in failure to meet developmental and societal standards for independent living and social responsibility. Support will be needed to function in areas such as communication,

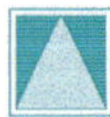

Table 3-1.
Intellectual Developmental Disorder (Intellectual Disability)/Disorders of Intellectual Development

	DSM-5-TR	ICD-10	ICD-11
Diagnostic Name	Intellectual Developmental Disorder (Intellectual Disability)	Mental Retardation	Disorders of Intellectual Development
Symptoms	• Deficits in reasoning, abstraction, judgment, learning • Deficits in adaptive functioning causing failure to meet developmental milestones for independence and social functioning • Deficits arise during the developmental period	An arrest or incomplete development of ≥1 of the skills contributing to overall intelligence: cognitive, language, motor, and social abilities	• The presence of significant limitations in intellectual functioning across various domains such as perceptual reasoning, working memory, processing speed, and verbal comprehension • The presence of significant limitations in adaptive behavior, which refers to the set of conceptual, social, and practical skills that have been learned and are performed by people in their everyday lives • Onset occurs during the developmental period
Severity specifiers	**Mild** **Moderate** **Severe** **Profound**	**Mild** **Moderate** **Severe** **Profound**	**Mild** **Moderate** **Severe** **Profound**
Comments	**Unspecified diagnosis.** Unspecified Intellectual Developmental Disorder (Intellectual Disability) for persons >5 yr, and assessment is difficult or impossible due to sensory or other physical impairments		**Disorder of Intellectual Development, Provisional.** Assigned when there is evidence of a Disorder of Intellectual Development but the individual is an infant or child under the age of 4, making it difficult to ascertain whether the observed impairments represent a transient delay Disorders of Intellectual Development, Unspecified

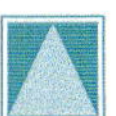

Table 3-2.
Developmental Characteristics of Intellectual Developmental Disorder (Intellectual Disability)

Level of Intellectual Disability	Preschool Age (0–5 yr) Maturation and Development	School Age (6–20 yr) Training and Education	Adult (21 yr and Above) Social and Vocational Adequacy
Profound	Gross disability; minimal capacity for functioning in sensorimotor areas; needs nursing care; constant aid and supervision required	Some motor development present; may respond to minimal or limited training in self-help	Some motor and speech development; may achieve very limited self-care; needs nursing care
Severe	Poor motor development; speech minimal; generally unable to profit from training in self-help; little or no communication skills	Can talk or learn to communicate; can be trained in elemental health habits; profits from systematic habit training; unable to profit from vocational training	May contribute partially to self-maintenance under complete supervision; can develop self-protection skills to a minimal useful level in controlled environment
Moderate	Can talk or learn to communicate; poor social awareness; fair motor development; profits from training in self-help; can be managed with moderate supervision	Can profit from training in social and occupational skills; unlikely to progress beyond second-grade level in academic subjects; may learn to travel alone in familiar places	May achieve self-maintenance in unskilled or semiskilled work under sheltered conditions; needs supervision and guidance when under mild social or economic stress
Mild	Can develop social and communication skills; minimal retardation in sensorimotor areas; often not distinguished from normal until later age	Can learn academic skills up to approximately sixth-grade level by late teens; can be guided toward social conformity	Can usually achieve social and vocational skills adequate for minimal self-support but may need guidance and assistance when under unusual social or economic stress

school, work, and community. (3) Onset of the intellectual and adaptive deficits emerges during the developmental period. Table 3-2 presents an overview of developmental levels in communication, academic functioning, and vocational skills expected of persons with various degrees of intellectual disability.

On a standardized test of intelligence using a mean of 100 as an average score and a standard deviation of 15, this means a score that is two standard deviations below the mean. Typically, this is an intellectual score of 65 to 75 (with a margin of error + or −5 points). Adaptive functioning can be measured using a standardized scale, such as the *Vineland Adaptive Behavior Scale.* This scale scores communications, daily living skills, socialization, and motor skills (up to 4 years, 11 months) and generates an adaptive behavior composite that correlates with the expected skills at a given age.

Approximately 85% of individuals who have IDD fall within the DSM-5-TR mild intellectual disability category. This category typically includes an IQ between 50 and 70 and an adaptive function severity in the mild range. Adaptive functions include skills such as communication, self-care, social skills, work, leisure, and understanding of safety. Genetic, environmental, and psychosocial factors all influence intellectual disability. A multitude of environmental and developmental factors, including subclinical lead intoxication and prenatal exposure to drugs, alcohol, and other toxins, can contribute to intellectual disability. Specific genetic syndromes associated with intellectual disability such as fragile X syndrome, Down syndrome, and Prader–Willi syndrome have characteristic patterns of social, linguistic, and cognitive development and typical behavioral manifestations.

DEGREES OF SEVERITY OF INTELLECTUAL DEVELOPMENTAL DISORDER (INTELLECTUAL DISABILITY)

DSM-5-TR classifies the severity levels of IDD as mild, moderate, severe, and profound. "Borderline intellectual functioning," is listed in DSM-5-TR as a condition that may be the focus of clinical attention and is defined as a condition that is used when an individual's level of intellectual function is the focus of clinical attention and does not meet criteria for mild intellectual disability.

Mild IDD represents approximately 85% of persons with intellectual disabilities. Children with mild intellectual disabilities often are not identified until the first or second grade, when academic demands increase. By late adolescence, they often acquire academic skills at approximately a sixth-grade level. Specific causes for intellectual disability are often unidentified in this group. Many adults with mild intellectual disabilities can live independently with appropriate support and raise their

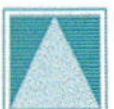

Table 3-3.
Global Developmental Delay

	DSM-5-TR	ICD-10	ICD-11
Diagnostic name	Global Developmental Delay	Other Disorders of Psychological Development (Global Developmental Delay)	Disorders of Intellectual Development, Unspecified
Symptoms	Failure to meet developmental milestones before the age of 5, with an inability to perform full assessment of testing of intellectual functioning	Classified as an unspecified disorder	

own families. IQ for this level of adaptive function may typically range from 50 to 70.

Moderate IDD represents about 10% of persons with intellectual disabilities. Most children with a moderate intellectual disability acquire language and can communicate adequately during early childhood. They are challenged academically and often are not able to achieve above a second- to third-grade level. During adolescence, socialization difficulties often set these persons apart, and a great deal of social and vocational support is beneficial. As adults, individuals with moderate intellectual disability may be able to perform semiskilled work under appropriate supervision. IQ for this level of adaptive function may typically range from 35 to 50.

Severe IDD represents about 4% of individuals with intellectual disabilities. They may be able to develop communication skills in childhood and often can learn to count as well as recognize words that are critical to functioning. In this group, the cause for the IDD is more likely to be identified than in milder forms of intellectual disability. In adulthood, persons with severe intellectual disability may adapt well to supervised living situations, such as group homes, and may be able to perform work-related tasks under supervision. IQ in individuals with this level of adaptive function may typically range from 20 to 35.

Profound IDD constitutes approximately 1% to 2% of individuals with intellectual disabilities. Most individuals with profound IDD have identifiable causes for their condition. Children with profound intellectual disabilities may be taught some self-care skills and learn to communicate their needs, given the appropriate training. IQ in individuals with this level of adaptive function may typically be less than 20.

The DSM-5-TR includes a disorder called Global Developmental Delay which is used for a child under the age of 5 years who has not met developmental milestone expectations in several areas of intellectual function and is unable to participate in testing to determine their severity (Table 3-3). "Unspecified Intellectual Disability" (intellectual developmental disorder) in DSM-5-TR is reserved for individuals over the age of 5 years with intellectual disability who are difficult or impossible to evaluate with standard assessments due to sensory or physical impairments such as blindness or deafness, or concurrent mental disorders.

CLINICAL FEATURES

Mild IDD may not be recognized or diagnosed in a child until school challenges the child's social and communication skills. Cognitive deficits include reduced ability to abstract and egocentric thinking, both of which become more readily evident as a child reaches middle childhood. Children with milder forms of intellectual disabilities may function academically at the high elementary level and may acquire vocational skills sufficient to support themselves in some cases; however, social assimilation may be problematic. Communication deficits, poor self-esteem, and dependence may further contribute to a relative lack of social spontaneity.

Moderate IDD is significantly more likely to be observed at a younger age since communication skills develop more slowly, and social isolation may ensue in the elementary school years. Academic achievement is usually limited to the middle-elementary level. Children with moderate IDD benefit from individual attention focused on the development of self-help skills. However, these children are aware of their deficits and often feel alienated from their peers and frustrated by their limitations. They continue to require a relatively high level of supervision but can become competent at occupational tasks in supportive settings.

Severe IDD is typically evident in the preschool years; affected children have minimal speech and impaired motor development. Some language development may occur in the school-age years. By adolescence, if the language has not improved significantly, nonverbal forms of communication may have evolved. Behavioral approaches are useful means to promote some self-care, although those with severe intellectual disabilities generally need extensive supervision.

Children with profound IDD require constant supervision and are severely limited in both communication and motor skills. By adulthood, some speech development may be present, and simple self-help skills may be acquired. Clinical features frequently observed in populations with intellectual disability, either in isolation or as part of a mental disorder, include hyperactivity, low frustration tolerance, aggression, affective instability, repetitive and stereotypic motor behaviors, and self-injurious behaviors. Self-injurious behaviors occur more frequently and with higher intensity in more severe intellectual disability. See Table 3-4 for a description of syndromes with IDD and behavioral phenotypes.

Liam was a healthy, full-term infant born to a mother whose pregnancy was without problems. At birth, he was noted to have unusually large ears and strabismus, which did not concern his pediatrician since both often resolve as a baby matures. Liam's parents were not worried about Liam's motor and verbal milestones because he was their first child and they believed he was developing typically. Liam was able to sit by himself at 10 months and started walking on his own at 18 months. Liam spoke his first words at 20 months. Liam's parents were concerned about his very high activity level by the time he was 2½ years of age, however, the pediatrician reassured them that boys of his age are often very active.

When Liam was 3 years old, his preschool teacher reported to his parents that he was hyperactive compared to the rest of his class and disruptive and aggressive toward the other children. Liam was unable to participate in the circle activities with the other children. Instead, he ran around the classroom, prompting his parents to obtain a developmental evaluation. Liam's evaluation showed some delays in cognitive, linguistic, and motor functioning. Liam was inattentive, socially awkward, and anxious, and he displayed poor eye contact. Liam was enrolled in a special kindergarten and remained in a combination of special education and mainstreamed classes throughout his academic life.

At 7 years of age, Liam was evaluated by a psychologist for intellectual function using the Wechsler Intelligence Scale for Children (WISC-V) and a Vineland Scale for Adaptive Function to measure his adaptive skills. Liam was found to have mild intellectual disability. Liam displayed some scatter in the results of his testing with close to normal functioning in short-term memory and pronounced deficits in long-term memory, expressive language, and visual–spatial functioning. Liam struggled with writing tasks and arithmetic but loved to play with LEGOs and build structures. Liam was evaluated and met the criteria for attention-deficit/hyperactivity disorder and was prescribed Concerta, which was beneficial at a dose of 54 mg/d. As Liam continued to grow and develop, he displayed transient, intense interests in unusual items, such as vacuum cleaners and fans. When Liam entered the fourth grade at age 9 years, he began to have more difficulty socially, and peers bullied him for being "weird," for being enrolled in special education, for his long head and big ears. Liam's parents became aware that Liam had intellectual disability, but none of his doctors were able to tell them why.

During the fourth grade, Liam's parents happened to watch a television documentary on genetic causes of intellectual disability. They were overwhelmed by the similarities between Liam and one of the children described in the program. They later described the experience as a "jolt." They had always accepted Liam's quirks and had stopped pushing their doctors for reasons "why" when Liam had intellectual and social difficulties. After watching the documentary, Liam's parents immediately called their pediatrician and requested that Liam receive genetic testing. Within 8 weeks, Liam's genetic test confirmed a diagnosis of fragile X syndrome.

Although Liam's day-to-day life did not change dramatically after the fragile X diagnosis, his parents reported a big difference in their approach to his social skills deficits, restricted interests, odd preoccupations, and inattention. Liam's parents found a social skills therapeutic group for Liam, and they attended a parent support group for parents of children with fragile X syndrome. Knowing his diagnosis, Liam's parents were more supportive to him and worked hard to provide structured peer activities for him. Liam was prescribed a trial of sertraline, a selective serotonin reuptake inhibitor (SSRI), for anxiety, which decreased his social anxiety and facilitated activities with a few peers. Liam's parents reported a mixture of feeling sad that he had a genetic disorder and also relief in finally knowing and understanding how to support him. Liam's parents were energized by Liam's positive responses to treatments for his attentional and anxiety symptoms and were pleased with his recent increased interest in sharing activities with classmates and peers.

A negative self-image and poor self-esteem are not infrequent associated features of mildly and moderately intellectually disabled persons who are aware of their social and academic differences from others. Given their experience of repeated failure and disappointment in being unable to meet their parents' and society's expectations, they may also fall progressively behind younger siblings. Communication difficulties further increase their vulnerability to feelings of ineptness and frustration. Inappropriate behaviors, such as withdrawal, are common. The perpetual sense of isolation and inadequacy is related to feelings of anxiety, anger, dysphoria, and depression. Parents of children with intellectual disability who develop an understanding and obtain education regarding intellectual disability will be able to offer their children greater support and be more able to seek appropriate social and educational opportunities for them.

DIAGNOSIS

The diagnosis of IDD occurs after obtaining the history, using information from a standardized intellectual assessment, and a standardized measure of adaptive function indicating that a child is significantly below the expected level in both areas. The severity of the intellectual disability is determined based on the level of adaptive function. A history and psychiatric interview are useful in obtaining a longitudinal picture of the child's development and functioning. Examination of physical signs, neurologic abnormalities, and in some cases, laboratory tests, can help ascertain the cause and prognosis.

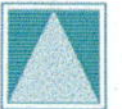

Table 3-4.
Syndromes with Intellectual Disability and Behavioral Phenotypes

Disorder	Pathophysiology	Clinical Features and Behavioral Phenotype
Down syndrome	Trisomy 21, 95% nondisjunction, approximately 4% translocation; 1/1,000 live births: 1:2,500 in women less than 30 yr old, 1:80 over 40 yr old, 1:32 at 45 yr old; possible overproduction of β-amyloid due to defect at 21q21.1	Hypotonia, upward-slanted palpebral fissures, midface depression, flat wide nasal bridge, simian crease, short stature, increased incidence of thyroid abnormalities, and congenital heart disease Passive, affable, hyperactivity in childhood, stubborn; verbal > auditory processing, increased risk of depression, and dementia of the Alzheimer type in adulthood
Fragile X syndrome	Inactivation of *FMR-1* gene at X q27.3 due to CGG base repeats, methylation; recessive; 1:1,000 male births, 1:3,000 female; accounts for 10–12% of intellectual disability in males	Long face, large ears, midface hypoplasia, high arched palate, short stature, macro-orchidism, mitral valve prolapse, joint laxity, strabismus Hyperactivity, inattention, anxiety, stereotypies, speech and language delays, IQ decline, gaze aversion, social avoidance, shyness, irritability, learning disorder in some females; mild intellectual disability in affected females, moderate to severe in males; verbal IQ > performance IQ
Prader–Willi syndrome	Deletion in 15q12 (15q11–15q13) of paternal origin; some cases of maternal uniparental disomy; dominant 1/10,000 live births; 90% sporadic; candidate gene: small nuclear ribonucleoprotein polypeptide (SNRPN)	Hypotonia, failure to thrive in infancy, obesity, small hands and feet, micro-orchidism, cryptorchidism, short stature, almond-shaped eyes, fair hair and light skin, flat face, scoliosis, orthopedic problems, prominent forehead and bitemporal narrowing Compulsive behavior, hyperphagia, hoarding, impulsivity, borderline to moderate intellectual disability, emotional lability, tantrums, excess daytime sleepiness, skin picking, anxiety, aggression
Angelman syndrome	Deletion in 15q12 (15q11–15q13) of maternal origin; dominant; frequent deletion of γ-aminobutyric acid (GABA) B-3 receptor subunit, prevalence unknown but rare, estimated 1/20,000–1/30,000	Fair hair and blue eyes (66%); dysmorphic faces including wide smiling mouth, thin upper lip, and pointed chin; epilepsy (90%) with characteristic EEG; ataxia; small head circumference, 25% microcephalic Happy disposition, paroxysmal laughter, hand flapping, clapping; profound intellectual disability; sleep disturbance with nighttime waking; possible increased incidence of autistic features; anecdotal love of water and music
Cornelia de Lange syndrome	Lack of pregnancy-associated plasma protein A (PAPPA) linked to chromosome 9q33; similar phenotype associated with trisomy 5p, ring chromosome 3; rare (1/40,000–1/100,000 live births); possible association with 3q26.3	Continuous eyebrows, thin downturned upper lip, microcephaly, short stature, small hands and feet, small upturned nose, anteverted nostrils, malformed upper limbs, failure to thrive Self-injury, limited speech in severe cases, language delays, avoidance of being held, stereotypic movements, twirling, severe to profound intellectual disability
Williams syndrome	1/20,000 births; hemizygous deletion that includes elastin locus chromosome 7q11–23; autosomal dominant	Short stature, unusual facial features including broad forehead, depressed nasal bridge, stellate pattern of the iris, widely spaced teeth, and full lips; elfin-like facies; renal and cardiovascular abnormalities; thyroid abnormalities; hypercalcemia Anxiety, hyperactivity, fears, outgoing, sociable, verbal skills > visual–spatial skills
Cri-du-chat syndrome	Partial deletion 5p; 1/50,000; region may be 5p15.2	Round face with hypertelorism, epicanthal folds, slanting palpebral fissures, broad flat nose, low-set ears, micrognathia; prenatal growth retardation; respiratory and ear infections; congenital heart disease; gastrointestinal abnormalities Severe intellectual disability, infantile catlike cry, hyperactivity, stereotypies, self-injury
Smith–Magenis syndrome	Incidence unknown, estimated 1/25,000 live births; complete or partial deletion of 17p11.2	Broad face; flat midface; short, broad hands; small toes; hoarse, deep voice Severe intellectual disability; hyperactivity; severe self-injury including hand biting, head banging, and pulling out finger and toenails; stereotyped self-hugging; attention seeking; aggression; sleep disturbance (decreased REM)

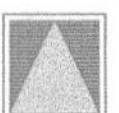

Table 3-4.
Syndromes with Intellectual Disability and Behavioral Phenotypes (Continued)

Disorder	Pathophysiology	Clinical Features and Behavioral Phenotype
Rubinstein–Taybi syndrome	1/250,000, approximate male = female; sporadic; likely autosomal dominant; documented microdeletions in some cases at 16p13.3	Short stature and microcephaly, broad thumb and big toes, prominent nose, broad nasal bridge, hypertelorism, ptosis, frequent fractures, feeding difficulties in infancy, congenital heart disease, EEG abnormalities, seizures Poor concentration, distractible, expressive language difficulties, performance IQ > verbal IQ; anecdotally happy, loving, sociable, responsive to music, self-stimulating behavior; older patients have mood lability and temper tantrums
Tuberous sclerosis complex 1 and 2	Benign tumors (hamartomas) and malformations (hamartias) of central nervous system (CNS), skin, kidney, heart; dominant; 1/10,000 births; 50% TSC 1, 9q34; 50% TSC 2, 16p13	Epilepsy, autism, hyperactivity, impulsivity, aggression; spectrum of intellectual disability from none (30%) to profound; self-injurious behaviors, sleep disturbances
Neurofibromatosis type 1 (NF1)	1/2,500–1/4,000; male = female; autosomal dominant; 50% new mutations; more than 90% paternal NF1 allele mutated; *NFl* gene 17q11.2; gene product is neurofibromin thought to be tumor suppressor gene	Variable manifestations; café-au-lait spots, cutaneous neurofibromas, Lisch nodules; short stature and macrocephaly in 30–45% Half with speech and language difficulties; 10% with moderate to profound intellectual disability; verbal IQ > performance IQ; distractible, impulsive, hyperactive, anxious; possibly associated with increased incidence of mood and anxiety disorders
Lesch–Nyhan syndrome	Defect in hypoxanthine guanine phosphoribosyl-transferase with accumulation of uric acid; Xq26–27; recessive; rare (1/10,000–1/38,000)	Ataxia, chorea, kidney failure, gout Often severe self-biting behavior, aggression, anxiety, mild to moderate intellectual disability
Galactosemia	Defect in galactose-1-phosphate uridyltransferase or galactokinase or empiramase, autosomal recessive; 1/62,000 births in the United States	Vomiting in early infancy, jaundice, hepatosplenomegaly; later cataracts, weight loss, food refusal, increased intracranial pressure and increased risk for sepsis, ovarian failure, failure to thrive, renal tubular damage Possible intellectual disability, even with treatment, visuospatial deficits, language disorders, reports of increased behavioral problems, anxiety, social withdrawal, and shyness
Phenylketonuria	Defect in phenylalanine hydroxylase (PAH) or cofactor (biopterin) with accumulation of phenylalanine; approximately 1/11,500 births; varies with geographical location; gene for PAH, 12q22–24.1; autosomal recessive	Symptoms absent neonatally, later development of seizures (25% generalized), fair skin, blue eyes, blond hair, rash Untreated: mild to profound intellectual disability, language delay, destructiveness, self-injury, hyperactivity
Hurler syndrome	1/100,000; deficiency in α-L-iduronidase activity; autosomal recessive	Early onset; short stature, hepatosplenomegaly; hirsutism, corneal clouding, death before age 10 yr, dwarfism, coarse facial features, recurrent respiratory infections Moderate to severe intellectual disability, anxious, fearful, rarely aggressive Hyperactivity, intellectual disability by 2 yr; speech delay; loss of speech at 8–10 yr; restless, aggressive, inattentive, sleep abnormalities; apathetic, sedentary with disease progression
Fetal alcohol syndrome	Maternal alcohol consumption (trimester III > II > I); 1/3,000 live births in Western countries; 1/300 with fetal alcohol effects	Microcephaly, short stature, midface hypoplasia, short palpebral fissure, thin upper lip, retrognathia in infancy, micrognathia in adolescence, hypoplastic long or smooth philtrum Mild to moderate intellectual disability, irritability, inattention, memory impairment

History

When we take the history, which may elucidate pathways to IDD, we should pay particular attention to the mother's pregnancy, labor, and delivery; the presence of a family history of intellectual disability; consanguinity of the parents; and known familial hereditary disorders that may impact intellectual functioning.

Laboratory Examination

Laboratory tests that may elucidate the causes of intellectual disability include chromosomal analysis, urine and blood testing for metabolic disorders, and neuroimaging. Chromosomal abnormalities are the most commonly known cause of intellectual disability.

Chromosome Studies. When multiple physical anomalies, developmental delays, and intellectual disability present together, chromosome analysis may be useful in elucidating their etiology. Current techniques can identify chromosomal regions with specific fluorescent in situ hybridization (FISH) markers, enabling the identification of microscopic deletions in up to 7% of persons with moderate to severe intellectual disability. A history of growth retardation, the presence of microcephaly, a family history of intellectual disability, short stature, hypertelorism, and other facial abnormalities increase the risk of finding subtelomeric defects.

Amniocentesis, in which clinicians remove a small amount of amniotic fluid from the amniotic cavity transabdominally at about 15 weeks of gestation, has been useful for diagnosing prenatal chromosomal abnormalities. Its use is considered when an increased fetal risk exists, such as with increased maternal age. Amniotic fluid cells, mostly fetal in origin, are cultured for cytogenetic and biochemical studies.

Chorionic villi sampling (CVS) is a screening technique to determine fetal chromosomal abnormalities. It is done at 8 to 10 weeks of gestation, 6 weeks earlier than amniocentesis. The results are available in a short time, within hours or days.

A noninvasive blood test called MaterniT21 is a proprietary prenatal test that detects abnormalities of chromosomes 21, 18, 13, X, and Y. It is highly specific for Down syndrome. There is a slight risk of miscarriage.

Urine and Blood Analysis. Lesch–Nyhan syndrome, galactosemia, phenylketonuria (PKU), Hurler syndrome, and Hunter syndrome are examples of disorders characterized by an intellectual disability that we can identify through assays of the appropriate enzyme or organic or amino acids. Enzymatic abnormalities in chromosomal disorders, such as Down syndrome, promise to become useful diagnostic tools.

Electroencephalography. Whenever considering a seizure disorder, we should request electroencephalography (EEG). "Nonspecific" EEG changes, characterized by slow frequencies with bursts of spikes and sharp or blunt wave complexes, are found with higher frequency among populations with intellectual disability than in the general population; however, these findings do not elucidate specific diagnoses.

Neuroimaging. Neuroimaging studies with populations of intellectually disabled patients using either computerized tomography (CT) or magnetic resonance imaging (MRI) have found high rates of abnormalities in those patients with microcephaly, significant delay, cerebral palsy, and profound disability. Among patients with intellectual disability, seizures, microcephaly, or macrocephaly, loss of previously acquired skills, or neurologic signs such as dystonia, spasticity, or altered reflexes all are indications for neuroimaging.

Although clinically not diagnostic, neuroimaging studies are currently also utilized to gather data that may eventually uncover biologic mechanisms contributing to intellectual disability. Structural MRI, functional MRI (fMRI), and diffusion tensor imaging (DTI) are useful in current research. For example, current data suggest that individuals with fragile X syndrome and concurrent attentional deficits are also more likely to show aberrant frontal–striatal pathways on MRI than those patients without attentional problems. MRI is also useful to elucidate myelination patterns. MRI studies can also provide a baseline for comparison of a later, potentially degenerative process in the brain.

Hearing and Speech Evaluations. We should evaluate a patient's hearing and speech routinely. Speech development may be the most reliable criterion in investigating intellectual disability. Various hearing impairments often occur in persons who are intellectually disabled, but in some instances, hearing impairments can simulate intellectual disability. The commonly used methods of hearing and speech evaluation, however, require the patient's cooperation and, thus, are often unreliable in severely disabled persons.

DIFFERENTIAL DIAGNOSIS

By definition, IDD must begin in the developmental period. In some cases, environmental factors such as child maltreatment can contribute to reversible delays in development, which can appear to be an intellectual disability. However, these delays may be overcome by nurturing caregivers and a stimulating environment. Sensory disabilities, especially deafness and blindness, can be mistaken for intellectual disability when a lack of awareness of the sensory deficit leads to inappropriate testing. Expressive and receptive speech disorders may give the impression of intellectual disability in a child of average intelligence, and cerebral palsy may be mistaken for intellectual disability. Chronic, debilitating medical diseases may depress and delay a child's functioning and achievement despite average intelligence. Seizure disorders, especially uncontrolled, may contribute to persisting intellectual disability. Specific syndromes leading to isolated handicaps such as failure to read (alexia), failure to write (agraphia), or failure to communicate (aphasia) may occur in a child of average and even superior intelligence. Children with learning disorders (which can coexist with intellectual disability) experience a delay or failure of development in a specific area, such as reading or mathematics, but they usually develop in other areas. In contrast, children with IDD show delays in most areas of development.

IDD and autism spectrum disorder (ASD) can coexist. Divergent rates of intellectual disability in youth with ASD have been reported in epidemiologic studies over the past few decades. In the early 2000s, a large epidemiologic study reported that an IQ < 70 was present in 50% of children with ASD. A more recent epidemiologic study in 2014 by J. Baio and colleagues in the Autism and Developmental Disabilities Monitoring Network of 8-year-olds with ASD reported that only 31% of those youth with ASD evidenced an IQ < 70. This study reported that 25% of children with ASD showed evidence of an IQ in the range of 71 to 85, and 44% had IQ scores in the average to above average range (IQ ≥ 85). Also, epidemiologic data indicate that ASD occurs in approximately 10% of persons with IDD. Children with ASD have relatively more severe impairment in social relatedness and language than other children with the same level of intellectual disability.

COMORBIDITY

Many psychiatric disorders occur more commonly in children and adolescents with intellectual disabilities, including depressive disorders, attention-deficit disorders, anxiety disorders, and neurologic disorders.

Attention-Deficit/Hyperactivity Disorder

Estimates of attention-deficit/hyperactivity disorder (ADHD) and ADHD-like symptoms among children with intellectual disabilities, genetic disorders, and global developmental delay are estimated to be significantly higher than rates in the community.

Neurologic Disorders

Seizure disorders occur more frequently in individuals with IDD than in the general population, and prevalence rates for seizures increase proportionally to the severity level of intellectual disability. A review of psychiatric disorders in children and adolescents with intellectual disability and epilepsy found that approximately one-third had comorbid ASD. The combination of intellectual disability, epilepsy, and ASD may occur in 0.07% of the general population.

COURSE AND PROGNOSIS

Although the underlying intellectual impairment does not improve, in most cases of IDD, the level of adaptation increases with age and can be influenced positively by an enriched and supportive environment. In general, persons with mild and moderate intellectual disabilities have the most flexibility in adapting to various environmental conditions. Comorbid psychiatric disorders negatively impact overall prognosis. When psychiatric disorders co-occur with IDD, standard treatments for comorbid mental disorders are often beneficial; however, less robust responses and increased vulnerability to side effects of psychopharmacologic agents are common.

TREATMENT

Interventions for children and adolescents with IDD incorporate an assessment of social, educational, psychiatric, and environmental needs. Intellectual disability is associated with a variety of comorbid psychiatric disorders that often require specific treatment, in addition to psychosocial support. Of course, when preventive measures are available, the optimal approach includes primary, secondary, and tertiary interventions.

Prevention

Primary Prevention. Primary prevention comprises actions taken to eliminate or reduce the conditions that lead to the development of various forms of intellectual disability, as well as associated disorders. For example, screening babies for PKU, and administrating a low phenylalanine diet when PKU is present, significantly alters the emergence of intellectual disability in those affected children. Additional primary prevention steps include education of the general public about strategies to prevent intellectual disability, such as abstinence from alcohol during pregnancy, continuing efforts of health professionals to ensure and upgrade public health policies, and legislation to provide optimal maternal and child health care. Family and genetic counseling help reduce the incidence of intellectual disability in a family with a history of a genetic disorder.

Secondary and Tertiary Prevention. Prompt attention to medical and psychiatric complications of intellectual disability can diminish their course (secondary prevention) and minimize the sequelae or consequent disabilities (tertiary prevention). Hereditary metabolic and endocrine disorders, such as PKU and hypothyroidism, can be treated effectively in an early stage by dietary control or hormone replacement therapy.

Psychosocial Interventions

Educational Interventions. Educational settings for children with intellectual disabilities should include a comprehensive program that addresses academics and training in adaptive skills, social skills, and vocational skills. Particular attention should focus on communication and efforts to improve the quality of life.

Behavioral and Cognitive-Behavioral Interventions. The difficulties in adaptation among populations with various intellectual disabilities are widespread and so varied that several interventions alone or in combination may be beneficial. Behavior therapy has been used for many years to shape and enhance social behaviors and to control and minimize aggressive and destructive behaviors. Positive reinforcement for desired behaviors and benign punishment (e.g., loss of privileges) for objectionable behaviors has been helpful. Cognitive-behavioral therapy, such as dispelling false beliefs and relaxation exercises with self-instruction, has also been recommended for intellectually disabled persons who can follow the instructions. Psychodynamic therapy has been used with patients and their families to decrease conflicts about expectations that result in persistent anxiety, rage, and depression. Psychiatric treatment modalities require modifications that take into consideration the patient's level of intelligence.

Family Education. One of the most critical areas that we can address is educating the family of a child or adolescent with intellectual disability about ways to enhance competence and self-esteem while maintaining realistic expectations for the patient. The family often finds it challenging to balance the fostering of independence and the providing of a nurturing and supportive environment for an intellectually disabled child, who is likely to experience some rejection and failure outside the family context. The parents may benefit from continuous counseling or family therapy and should be allowed opportunities to express their feelings of guilt, despair, anguish, recurring denial, and anger about their child's disorder and future. We should give the parents all the necessary and current medical information regarding causes, treatment, and other pertinent areas (e.g., specialized training and the correction of sensory deficits).

Social Intervention. One of the most prevalent problems among persons with an intellectual disability is a sense of social isolation and social skills deficits. Thus, improving the quantity and quality of social competence is a critical part of their care. Special Olympics International is the most extensive recreational sports program geared for this population. In addition to providing a forum to develop physical fitness, Special Olympics also enhances social interactions, friendships, and (hopefully) general self-esteem.

Psychopharmacologic Interventions

Pharmacologic approaches to the treatment of behavioral and psychological symptoms in children with an intellectual disability follow the paradigms of the evidence-based literature on treatment for all children with psychiatric disorders. However, given the paucity of randomized trials in the childhood intellectual disability population, an empirical approach must also be taken.

Treating Comorbid Disorders and Symptoms

AGGRESSION, IRRITABILITY, AND SELF-INJURIOUS BEHAVIOR. Antipsychotic medicine may be useful for reducing self-injurious and aggressive behaviors toward others. Among the antipsychotics, both aripiprazole and risperidone had reasonable effect sizes in multiple studies. However, we should view these findings cautiously, as many of the studies had significant methodologic limitations. Overall, the consensus seems to be that antipsychotics are helpful in the short term. Among them, aripiprazole and risperidone were studied in the majority of studies and show effect sizes in the moderate to large range. There is little evidence on the long-term use of these medications. Given the significant side effects (weight gain, sedation, cardiovascular risks, extrapyramidal side effects, and increased prolactin levels, which are of particular concern in children), caution should be taken when continuing medications in this class beyond an acute crisis.

Other medications, such as anticonvulsants and antioxidants, may be helpful; however, the data are not conclusive. GABA analogs, such as piracetam, may have promise, but the supportive data are limited.

ATTENTION-DEFICIT/HYPERACTIVITY DISORDER. The existing data for the treatment of ADHD and ADHD-like symptoms in youth with subaverage intelligence and developmental disorders suggest that agents, particularly stimulants used to treat ADHD in typically developing children, provide some degree of benefit to children with intellectual disability and ADHD. However, these children experience more side effects than ADHD children without an intellectual disability. Thus, recommendations regarding the treatment of ADHD in children and adolescents with comorbid intellectual disability include close monitoring for side effects. Studies of methylphenidate treatment in those with mild IDD and ADHD show significant improvement in the ability to maintain attention and to stay focused on tasks. Methylphenidate treatment studies have not shown evidence of long-term improvement in social skills or learning.

In addition to stimulants and antipsychotics, clonidine has been used clinically in this population, especially to ameliorate hyperactivity and impulsivity. Although there are scant data, clinical ratings by parents and clinicians suggest its efficacy. Atomoxetine may also help for this population.

DEPRESSIVE DISORDERS. The identification of depressive disorders, including disruptive mood dysregulation disorder, among individuals with intellectual disabilities requires careful evaluation since they are easy to miss when aggressive behaviors are prominent. There have been anecdotal reports of disinhibition in response to

SSRIs in intellectually disabled individuals with ASD. Given the relative safety of SSRI antidepressants, it is reasonable to try them when a child with an intellectual disability is depressed.

STEREOTYPICAL MOTOR MOVEMENTS. Antipsychotic medications are used in the treatment of repetitive self-stimulatory behaviors in children with intellectual disability when these behaviors are either harmful to the child or disruptive. Anecdotal reports indicate that these agents may diminish self-stimulatory behaviors; however, there is no improvement seen in adaptive behavior. Obsessive-compulsive symptoms often overlap with the repetitive stereotypical behaviors seen in children and adolescents with intellectual disability, particularly in those with comorbid ASD. SSRIs such as fluoxetine, fluvoxamine, paroxetine, and sertraline have efficacy for treating obsessive-compulsive symptoms in children and adolescents. There are no FDA-approved medications for stereotyped movement disorders, and although SSRI medications are theorized to be helpful for stereotyped motor movements, behavioral interventions remain the first line of treatment for these symptoms.

INTERMITTENT EXPLOSIVE DISORDER. Antipsychotic medications are used for the treatment of intermittent explosive disorder when the behaviors are severe enough to cause potential harm to the child or others. As with the treatment of aggression, there is a need for more data investigating this use. β-Adrenergic receptor antagonists (β-blockers), such as propranolol, have been anecdotally reported to result in fewer explosive rages in some children with intellectual disability and ASD.

Services and Support for Children with Intellectual Disability

Early Intervention. Early intervention programs serve individuals for the first 3 years of life. Such services are generally provided by the state and begin with a specialist visiting the home for several hours per week. Since the passage of Public Law 99–457, the Education of the Handicapped Amendments of 1986, the emphasis is on early intervention services for the entire family. Agencies are required to develop an Individualized Family Service Plan (IFSP) for each family, which identifies specific interventions to best help the family and child.

School. From ages 3 to 21 years, school is responsible by law to provide appropriate educational services to children and adolescents with intellectual disability in the United States. Two laws codified these mandates, Public Law 94–142, the Education for all Handicapped Children Act of 1975, and the IDEA of 1990. Through these laws, public schools must develop and provide an individualized educational program for each student with intellectual disability, determined at a meeting designated as the Individualized Education Plan (IEP) with school personnel and the family. Schools should educate the children in the "least restrictive environment" that will allow the child to learn.

Supports. A wide variety of organized groups and services are available for children with IDD and their families. These include short-term respite care, which allows families a break and is generally set up by state agencies. Other programs include the Special Olympics, which allows children with intellectual disabilities to participate in team sports and sports competitions. Many organizations also exist for families who wish to connect with others who have children with intellectual disabilities.

EPIDEMIOLOGY

The prevalence of intellectual disability at any one time is estimated to range from 1% to 3% of the population in Western societies. The incidence of intellectual disability is difficult to calculate because mild disabilities may be unrecognized until middle childhood. In some cases, even when the intellectual function is limited, adaptive social skills may not be challenged until late childhood or early adolescence. The highest incidence of intellectual disability is reported in school-age children, with a peak at ages 10 to 14 years. Intellectual disability is about 1.5 times more common among males than females.

Prevalence

Epidemiologic surveys indicate that up to two-thirds of children and adults with intellectual disabilities have comorbid psychiatric disorders, and this rate is several times higher than that in community samples without intellectual disability. The prevalence of psychopathology appears to correlate with the severity of the intellectual disability; the more severe the intellectual disability, the higher the risk for coexisting psychiatric disorders. An epidemiologic study found that 40.7% of intellectually disabled children between 4 and 18 years of age met the criteria for at least one additional psychiatric disorder.

The severity of intellectual disability influences the risk of particular comorbid psychiatric disorders. Disruptive and conduct-disorder behaviors occur more frequently in those diagnosed with mild intellectual disability. In contrast, those with more severe intellectual disabilities are more likely to meet criteria for ASD and exhibit symptoms such as self-stimulation and self-mutilation. Comorbidity of psychiatric disorders with intellectual disability in children do not appear to correlate with age or gender.

Psychiatric disorders among persons with intellectual disabilities vary and include mood disorders, schizophrenia, ADHD, and conduct disorder. Children diagnosed with severe intellectual disabilities have an unusually high rate of comorbid ASD. Approximately 2% to 3%

of those with an intellectual disability meet diagnostic criteria for schizophrenia, which is several times higher than the rate for the general population. Up to 50% of children and adults with intellectual disabilities meet the criteria for a mood disorder as measured on an appropriate depression scale. However, a limitation of these studies is that these instruments are not standardized within intellectual disability populations. Frequent psychiatric symptoms that occur in children with intellectual disability, outside the context of a full psychiatric disorder, include hyperactivity and short attention span, self-injurious behaviors (e.g., head-banging and self-biting), and repetitive stereotypical behaviors (hand-flapping and toe-walking). In children and adults with milder forms of intellectual disability, negative self-image, low self-esteem, poor frustration tolerance, interpersonal dependence, and a rigid problem-solving style are frequent.

ETIOLOGY

Etiologic factors in IDD can be genetic, developmental, environmental, or a combination. Genetic causes include chromosomal and inherited conditions; developmental and environmental factors include prenatal exposure to infections and toxins; and environmental or acquired factors include prenatal trauma (e.g., prematurity) and sociocultural factors. The severity of intellectual disability may relate to the timing and duration of a given trauma as well as to the degree of exposure to the central nervous system (CNS). In about three-fourths of persons diagnosed with severe intellectual disability there is an identifiable cause, whereas the etiology is apparent in only about half of those diagnosed with mild intellectual disability. No cause is known for three-fourths of persons with intellectual disability with an IQ between 70 and 80 and variable adaptive functioning. Among chromosomal disorders, Down syndrome and fragile X syndrome are the most common disorders that usually produce at least moderate intellectual disability. A prototype of a metabolic disorder associated with an intellectual disability is PKU. Deprivation of nutrition, nurturance, and social stimulation can potentially contribute to the development of at least mild forms of intellectual disability. Current knowledge suggests that genetic, environmental, biologic, and psychosocial factors work additively to the emergence of intellectual disability.

Genetic Etiologic Factors in Intellectual Disability

Single-Gene Causes. One of the most well-known single-gene causes of intellectual disability is fragile X syndrome, a mutation of the *FMR1* gene. It is the most common and first X-linked gene to be identified as a direct cause of intellectual disability. Abnormalities in autosomal chromosomes are frequently associated with intellectual disability. In contrast, aberrations in sex chromosomes can result in characteristic physical syndromes that do not include intellectual disability (e.g., Turner syndrome with XO and Klinefelter syndrome with XXY, XXXY, and XXYY variations). Some children with Turner syndrome have average to superior intelligence. An agreement exists on a few predisposing factors for chromosomal disorders—among them, advanced maternal age, increased age of the father, and x-ray radiation.

Visible and Submicroscopic Chromosomal Causes of Intellectual Disability. Trisomy 21 (Down syndrome) is a prototype of a cytogenetically visible abnormality that accounts for about two-thirds of the 15% of intellectual disability attributable to visible abnormal cytogenetics. Other microscopically visible chromosomal abnormalities associated with intellectual disability include deletions, translocations, and supernumerary marker chromosomes. Typically, microscopic chromosome analysis can identify abnormalities of 5 to 10 million base pairs or higher.

Submicroscopic identification requires the use of microarrays that can identify losses of chromosomal segments too small to be picked up by light microscopy. The altered copy number variants (CNVs) in submicroscopic segments of the chromosome are associated with up to 13% to 20% of cases of intellectual disability. That is, the genes associated with a particular developmental abnormality are in the critical regions of the pathogenic CNVs.

Genetic Intellectual Disability and Behavioral Phenotype

Specific and predictable behaviors are associated with certain genetically based cases of intellectual disability. These behavioral phenotypes are a syndrome of observable behaviors that occur with a significantly higher probability than expected among those individuals with a specific genetic abnormality.

Examples of behavioral phenotypes occur in genetically determined syndromes such as fragile X syndrome, Prader–Willi syndrome, and Down syndrome, in which we can expect specific behavioral manifestations. Persons with fragile X syndrome have incredibly high rates (up to three-fourths of those studied) of ADHD. High rates of aberrant interpersonal behavior and language function often meet the criteria for autistic disorder and avoidant personality disorder. Prader–Willi syndrome is almost always associated with compulsive eating disturbances, hyperphagia, and obesity. Socialization is an area of weakness, especially in coping skills. Externalizing behavior problems—such as temper tantrums, irritability, and arguing—seem to be heightened in adolescence.

Down Syndrome. The etiology of Down syndrome, known to be caused by an extra copy of the entire chromosome 21, makes it one of the more complicated disorders. The original description of Down syndrome, first made by the English physician Langdon Down in 1866, was based on physical characteristics associated with subnormal mental functioning. Since then, Down syndrome has been the most investigated and most discussed syndrome in intellectual disability. Recent data have suggested that Down syndrome may be more amenable to postnatal interventions to address the cognitive deficits that it produces than was previously thought. Although still in the early stages of animal research, data from experiments with one mouse model, the Ts65Dn, indicate that pharmacologic interventions may influence learning and memory deficits known to occur in Down syndrome.

Phenotypically, children with Down syndrome have characteristic physical attributes, including slanted eyes, epicanthal folds, and a flat nose. Figure 3-1 illustrates the typical features.

There are three types of chromosomal aberrations in Down syndrome, which complicate the diagnosis. They are:

1. Patients with trisomy 21 (three chromosomes 21, instead of the usual two) represent the overwhelming majority; they have 47 chromosomes, with an extra chromosome 21. The mothers' karyotypes are normal. A nondisjunction during meiosis, occurring for unknown reasons, is held responsible for the disorder.
2. Nondisjunction occurring after fertilization in any cell division results in mosaicism, a condition in which there are both normal and trisomic cells in various tissues.
3. In translocation, a fusion occurs of two chromosomes, usually 21 and 15, resulting in a total of 46 chromosomes, despite the presence of an extra chromosome 21. The disorder, unlike trisomy 21, is usually inherited, and the translocated chromosome may occur in unaffected parents and siblings. The asymptomatic carriers have only 45 chromosomes.

Approximately 6,000 babies are affected with Down syndrome in the United States annually, which makes the incidence of Down syndrome 1 in every 700 births, or 15 per 10,000 live births. For women older than 32 years of age, the risk of having a child with Down syndrome (trisomy 21) is about 1 in 100 births. The risk is 1 in 400 at age 35, and about 1 in 100 at age 40. Most children with Down syndrome are mildly to moderately intellectually disabled, with a minority having an IQ above 50. Cognitive development appears to progress normally from birth to 6 months of age; IQ scores gradually decrease from near normal at 1 year of age to about 30 to 50 as development proceeds. The decline in intellectual function may not be readily apparent. Infant tests may not reveal the full extent of the deficits. According to anecdotal clinical reports, children with Down syndrome are typically placid, cheerful, and cooperative and adapt quickly at home. With adolescence, the picture changes: youth with Down syndrome may experience more social and emotional difficulties and behavior disorders, and there is an increased risk for psychotic disorders.

In Down syndrome, language function is a relative weakness, whereas sociability and social skills, such as interpersonal cooperation and conformity with social conventions, are relative strengths. Children with Down syndrome typically manifest deficits in scanning the environment; they are more likely to focus on a single stimulus, leading to difficulty noticing environmental changes. A variety of comorbid psychiatric disorders emerge in persons with Down syndrome; however, the rates appear to be lower than in children with intellectual disability and ASD.

The diagnosis of Down syndrome is relatively simple in an older child, but it is often tricky in newborn infants. The most important signs in a newborn include general hypotonia; oblique palpebral fissures; abundant

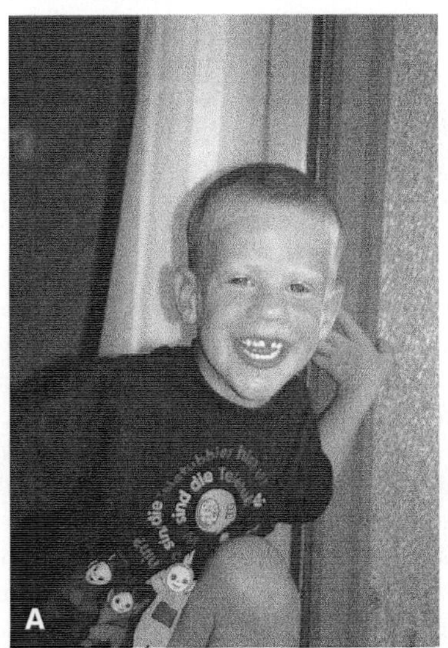

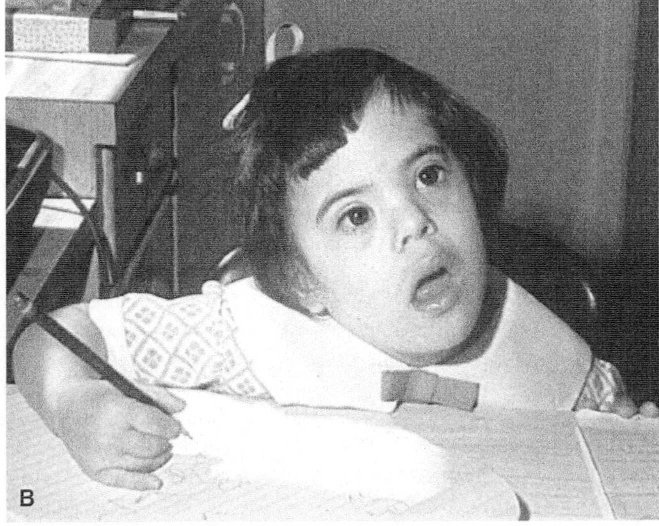

FIGURE 3-1. **A:** Down Syndrome. (Bryke CR, Raca G. Genetic and developmental disorders. In: Strayer DS, Saffitz JE, Rubin E, eds. *Rubin's Pathology*. 8th ed. Wolters Kluwer; 2020:247–323.) **B:** Fragile X Syndrome. (Schaaf CP, Zschocke J, Potocki L. *Human Genetics: From Molecules to Medicine*. Lippincott Williams & Wilkins; 2012.)

neck skin; a small, flattened skull; high cheekbones; and a protruding tongue. The hands are broad and thick, with a single palmar transversal crease, and the little fingers are short and curved inward. Moro reflex is weak or absent. More than 100 signs or stigmata may occur in Down syndrome, but rarely all in one person. Commonly occurring physical problems in Down syndrome include cardiac defects, thyroid abnormalities, and gastrointestinal problems. Life expectancy was once drastically limited to about the age of 40. However, it is now significantly increased, although still shorter than those without intellectual disability.

Down syndrome includes deterioration in language, memory, self-care skills, and problem solving by the third decade of life. Postmortem studies of individuals with Down syndrome older than age 40 have shown a high incidence of senile plaques and neurofibrillary tangles, similar to those seen in Alzheimer disease. Neurofibrillary tangles are known to occur in a variety of degenerative diseases, whereas senile plaques seem to be found most often in Alzheimer disease and Down syndrome.

Fragile X Syndrome. Fragile X syndrome is the second most common single cause of intellectual disability. The syndrome results from a mutation on the X chromosome at what is known as the fragile site (Xq27.3). The fragile site occurs in only some cells, and it may be absent in asymptomatic males and female carriers. Much variability is present in both genetic and phenotypic expression. Fragile X syndrome occurs in about 1 in every 1,000 males and 1 in every 2,000 females. The typical phenotype includes a large, long head and ears, short stature, hyperextensible joints, and postpubertal macro-orchidism (see Fig. 3-1). Associated intellectual disability ranges from mild to severe. The behavioral profile of persons with the syndrome includes a high rate of ADHD, learning disorders, and ASD. Deficits in language function include rapid perseverative speech with abnormalities in combining words into phrases and sentences. Persons with Fragile X syndrome seem to have relatively strong skills in communication and socialization; their intellectual functions seem to decline in the pubertal period. Often, female carriers are less impaired than males with Fragile X syndrome, but females can also manifest the typical physical characteristics and may have a mild intellectual disability.

Prader–Willi Syndrome. Prader–Willi syndrome likely results from a small deletion involving chromosome 15, occurring sporadically. Its prevalence is less than 1 in 10,000. Persons with the syndrome exhibit compulsive eating behavior and often obesity, intellectual disability, hypogonadism, small stature, hypotonia, and small hands and feet.

Cat's Cry (Cri-du-Chat) Syndrome. Children with cat's cry syndrome have a deletion in chromosome 5. They are typically severely intellectually disabled and show many signs often associated with chromosomal aberrations, such as microcephaly, low-set ears, oblique palpebral fissures, hypertelorism, and micrognathia. The characteristic cat-like cry that gave the syndrome its name is caused by laryngeal abnormalities that gradually change and disappear with increasing age.

Phenylketonuria. Ivar Asbjörn Fölling first described PKU in 1934 as an inborn error of metabolism. PKU is transmitted as a recessive autosomal mendelian trait and occurs in about 1 of every 10,000 to 15,000 live births. For parents who have already had a child with PKU, the chance of having another child with PKU is 20% to 25% of successive pregnancies. PKU is reported predominantly in persons of North European origin; a few cases may occur in African Americans, Yemenite Jews, and Asians. The underlying metabolic defect in PKU is an inability to convert phenylalanine, an essential amino acid, to paratyrosine because of the absence or inactivity of the liver enzyme phenylalanine hydroxylase, which catalyzes the conversion. Therefore, PKU is mostly preventable with a screening for it, which, if positive, should be followed with a low phenylalanine diet. Other types of hyperphenylalaninemia exist but are rare and often fatal.

Most patients with PKU are severely intellectually disabled, but some have borderline or average intelligence. Eczema, vomiting, and convulsions occur in about one-third of all patients. Although the clinical picture varies, typically, children with PKU are reported to be hyperactive and irritable. They frequently exhibit temper tantrums and often display bizarre movements of their bodies and upper extremities, including twisting hand mannerisms. Verbal and nonverbal communication is commonly severely impaired or nonexistent. The child has reduced coordination, and they have many perceptual difficulties.

Currently, the Guthrie inhibition assay is a widely applied screening test using a bacteriologic procedure to detect phenylalanine in the blood. In the United States, screening newborn infants for PKU is routine. Early diagnosis is essential because a low-phenylalanine diet, in use since 1955, significantly improves both behavior and developmental progress. The best results seem to be obtained with early diagnosis, and the start of dietary treatment before the child is 6 months of age. Dietary treatment, however, is not without risk. Phenylalanine is an essential amino acid, and its omission from the diet can lead to severe complications such as anemia, hypoglycemia, or edema. The dietary treatment of PKU continues indefinitely. Children who receive a diagnosis before the age of 3 months and have an optimal dietary regimen may have average intelligence. A low-phenylalanine diet does not reverse intellectual disability in untreated older children and adolescents with PKU, but the diet does decrease irritability and abnormal EEG changes and does increase social responsiveness and attention span. The parents of children with PKU and some of the children's unaffected siblings are heterozygous carriers.

Rett Syndrome. Rett syndrome, a form of ASD not included in the DSM-5-TR, is believed to be caused by a dominant X-linked gene. It is degenerative and affects only females. In 1966, Andreas Rett reported on 22 girls with a severe progressive neurologic disability. Deterioration in communications skills, motor behavior, and social functioning starts at about 1 year of age. Symptoms include ataxia, facial grimacing, teeth-grinding, and loss of speech. Intermittent hyperventilation and a disorganized breathing pattern are characteristic while the child is awake. Stereotypical hand movements, including hand-wringing, are typical. Progressive gait disturbance, scoliosis, and seizures occur. Severe spasticity is usually present in middle childhood. Cerebral atrophy occurs with decreased pigmentation of the substantia nigra, which suggests abnormalities of the dopaminergic nigrostriatal system.

Associated features include seizures in up to 75% of affected children and disorganized EEG findings with some epileptiform discharges in almost all young children with Rett syndrome, even in the absence of clinical seizures. An additional associated feature is irregular respiration, with episodes of hyperventilation, apnea, and breath-holding. Disorganized breathing occurs in most patients while they are awake; during sleep, the breathing usually normalizes. Many patients with Rett syndrome also have scoliosis. As the disorder progresses, muscle tone seems to change from an initial hypotonic condition to spasticity to rigidity.

Although children with Rett syndrome may live for well over a decade after the onset of the disorder, after 10 years, many patients are wheelchair-bound, with muscle wasting, rigidity, and virtually no language ability. Long-term receptive and expressive communication and socialization abilities remain at a developmental level of less than 1 year.

Lena was born as a full-term and healthy baby after an uncomplicated pregnancy. A chorionic villus sampling (CVS) was obtained because of her mother's age of 41 years, and the findings were normal. At birth, Lena received good Apgar scores, and her weight, height, and head circumference were all near the 50th percentile. Lena's development during the first months of life was unremarkable. At approximately 8 months of age, Lena's development seemed to slow down, and her interest in engaging with her parents and others seemed to decline. Lena's developmental milestones did not progress and then became markedly delayed. Lena was just starting to walk on her second birthday and had no words. Evaluation at that time revealed that head growth had decelerated. Lena began to display self-stimulatory behaviors, and in addition, marked cognitive and communicative delays were noted on formal testing. Lena began to have seizures, and EEG revealed that she had epileptiform discharges even when she was not having a clinical seizure. Lena began to lose purposeful hand movements and developed unusual stereotypical hand-washing behaviors. By age 6, Lena's abnormal hand movements were prominent. Subsequently, Lena developed truncal ataxia and breath-holding spells, and her motor skills further deteriorated. A diagnosis of Rett syndrome was made. (Adapted from Fred Volkmar, M.D.)

Neurofibromatosis. Also called *von Recklinghausen* disease, neurofibromatosis is the most common of the neurocutaneous syndromes caused by a single dominant gene, which may be inherited or occur as a new mutation. The disorder occurs in about 1 of 5,000 births and is characterized by café-au-lait spots on the skin and by neurofibromas, including optic gliomas and acoustic neuromas, caused by abnormal cell migration. Mild intellectual disability occurs in up to one-third of those with the disease.

Tuberous Sclerosis. Tuberous sclerosis is the second most common of the neurocutaneous syndromes; a progressive intellectual disability occurs in up to two-thirds of all affected persons. It occurs in about 1 of 15,000 persons who inherit it through autosomal dominant transmission. Seizures are present in all those with intellectual disability and in two-thirds of those without. Infantile spasms may occur as early as 6 months of age. The phenotypic presentation includes adenoma sebaceum and ash-leaf spots, identifiable with a slit lamp.

Childhood Disintegrative Disorder. The previous diagnosis of childhood disintegrative disorder, now included in ASD, is characterized by marked regression in several areas of functioning after at least 2 years of apparently normal development. Childhood disintegrative disorder, also called *Heller syndrome* and *disintegrative psychosis,* was described in 1908 as a deterioration over several months of intellectual, social, and language function occurring in 3- and 4-year-olds with previously normal function. After the deterioration, the children closely resembled children with autistic disorder.

Tim's neonatal and early development was typical. By age 2 years, Tim had developed language and could speak in short sentences, and his development appeared to be proceeding typically. At 3½ years of age, Tim suddenly regressed, and his parents thought it was a transient reaction to the birth of his younger sister. Tim's regressed development persisted, however, and he lost much of his language skills and stopped using the bathroom as he had been previously trained to do. Tim became more withdrawn and less interested in social interaction, exhibiting various self-stimulatory behaviors such as waving his hand repeatedly. A comprehensive pediatric examination and workup did not reveal the onset of medical illness that might account for this developmental regression. Behaviorally, Tim exhibited features of ASD. At follow-up at age 12, he spoke only an occasional single word and had severe intellectual disability. Tim was then diagnosed with childhood disintegrative disorder, a form of ASD. (Adapted from Fred Volkmar, M.D.)

Lesch–Nyhan Syndrome. Lesch–Nyhan syndrome is a rare disorder caused by a deficiency of an enzyme involved in purine metabolism. The disorder is X-linked; patients have intellectual disability, microcephaly, seizures, choreoathetosis, and spasticity. The syndrome is also associated with severe compulsive self-mutilation by biting the mouth and fingers. Lesch–Nyhan syndrome is another example of a genetically determined syndrome with a specific, predictable behavioral pattern.

Adrenoleukodystrophy. The most common of several disorders of sudanophilic cerebral sclerosis, adrenoleukodystrophy is characterized by diffuse demyelination of the cerebral white matter resulting in visual and intellectual impairment, seizures, spasticity, and progression to death. Adrenocortical insufficiency accompanies cerebral degeneration. A sex-linked gene located on the distal end of the long arm of the X chromosome transmits the disorder. The clinical onset is generally between 5 and 8 years of age, with early seizures, disturbances in gait, and mild intellectual impairment. Abnormal pigmentation reflecting adrenal insufficiency sometimes precedes the neurologic symptoms, and attacks of crying are frequent. Spastic contractures, ataxia, and swallowing disturbances are also frequent. Although the course is often rapidly progressive, some patients may have a relapsing and remitting course.

Maple Syrup Urine Disease. The clinical symptoms of maple syrup urine disease appear during the first week of life. The infant deteriorates rapidly and has decerebrate rigidity, seizures, respiratory irregularity, and hypoglycemia. If untreated, maple syrup urine disease is usually fatal in the first months of life, and the survivors have a severe intellectual disability. Some variants have transient ataxia and only mild intellectual disability. Treatment follows the general principles established for PKU and consists of a diet deficient in the three involved amino acids—leucine, isoleucine, and valine.

Other Enzyme Deficiency Disorders. We have identified several enzyme deficiency disorders associated with intellectual disability and are adding more as discoveries are made, including Hartnup disease, galactosemia, and glycogen storage disease. Table 3-5 lists 30 significant disorders with inborn errors of metabolism, hereditary transmission patterns, defective enzymes, clinical signs, and relation to intellectual disability.

Acquired and Developmental Factors

Prenatal Period. Essential prerequisites for the overall development of the fetus include the mother's physical, psychological, and nutritional health during pregnancy. Many illnesses and conditions can affect fetal brain development, including uncontrolled diabetes, anemia, emphysema, hypertension, and long-term use of alcohol and narcotic substances. Maternal infections during pregnancy, especially viral infections, have been known to cause fetal damage and intellectual disability. The extent of fetal damage depends on several factors. These factors include the type and severity of the viral infection and the gestational age of the fetus.

Rubella (German Measles). Rubella has replaced syphilis as the primary cause of congenital malformations and intellectual disability caused by maternal infection. The children of affected mothers may show several abnormalities, including congenital heart disease, intellectual disability, cataracts, deafness, microcephaly, and microphthalmia. Timing is crucial because the extent and frequency of the complications are inversely related to the duration of the pregnancy at the time of maternal infection. When mothers become infected in the first trimester of pregnancy, 10% to 15% of the children are affected. This incidence rises to almost 50% when the infection occurs in the first month of pregnancy. Undetected subclinical forms of maternal infection can complicate the situation. Immunization can prevent maternal rubella.

Cytomegalic Inclusion Disease. In many cases, cytomegalic inclusion disease remains dormant in the mother. Some children are stillborn, and others have jaundice, microcephaly, hepatosplenomegaly, and radiographic findings of intracerebral calcification. Children with intellectual disability from the disease frequently have cerebral calcification, microcephaly, or hydrocephalus. Positive findings of the virus in throat and urine cultures and the recovery of inclusion-bearing cells in the urine all can confirm the diagnosis.

Syphilis. Syphilis in pregnant women was once the leading cause of various neuropathologic changes in their offspring, including intellectual disability. Today, the incidence of syphilitic complications of pregnancy fluctuates with the incidence of syphilis in the general population. Some recent alarming statistics from several major cities in the United States indicate that there is still no room for complacency.

Toxoplasmosis. The mother can transmit toxoplasmosis to the fetus. It causes mild or severe intellectual disability and, in severe cases, hydrocephalus, seizures, microcephaly, and chorioretinitis.

Herpes Simplex. The herpes simplex virus can be transmitted transplacentally, although the most common mode of infection is during birth. Microcephaly, intellectual disability, intracranial calcification, and ocular abnormalities may result.

Human Immunodeficiency Virus. Cognitive impairments are well known to be associated with the transmission of human immunodeficiency virus (HIV) from mothers to their babies. HIV may have both direct and indirect influences on the developing brain. A subset of infants born infected with HIV may develop progressive encephalopathy, intellectual disabilities, and seizures within the first year of life. Fortunately, over the last two decades, there has been a dramatic decrease in perinatal HIV transmission due to a combination of antiviral agents provided to mothers during pregnancy and delivery, obstetric interventions that reduce risk, and administration of zidovudine (ZDV) as prophylaxis for

Table 3-5. Inborn Errors of Metabolism

Category	Gene/Disease	Prevalence	Inheritance Pattern	Cognitive Symptoms	Other Symptoms or Complications	Treatment
Disorders of Amino Acid Metabolism	**PAH** (Phenylketonuria)	1 in 10,000	Autosomal recessive	Intellectual disability and behavioral problems if untreated. Early dietary management can prevent impairment	Seizures, eczema	Phenylalanine-restricted diet, sapropterin (BH4), pegvaliase for adults
	CBS (Homocystinuria)	1 in 200,000	Autosomal recessive	Cognitive impairment	Thrombosis, lens dislocation, skeletal abnormalities, marfanoid features	Methionine-restricted diet, pyridoxine (vitamin B6), betaine, folate, vitamin B12
	BCKDHA (Maple syrup urine disease) (also could be caused by **BCKDHB**, **DBT**, or **DLD** genes)	1 in 185,000	Autosomal recessive	Intellectual disability	Metabolic crisis, encephalopathy	Dietary restriction of branched-chain amino acids, thiamine supplementation in thiamine-responsive cases
	FAH (Tyrosinemia type I)	Rare	Autosomal recessive	Cognitive impairment	Liver failure, renal dysfunction, risk of hepatocellular carcinoma if not treated	Nitisinone (NTBC), tyrosine and phenylalanine-restricted diet, liver transplantation in severe cases
Disorders of Carbohydrate Metabolism	**GALT** (Galactosemia)	1 in 60,000	Autosomal recessive	Intellectual disability	Liver dysfunction, cataracts, ovarian failure	Galactose-restricted diet, calcium supplementation
	GALK (Galactokinase deficiency)	Rare	Autosomal recessive	Usually normal cognition	Cataracts	Lactose/galactose-restricted diet
	GALE (UDP galactose epimerase deficiency)	Rare	Autosomal recessive	Variable cognitive impairment depending on severity of the disease	Liver dysfunction	Galactose restriction (severity-dependent)
	ALDOB (Hereditary fructose intolerance)	Rare	Autosomal recessive	Cognitive impairment	Hypoglycemia, liver dysfunction	Fructose, sucrose, and sorbitol restriction
	GAA (Glycogen storage disease type II, Pompe disease)	1 in 40,000	Autosomal recessive	Variable developmental delay, mainly in infantile-onset. Adult-onset usually benign	Hypotonia, cardiomyopathy in infantile form	Enzyme replacement therapy with alglucosidase alfa, supportive care
	G6PC (Glycogen storage disease type I)	1 in 100,000	Autosomal recessive	Cognitive impairment	Hypoglycemia, hepatomegaly	Continuous cornstarch therapy, frequent feedings, uncooked cornstarch
	PYGM (Glycogen storage disease type V, McArdle disease)	Rare	Autosomal recessive	Usually normal cognition	Muscle pain, exercise intolerance	Glucose before exercise, moderate aerobic conditioning

(continued)

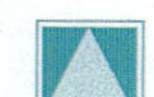

Table 3-5.
Inborn Errors of Metabolism (Continued)

Category	Gene/Disease	Prevalence	Inheritance Pattern	Cognitive Symptoms	Other Symptoms or Complications	Treatment
Disorders of Fatty Acid Metabolism	**ACADM** (Medium-chain acyl-CoA dehydrogenase deficiency)	1 in 15,000	Autosomal recessive	Usually normal, metabolic crises may affect development	Hypoglycemia, liver dysfunction	Avoidance of fasting, medium-chain triglyceride (MCT) oil, L-carnitine supplementation
	ACADVL (Very long–chain acyl-CoA dehydrogenase deficiency)	1 in 42,500 to 120,000	Autosomal recessive	Cognitive impairment	Cardiomyopathy, liver dysfunction	Avoidance of fasting, MCT oil, low-fat/high-carbohydrate diet
	HADHA (Long-chain 3-hydroxyacyl-CoA dehydrogenase deficiency)	1 in 110,000	Autosomal recessive	Cognitive impairment	Retinopathy, peripheral neuropathy	MCT oil, low-fat/high-carbohydrate diet, avoidance of fasting
	HADHA, HADHB (Trifunctional protein deficiency)	Rare	Autosomal recessive	Cognitive impairment	Retinopathy, peripheral neuropathy	MCT oil, low-fat/high-carbohydrate diet, avoidance of fasting
	SLC22A5 (Carnitine transporter deficiency)	1 in 20,000 to 120,000	Autosomal recessive	Cognitive impairment	Low total and free carnitine levels	L-carnitine supplementation
	SLC25A20 (Carnitine-acylcarnitine translocase deficiency)	Rare	Autosomal recessive	Cognitive impairment	Elevated C16–, C16:1–, C18, C18:1–acylcarnitines	Avoidance of fasting, low-fat/high-carbohydrate diet, MCT oil
	CPT1A (Carnitine palmitoyltransferase 1A deficiency)	1 in 500,000	Autosomal recessive	Variable cognitive impairment (Arctic variant often benign). Repeated untreated episodes can cause permanent brain damage	Hypoketotic hypoglycemia, hepatic encephalopathy, liver failure	Avoidance of fasting, high-carbohydrate diet, MCT supplementation
	CPT2 (Carnitine palmitoyltransferase 2 deficiency)	Rare	Autosomal recessive	Cognitive impairment	Recurrent rhabdomyolysis, muscle pain, myoglobinuria (in adult form)	Avoidance of fasting, carbohydrate loading before exercise, MCT supplement
Disorders of Purine and Pyrimidine Metabolism	**HPRT1** (Lesch–Nyhan syndrome)	1 in 380,000	X-linked recessive	Severe intellectual disability	Self-mutilation, kidney stones	Allopurinol, behavioral management, physical restraints
	ADA (Adenosine deaminase deficiency)	Rare	Autosomal recessive	Cognitive impairment	Severe combined immunodeficiency	Enzyme replacement therapy, hematopoietic stem cell transplantation, gene therapy
Urea Cycle Disorders	**OTC** (Ornithine transcarbamylase deficiency)	1 in 80,000	X-linked	Confusion, lethargy during hyperammonemia episodes	Hyperammonemia, vomiting. Female presentation more variable.	Protein restriction, ammonia scavengers (sodium benzoate, sodium phenylbutyrate), arginine supplementation
	ASS1 (Citrullinemia type I)	1 in 57,000	Autosomal recessive	Cognitive impairment	Hyperammonemia, liver dysfunction	Protein restriction, ammonia scavengers, arginine supplementation

Lysosomal Storage Disorders	**GLA** (Fabry disease)	1 in 40,000 males	X-linked	Cognitive impairment, depression	Pain, kidney failure, heart disease. Female presentation more variable due to X-inactivation patterns	Enzyme replacement therapy (agalsidase), chaperone therapy (migalastat)
	GBA (Gaucher disease)	1 in 40,000	Autosomal recessive	Mild cognitive impairment in type I, other types more severe	Enlarged liver and spleen, bone pain	Enzyme replacement therapy, substrate reduction therapy
	IDUA (MPS I—Hurler, Hurler–Scheie, Scheie)	1 in 100,000	Autosomal recessive	Cognitive impairment if not treated	Hepatosplenomegaly, skeletal abnormalities	Enzyme replacement therapy, hematopoietic stem cell transplantation
	IDS (MPS II—Hunter)	1 in 100,000 males	X-linked	Cognitive impairment if not treated	Hepatosplenomegaly, skeletal abnormalities	Enzyme replacement therapy (idursulfase)
	SGSH (MPS III—Sanfilippo)	Rare	Autosomal recessive	Cognitive impairment	Behavioral problems, sleep disturbances	Supportive care, clinical trials for enzyme replacement therapy
	GALNS (MPS IV—Morquio)	Rare	Autosomal recessive	Usually normal cognition	Skeletal abnormalities, corneal clouding	Enzyme replacement therapy (elosulfase alfa)
	ARSB (MPS VI—Maroteaux-Lamy)	Rare	Autosomal recessive	Usually normal cognition	Skeletal abnormalities, corneal clouding	Enzyme replacement therapy (galsulfase)
	GUSB (MPS VII—Sly)	Rare	Autosomal recessive	Variable cognitive impairment	Hepatosplenomegaly, skeletal abnormalities	Enzyme replacement therapy (vestronidase alfa)
	HYAL1 (MPS IX—Natowicz)	Rare	Autosomal recessive	Cognitive impairment	Skeletal abnormalities, joint stiffness	Supportive care
	HEXA (GM2 gangliosidosis type I—Tay–Sachs)	1 in 360,000	Autosomal recessive	Severe intellectual disability in classic infantile form. Juvenile and adult-onset forms less severe.	Progressive neurodegeneration	Supportive care, substrate reduction therapy in trials
	HEXB (GM2 gangliosidosis type II—Sandhoff)	Rare	Autosomal recessive	Severe intellectual disability	Progressive neurodegeneration	Supportive care, substrate reduction therapy in trials
	GLB1 (GM1 gangliosidosis)	Rare	Autosomal recessive	Severe intellectual disability	Hepatosplenomegaly, skeletal abnormalities, progressive neurodegeneration (particularly infantile form)	Supportive care
	GALC (Krabbe disease)	1 in 100,000	Autosomal recessive	Severe intellectual disability	Progressive neurodegeneration if not treated	Hematopoietic stem cell transplantation (early intervention)
	ARSA (Metachromatic leukodystrophy)	1 in 40,000	Autosomal recessive	Behavioral changes, Severe intellectual disability	Progressive neurodegeneration, motor regression	Hematopoietic stem cell transplantation (early intervention), gene therapy in trials
Mitochondrial Disorders	**MT-TL1** (MELAS syndrome)	Rare	Mitochondrial (Maternal Inheritance)	Stroke-like episodes, dementia	Muscle weakness, lactic acidosis	L-arginine, coenzyme Q10, dietary modifications, supportive care
	MT-ND1 (Leber hereditary optic neuropathy). Other mitochondrial genes may also cause	Rare	Mitochondrial (Maternal Inheritance).	Vision loss	Cardiac arrhythmias	Idebenone, coenzyme Q10, avoiding triggers

(continued)

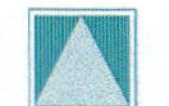

Table 3-5.
Inborn Errors of Metabolism (Continued)

Category	Gene/Disease	Prevalence	Inheritance Pattern	Cognitive Symptoms	Other Symptoms or Complications	Treatment
	PDHA1 (Pyruvate dehydrogenase deficiency)	Rare	X-linked (most cases)	Cognitive impairment	Lactic acidosis, muscle weakness	Ketogenic diet, thiamine supplementation
	SUCLG1 (Mitochondrial DNA depletion syndromes)	Rare	Autosomal recessive	Cognitive impairment	Muscle weakness, liver dysfunction	Supportive care, nutritional supplements
	Multiple genes (Cytochrome C oxidase deficiency [COX], Complex IV deficiency)	Rare	Varies (autosomal/ mitochondrial)	Cognitive impairment	Muscle weakness, liver dysfunction	Coenzyme Q10, riboflavin, supportive care
	TYMP (Mitochondrial neuro-gastrointestinal encephalopathy syndrome—MNGIE)	Rare	Autosomal recessive	Cognitive impairment	Gastrointestinal dysmotility, muscle weakness	Supportive care, allogenic hematopoietic stem cell transplantation
Peroxisomal Disorders	**PEX1** (Zellweger spectrum disorders ranging from classic Zellweger syndrome to milder forms [Refsum disease])	1 in 50,000	Autosomal recessive	Severe intellectual disability	Liver dysfunction, hearing loss, hypotonia, seizures	Supportive care, DHA supplementation, primary bile acid therapy
	AGPS (RCDP type III)	Rare	Autosomal recessive	Severe intellectual disability	Skeletal abnormalities, cataracts	Supportive care
	FAR1 (RCDP type IV)	Rare	Autosomal recessive	Severe intellectual disability	Skeletal abnormalities, cataracts	Supportive care
	ACOX1 (Acyl CoA oxidase 1 deficiency)	Rare	Autosomal recessive	Cognitive impairment	Liver dysfunction, hypotonia	Supportive care
	AMACR (Alpha-methylacyl-CoA racemase deficiency)	Rare	Autosomal recessive	Cognitive impairment	Liver dysfunction, hypotonia	Supportive care
	SCPX (Sterol carrier protein X deficiency)	Rare	Autosomal recessive	Cognitive impairment	Liver dysfunction, hypotonia	Supportive care
	ABCD1 (X-linked adrenoleukodystrophy)	1 in 20,000 males	X-linked	Cognitive decline	Adrenal insufficiency, progressive neurologic deterioration. Phenotypic spectrum includes adrenomyeloneuropathy with later onset and slower progression	Lorenzo's oil, steroid replacement, hematopoietic stem cell transplantation (early intervention)
Disorders of Trace Metal Metabolism	**ATP7B** (Wilson disease)	~1 in 30,000	Autosomal recessive	Cognitive decline, personality changes	Liver dysfunction, tremor, dystonia, Kayser–Fleischer rings	Chelation (penicillamine or trientine), zinc, liver transplant
	ATP7A (Menkes disease)	~1 in 100,000 males	X-linked recessive	Severe intellectual disability	Seizures, kinky hair, failure to thrive, hypotonia	Copper histidine injections (early), supportive care
	CP (Aceruloplasminemia)	Very rare	Autosomal recessive	Dementia, psychiatric symptoms	Diabetes, retinal degeneration, brain and liver iron overload	Iron chelation (e.g., deferox-amine), antioxidants, supportive

6 weeks to newborns exposed to HIV. In the United States, the annual number of HIV infections through perinatal transmission has declined about 40% over the last 5 years and is dramatically less than in the 1990s when the transmission was at its peak. In 2015, the rates were less than 1% in white and Hispanic/Latino HIV-infected mothers. However, that rate is about five times greater in African American mothers with HIV. Vertical transmission of HIV from mother to child around the world, especially in Africa, is also considerable.

Fetal Alcohol Syndrome. Fetal alcohol syndrome (FAS) results from prenatal alcohol exposure and can lead to a wide range of problems in the newborn. According to the Centers for Disease Control and Prevention, FAS in the United States occurs at a rate ranging from 0.2 to 1.5 per 1,000 live births. FAS is one of the leading preventable causes of intellectual disability and physical disabilities. Table 3-6 lists the typical characteristics of FAS (Fig. 3-2).

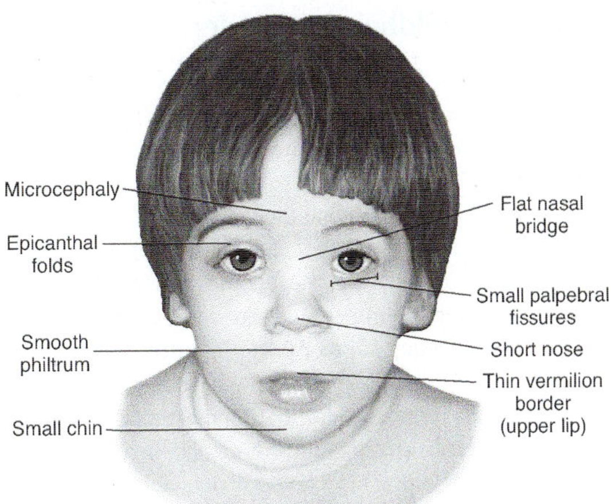

FIGURE 3-2. Physical features of fetal alcohol syndrome. (Stanfill AG. Genetic and congenital disorders. In: Norris TL, ed. *Porth's Essentials of Pathophysiology*. 5th ed. Wolters Kluwer; 2020:75–93.)

Prenatal Drug Exposure. Prenatal exposure to opioids, such as heroin, often results in infants who are small for their gestational age, with head circumference below the 10th percentile and withdrawal symptoms that appear within the first 2 days of life. The withdrawal symptoms of infants include irritability, hypertonia, tremor, vomiting, a high-pitched cry, and an abnormal sleep pattern. Seizures are unusual, but the withdrawal syndrome can be life-threatening to infants if it is untreated. Diazepam, phenobarbital, chlorpromazine, and paregoric have been used to treat neonatal opioid withdrawal. The long-term sequelae of prenatal opioid exposure are not fully known; the children's developmental milestones and intellectual functions may be within the normal range, but they have an increased risk for impulsivity and behavioral problems. Infants prenatally exposed to cocaine are at high risk for low birth weight and premature delivery. In the early neonatal period, they may have transient neurologic and behavioral abnormalities, including abnormal results on EEG studies, tachycardia, poor feeding patterns, irritability, and excessive drowsiness. The physiologic and behavioral abnormalities are from cocaine intoxication, not withdrawal, as cocaine excretion may take up to a week after.

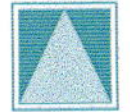

Table 3-6.
Characteristics of Fetal Alcohol Syndrome

Characteristics of Fetal Alcohol Syndrome
Growth retardation of prenatal origin (height, weight)
Facial dysmorphism
Microcephaly (head circumference below the third percentile)
Hypertelorism (large distance between eyes)
Microphthalmia (small eyeballs)
Short palpebral fissures
Inner epicanthal folds
Midface hypoplasia (underdevelopment)
Smooth or short philtrum
Thin upper lip
Short, turned-up nose
Cardiac defects
Central nervous system (CNS) manifestations
Delayed development
Hyperactivity
Attention deficits
Learning disabilities
Intellectual deficits
Seizures

Complications of Pregnancy. Toxemia of pregnancy and uncontrolled maternal diabetes present hazards to the fetus and can potentially result in intellectual disability. Maternal malnutrition during pregnancy often results in prematurity and other obstetrical complications. Vaginal hemorrhage, placenta previa, premature separation of the placenta, and prolapse of the cord can damage the fetal brain by causing anoxia.

Perinatal Period. Some evidence indicates that premature infants and infants with low birth weight are at high risk for neurologic and subtle intellectual impairments that may not be apparent until their school years. Infants who sustain intracranial hemorrhages or show evidence of cerebral ischemia are especially vulnerable to cognitive abnormalities. The degree of neurodevelopmental impairment generally correlates with the severity of the intracranial hemorrhage. Recent studies have documented that, among children with low birth weight (less than 1 kg), 20% had significant disabilities, including cerebral palsy, intellectual disability, autism, and low intelligence with severe learning problems. Very premature children and those who had intrauterine growth retardation were at high risk for developing both social problems and academic difficulties. Socioeconomic deprivation can also affect the adaptive function of these vulnerable infants. Early intervention may improve their cognitive, language, and perceptual abilities.

Acquired Childhood Disorders

Infection. The most severe infections affecting cerebral integrity are encephalitis and meningitis. The universal use of the measles vaccine virtually eliminated measles encephalitis. However, a recent refusal by some individuals and communities to vaccinate their children has increased the risk of this as well as subacute sclerosing panencephalitis, a rare and usually fatal degenerative disease that can occur years after the infection. Antibacterial agents have reduced the incidence of other bacterial infections, at least in the developed world. Viruses now cause most episodes of encephalitis. Sometimes a clinician must retrospectively consider a probable encephalitic component in a previously unknown illness with a high fever. A delayed diagnosis of meningitis, even when followed by antibiotic treatment, can seriously affect a child's cognitive development. Thrombotic and purulent intracranial phenomena secondary to septicemia are rarely seen today except in small infants.

Head Trauma. The best-known causes of head injury in children that produce developmental handicaps, including seizures, are motor vehicle accidents (household accidents are the most common cause of head injuries, such as falls from tables, open windows, and on stairways). Child maltreatment is a frequent cause of head traumas or intracranial trauma such as bleeding due to "shaken baby" syndrome.

Asphyxia. Brain damage due to asphyxia associated with near-drowning is not an uncommon cause of intellectual disability.

Long-Term Exposures. Long-term exposure to lead is a well-established cause of compromised intelligence and learning skills. Intracranial tumors of various types and origins, surgery, and chemotherapy can also adversely affect brain function.

Environmental and Sociocultural Factors

Mild intellectual disability is associated with significant deprivation of nutrition and nurturance. Children who have endured these conditions are at risk for a host of psychiatric disorders, including mood disorders, posttraumatic stress disorder (PTSD), and attentional and anxiety disorders. A prenatal environment compromised by poor medical care and poor maternal nutrition may be contributing factors in the development of mild intellectual disability. Teenage pregnancies are at risk for mild intellectual disability in the baby due to the increased risk of obstetrical complications, prematurity, and low birth weight. Poor postnatal medical care, malnutrition, exposure to toxic substances such as lead, and potential physical trauma are additional risk factors for mild intellectual disabilities. Child neglect and inadequate caretaking may deprive an infant of both physical and emotional nurturance, leading to failure to thrive syndromes.

Further Readings

Aishworiya R, Valica T, Hagerman R, Restrepo B. An update on psychopharmacological treatment of autism spectrum disorder. *Neurotherapeutics*. 2022;19(1):248–262.

Allen J, Molloy E, McDonald D. Severe neurological impairment: a review of the definition. *Dev Med Child Neurol*. 2020;62(3):277–282.

Arnold LE, Farmer C, Kraemer HC, et al. Moderators, mediators, and other predictors of risperidone response in children with autistic disorder and irritability. *J Child Adolesc Psychopharmacol*. 2010;20:83–93.

Beqiraj L, Denne LD, Hastings RP, Paris A. Positive behavioural support for children and young people with developmental disabilities in special education settings: a systematic review. *J Appl Res Intellect Disabil*. 2022;35(3):719–735.

Baio J, Wiggins L, Christensen DL, et al. Prevalence of autism spectrum disorder among children aged 8 years—Autism and Developmental Disabilities Monitoring Network, 11 sites, United States, 2014. *MMWR Surveill Summ*. 2018;67(6):1–23.

Chiurazzi P, Kiani AK, Miertus J, et al. Genetic analysis of intellectual disability and autism. *Acta Biomed*. 2020;91(13-S):e2020003.

Ellison JW, Rosengeld JA, Shaffer LG. Genetic basis of intellectual disability. *Annu Rev Med*. 2013;64:441–450.

Gothelf D, Furfaro JA, Penniman LC, Glover GH, Reiss AL. The contribution of novel brain imaging techniques to understanding the neurobiology of intellectual disability and developmental disabilities. *Ment Retard Dev Disabil Res Rev*. 2005;11:331–339.

Hageman JR, Alcocer Alkureishi L. Developmental disabilities awareness. *Pediatr Ann*. 2023;52(4):e122–e123.

Ismail S, Buckley S, Budacki R, Jabbar A, Gallicano GI. Screening, diagnosing and prevention of fetal alcohol syndrome: is this syndrome treatable? *Dev Neurosci*. 2010;32:91–100.

McConkey R, Samadi SA, Mahmoodizadeh A, Taggart L. The use of psychotropic medication in Iranian children with developmental disabilities. *Int J Environ Res Public Health*. 2021;18(8):4120.

McLaren JL, Lichtenstein JD. The pursuit of the magic pill: the overuse of psychotropic medications in children with intellectual and developmental disabilities in the USA. *Epidemiol Psychiatr Sci*. 2019;28(4):365–368.

Modula MJ, Sumbane GO. Families' experiences on safety needs of children with intellectual disability. *Int J Environ Res Public Health*. 2022;19(22):15246.

Obi O, Braun KVN, Baio J, Drews-Botsch C, Devine O, Yeargin-Allsopp M. Effect of incorporating adaptive functioning scores on the prevalence of intellectual disability. *Am J Intellect Dev Disabil*. 2011;116:360–370.

Olusanya BO, Smythe T, Ogbo FA, Nair MKC, Scher M, Davis AC. Global prevalence of developmental disabilities in children and adolescents: a systematic umbrella review. *Front Public Health*. 2023;11:1122009.

Reyes M, Croonenberghs J, Augustybs I, Eerdekens M. Long-term use of risperidone in children with disruptive behavior disorders and subaverage intelligence: efficacy, safety, and tolerability. *J Child Adolesce Psychopharmacol*. 2006;16:260–272.

Rowles BM, Findling RL. Review of pharmacotherapy options for the treatment of attention-deficit/hyperactivity disorder (ADHD) and ADHD-like symptoms in children and adolescents with developmental disorders. *Dev Disabil Res Rev*. 2010;16:273–282.

Sajewicz-Radtke U, Jurek P, Olech M, Łada-Maśko AB, Jankowska AM, Radtke BM. Heterogeneity of cognitive profiles in children and adolescents with Mild Intellectual Disability (MID). *Int J Environ Res Public Health*. 2022;19(12):7230.

Stuart H. United Nations convention on the rights of persons with disabilities: a roadmap for change. *Curr Opin Psychiatry*. 2012;25:365–369.

Sturgeon X, Le T, Ahmed MM, Gardiner KJ. Pathways to cognitive deficits in Down syndrome. *Prog Brain Res*. 2012;197:73–100.

United Nations General Assembly. *Convention on the Rights of Persons with Disabilities (CRPD)*. United Nations; 2006.

Wijetunge LS, Chatterji S, Wyllie DJ, Kind PC. Fragile X syndrome: from targets to treatments. *Neuropharmacology*. 2013;68:83–96.

Wolstencroft J, Wicks F, Srinivasan R, et al; IMAGINE Study. Neuropsychiatric risk in children with intellectual disability of genetic origin: IMAGINE, a UK national cohort study. *Lancet Psychiatry*. 2022;9(9):715–724.

Yoshida K, Koyama E, Zai CC, et al. Pharmacogenomic studies in intellectual disabilities and autism spectrum disorder: a systematic review. *Can J Psychiatry*. 2021;66(12):1019–1041.

4 Communication Disorders

Communication disorders range from mild delays in acquiring language to expressive or mixed receptive–expressive disorders, phonologic disorders, and stuttering, which may remit spontaneously or persist into adolescence or even adulthood. Language delay is one of the most common very early childhood developmental delays, affecting up to approximately 7% of 5-year-olds. The rates of language disorders are understandably higher in preschoolers than in school-age children; rates were close to 20% of 4-year-olds in the Early Language in Victoria Study (ELVS). To communicate effectively, children must master multiple aspects of language—the ability to understand and express ideas—using words and speech to express themselves in vernacular language. In DSM-5-TR, Language Disorder includes both expressive and mixed receptive–expressive problems. DSM-5-TR speech disorders include Speech Sound Disorder (formerly known as Phonologic Disorder) and Childhood-Onset Fluency Disorder (Stuttering). Children with expressive language deficits have difficulties expressing their thoughts with words and sentences at a level of sophistication expected for their age and developmental level in other areas. These children may struggle with a limited vocabulary, speak in sentences that are short or ungrammatical, and often present descriptions of situations that are disorganized, confusing, and infantile. They may be slow to develop an understanding and a memory of words compared with others their age. Children with language disorders are at higher risk for developing reading difficulties. Current expert consensus considers reading comprehension impairment a form of language impairment, distinct from other reading deficits such as dyslexia.

Language and speech are pragmatically intertwined despite the distinct categories of language disorders and speech disorders in DSM-5-TR. Language competence spans four domains: phonology, grammar, semantics, and pragmatics. *Phonology* refers to the ability to produce sounds that constitute words in a given language and the skills to discriminate the various phonemes (sounds made by a letter or group of letters in a language). A child must be able to produce the sounds of a word to imitate them. *Grammar* designates the organization of words and the rules for placing words in an order that makes sense in that language. *Semantics* refers to the organization of concepts and the acquisition of words themselves. A child draws from a mental list of words to produce sentences. Children with language impairments exhibit a wide range of semantics difficulties, including acquiring new words, storing and organizing known words, and retrieval. Speech and language evaluations that are sufficiently broad to test all other skill levels will be more accurate in evaluating a child's remedial needs. *Pragmatics* is a branch of linguistics that concentrates on the skill of using language. It involves understanding the context of one's speech and how to interact and converse. It requires understanding the literal meaning of a sentence and the speaker's intention. By age 2, toddlers without speech or language delay may know a few words or up to 200 words, and by age 3 years, most children understand the basic rules of language and can converse effectively. Overviews typical language and nonverbal development milestones.

Over the last decade, there have been an increasing number of investigative studies of speech and language interventions with positive outcomes identified in numerous areas of language. These include improvements in expressive vocabulary, syntax usage, and overall phonologic development. Most interventions are targeted strategies for the child's particular deficit and are delivered by speech and language therapists.

LANGUAGE DISORDER

Language disorder consists of difficulties acquiring and using language across many modalities, including spoken and written, due to deficits in comprehension or production based on both expressive and receptive skills. These deficits include reduced vocabulary, limited abilities in forming sentences using the rules of grammar, and impairments in conversing based on difficulties using vocabulary to connect sentences in descriptive ways. Table 4-1 lists the approaches to diagnosing language disorders.

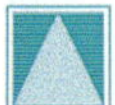

Table 4-1.
Language Disorder

	DSM-5-TR	ICD-10	ICD-11
Diagnostic name	Language Disorder	Specific Developmental Disorders of Speech and Language	Developmental Language Disorder
Duration	Onset in the early developmental period	Onset in the early developmental period	Onset in the early developmental period
Symptoms	• Reduced vocabulary • Limited sentence structure • Impairments in discourse • Difficulties are substantially below that expected for that age group	General category that includes the communication disorders listed below, including articulation, expressive and receptive disorders	Persistent deficits in the acquisition, understanding, production, or use of language (spoken or signed) beyond that expected for the age. This includes deficits in the following: • Phonologic awareness • Syntax, morphology, or grammar • Semantics • Narrative or conversational discourse • Pragmatics
Required number of symptoms	Any of the above		Any of the above
Psychosocial Consequences	Limitations in communication affect social, academic, and occupational functioning		Limitations in communication affect social, academic, and occupational functioning
Exclusions	Sensory impairment, motor dysfunction, or medical or neurologic condition		Disorders of intellectual development, autism spectrum disorder, other neurodevelopmental disorder, Sensory impairment, motor dysfunction, or medical or neurologic condition
Symptoms Specifiers			With impairment of receptive and expressive language With impairment of mainly expressive language With impairment of mainly pragmatic language With other specified language impairment

Expressive Language Deficits

Expressive language deficits occur when a child demonstrates a selective deficit in expressive language development relative to receptive language skills and nonverbal intellectual function. Infants and young children with typically developing expressive language will laugh and coo by about 6 months of age, babble and verbalize syllables such as *mama* or *dada* by about 9 months, and by 1 year, babies imitate vocalizations and can often speak at least one word. Expressive speech and language generally continue to develop stepwise so that at a year and a half, children typically can say a handful of words, and by 2 years, children generally combine words into simple sentences. By 2½ years, children can name actions in a picture and make themselves understood about half the time through verbalizations. By 3 years, most children can speak understandably, name a color, and describe what they see with several adjectives. At 4 years, children typically can name at least four colors and converse understandably. In the early years, before entering preschool, proficiency in vocabulary and language usage is highly variable and influenced by the amount and quality of verbal interactions with family members. After beginning school, the level of verbal engagement can significantly impact a child's language skills. A child with expressive language deficits may demonstrate a verbal intellectual level that appears depressed compared with the child's overall IQ. A child with expressive language problems will likely function below the expected levels of acquired vocabulary, correct tense usage, complex sentence constructions, and word recall. Children with expressive language deficits often present verbally as younger than their age. Language disability can be acquired during childhood (e.g., secondary to a trauma or a neurologic disorder), although less frequently, or it can be developmental; it is usually congenital without an apparent cause. Most childhood language disorders fall into the developmental category. In either case, deficits in receptive skills (language comprehension) or expressive skills (ability to use language) can occur. Expressive language disturbance often appears without comprehension difficulties, whereas receptive dysfunction generally diminishes proficiency in language expression. Children with expressive language disturbance alone have better prognoses and less interference with learning than children with mixed receptive–expressive language disturbances.

Although language use depends on expressive and receptive skills, the deficits in a given individual may be severe in one area and hardly impaired at all in the other. Thus, language disorders can exist in children with expressive language disturbance without receptive language problems, or both receptive and expressive language syndromes can be present. Expressive skills are also impaired when receptive skills are sufficiently impaired to warrant a diagnosis. In DSM-5-TR, a language disorder is not limited to developmental language disabilities; it also includes acquired forms of language disturbances. To meet the DSM-5-TR criteria for language disorder, patients must have scores on standardized expressive or receptive language measures markedly below those of standardized nonverbal IQ subtests and standardized tests.

Clinical Features. Children with expressive language deficits are vague when telling a story and use filler words such as "stuff" and "things" instead of naming specific objects.

The essential feature of expressive deficits in language disorder is marked impairment in the development of age-appropriate expressive language, which results in verbal or sign language markedly below the expected level given a child's nonverbal intellectual capacity. Language understanding (decoding) skills remain relatively intact. When severe, the disorder becomes recognizable by about 18 months, when a child fails to utter spontaneously or even echo single words or sounds. Even simple words, such as "Mama" and "Dada," are absent from the child's active vocabulary, and the child points or uses gestures to indicate desires. The child seems to want to communicate, maintains eye contact, relates well to the mother, and enjoys games such as pat-a-cake and peek-a-boo. The child's vocabulary is severely limited. At 18 months, the child may only point at common objects when they are named.

When a child with expressive language deficits begins to speak, language impairment gradually becomes apparent. Articulation is often immature; numerous articulation errors occur but are inconsistent, particularly with such sounds as *th, r, s, z, y,* and *l,* which the child either omits or substitutes with other sounds.

By the age of 4 years, most children with expressive language disturbance can speak in short phrases but may have difficulty retaining new words. After beginning to speak, they acquire language more slowly than most children. Their use of various grammatical structures is also markedly below the age-expected level, and they may have delayed milestones. Emotional problems involving poor self-image, frustration, and depression may develop in school-age children.

Diagnosis. We should diagnose a language disorder of the expressive disturbance type when a child has a selective deficit in language skills and is functioning well in nonverbal areas. Markedly below–age-level verbal or sign language, accompanied by a low score on standardized expressive verbal tests, is diagnostic of expressive deficits in language disorder. Although expressive language deficits often occur in children with autism spectrum disorders, these disturbances also frequently occur in the absence of autism spectrum disorder and are characterized by the following features: limited vocabulary, simple grammar, and variable articulation. "Inner language" or the appropriate use of toys and household objects is present. One assessment tool, the *Carter Neurocognitive Assessment,* itemizes and quantifies skills in social awareness, visual attention, auditory comprehension, and vocal communication even when there are compromised expressive language and motor skills in very young children—up to 2 years of age. Also, we should administer standardized expressive language and nonverbal intelligence tests. Observations of children's verbal and sign language patterns in various settings (e.g., schoolyard, classroom, home, and playroom) and during interactions with other children help ascertain the severity and specific areas of a child's impairment and aid in early detection of behavioral and emotional complications. Family history should include the presence or absence of expressive language disorder among relatives.

Damien was a friendly, alert, and hyperactive 2-year-old whose expressive vocabulary was limited to only two words (*mama, daddy*). He used these words one at a time in inappropriate situations. Damien supplemented his infrequent verbal communications with pointing and simple gestures to request desired objects or actions. He could not communicate for other purposes (e.g., commenting or protesting). Damien appeared to develop typically in other areas, especially in gross motor skills, although his fine motor skills were also poor. Damien sat, stood, walked, and played happily with other children, enjoying activities and toys appropriate for 2-year-olds. Although he had a history of frequent ear infections, a recent hearing test revealed normal hearing. Despite his expressive limitations, Damien exhibited age-appropriate comprehension of the names of familiar objects and actions and simple verbal instructions (e.g., "Put that down." "Get your shirt." "Clap your hands."). However, his hyperactivity and impulsivity often required multiple directions to complete a simple task.

Despite Damien's slow start in language development, his pediatrician had reassured his parents that most of the time, toddlers like Damien spontaneously overcome their initial slow start in language development. Fortunately, Damien's language delay spontaneously remitted by the time he entered preschool at 3½ years of age, although he showed symptoms of an attention-deficit/hyperactivity disorder.

Trina was a friendly, active 5½-year-old who presented with a language disorder. Despite her language deficits, she was well-liked in kindergarten and played with many classmates. Trina struggled during an activity in which each student recounted the story of Goldilocks and the Three Bears; Trina started to say, "Bears live in woods and eat soup. Someone sleeps in the bed."

Trina's story was characteristic of expressive language deficits at her age, including short, incomplete sentences; simple sentence structures; omission of grammatical function words (e.g., *is* and *the*) and inflectional endings (e.g., possessives and present tense verbs); problems in question formation; and incorrect use of pronouns (e.g., *her* for *she*). Trina, however, understood the story as well as her classmates. Trina also demonstrated adequate comprehension skills in her kindergarten classroom, where she readily followed the teacher's multistep verbal instructions (e.g., "After you write your name in the top left corner of your paper, get your crayons and scissors, put your library books under your chair, and line up at the back of the room.").

Jimmy was a quiet but playful 8-year-old boy whose expressive language problems had improved over time and were no longer obvious in play with peers. Jimmy's expressive deficits, however, were still impairing him in tasks involving abstract use of language, and he was struggling in his third-grade academic work. Jimmy's explanation of a recent science experiment lacked appropriate detail because he could not find the words to describe them: "The teacher put some liquid stuff in some jars. He poured it, and it turned blue. The other one made it white." Although each sentence was grammatical, his explanation was difficult to follow because he was too vague and was unable to give any details about what the experiment showed. Jimmy especially had problems in word-finding, relying on vague and nonspecific terms, such as *thing, stuff,* and *got.*

In the first and second grades, Jimmy could keep up with his classmates in reading, writing, and other academic skills. By third grade, however, the increasing demands for verbal and written work were beyond his abilities. Jimmy's written work was disorganized and lacked specific details. Classmates began to tease him about his difficulties and reacted aggressively, often leading to physical fighting. Jimmy received speech and language therapy and showed relatively good spoken language comprehension, including classroom teaching concerning abstract concepts. Jimmy was able to comprehend, and understood sentences and concepts that were grammatically and conceptually complex, "The car the truck hit had already been dented by a previous accident."

PATHOLOGY AND LABORATORY EXAMINATION. Children with speech and language disorders should have an audiogram to rule out hearing loss.

Course and Prognosis. The prognosis for expressive language disturbance worsens the longer it persists in a child; the prognosis also depends on the disorder's severity. Studies of infants and toddlers who are "late talkers" concur that 50% to 80% of these children master language skills that are within the expected level during the preschool years. Most children with language delays later catch up in their preschool years. Other comorbid disorders may influence the outcome of expressive language deficits. If children do not develop mood disorders or disruptive behavior problems, the prognosis is better. The rapidity and extent of recovery depend on the severity of the disorder, the child's motivation to participate in speech and language therapy, and the timely initiation of therapeutic interventions. The presence or absence of hearing loss or intellectual disability impedes remediation and leads to a worse prognosis. Up to 50% of children with mild expressive language disorder recover spontaneously without any sign of language impairment, but those children with a severe expressive speech disorder may persist in exhibiting some symptoms into middle childhood or later.

Current literature shows that children with poor comprehension, articulation, or academic performance tend to have problems in these areas at follow-up 7 years later. There is also an association between particular language impairment profiles and persistent mood and behavior problems. Children with poor comprehension associated with expressive difficulties seem more socially isolated and impaired concerning peer relationships.

Differential Diagnosis. Language disorders are associated with various psychiatric disorders, including other learning disorders and attention-deficit/hyperactivity disorder (ADHD), and in some cases, the language disorder is challenging to separate from another dysfunction. In mixed receptive–expressive language disorder, language comprehension (decoding) is markedly below the expected age-appropriate level, whereas in expressive language disorder, language comprehension remains within normal limits.

In autism spectrum disorders, children often have impaired language, symbolic and imagery play, appropriate use of gestures, or the capacity to form typical social relationships. In contrast, children with expressive language disorder become very frustrated with their disorder and are usually highly motivated to make friends despite their disability.

Children with acquired aphasia or dysphasia have a history of early normal language development; the disordered language had its onset after head trauma or other neurologic disorders (e.g., a seizure disorder). Children with selective mutism have normal language development. Often, these children speak only in front of family members (e.g., mother, father, and siblings). Children affected by selective mutism are socially anxious and withdrawn outside the family. Table 4-2 lists the differential diagnosis for language disorders.

Comorbidity. Children with language disorders have above-average rates of comorbid psychiatric disorders.

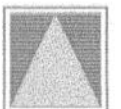

Table 4-2.
Differential Diagnosis of Language Disorder

Disorder	Receptive Language	Expressive Language	Onset Pattern	Associated Features	Distinctive Features
Language disorder	Often impaired (esp. in mixed type)	Impaired	Early developmental period	May co-occur with ADHD, learning disorders; impairs social/academic function	Must be significantly below age expectations in standardized or functional assessments
Speech sound disorder	Normal	Errors in sound production	Early developmental period	May co-occur with language disorder	Impaired articulation, not comprehension or word usage
Autism spectrum disorder	Often impaired	Often impaired	Early developmental period	Disturbed social interaction, limited communicative intent, repetitive behaviors	Social communication deficits are core; concurrent diagnosis possible if language deficits are more severe
Intellectual developmental disorder	Impaired in proportion to cognitive ability	Impaired in proportion to cognitive ability	Early developmental period	Global developmental delays	All areas (receptive, expressive, nonverbal IQ) significantly below age expectations
Selective mutism	Normal	Limited due to anxiety	Onset typically by age 5	Marked social anxiety; speech restricted to familiar settings	Receptive and nonverbal skills intact; expressive limitation is situational
Hearing impairment	Impairment depends on the severity of hearing loss	May appear disordered	Congenital or acquired	Audiometric testing confirms impairment	Language deficits stem from lack of auditory input
Acquired aphasia/ dysphasia (e.g., TBI, CVA)	Initially normal; then impaired	Initially normal; then impaired	Postinjury onset	Head trauma, seizures, stroke, infection, anoxia, toxin exposure	Sudden regression; may spare basic language but impair complex discourse and pragmatic communication
Landau–Kleffner syndrome	Declines after normal development	Declines after normal development	Ages 3–7 yr	EEG abnormalities; seizures (esp. during sleep); behavioral issues like hyperactivity or depression	Abrupt or gradual loss of language; no hearing loss despite parental suspicion
Environmental deprivation		May be impaired due to limited stimulation	May be impaired	Variable; often gradual	Low language exposure; poor stimulation environment
Specific learning disorder (written expression or reading)	Typically intact	May be impaired in sentence structure, vocabulary, and grammar	School-age onset	Reading and writing difficulties	Co-occurrence with language disorder is common; requires screening
Second language acquisition (normal variant)	Normal for age/ experience	Errors common in second language learning	When learning a new language	Errors context-specific; influenced by native language	Not a disorder; requires culturally and linguistically informed evaluation

In one large study of children with speech and language disorders, the most common comorbid disorders were ADHD (19%), anxiety disorders (10%), oppositional defiant disorder, and conduct disorder (7% combined). Children with expressive language disorder are also at higher risk for a speech disorder, receptive difficulties, and other learning disorders. Many disorders—such as reading, developmental coordination, and other communication disorders—are associated with expressive language disturbance. Children with expressive language disturbance often have some receptive impairment, although not always sufficiently significant for the diagnosis of language disorder on this basis. Speech sound disorder, formerly known as phonologic disorder, is commonly found in young children with a language disorder, and neurologic abnormalities exist in some children, including soft neurologic signs, depressed vestibular responses, and EEG abnormalities.

Treatment. The primary goals for early childhood speech and language treatment are to guide children and their parents toward greater production of meaningful language. There is more data to support improvements through speech and language interventions for expressive language deficits in young school-age children with primary deficits than in preschool children. A study investigating Parent–Child Interaction Therapy (PCIT) for school-age children with expressive language impairment found that PCIT was particularly efficacious in improving a child's verbal initiation, mean length of utterances, and the proportion of child-to-parent utterances. A large-scale randomized trial of a yearlong intervention targeting preschoolers with language delay in Australia found that a community-based program did not affect language acquisition in 2- and 3-year-olds. Given the high rate of spontaneous remission of language deficits in preschoolers and the less robust effects of interventions for young children, treatment for expressive language disorder is generally not initiated unless it persists after the preschool years. Various techniques may help a child improve their use of such parts of speech as pronouns, correct tenses, and question forms. Direct interventions use a speech and language pathologist who works directly with the child. Mediated interventions have also been efficacious in which a speech and language professional teaches a child's teacher or parent how to promote therapeutic language techniques. Language therapy also works on using words to improve communication strategies and social interactions. Such therapy consists of behaviorally reinforced exercises and training with phonemes (sound units), vocabulary, and sentence construction. The goal is to increase the number of phrases using block-building methods and conventional speech therapies.

Etiology. The specific causes of the expressive components of language disorder are likely to be multifactorial. Scant data are available on the specific brain structure of children with a language disorder. However, limited MRI studies suggest that language disorders are associated with diminished left–right brain asymmetry in the perisylvian and planum temporale regions. Results of one small MRI study suggested possible inversion of brain asymmetry (right > left). Left-handedness or ambilaterality is more frequently associated with expressive language problems than right-handedness. Evidence shows that language disorders occur more frequently within some families, and several studies of twins show significant concordance for monozygotic twins for language disorders. Environmental and educational factors also likely contribute to developmental language disorders.

Mixed Receptive and Expressive Deficits

Children with both receptive and expressive language impairment may have impaired ability in sound discrimination, deficits in auditory processing, or poor memory for sound sequences. Children with mixed receptive–expressive disturbance have impaired skills in the expression and reception (understanding and comprehension) of spoken language. The expressive difficulties in these children may be similar to those of children with only expressive language disturbance, characterized by limited vocabulary, use of simple sentences, and short sentence usage. Children with receptive language difficulties may be experiencing additional deficits in basic auditory processing skills, such as discriminating between sounds, rapid sound changes, the association of sounds and symbols, and the memory of sound sequences. These deficits may lead to a whole host of communication barriers for a child, including a lack of understanding of questions or directives from others or an inability to follow the conversations of peers or family members. Teachers or parents may initially misattribute communication difficulties to behavioral problems, delaying recognizing the actual diagnosis.

We can measure the essential features of mixed receptive–expressive language disturbance on standardized tests; both receptive (comprehension) and expressive language development scores fall substantially below those obtained from standardized measures of nonverbal intellectual capacity. Language difficulties must be sufficiently severe to impair academic achievement or daily social communication.

Clinical Features. The essential clinical feature of this language disturbance is a significant impairment in both language comprehension and expression. In the mixed type, expressive impairments are similar to expressive language disturbance but can be more severe. The clinical features of the receptive component of the disorder typically appear before the age of 4 years. Severe forms are apparent by the age of 2 years; mild forms may not become evident until age 7 (second grade) or older when language becomes complex. Children with language disorder characterized by mixed receptive–expressive disturbance show markedly delayed and below-normal ability to comprehend (decode) verbal or sign language; however, they have age-appropriate nonverbal intellectual capacity. Patients with receptive dysfunction are also impaired in verbal or sign expression (encoding) of language. Children between 18 and 24 months with mixed receptive–expressive language disturbance cannot spontaneously utter a single phoneme or mimic another person's words.

Many children with mixed receptive–expressive language deficits have auditory sensory difficulties and compromised ability to process visual symbols, such as explaining the meaning of a picture. They have deficits in integrating auditory and visual symbols—for example, recognizing the common attributes of a toy truck and a toy passenger car. Whereas at 18 months, a child with expressive language deficits only comprehends simple commands and can point to familiar household objects when told to do so, a child of the same age with mixed receptive–expressive language disturbance typically cannot either point to everyday objects or obey simple commands. A child with mixed receptive–expressive language deficits may appear deaf. They respond appropriately to sounds from the environment but not to spoken language. If the child later starts to speak, the speech contains numerous articulation errors, such as omissions, distortions, and substitutions of phonemes. Language acquisition is much slower for children with mixed receptive–expressive language disturbance than for other children of the same age.

Children with mixed receptive–expressive language disturbance have difficulty recalling early visual and auditory memories and recognizing and reproducing symbols in a proper sequence. Some children with mixed receptive–expressive language deficits have a partial hearing defect for true tones, an increased threshold of auditory arousal, and an inability to localize sound sources. Seizure disorders and reading disorders are more common among the relatives of children with mixed receptive–expressive problems than in the general population.

Diagnosis. Children with mixed receptive–expressive language deficits develop language more slowly than their peers and have trouble understanding conversations that peers can follow. In mixed receptive–expressive language disorder, receptive dysfunction coexists with expressive dysfunction. Therefore, we should give standardized tests for receptive and expressive language abilities to anyone suspected of having a language disorder with mixed receptive–expressive disturbance.

A markedly below-expected level of comprehension of verbal or sign language with intact age-appropriate nonverbal intellectual capacity, confirmation of language difficulties by standardized receptive language tests, and the absence of autism spectrum disorder confirm the diagnosis of mixed receptive–expressive language deficits; however, in DSM-5-TR, these deficits are included in the diagnosis of language disorder.

PATHOLOGY AND LABORATORY EXAMINATION. All children thought to have mixed receptive–expressive language disturbance should have an audiogram to rule out or confirm the presence of deafness or auditory deficits. A history of the child and family and observation of the child in various settings help to clarify the diagnosis.

Tony was a cheerful 3-year-old who did not yet use spoken words and did not respond to simple commands without gestures. He made his needs known with vocalizations and gestures (e.g., showing or pointing), such as those typically used by younger children. Tony understood the names of familiar people and objects (e.g., *mommy, daddy, cat, bottle,* and *cookie*). Compared with other children his age, he had better receptive understanding than expression but still exhibited less comprehension of vocabulary and showed limited understanding of simple verbal directions (e.g., "Get your ball," "Close your eyes."). Tony's motor and play skills were well-developed for his age. He was well-coordinated, active, and interested in other children's activities at his daycare.

Ashley was a shy, reserved 5-year-old who grew up in a bilingual home. Ashley's parents and older siblings spoke English and Mandarin proficiently. Her grandparents, who lived in the same home, spoke only Mandarin. Ashley began to understand and speak both languages later than her older siblings had. Throughout her preschool years, Ashley slowly developed comprehension and expression in both English and Mandarin. When she started kindergarten, Ashely understood fewer English words than her classmates. Ashely could not follow complicated classroom instructions, particularly those involving words for time concepts (e.g., *tomorrow, before,* or *day*) and space (e.g., *behind, next to,* or *under*). Ashley was better at matching one of several pictures to a syntactically complex sentence that she had heard (e.g., "It was not the train she was waiting for." "Because he had already completed his work, he was not kept after school."). Ashley played with other children but rarely tried to speak with them, which led to her classmates preferring other playmates. Ashley often played alone, limiting her opportunities to learn and practice her language skills with peers. Ashley also showed limited receptive and expressive skills in Mandarin, as revealed by an assessment conducted with the assistance of an interpreter. Ashley's nonverbal cognitive and motor skills were within the normal range for her age. Ashley was quite proficient in solving spatial and numerical problems, especially when they were presented on paper and were not word problems.

Mark received a diagnosis of Language Disorder based on mixed receptive–expressive deficits when he was a preschooler. By 7 years of age, he had also received the comorbid diagnoses of reading disorder and ADHD. This combination of language, reading, and attention problems made it virtually impossible for Mark to succeed in school, although he could engage his peers during free play. His comprehension and attention difficulties limited his ability to understand and learn valuable information or to follow classroom instructions or discussions. Mark fell further and further behind his classmates. He was also disadvantaged because he could read only a few familiar words. This disadvantage meant that Mark was neither motivated nor able to learn academic information outside the classroom by reading. Mark received tutoring and speech and language interventions, and despite some improvements, he continued to lag behind his classmates academically. Despite his academic problems, however, Mark made friends during sports activities in which he excelled and continued to show nonverbal intellectual skills within the average range.

Differential Diagnosis. Children with language disorder characterized by mixed receptive–expressive deficits have a language comprehension and production deficit. The receptive deficit may be overlooked initially because the expressive language deficit may be more prominent. In expressive language disturbance alone, spoken language comprehension (decoding) remains within age norms. Children with speech sound disorder and child-onset fluency disorder (stuttering) have normal expressive and receptive language competence despite the speech impairments.

Most children with mixed receptive–expressive language disturbance have a history of variable and inconsistent responses to sounds; they respond more often to environmental sounds than speech sounds (Table 4-2). We should also rule out intellectual disability, selective mutism, acquired aphasia, and autism spectrum disorder.

Comorbidity. Children with mixed receptive–expressive deficits are at high risk for additional speech and language disorders, learning disorders, and additional psychiatric disorders. About half of children with these deficits also have pronunciation difficulties leading to speech sound disorder, and about half also have a reading disorder. These rates are significantly higher than the comorbidity found in children with only expressive language problems. ADHD is present in at least one-third of children with mixed receptive–expressive language disturbances.

Course and Prognosis. The overall prognosis for language disorder with mixed receptive–expressive disturbance is less favorable than that for expressive language disturbance alone. When the mixed disorder is identified in a young child, it is usually severe, and the short-term prognosis is poor. Language develops rapidly in early childhood, and young children with the disorder may appear to be falling behind. Given the likelihood of comorbid learning disorders and other mental disorders, there is a guarded prognosis. Young children with severe mixed receptive–expressive language deficits are likely to have learning disorders in the future. In children with mild versions, it may take several years to identify the mixed disorder, and the disruption in everyday life may be less overwhelming than that in severe forms of the disorder. Over the long run, some children with mixed receptive–expressive language disturbance achieve close to normal language functions. The prognosis for children with mixed receptive–expressive language disturbances varies widely and depends on the nature and severity of the damage.

Treatment. Given the complexities of having both deficits, children with mixed receptive–expressive language disturbance should have a comprehensive speech and language evaluation. Some controversy exists as to whether remediation of receptive deficits before expressive deficits improves the overall efficacy of treatment. A literature review indicates that it is not more beneficial to address receptive deficits before expressive, and, in some cases, remediation of expressive language may reduce or eliminate the need for receptive language remediation. Thus, current recommendations are to address both simultaneously or provide interventions for the expressive component first, then address the receptive language. Preschoolers with mixed receptive–expressive language problems optimally receive interventions to promote social communication, literacy, and oral language. The optimal intervention for children at the kindergarten level includes direct teaching of key prereading skills and social skills training. An essential early goal of interventions for young children with mixed receptive–expressive language disturbance is the achievement of rudimentary reading skills, in that these skills are protective against the academic and psychosocial ramifications of falling behind early on in reading. Some language therapists favor a low-stimuli setting, giving children individual linguistic instruction. Others recommend integrating speech and language instruction into a varied setting with several children with whom they teach several language structures simultaneously. A child with receptive and expressive language deficits often benefits from a small, special educational setting that allows more individualized learning.

Psychotherapy may be helpful for children with mixed language disorder who have associated emotional and behavioral problems. We should pay particular attention to evaluating the child's self-image and social skills. Family counseling in which parents and children can develop more effective, less frustrating communication methods may be beneficial.

Epidemiology. Mixed receptive–expressive language deficits occur less frequently than expressive deficits; however, epidemiologic data regarding specific prevalence rates are scant. The language disturbance is believed to occur in about 5% of preschoolers and persists in about 3% of school-age children. It is less common than expressive language disturbance. Mixed receptive–expressive language disorder is likely twice as prevalent in boys as in girls.

Etiology. Language disorders most likely have multiple determinants, including genetic factors, developmental brain abnormalities, environmental influences, neurodevelopmental immaturity, and auditory processing features in the brain. As with expressive language disturbance alone, there is evidence of familial aggregation of mixed receptive–expressive language deficits. Twin studies implicate a genetic contribution to this disorder, but there is no proven mode of genetic transmission. Some studies of children with various speech and language disorders have also shown cognitive deficits, notably slower processing of tasks involving naming objects and fine motor tasks. Slower myelinization of neural pathways may account for the slow processing in children with developmental language disorders. Several studies suggest an underlying impairment of auditory discrimination because most children with the disorder are more responsive to environmental sounds than speech sounds.

SPEECH SOUND DISORDER

Children with speech sound disorder have difficulty pronouncing speech sounds correctly due to omissions, distortions of sounds, or atypical pronunciation. Formerly called phonologic disorder, typical speech disturbances in speech sound disorder include omitting the last sounds of the word (e.g., saying *mou* for *mouse* or *drin* for *drink*) or substituting one sound for another (saying *bwu* instead of *blue* or *tup* for *cup*). Distortions in sounds can occur when children allow too much air to escape from the side of their mouths while saying sounds like *sh* or producing sounds like *s* or *z* with their tongue protruding. Speech sound errors can also occur in patterns because a child has an interrupted airflow instead of a steady airflow, preventing their pronouncing words (e.g., *pat* for *pass* or *bacuum* for *vacuum*). Children with speech sound disorder can be mistaken for younger children because of their difficulties in producing speech sounds correctly. We diagnose a speech sound disorder by comparing the skills of a given child with the expected skill level of others of the same age. The disorder results in errors in whole words because of incorrect pronunciation of consonants, substitution of one sound for another, omission of entire phonemes, and, in some cases, dysarthria (slurred speech because of incoordination of speech muscles) or dyspraxia (difficulty planning and executing speech). Speech sound development likely depends on linguistic and motor development, which we must integrate to produce sounds.

Speech sound disturbances such as dysarthria and dyspraxia are not diagnosed as speech sound disorders if they are known to have a neurologic basis, according to DSM-5-TR. Thus, speech sound abnormalities accounted for by cerebral palsy, cleft palate, deafness or hearing loss, traumatic brain injury, or neurologic conditions are not diagnosed as speech sound disorder. Articulation difficulties not associated with a neurologic condition are the most common components of speech sound disorder in children. Articulation deficits include poor articulation, sound substitution, and speech sound omission, and give the impression of "baby talk." Typically, these deficits are not caused by anatomical, structural, physiologic, auditory, or neurologic abnormalities. They vary from mild to severe and result in speech that ranges from entirely intelligible to unintelligible.

Clinical Features

Children with speech sound disorder have a delay in, or are incapable of, producing accurate speech sounds typical for their age, intelligence, and dialect. The sounds are often substitutions—for example, the use of *t* instead of *k*—and omissions, such as leaving off the final consonants of words. We can usually recognize speech sound disorder in early childhood. We can recognize it in severe cases between 2 and 3 years of age. In less severe cases, the disorder may not be apparent until the age of 6 years. A child's articulation is disordered when it is significantly behind most children at the same age, intellectual, and educational levels.

A single speech sound (i.e., phoneme) may be affected in very mild cases. When a single phoneme is affected, it is usually acquired late in normal language acquisition. The speech sounds most frequently misarticulated are also those acquired late in the developmental sequence, including *r, sh, th, f, z, l,* and *ch.* In severe cases and young children, sounds such as *b, m, t, d, n,* and *h* may be mispronounced. One of many speech sounds may be affected, but vowel sounds are not among them.

Children with speech sound disorder cannot articulate specific phonemes correctly and may distort, substitute, or even omit the affected phonemes. With omissions, the phonemes are absent entirely—for example, *bu* for *blue, ca* for *car,* or *whaa for what's that.* With substitutions, children may replace difficult phonemes with incorrect ones—for example, *wabbit* for *rabbit, fum* for *thumb*, or *whath dat* for *what's that.* With distortions, the child may approximate the correct phoneme but articulate it incorrectly. Rarely, additions (usually of the vowel uh) occur—for example, *puhretty* for *pretty, what's uh that uh* for *what's that.*

Omissions are the most severe type of misarticulation, with substitutions being the most serious and distortions being the least severe type. Omissions, most frequent in young children's speech, usually occur at the ends of words or in clusters of consonants (ka for car, scisso for scissors). Distortions, found mainly in older children's speech, result in a sound not part of the speaker's dialect. Distortions may be the last type of misarticulation remaining in the speech of children whose articulation problems have mostly remitted. The most common types of distortions are the lateral slip—in which a child pronounces *s* sounds with the airstream going across the tongue, producing a whistling effect—and the palatal or lisp—in which the *s* sound, formed with the tongue too close to the palate, produces a *ssh* sound effect.

The misarticulation of children with speech sound disorder is often inconsistent and random. A child may pronounce a phoneme correctly one time and incorrectly another time. Misarticulating is most common at the ends of words, in long and syntactically complex sentences, and during rapid speech.

Omissions, distortions, and substitutions also usually occur in the speech of young children learning to talk. However, whereas young, typically speaking children soon replace their misarticulating, children with speech sound disorder do not. Even as children with articulation problems grow and finally acquire the correct phoneme, they may use it only in newly acquired words and may not correct the words learned earlier that they have been mispronouncing for some time.

Most children eventually outgrow speech sound disorder, usually by the third grade. After the fourth grade, however, spontaneous recovery is unlikely, so it is essential to try to remediate the disorder before the development of complications. Often, beginning kindergarten or school precipitates the improvement when recovery from speech sound disorder is spontaneous. Children without spontaneous improvement by the third or fourth grade should have speech therapy. Speech therapy should be initiated at an early age for children whose articulation is significantly unintelligible and who are troubled by their inability to speak clearly.

Children with speech sound disorder may have various social, emotional, and behavioral problems, mainly when comorbid expressive language problems are present. Children with chronic expressive language deficits and severe articulation impairment are the ones most likely to suffer from psychiatric problems.

Jose was a talkative, likable 3-year-old with virtually unintelligible speech despite excellent receptive language skills and normal hearing. Jose's level of expressive language development was difficult to quantify due to his very poor pronunciation. The rhythm and melody of his speech suggested that he was trying to produce sentences, but his words could not be deciphered. Jose made only a few vowels (*/ee/*, */ah/*, and */oo/*), some early developing consonants (*/m/*, */n/*, */d/*, */t/*, */p/*, */b/*, */h/*, and */w/*), and limited syllables. This reduced sound repertoire made many spoken words indistinguishable (e.g., he said *bahbah* for *bottle*, *baby*, and *bubble*, and he used *nee* for *knee*, *need*, and *Anita* [his sister]). Moreover, he consistently omitted consonant sounds at the end of words and in consonant cluster sequences (e.g., */tr-/*, */st-/*, */-nt/*, and */-mp/*). Understandably, Jose occasionally reacted with frustration and tantrums to his difficulties understanding his needs.

Liam was a happy 5-year-old with difficulty pronouncing sounds in preschool, which persisted into kindergarten. His language comprehension skills and hearing were typical of his age. Liam showed mild expressive language problems in using certain grammatical features (e.g., pronouns, auxiliary verbs, and past-tense word endings) and formulating sentences. Liam was able to produce all vowel sounds correctly and most of the early-developing consonants, but he was inconsistent in his attempts to produce later-developing consonants (e.g., */r/*, */l/*, */s/*, */z/*, */sh/*, */th/*, and */ch/*). Sometimes, he omitted them; sometimes, he substituted other sounds for them (e.g., */w/* for */r/* or */f/* for */th/*); occasionally, he even produced them correctly. Liam had particular problems in correctly producing consonant cluster sequences and multisyllabic words. Cluster sequences had omitted or incorrect sounds (e.g., *blue* might be produced as *bue* or *bwue*, and *hearts* as *hots* or *hars*). Multisyllabic words omitted syllables (e.g., *efant* for *elephant* and *getti* for *spaghetti*), and sounds were mispronounced or transposed (e.g., *aminal* for *animal* and *lemon* for *melon*). Strangers were unable to understand most of Liam's speech. Liam tried to speak more slowly and clearly than usual when asked to repeat something, which often did not clarify his intended words.

Emily was a talkative and hyperactive 7-year-old with a history of significant speech delay. She received speech and language therapy and overcame many earlier speech errors during preschool and early school. However, a few late-developing sounds (*/r/*,*/l/*, and */th/*) continued challenging her. Emily often substituted */f/* or */d/* for*/th/*and produced */w/* for */r/* and */l/*. Overall, her speech was easily understood despite these minor errors. Emily became angry and somewhat aggressive with her peers because of the teasing she occasionally still received from her classmates about her speech.

Diagnosis

The essential feature of speech sound disorder is a child's delay or failure to produce developmentally expected speech sounds, especially consonants, resulting in sound omissions, substitutions, and distortions of phonemes. A rough guideline for clinical assessment of children's articulation is that normal 3-year-olds correctly articulate *m, n, ng, b, p, h, t, k, q,* and *d;* ordinary 4-year-olds correctly articulate *f, y, ch, sh,* and *z;* and typical 5-year-olds correctly articulate *th, s, and r.*

Structural or neurologic abnormalities cannot account for speech sound disorder; typically, normal language development accompanies it. Table 4-3 lists the diagnostic approaches to speech sound disorder.

Differential Diagnosis

The differential diagnosis of speech sound disorder includes carefully determining symptoms, severity, and possible medical conditions that might produce the symptoms.

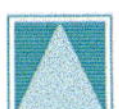

Table 4-3. Speech Sound Disorder

	DSM-5-TR	ICD-10	ICD-11
Diagnostic name	Speech Sound Disorder	Expressive Language Disorder	Developmental Speech Sound Disorder
Duration	Onset in the early developmental period		Onset in the early developmental period
Symptoms	Difficulty with speech sound production (articulation of phonemes)	The child's ability to use expressive spoken language is markedly below the appropriate level for its mental	Persistent errors of pronunciation, articulation, or phonology
Psychosocial Consequences	Limitations in communication affect social, academic, and occupational functioning		Limitations in communication affect social, academic, and occupational functioning
Exclusions	Not due to congenital/ acquired conditions affecting speech (cerebral palsy, cleft palate), sensory impairment, or other medical or neurologic condition		Not due to congenital/acquired conditions affecting speech (cerebral palsy, cleft palate), sensory impairment, or other medical or neurologic condition

First, we must determine that the misarticulating is sufficiently severe to impair the child rather than a normative developmental process of learning to speak. Second, we must determine that no physical abnormalities account for the articulation errors and must rule out neurologic disorders that may cause dysarthria, hearing impairment, mental retardation, and pervasive developmental disorders. Third, we must obtain an evaluation of receptive and expressive language to determine that the speech difficulty is not solely attributable to the disorders, as mentioned earlier.

Neurologic, oral structural, and audiometric examinations may be necessary to rule out physical factors that cause specific articulation abnormalities. Children with dysarthria, a disorder caused by structural or neurologic abnormalities, differ from children with speech sound disorder in that dysarthria is less likely to remit spontaneously and may be more difficult to remediate. Drooling, slow or uncoordinated motor behavior, abnormal chewing or swallowing, and awkward or slow protrusion and retraction of the tongue indicate dysarthria. A slow speech rate also indicates dysarthria (Table 4-4).

Comorbidity

More than half of children with speech sound disorder have some difficulty with language. The disorders most commonly present with speech sound disorders are language, reading, and developmental coordination disorders. Enuresis may also accompany the disorder. A delay in reaching speech milestones (e.g., first word and first sentence) occurs in some children with speech sound disorder, but most children begin speaking at the appropriate age. Children with both speech sound and language disorders are at the highest risk for attentional problems and specific learning disorders. Children with speech sound disorder in the absence of language disorder have a lower risk of comorbid psychiatric disorders and behavioral problems.

Course and Prognosis

Spontaneous remission of symptoms is common in children whose misarticulating involves only a few phonemes. Children who persist in exhibiting articulation problems after the age of 5 years may be experiencing a myriad of other speech and language impairments, so it is appropriate to perform a comprehensive evaluation at that time. Children older than 5 with articulation problems are at higher risk for auditory perceptual issues. Spontaneous recovery is rare after the age of 8 years. Some debate exists regarding the relationship between articulation problems and reading disorder or dyslexia. A recent study comparing children with phonologic problems, children with dyslexia, and those with both phonologic difficulties and dyslexia concluded that children with both disorders have distinct profiles and are comorbid disorders rather than one mixed disorder.

Treatment

Two main approaches can successfully improve speech sound difficulties. The first one, the *phonologic approach,* is usually chosen for children with extensive patterns of multiple speech sound errors that may include final consonant deletion or consonant cluster reduction. Exercises in this approach to treatment focus on the guided practice of specific sounds, such as final consonants, and when

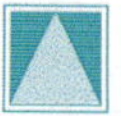

Table 4-4.
Differential Diagnosis of Speech Sound Disorder

Disorder (DSM-5-TR Term or Clinical Term)	Speech Severity	Physical Abnormalities	Neurologic Signs	Hearing or Language Impairment	Distinctive Features
Speech sound disorder	Must be severe enough to impair communication	No structural abnormalities	No signs of neurologic dysfunction	Not solely due to hearing or language disorder	Errors in sound production; may remit spontaneously
Speech disturbance due to neurologic condition (e.g., dysarthria)	May be severe	Often due to structural or neurologic abnormalities	Drooling, slow speech, poor coordination, abnormal chewing/swallowing, tongue issues	May co-occur	Persistent, with clear motor-speech abnormalities
Hearing loss (not DSM-5 disorder)	May contribute to articulation errors	No relevant abnormalities	No neurologic findings	Hearing loss present	Identified via audiometric testing
Intellectual disability (intellectual developmental disorder)	May present with articulation issues	No specific abnormalities	May show neurologic signs depending on etiology	Language delays common	Global developmental delays including cognition and communication
Autism spectrum disorder	May present with disordered or atypical speech	No specific abnormalities	May be present (e.g., motor stereotypies)	Often includes receptive and expressive language deficits	Speech issues part of broader social communication deficits
Developmental language disorder	Speech may appear disordered, but root is language	No structural abnormalities	No clear neurologic signs	Core deficits in expressive and/or receptive language	Grammar, vocabulary, and narrative structure impaired; may impact intelligibility

mastering that skill, extending the practice to use it in meaningful words and sentences. The other *traditional approach* is used for children who produce substitution or distortion errors in just a few sounds. In this approach, the child practices the production of the problem sound while we provide immediate feedback and cues concerning the correct placement of the tongue and mouth for improved articulation. Children who have errors in articulation because of abnormal swallowing resulting in tongue thrust and lisps should receive exercises to improve their swallowing patterns and, in turn, improve their speech. A speech-language pathologist typically provides speech therapy, yet parents can learn to provide adjunctive help by practicing techniques used in the treatment. Early intervention can be helpful because, for many children with mild articulation difficulties, even several months of intervention may be helpful in early elementary school. In general, when a child's articulation and intelligibility are noticeably different from peers by 8 years of age, speech deficits often lead to problems with peers, learning, and self-image, especially when the disorder is so severe that many consonants are misarticulated, and when errors involve omissions and substitutions of phonemes, rather than distortions.

Children with persistent articulation problems are likely to be teased or ostracized by peers and may become isolated and demoralized. Therefore, it is crucial to support children with phonologic disorders and, whenever possible, to support prosocial activities and social interactions with peers. Parental counseling and monitoring child–peer relationships and school behavior can help minimize social impairment in children with speech sound and language disorders.

Epidemiology

Epidemiologic studies suggest that the prevalence of speech sound disorder is at least 3% in preschoolers, 2% in children 6 to 7 years of age, and 0.5% in 17-year-old adolescents. Approximately 7% to 8% of 5-year-old children in one large community sample had speech sound production problems of developmental, structural, or neurologic origins. Another study found that up to 7.5% of children between 7 and 11 years had speech sound disorders. Of those, 2.5% had speech delay (deletion and substitution errors past the age of 4 years), and 5% had residual articulation errors beyond 8 years. Speech sound disorders occur much more frequently than disorders with a known structural or neurologic origin. Speech sound disorder is approximately two to three times more common in boys than in girls. It is also more common among first-degree relatives of patients with the disorder than in the general population. Although speech sound mistakes are quite common in children younger than 3 years of age, these mistakes are usually self-corrected by age 7 years. Misarticulating after the age of 7 years is likely to represent a speech sound disorder. The prevalence of speech sound disorders reportedly falls to 0.5% by mid to late adolescence.

Etiology

Contributing factors leading to speech disturbance may include perinatal problems, genetic factors, and auditory processing problems. Given the high rates of spontaneous remission in very young children, there may be a maturational delay in the developmental brain process underlying speech in some cases. The likelihood of neuronal cause is supported by the observation that children with speech sound disorder are also more likely to manifest "soft neurologic signs" as well as language disorder and a higher-than-expected rate of reading disorder. Data from twin studies implicate genetic factors, as they show concordance rates for monozygotic twins that are higher than chance.

Articulation disorders caused by structural or mechanical problems are rare. Articulation problems not caused by speech sound disorder could represent a neurologic impairment, such as dysarthria and apraxia or dyspraxia. Dysarthria results from an impairment in the neural mechanisms regulating the muscular control of speech. This impairment can occur in congenital conditions, such as cerebral palsy, muscular dystrophy, or head injury, or because of infectious processes. Apraxia or dyspraxia is characterized by difficulty in the execution of speech, even when no apparent paralysis or weakness of the muscles used in speech exists.

Environmental factors may play a role in speech sound disorder, but constitutional factors contribute most significantly. The high proportion of speech sound disorder in individual families implies a genetic component in developing this disorder. Developmental coordination disorder and coordination in the mouth (such as chewing and blowing the nose) may be associated.

CHILD-ONSET FLUENCY DISORDER (STUTTERING)

Child-onset fluency disorder (stuttering) usually begins during the first years of life and is characterized by disruptions in the normal flow of speech by involuntary speech motor events. Stuttering can include a variety of specific fluency disruptions, including sound or syllable repetitions, sound prolongations, dysrhythmic phonations, and complete blocking or unusual pauses between sounds and syllables of words. In severe cases, the stuttering may include accessory or secondary attempts to compensate, such as respiratory, abnormal voice phonations, or tongue clicks. Associated behaviors, such as eye blinks, facial grimacing, head jerks, and abnormal body movements, may be observed before or during the disrupted speech.

Early intervention is necessary because children who receive it can be more than seven times more likely to have complete resolution of their stuttering. In severe and some untreated cases, stuttering can become an entrenched pattern that is more challenging to remediate later in life and is associated with significant psychological and social distress. When stuttering becomes chronic, persisting into adulthood, the rate of concurrent social anxiety disorder is between 40% and 60%.

Diagnosis

Diagnosing childhood-onset fluency disorder (stuttering) is not difficult when the clinical features are apparent and well-developed, and each of the following four phases (described in the next section) is readily recognized. Diagnostic difficulties can arise when evaluating for stuttering in young children because some preschool children experience transient dysfluency. It may not be clear whether the nonfluent pattern is part of normal speech and language development or represents the initial stage of stuttering development. If incipient stuttering is suspected, the child should be referred to a speech therapist. Table 4-5 compares the approaches to diagnosing stuttering.

Clinical Features

Stuttering usually appears between 18 months and 9 years, with two sharp peaks of onset between 2 to 3.5 years and 5 to 7 years. Some, but not all, stutterers have other speech and language problems, such as phonologic disorder and expressive language disorder. Stuttering does not begin suddenly; it typically develops over weeks or months with a repetition of initial consonants, whole words that are usually the first words of a phrase, or long words. As the disorder progresses, the repetitions become more frequent, with consistent stuttering on the most important words or phrases. Even after it develops, stuttering may be absent during oral readings, singing, and talking to pets or inanimate objects.

There are four gradually evolving phases in the development of stuttering:

- **Phase 1** occurs during the preschool period. Initially, the difficulty tends to be episodic and appears between long interludes of normal speech for weeks or months. A high percentage of recovery from these periods of stuttering occurs. During this phase, children often stutter when excited or upset, when they seem to have a great deal to say, and under other conditions of communicative pressure.

Table 4-5.
Childhood-Onset Fluency Disorder (Stuttering)

	DSM-5-TR	ICD-10	ICD-11
Diagnostic name	Childhood-Onset Fluency Disorder (Stuttering)	Stuttering (stammering)	Developmental Speech Fluency Disorder
Duration	Onset of symptoms during the developmental period		Onset of symptoms during the developmental period
Symptoms	Fluency and speech abnormalities as evidenced by: • Repetition of sounds and/or syllables • Prolonging sounds or consonants • Using broken words • Blocking or pausing • Frequent word substitution (circumlocution) • Excess physical tension during word production • Repeating monosyllabic words	Speech is characterized by repetition or prolongation of sounds or words or by frequent pauses, resulting in disruption or normal flow or rhythm of speech	Frequent or pervasive disruption of the normal rhythmic flow and rate of speech, including: • Repetitions and prolongations in sounds, syllables, words, and phrases • Blocking (inaudible or silent fixations or inability to initiate sounds) • Word avoidance or substitutions
Psychosocial Consequences	Causing severe anxiety and/ or impairment in areas of functioning		Limitations in communication affect social, academic, and occupational functioning
Exclusions	Result of: • Speech-motor or sensory issues • Neurologic injury • Another medical condition • Another mental disorder Note: Later-onset cases after the developmental period are coded as "adult-onset fluency disorder"	Result of: Tic disorders	Disorder of Intellectual Development Disease of the Nervous System Sensory impairment Structural abnormality

- **Phase 2** usually occurs in the elementary school years. The disorder is chronic, with few, if any, intervals of normal speech. Affected children become aware of their speech difficulties and regard themselves as stutterers. In phase 2, the stuttering occurs mainly with the significant parts of speech—nouns, verbs, adjectives, and adverbs.
- **Phase 3** usually appears after the age of 8 years and up to adulthood, most often in late childhood and early adolescence. During phase 3, stuttering comes mainly in response to specific situations, such as reciting in class, speaking to strangers, making purchases in stores, and using the telephone. Some words and sounds are more complex than others.
- **Phase 4** typically appears in late adolescence and adulthood.

Stutterers show vivid, fearful anticipation of stuttering. Words, sounds, and situations can all be intimidating. Word substitutions and circumlocutions are common. Stutterers avoid situations requiring speech and show other evidence of fear and embarrassment.

Stutterers may have associated clinical features: vivid, fearful anticipation of stuttering; avoidance of particular words, sounds, or situations in which stuttering is anticipated; and eye blinks, tics, and tremors of the lips or jaw. Frustration, anxiety, and depression are common among those with chronic stuttering.

Differential Diagnosis

Normal speech dysfluency in preschool years is challenging to differentiate from incipient stuttering. Stuttering causes more nonfluencies, part-word repetitions, sound prolongations, and disruptions in voice airflow through the vocal tract. Children who stutter appear tense and uncomfortable with their speech pattern, unlike young children who are nonfluent in their speech but seem to be at ease. Spastic dysphonia is a stuttering-like speech disorder distinguished from stuttering by the presence of an abnormal breathing pattern.

Cluttering is a speech disorder characterized by erratic and dysrhythmic speech patterns of rapid and jerky spurts of words and phrases. In cluttering, those affected are usually unaware of the disturbance, whereas, after the initial phase of the disorder, stutterers are aware of their speech difficulties. Cluttering is often an associated feature of expressive language disturbance.

Comorbidity

Very young children who stutter typically show some delay in language development and articulation without additional speech and language disorders. Preschoolers and school-age children who stutter exhibit an increased incidence of social anxiety, school refusal, and other anxiety symptoms. Older children who stutter also do not necessarily have comorbid speech and language disorders but often manifest anxiety symptoms and disorders. When stuttering persists into adolescence, social isolation occurs more than in the general adolescent population. Stuttering is associated with abnormal motor movements, upper body tics, and facial grimaces. Other disorders that coexist with stuttering include phonologic disorder, expressive language disorder, mixed receptive–expressive language disorder, and ADHD.

Course and Prognosis

Stuttering is often long-term, with periods of partial remission lasting for weeks or months and exacerbations occurring most frequently when a child is under pressure to communicate. In children with mild cases, 50% to 80% recover spontaneously. School-age children who stutter chronically may have impaired peer relationships as a result of teasing and social rejection. These children may face academic difficulties, especially if they persistently avoid speaking in class. Stuttering is associated with anxiety disorders in chronic cases, and approximately half of individuals with persistent stuttering have social anxiety disorder.

Treatment

There are several evidence-based treatments for stuttering. One such treatment is the Lidcombe Program, which uses an operant conditioning model in which parents use praise for periods in which the child does not stutter and intervene when the child does stutter to request the child to self-correct the stuttered word. This treatment program is primarily administered at home by parents, under the supervision of a speech and language therapist. A second treatment program in clinical trials is a family-based PCIT that identifies stressors possibly associated with increased stuttering and aims to diminish these stressors. A third treatment under investigation in clinical trials relies on the knowledge that speaking each syllable in time to a particular rhythm has reduced stuttering in adults. This treatment program appears promising when administered early on to preschoolers.

Distinct forms of interventions have historically helped stuttering. The first approach, direct speech therapy, targets modification of the stuttering response to fluent-sounding speech by systematic steps and rules of speech mechanics that the person can practice. The other form of therapy for stuttering targets diminishing tension and anxiety during speech. These treatments may utilize breathing exercises and relaxation techniques to help children slow their speaking rate and modulate speech volume. Relaxation techniques use the premise that it is nearly impossible to be relaxed and stutter in the usual manner simultaneously—current interventions for stuttering use individualized combinations of behavioral distraction, relaxation techniques, and directed speech modification.

Stutterers who have a poor self-image, comorbid anxiety disorders, or depressive disorders are likely to require additional treatments with cognitive-behavioral therapy (CBT) or pharmacologic agents such as one of the selective serotonin reuptake inhibitor (SSRI) antidepressants.

An approach to stuttering proposed by the Speech Foundation of America is labeled self-therapy, based on the premise that stuttering is not a symptom but a behavior that can be modified. Stutterers can learn to control their difficulty partly by modifying their feelings about stuttering and attitudes toward it and partly by modifying the deviant behaviors associated with their stuttering blocks. The approach includes desensitizing, reducing the emotional reaction to and fears of stuttering, and substituting positive action to control the moment of stuttering.

Epidemiology

An epidemiologic survey of 3- to 17-year-olds derived from the United States National Health Interview Surveys reports that the prevalence of stuttering is approximately 1.6%. Stuttering is most common in young children and often resolves spontaneously as the child ages. The typical age of onset is 2 to 7 years of age, with 90% of children exhibiting symptoms by age 7. Approximately 65% to 80% of young children who stutter will likely have spontaneous remission over time. According to the DSM-5-TR, the rate dips to 0.8% by adolescence. Stuttering affects about three to four males and every one female. The disorder is significantly more common among family members of affected children than in the general population. Reports suggest that for male persons who stutter, 20% of their male children and 10% of their female children will also stutter.

Etiology

Converging evidence indicates that the cause of stuttering is multifactorial, including genetic, neurophysiologic, and psychological factors predisposing a child to have poor speech fluency. Although research evidence does not indicate that anxiety or conflicts cause stuttering or that persons who stutter have more psychiatric disturbances than those with other forms of speech and language disorders, stressful situations can exacerbate stuttering.

Other theories about the cause of stuttering include organic models and learning models. Organic models include those that focus on incomplete lateralization or abnormal cerebral dominance. Several EEG studies found that stuttering males had right hemispheric α-suppression across stimulus words and tasks; nonstutterers had left hemispheric suppression. Some studies of stutterers have noted an overrepresentation of lefthandedness and ambidexterity. Twin studies and striking gender differences indicate that stuttering has some genetic basis.

Learning theories about the cause of stuttering include the semantogenic theory, in which stuttering is a learned response to normative early childhood disfluencies. Another learning model focuses on classical conditioning, in which stuttering becomes conditioned by environmental factors. In the cybernetic model, speech is a process that depends on appropriate feedback for regulation; stuttering is hypothesized to occur because of a breakdown in the feedback loop. The observations that white noise reduces stuttering and delayed auditory feedback produces stuttering in regular speakers support the feedback theory.

The motor functioning of some children who stutter appears to be delayed or slightly abnormal. Observing difficulties in speech planning exhibited by some children who stutter suggests that higher-level cognitive dysfunction may contribute to stuttering. Although children who stutter do not routinely exhibit other speech and language disorders, family members of these children often show an increased incidence of a variety of speech and language disorders. Interacting variables, including genetic and environmental factors, likely cause stuttering.

SOCIAL (PRAGMATIC) COMMUNICATION DISORDER

Social (pragmatic) communication disorder is a newly added diagnosis to DSM-5 characterized by persistent deficits in verbal and nonverbal communication for social purposes in the absence of restricted and repetitive interests and behaviors. Observable deficits include difficulty understanding and following social rules of language, gesture, and social context. This deficit may limit a child's ability to communicate effectively with peers in academic settings and family activities. For successful social and pragmatic communication, a child or adolescent must integrate gestures, language, and the social context of a given interaction to infer its meaning correctly. Thus, the child or adolescent must understand another speaker's "intention" in communicating with verbal and nonverbal cues. This understanding requires that they understand the environmental and social context of the interaction. One of the reasons DSM-5 introduced the diagnosis of social (pragmatic) communication disorder was to include those children with social communication impairment who do not exhibit restrictive and repetitive interests and behaviors and, therefore, do not fulfill the criteria for autism spectrum disorders. Pragmatic communication encompasses the ability to infer meaning in a given communication by understanding the words used and integrating the phrases into their prior understanding of the social environment. Social (pragmatic) communication disorder is new; however, the concept of children with social communication deficits without repetitive and restrictive interests and behaviors has been identified for many years and is often associated with delayed language acquisition and language disorder.

Clinical Features

Social (pragmatic) communication disorder is an impaired ability to use verbal and nonverbal communication for social purposes effectively and occurs without restricted and repetitive interests and behaviors. Although the preceding deficits begin in the early developmental period, we would rarely make the diagnosis in a child younger than 4 years of age. In milder cases, the difficulties may not become apparent until adolescence, with increased language and social understanding demands. The deficits in social communication lead to impairment in function in social situations, in developing relationships, and in family and academic settings.

Diagnosis

According to the DSM-5-TR, all the following features must be present to meet diagnostic criteria: (1) Deficits in using appropriate communication, such as greeting or sharing information in a social situation or context. (2) Impaired ability to modulate the tone, level, or vocabulary used in social communication to match the listener and the situation, such as the inability to simplify communication when speaking to a young child. (3) Impaired ability to follow the rules for conversations, such as taking turns or rephrasing a statement for clarification, and failure to recognize and respond socially appropriately to verbal and nonverbal feedback. (4) Difficulty understanding statements that are not explicit, impaired ability to make inferences, understand humor, or interpret socially ambiguous stimuli.

The diagnosis of social (pragmatic) communication disorder can be difficult to distinguish from mild variants of autism spectrum disorder in which repetitive and restricted interests and behaviors are minimal. There are discrepant data regarding how many children previously diagnosed with autism would be excluded from the DSM-5-TR criteria, which now focus on only two symptom domains: social communication deficits and restricted repetitive interests and behaviors. In one study, only 60.6% of children who had previously met the criteria for autistic spectrum disorder in the previous edition of the DSM met DSM-5-TR criteria for autistic spectrum disorder. However, in another study, up to 91% of patients with autism continued to meet the same DSM-5-TR criteria.

The essential features of social (pragmatic) communication disorder are persistently impaired social pragmatic communication, resulting in limited effective communication, compromised social relationships, and academic or occupational achievement difficulties.

Table 4-6 lists the diagnostic approach to social (pragmatic) communication disorder.

Differential Diagnosis

The primary diagnostic consideration in social (pragmatic) communication disorder is autism spectrum disorder. The two disorders are most easily distinguished when the prominence of restricted and repetitive interests

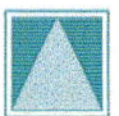

Table 4-6.
Social (Pragmatic) Communication Disorder

	DSM-5-TR	ICD-10	ICD-11
Diagnostic name	Social (Pragmatic) Communication Disorder	Developmental Disorder of Speech and Language, Unspecified	Listed as a specifier for Developmental Language Disorder (with impairment of mainly pragmatic language)
Symptoms	Difficulties with using verbal or nonverbal communication in social situations, as evidenced by: • Difficulty greeting others or sharing information with others • Difficulties matching tone or context in a conversation • Difficulty following social rules and expectations in conversations • Difficulties understanding implicit meaning in conversations Onset of symptoms in the early developmental period		
Psychosocial Consequences	Causing functional limitation		
Exclusions	Another medical or neurologic condition Autism spectrum disorder Intellectual disability or global developmental delay Another mental disorder		

and behaviors characteristic of autistic spectrum disorder is present. However, in many cases of autism, restrictive interests, and repetitive behaviors manifest more prominently in the early developmental period and are not apparent in older childhood. However, even when these features are not observable, if we can obtain them in the patient's history, we would diagnose autism rather than social (pragmatic) communication disorder. We should consider social (pragmatic) communication disorder only when restricted interests and repetitive behaviors have never been present. ADHD may overlap with a social (pragmatic) communication disorder in social communication disturbance; however, the core features of ADHD are not likely to be confused with autism spectrum disorder.

In some cases, however, the two disorders may coexist. Another childhood disorder with socially impairing symptoms that may overlap with social (pragmatic) communication disorder is social anxiety disorder. In social anxiety disorder, however, social communication skills are present but not manifested in feared social situations. Appropriate social communication skills are absent in social (pragmatic) communication disorder. Both social anxiety disorder and social (pragmatic) communication disorder may occur comorbidly, however, and children with social (pragmatic) communication disorder may be at higher risk for social anxiety disorder. Finally, intellectual disability may be confused with social (pragmatic) communication disorder in that social communication skills may be deficit in children with intellectual disability. We should only make a diagnosis of social (pragmatic) communication disorder when social communication skills are more severe than intellectual disability.

Comorbidity

Social (pragmatic) communication disorder is commonly associated with language disorder, consisting of diminished vocabulary for expected age, deficits in receptive skills, and impaired ability to use expressive language. ADHD is often concurrent with social (pragmatic) communication disorder. Specific learning disorders with impairments in reading and writing are also commonly comorbid disorders with social (pragmatic) communication disorder. Although some symptoms of social anxiety disorder may overlap with social (pragmatic) communication disorder, the full disorder of social anxiety disorder may emerge comorbidly with social (pragmatic) communication disorder.

Course and Prognosis

The course and outcome of social (pragmatic) communication disorder are highly variable and dependent on both the severity of the disorder and potential interventions administered. By age 5 years, most children demonstrate enough speech and language to discern the presence of deficits in social communication. However, in the milder forms of the disorder, social communication deficits may not be identified until adolescence, when language and social interactions are sufficiently complex that deficits stand out. Many children significantly improve over time; however, some early pragmatic deficits may cause lasting impairment in social relationships and academic progress. There is a newly growing body of investigations on therapeutic interventions that may affect future outcomes of social (pragmatic) communication disorder.

Treatment

There is little data to date to inform an evidence-based treatment for social (pragmatic) communication disorder or to sufficiently distinguish it from other disorders with overlapping symptoms, such as autism spectrum disorder, ADHD, and social anxiety disorder. A randomized controlled trial (RCT) of a social communication intervention explicitly directed at children with social (pragmatic) communication disorder aimed at three areas of communication: (1) social understanding and social interaction; (2) verbal and nonverbal pragmatic skills, including conversation; and (3) language processing, involving making inferences, and learning new words. Although the primary outcome measure in this study did not show significant differences for the intervention group versus the "treatment as usual" group, there were several ratings by parents and teachers demonstrating potential improvements in social communication skills after a 20-session intensive intervention for social (pragmatic) communication disorder. Continued investigation is necessary to validate the preceding results and promote evidence-based treatments for children with social (pragmatic) communication disorder.

Epidemiology

Estimating the prevalence of social (pragmatic) communication disorder is complex. Nevertheless, a body of literature has documented a profile of children who present with these persistent difficulties in pragmatic language and who do not meet the criteria for autism spectrum disorder.

Etiology

A family history of communication disorders, autism spectrum disorder, or specific learning disorder all appear to increase the risk for social (pragmatic) communication disorder. This increased risk suggests that genetic influences contribute to this disorder's development. The etiology of social (pragmatic) communication disorder, however, is likely to be multifactorial, and given its frequent comorbidity with both language disorder and ADHD, developmental and environmental influences are also likely to play a role.

UNSPECIFIED COMMUNICATION DISORDER

Disorders that do not meet the diagnostic criteria for any specific communication disorder fall into the category of unspecified communication disorder. An example is voice disorder, in which the patient has an abnormality in pitch, loudness, quality, tone, or resonance. The voice abnormality must be sufficiently severe to impair academic achievement or social communication to be a disorder. Operationally, speech production includes five interacting subsystems, including respiration (airflow from the lungs), phonation (sound generation in the larynx), resonance (shaping of the sound quality in the pharynx and nasal cavity), articulation (modulation of the sound stream into consonant and vowel sounds with the tongue, jaw, and lips), and suprasegmentals (speech rhythm, loudness, and intonation). These systems work together, and voice quality conveys information about the speaker's emotional, psychological, and physical status. Thus, voice abnormalities can cover a broad area of communication and indicate many different abnormalities.

Cluttering is not a disorder in the DSM-5-TR, but it is an associated speech abnormality in which a disturbed rate and rhythm of speech impair intelligibility. ICD-10 does include it as a behavioral disorder usually occurring in childhood or adolescence. ICD-11 lists it as an alternative term for Developmental Speech Fluency Disorder.

Cluttering speech is erratic and dysrhythmic and consists of rapid, jerky spurts inconsistent with standard phrasing patterns. The disorder usually occurs in children between 2 and 8 years of age; in two-thirds of cases, the patient recovers spontaneously by early adolescence. Cluttering is associated with learning disorders and other communication disorders.

Further Readings

Adams C, Lockton E, Freed J, et al. The Social Communication Intervention Project: a randomized controlled trial of the effectiveness of speech and language therapy for school-age children who have pragmatic and social communication problems with or without autism spectrum disorder. *Int J Lang Commun Disord.* 2012;47:233–244.

Allen J, Marshall CR. Parent-Child Interaction Therapy (PCIT) in school-aged children with specific language impairment. *Int J Lang Commun Disord.* 2011;46:397–410.

Bressman T, Unspecified communication disorder. In: Boland RJ, Verduin ML, eds. *Kaplan & Sadock's Comprehensive Textbook of Psychiatry.* 11th ed. Wolters Kluwer; 2024.

Cantwell DP, Baker LP. *Psychiatric and Developmental Disorders in Children with Communication Disorders.* American Psychiatric Press; 1991.

Gibson J, Adams C, Lockton E, Green J. Social communication disorder outside autism? A diagnostic classification approach to delineating pragmatic language impairment, high functioning autism and specific language impairment. *J Child Psychol Psychiatry.* 2013;54:1186–1197.

Huerta M, Bishop SL, Duncan A, Hus V, Lord C. Application of DSM-5 criteria for autism spectrum disorder to three samples of children with DSM-IV diagnoses of pervasive developmental disorders. *Am J Psychiatry.* 2012;169:1056–1064.

Jones M, Onslow M, Packman A, et al. Extended follow-up of a randomized controlled trial of the Lidcombe Program of Early Stuttering Intervention. *Int J Lang Commun Disord.* 2008;43:649–661.

Kant T, Koyama E, Ashraf M, Kennedy JL. Language disorder In: Boland RJ, Verduin ML, eds. *Kaplan & Sadock's Comprehensive Textbook of Psychiatry.* 11th ed. Wolters Kluwer; 2024.

Kass M, Kim YS, Leventhal B. Social (pragmatic) communication disorder. In: Boland RJ, Verduin ML, eds. *Kaplan & Sadock's Comprehensive Textbook of Psychiatry.* 11th ed. Wolters Kluwer; 2024.

Koyama E, Ashraf M, Kant T, Kennedy JL. Speech sound disorder. In: Boland RJ, Verduin ML, eds. *Kaplan & Sadock's Comprehensive Textbook of Psychiatry.* 11th ed. Wolters Kluwer; 2024.

Koyama E, Ashraf M, Kennedy JL, Kant T. Stuttering. In: Boland RJ, Verduin ML, eds. *Kaplan & Sadock's Comprehensive Textbook of Psychiatry*. 11th ed. Wolters Kluwer; 2024.

Latterman C, Euler HA, Neumann K. A randomized control trial to investigate the impact of the lidcombe program on early stuttering in German-speaking preschoolers. *J Fluency Disord*. 2008;33: 52–65.

Law J, Dennis JA, Charlton JJV. Speech and language therapy interventions for children with primary speech and/or language delay or disorder. *Cochrane Database Syst Rev*. 2017;(1):CD012490.

McPartland JC, Reichow B, Volkmar FR. Sensitivity and specificity of the proposed DMS-5 diagnostic criteria for autism spectrum disorder. *J Am Acad Child Adolesc Psychiatry*. 2012;51:368–383.

Millard SK, Nicholas A, Cook FM. Is parent-child interaction therapy effective in reducing stuttering? *J Speech Lang Hear Res*. 2008;51: 636–650.

Norbury CF. Practitioner review: social (pragmatic) communication disorder conceptualization, evidence and clinical implications. *J Child Psychol Psychiatry*. 2014;55(3):204–216.

Onslow M, O'Brien S. Management of childhood stuttering. *J Paediatr Child Health*. 2013;49:E112–E115.

Petursdottir AI, Carr JE. A review of recommendations for sequencing receptive and expressive language instruction. *J Appl Behav Anal*. 2011; 44:859–876.

Ramus F, Marshall CR, Rosen S, van der Lely HKJ. Phonological deficits in specific language impairment and developmental dyslexia: towards a multidimensional model. *Brain*. 2012;136:630–645.

Reilly S, Wake M, Ukoumunne OC, et al. Predicting language outcomes at 4 years of age: findings from early language in Victoria study. *Pediatrics*. 2010;126:e1530–e1537.

Reisinger LM, Cornish KM, Fombonne E. Diagnostic differentiation of autism spectrum disorders and pragmatic language impairment. *J Autism Dev Disord*. 2011;41:1694–1704.

Snowling MJ, Hulme C. Interventions for children's language and literacy difficulties. *Int J Commun Discord*. 2012;47:27–34.

Trajkovski N, Andrews C, Onslow M, O'Brian S, Packman A, Menzies R. A phase II trial of the Westmead Program: syllable-timed speech treatment for pre-school children who stutter. *Int J Speech Lang Pathol*. 2011;13:500–509.

Wake M, Levickis P, Tobin S, et al. Improving outcomes of preschool language delay in the community: protocol for the language for learning randomized controlled trial. *BMC Pediatr*. 2012;12:96.

Wake M, Tobin S, Girolametto L, et al. Outcomes of population based language promotion for slow to talk toddlers at ages 2 and 3 years: Let's Learn Language cluster randomised clinical trial. *BMJ*. 2011;343:d4741.

Yaruss JS, Coleman CE, Quesal RW. Stuttering in school-age children: a comprehensive approach to treatment. *Lang Speech Hear Serv Sch*. 2012;43:536–548.

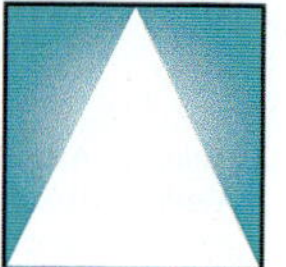

5 Autism Spectrum Disorder

Autism spectrum disorder (ASD) describes a wide range of impairments in social communication and interaction and restricted and/or repetitive behaviors or interests. Symptoms must be present in the early developmental period. All three of the symptoms in the "persistent deficits in social communication and social interaction" criterion, and at least two symptoms in the "restricted, repetitive patterns of behavior, interests or activities" criterion are necessary to meet the diagnosis of ASD according to DSM-5-TR. According to DSM-5-TR, symptoms of ASD must cause functional impairment, and the symptoms are not better explained by intellectual disability alone. ASD is a phenotypically heterogeneous group of neurodevelopmental syndromes, with polygenic heritability. In 2013, with the release of the DSM 5th edition, five disorders with overlapping symptoms were reclassified by the American Psychiatric Association as ASD; these included: autistic disorder, Asperger disorder, childhood disintegrative disorder, Rett syndrome, and pervasive developmental disorder not otherwise specified. These differ by the level of severity, specific syndrome, and in some cases underlying pathology. The ICD-10 diagnosis Pervasive Disorder of Development includes similar criteria as does the ICD-11 ASD. However, the recent clinical consensus has shifted the conceptualization of ASD toward a continuum model in which heterogeneity of symptoms is inherent in the disorder. Prior to DSM-5, an additional criterion of at least one symptom demonstrating qualitative impairment of communication was necessary for the diagnosis of Autistic Disorder. The DSM-5 collapsed the core diagnostic impairments into two domains: deficits in social communication, and restricted and repetitive behaviors. Aberrant language development and usage are no longer considered a core feature of ASD. This diagnostic change is based, in part, on studies in siblings with diagnoses of autistic disorder, suggesting that symptom domains may be transmitted separately and that aberrant language development and usage is not a defining feature, but an associated feature in some individuals with ASD. ASD is typically evident during the second year of life, and in some cases, a lack of developmentally appropriate interest in social interactions may be noted even in the first year. Some studies suggest that a decline in social interaction may ensue between the first and second years of life. In milder cases, core impairments in ASD may not be identified for several more years. Although language impairment is not a core diagnostic criterion in ASD, clinicians and parents share concerns about a child who, by 12 to 18 months, has not developed any language, and delayed language accompanied by diminished social behavior are frequently the heralding symptoms in ASD. In up to 25% of cases of ASD, some language develops and is subsequently lost. ASD in children with normal intellectual function and mild impairment in language function may not be identified until middle childhood when both academic and social demands increase. Children with ASD often exhibit intense, idiosyncratic interest in a narrow range of activities, resist change, and do not respond to their social environment typically compared to their peers. Approximately one-third of children who meet the DSM-5 criteria for ASD show intellectual disability.

Diagnoses of the five disorders that were previously recognized as distinct before DSM-5 are no longer used, and those diagnoses are currently folded into the ASD diagnosis in DSM-5-TR. The previous *Rett disorder* occurred exclusively in females and is characterized by normal development for at least 6 months, followed by stereotyped hand movements, a loss of purposeful motions, diminishing social engagement, poor coordination, and decreasing language use. In the formerly labeled *childhood disintegrative disorder,* development progresses normally for approximately 2 years, after which the child shows a loss of previously acquired skills in two or more of the following areas: language use, social responsiveness, play, motor skills, and bladder or bowel control. The former *Asperger disorder* is an impairment in social relatedness and repetitive and stereotyped patterns of behavior without delay or marked aberrant language development and usage. In Asperger disorder, cognitive abilities and significant adaptive skills are age-appropriate, although social communication is impaired. A survey of children undertaken with the former ASDs revealed that the average age of diagnosis was 3.1 years for children with autistic disorder, 3.9 years for children diagnosed with pervasive developmental disorder not otherwise specified, and 7.2 years for those youth with Asperger disorder. Children with ASD who exhibited severe language deficits received an ASD diagnosis, on average, a year earlier than children without impairment in language. Children with ASD who exhibited repetitive behaviors such as hand-flapping, toe-walking, and odd play were diagnosed with ASDs at a younger age than those who did not exhibit such behaviors. The current DSM-5-TR ASD criteria provide specifiers for the level of support needed based on the severity of the main domains of impairment, and also specifiers for the presence or absence of language impairment and intellectual impairment.

DIAGNOSIS AND CLINICAL FEATURES

Table 5-1 describes the DSM-5-TR, ICD-10, and ICD-11 diagnostic approaches to ASD.

Core Symptoms of Autism Spectrum Disorder

Persistent Deficits in Social Communication and Interaction. Children with ASD characteristically do not conform to the expected level and quality

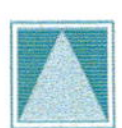

Table 5-1.
Autism Spectrum Disorder

	DSM-5-TR	ICD-10	ICD-11
Diagnostic name	Autism Spectrum Disorder	Childhood Autism	Autism Spectrum Disorder
Symptoms	Symptoms of difficulties/deficits in social interaction, as evidenced by: • Deficits in emotional reciprocity or failure to respond appropriately in social interactions • Deficits in nonverbal communication, eye contact, body language/gesturing, and/or facial expression • Deficits in forming, developing, or maintaining relationships or friendships Restricted and/or repetitive behaviors or interests, such as in: • Stereotyped motor movements • Inflexibility with regard to daily routines or rituals • Restricted or fixed interests • Hyper- or hyporeactivity to sensations or sensory stimuli Symptoms present in the early developmental period	Pervasive disorder of development involving • Abnormal development present before the age of 3 • Abnormal social functioning, communication, and repetitive/restricted behaviors	Persistent deficits in initiating and sustaining social communication and interactions outside the range for that age. May include limitations in: • Understanding or responding to verbal or nonverbal communication • Understanding or using language in a social context • Social awareness • Ability to imagine or respond to feelings • Mutual sharing of interests • Ability to make and sustain peer relationships Persistent restricted, repetitive, and inflexible patterns of behavior, interests, or activities that are inappropriate or excessive for the social context. These may include persistent: • Lack of adaptability to new experiences or circumstances • Inflexible adherence to routines • Excess adherence to rules • Excess and persistent ritualized patterns of behavior • Repetitive and stereotyped motor movement • Preoccupation with ≥1 special interests, parts of objects, or stimuli • Hyper- or hyposensitivity to sensory stimuli or unusual interest in the stimuli
Required number of symptoms	All three of the above criteria met		
Psychosocial consequences	Marked impairment in functioning		Marked impairment in functioning
Exclusions	Result of: • Intellectual disability • Global developmental delay		Rett syndrome

(continued)

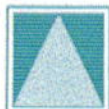

Table 5-1.
Autism Spectrum Disorder (Continued)

	DSM-5-TR	ICD-10	ICD-11
Symptoms specifiers	With or without accompanying intellectual impairment With or without accompanying language impairment Associated with another neurodevelopmental, mental, or behavioral disorder With catatonia		With or without accompanying intellectual impairment With or without accompanying language impairment • with mild or no impairment of functional language • with impaired functional language • with complete, or almost complete, absence of functional language
Severity specifiers	For social impairment: **Mild, Moderate, Severe** For behavior patterns: **Mild, Moderate, Severe**		
		NOTE: Atypical autism—symptoms do not meet all diagnostic criteria for childhood autism NOTE: Asperger Syndrome—difficulties in social interaction similar to that found in Autism, in addition to restricted interests; however, no deficits in language or cognition are seen	

of reciprocal social skills and spontaneous nonverbal social interactions. Infants with ASD may not develop a social smile, and as older babies may not reach up to indicate desire to be picked up by a primary caregiver or attachment figure. Less frequent and poor eye contact is common during childhood and adolescence compared to other children. The social development of children with ASD is characterized by atypical attachment behavior. For example, children with ASD may not explicitly acknowledge or differentiate the most influential persons in their lives—parents, siblings, and teachers—and on the other hand, may not react as strongly to being left with a stranger compared to other children of their age. Children with ASD often feel and display extreme anxiety when someone disrupts their usual routine. By the time children with this disorder reach school age, their social skills may have increased, and social withdrawal may be less obvious, particularly in children without intellectual disability, deficits in spontaneous play with peers and in subtle social abilities that promote developing friendships may be palpable. The social behavior of children with ASD is often awkward and may be inappropriate. In school-age children, social impairments may emerge in the form of awkward conversation, fewer shared interests with same age peers, and fewer body and facial gestures during conversations. Cognitively, children with ASD are frequently more skilled in visual–spatial tasks than in tasks requiring skill in verbal reasoning.

One area of particular difficulty in children with ASD is an impaired ability to infer or recognize the feelings or emotional state of peers and adults around them. The limited ability to recognize and surmise the emotional state of others (theory of mind) leads to difficulty with making attributions about the motivation or intentions of others and difficulty developing empathy. The compromised capacity for "theory of mind" limits children with ASD in interpreting the social behavior of others and exacerbates their poor social reciprocation.

Individuals with ASD generally desire friendships, and higher-functioning children may be aware that their poor skills in responding to the emotions and feelings of their peers are significant obstacles in making and keeping friends. Children with ASD are often shunned by peers, who are seeking to share mainstream activities and experience children with ASD as awkward and alienating. Adolescents and adults with ASD often desire romantic relationships, and for some, their increase in social competence and skills over time enables them to develop long-term relationships.

Restricted, Repetitive Patterns of Behavior, Interests, and Activities. From the first years of life in a child with ASD, developmentally expected exploratory play is restricted and muted. They may not use toys and objects in a typical manner. Instead, they often manipulate the toys in a ritualistic manner, with fewer symbolic features. Children with ASD typically don't show the level of imitative play or abstract pantomime that other children of their age exhibit spontaneously. The activities and play of children with ASD may appear more rigid, repetitive, and monotonous than their peers. Ritualistic and compulsive behaviors are common in early and middle childhood. Children with ASD often seem to enjoy spinning, banging objects, or watching water flow. Compulsive behaviors are not uncommon among children with ASD, such as lining up objects, and not infrequently a child with ASD may exhibit a strong attachment to a particular inanimate object. Children with ASD who are severely intellectually disabled have increased rates of self-stimulatory and self-injurious behaviors. Stereotypies, mannerisms, and grimacing emerge most frequently when a child with ASD is in a less-structured situation. Children with ASD often find transitions and change intimidating. Moving to a new house, rearranging furniture in a room, or even a change such as eating a meal before a bath when the reverse was the routine, may evoke panic, fear, or temper tantrums in a child with ASD.

Associated Physical Characteristics. At first glance, children with ASD do not show any particular physical signs indicating the disorder. Children with ASD, overall, do exhibit higher rates of minor physical anomalies, such as ear malformations, and others that may reflect abnormalities in fetal development of those organs along with parts of the brain.

A higher-than-expected number of children with ASD do not show early handedness and lateralization and remain ambidextrous longer than most children establish cerebral dominance. Children with ASD may have a higher incidence of abnormal dermatoglyphics (e.g., fingerprints) than those in the general population. This finding may suggest a disturbance in neuroectodermal development.

Associated Behavioral Symptoms that May Occur in Autism Spectrum Disorder

Disturbances in Language Development and Usage. Deficits in language development and difficulty using language to communicate ideas are no longer among the core criteria for diagnosing ASD; however, they occur in a significant subset of those individuals with ASD. Overall, approximately 20% to 25% of children with ASD may have language acquisition delays and/or difficulties with pragmatic use of language. Some children with ASD are not merely reluctant to speak, and their speech abnormalities do not result from a lack of motivation. Language deviance, as much as language delay, is characteristic of more severe subtypes of ASD. Children with more severe forms of ASD have significant difficulty putting meaningful sentences together, even when they have extensive vocabularies. When children with ASD with delayed language learn to converse fluently, their conversations may impart information without typical prosody or inflection.

In the first year of life, a typical pattern of babbling may be minimal or absent. Some children with ASD vocalize noises—clicks, screeches, or nonsense syllables—in a stereotyped fashion, without a seeming intent of communication. Unlike most young children, who generally have better receptive language skills than expressive ones, children with ASD may express more than they understand. Words and even entire sentences may drop in and out of a child's vocabulary. It is not atypical for a child with ASD to use a word once and then not use it again for a week, a month, or years. Children with ASD may exhibit speech that contains echolalia, both immediate and delayed, or stereotyped phrases that seem out of context. These language patterns are frequently associated with pronoun reversals. A child with autistic disorder might say, "You want the toy" when she means that she wants it. Difficulties in articulation are also common. Many children with autistic disorder use peculiar voice quality and rhythm. About 25% of children with more severe forms of ASD never develop useful speech. Some of the brightest children show a particular fascination with letters and numbers. Children with ASD sometimes excel in specific tasks or have special abilities; for example, a child may learn to read fluently at preschool age (hyperlexia), often astonishingly well. Very young children with ASD who can read many words, however, have little comprehension of the words read.

Intellectual Disability. Rates of intellectual disability in epidemiologic studies of youth with ASD have varied with the specific samples surveyed in the study and time frame. According to the Centers for Disease Control and Prevention (CDC) in 2023, about 31% of youth with ASD have an intellectual disability with an IQ <70 and limitations in adaptive function leading to interference with everyday life. Approximately 44% have IQ scores in the average to above average range. Approximately 25% of children with ASD have intellectual function in the low average range. About 10% of children with ASD have severe to profound intellectual disability. The IQ scores of children with ASD and intellectual disability tend to reflect relatively lower scores in verbal sequencing and abstraction skills, with relative strengths in visuospatial or rote memory skills. This finding highlights the importance of deficits in language-related functions in youth with ASD.

Irritability. Broadly defined, irritability includes aggression, self-injurious behaviors, and severe temper tantrums. These phenomena are common in children and adolescents with ASD. Severe temper tantrums may be difficult to subdue, and self-injurious behaviors are often problematic to control. Everyday situations can cause these symptoms in which one would expect a youth to transition from one activity to another, sit in a classroom setting, or remain still when they desire to run around. In children with ASD who are lower functioning and have intellectual deficits, aggression may emerge unexpectedly without an obvious trigger or purpose, and self-injurious behaviors such as head banging, skin picking, and biting oneself may also occur.

Instability of Mood and Affect. Some children with ASD exhibit sudden mood changes, with bursts of laughing or crying without an apparent reason. It is difficult to learn more about these episodes if the child cannot express the thoughts related to the affect.

Response to Sensory Stimuli. Children with ASD may overrespond to some stimuli and under respond to other sensory stimuli (e.g., to sound and pain). It is not uncommon for a child with ASD to at times show little response to a normal speaking voice; on the other hand, the same child may show intent interest in the sound of a wristwatch or running water. Some children have a heightened pain threshold or an altered response to pain. Some children with ASD do not respond to an injury by crying or seeking comfort. Some youth with ASD perseverate on a sensory experience; for example, they frequently hum a tune or sing a song or commercial jingle before saying words or using speech. It is frequent to observe children and adolescents with ASD repetitively engaging in vestibular stimulation such as spinning, swinging, and up-and-down movements.

Hyperactivity and Inattention. Hyperactivity and inattention are both common symptoms in children with ASD. Periods of lower than average activity level may alternate with hyperactivity. Short attention span and poor ability to focus on a task may interfere with daily functioning.

Precocious Skills. Some individuals especially with higher functioning ASD display precocious or splinter skills of high proficiency, such as prodigious rote memories or calculating abilities beyond the capabilities of their conventional peers. Other potential precocious abilities in some children with ASD include hyperlexia, an early ability to read well (even when they cannot understand the meaning of what is read), memorizing and reciting, and musical abilities (singing or playing tunes or recognizing musical pieces).

Insomnia. Insomnia is a frequent sleep problem among children and adolescents with ASD, estimated to occur in about 40% to 80% of school-age children.

Minor Infections and Gastrointestinal Symptoms. Young children with ASD may have a higher-than-expected incidence of upper respiratory infections and other minor infections. They may also have febrile seizures. Others do not become febrile when they have a minor infection, and may not display the typical malaise. Children with ASD are at high risk for many gastrointestinal symptoms. These include such symptoms as excessive burping, constipation, and loose bowel movements. In other children, behavior problems and relatedness seem to improve noticeably during a minor illness, and in some, such changes in behavior are a clue to physical illness.

Assessment Tools

A standardized instrument that can be very helpful in eliciting comprehensive information, associated with ASD. The Autism Diagnostic Observation Schedule-2 (ADOS-2) elicits information with respect to communication, social interaction, play, and restricted and repetitive behaviors. In conjunction with a clinical diagnosis, the ADOS-2 is highly sensitive for endorsing ASD.

Jessie was the second child born to parents in their early 40s who were computer programmers. As an infant, Jessie was relatively placid. His parents noted but were not concerned that, in contrast to his older brother who smiled at 2 months, Jessie did not develop a social smile by 4 months. Jessie's parents were comforted by his appropriate motor skills development and healthy appetite and weight gain. Jessie's parents first became concerned about his development when he was 18 months of age and still not speaking words, whereas his brother had some words at 12 months, and by 18 months, his brother could put two words together. In his daycare, where he spent the day while his parents worked, the daycare workers noted that, in comparison to other toddlers in his daycare, Jessie seemed less interested in social interaction and did not participate in social games with the other toddlers and daycare workers. Jessie would become extremely upset if his usual daycare worker was not present and would tantrum until the daycare called his mother to bring him home. Jessie's pediatrician initially reassured his parents that he was just a "late talker" and would catch up. When Jessie was 24 months old and still not speaking, he was referred for a developmental evaluation. At 24 months, motor skills were age-appropriate. Jessie's language and social development, however, were noticeably delayed; he was noted to get extremely upset if his daily routine was changed and he was unusually sensitive to aspects of the inanimate environment. Jessie's play skills were quite limited, and he played with toys in repetitive and idiosyncratic ways. At 3 years of age, Jessie received a developmental assessment using measures of, intellectual function and adaptive function and the Autism Diagnostic Observation Schedule, Second Edition (ADOS-2) was administered. Genetic screening and chromosome analysis were also obtained on Jessie.

Jessie was diagnosed with ASD, and he started a special education program and over time gradually began to speak in words and sentences. His speech was extremely literal and characterized by robotic-sounding speech alternating with sing-song speech. Jessie displayed pronoun reversals, such as saying "you want something" when he meant "I want something," and recurrent echolalia in which he repeated a phrase that was recently spoken to him. Jessie was able to make his needs known verbally, although his language was odd. As Jessie grew older, other children began to avoid playing with him, partly because he didn't use phrases typical for his peers and seemed to be a know-it-all at other times. Jessie pursued mainly solo activities and remained isolated. By age 5 years, Jessie was clingy and attached to his mother and often became anxious and upset when she went out, exhibiting severe tantrums. Jessie displayed several self-stimulatory behaviors, such as waving his fingers in front of his eyes and rocking his body. Intelligence testing revealed a full-scale IQ in the average range with relative weakness in the verbal subtests compared to the performance subtests. When he was 5 years old, Jessie began Applied Behavior Analysis (ABA) therapy to help him improve communication skills, social skills, and reduce tantrum behaviors. Jessie benefited from ABA when he was 5 years old, but by the time he was in fourth grade, Jessie began to have severe behavioral outbursts at school and at home under the pressure of the social and academic demands at school. Jessie was unable to complete his classwork and would get out of his seat and wander around the classroom. When his teacher would insist that he remain seated, he would begin to tantrum inappropriately for his age. Jessie would sometimes begin screaming so loudly that he had to leave the classroom. He would then become upset, aggressive, and throw all of his books off his desk in a rage, sometimes inadvertently hitting other students. It often took him up to 2 hours to calm down. At home, Jessie would fly into a tantrum if anyone moved his things, and he would become belligerent when asked to do anything that was not an expected part of his daily routine. By the time Jessie had completed the fifth grade, it became clear that he was barely manageable in his school setting. At 10 years old, Jessie was evaluated by a child and adolescent psychiatrist who recommended a social skills group for him and prescribed Concerta, hoping to mitigate his impulsivity and tantrum behaviors. Jessie's tantrums became less frequent and less severe. He seemed calmer and did not become physically out of control during tantrums. Jessie continued in middle school in a combination of special education classes and regular classes. Jessie's social skills group was helpful in terms of teaching him how to approach peers in ways that would lead to less rejection. Jessie had made some acquaintances, however, by the eighth grade, the impending move to high school had caused a decompensation and he became irritable, belligerent, angry, and defiant. It was difficult to manage him at home and in school, and his tantrums now potentially caused a danger to himself and others. He was reevaluated by his child and adolescent psychiatrist and a small dose of risperidone was added to the Concerta, which seemed to keep him calmer and more functional. When Jessie started high school, he made two acquaintances similar to himself who would come to his home and play video games with him. Jessie often played online computer games with virtual peers. Jessie knew that he was different from typical students, but he was able to find some peers within the virtual gaming world. Jessie continued in high school with a combination of special and regular education and made plans to attend a community college and live at home for the first year after high school. (Adapted from Fred Volkmar, M.D.)

DIFFERENTIAL DIAGNOSIS

Disorders to consider in the differential diagnosis of ASD include social (pragmatic) communication disorder, the newly described DSM-5 communication disorder; schizophrenia with childhood-onset; congenital deafness or severe hearing disorder; and psychosocial deprivation. It is also challenging to make the diagnosis of ASD because of its potentially overlapping symptoms with childhood schizophrenia, intellectual disability syndromes with behavioral symptoms, and language disorders. Given the many concurrent problems often encountered in ASD, Michael Rutter and Lionel Hersov suggested a stepwise approach to the differential diagnosis.

Social (Pragmatic) Communication Disorder

Patients with this disorder, which is within the category of language disorders, have difficulty with typical storytelling and understanding the rules of social communication through language, exemplified by a lack of conventional greeting of others, taking turns in a conversation, and responding to verbal and nonverbal cues of a listener. Other forms of language impairment may accompany social communication disorder, such as delay in learning language or expressive and receptive difficulties. Social communication disorder occurs with higher frequency in relatives of individuals with ASD, which increases the difficulty in discriminating this disorder from ASD. Although relationships may be negatively affected by social communication disorder, this disorder does not include restricted or repetitive behaviors and interests, as ASD does.

Childhood-Onset Schizophrenia

Schizophrenia is rare in children younger than 12 years and almost nonexistent before the age of 5 years. Characterized by hallucinations or delusions, childhood-onset schizophrenia has a lower incidence of seizures and intellectual disability, and poor social skills. Table 5-2 compares ASD and schizophrenia with childhood onset.

Intellectual Disability with Behavioral Symptoms

Children with intellectual disability but without a diagnosis of ASD may exhibit behavioral symptoms that

Table 5-2.
Autism Spectrum Disorder versus Childhood-Onset Schizophrenia

Criteria	Autism Spectrum Disorder	Schizophrenia (with Onset before Puberty)
Age of onset	Early developmental period	Rarely under the age of 5
Incidence	1%	<1 in 10,000
Sex ratio (M:F)	4:1	1.67:1 (slight preponderance of males)
Family history of schizophrenia	Not increased	Likely Increased
Prenatal and perinatal complications	Increased	Not increased
Behavioral characteristics	Poor social relatedness; may have aberrant language, speech or echolalia; stereotyped phrases; may have stereotypies, repetitive behaviors	Hallucinations and delusions; thought disorder
Adaptive functioning	Impaired	Deterioration in functioning
Level of intelligence	Wide range, may be intellectually disabled (30%)	Usually within normal range, may be low average normal
Pattern of IQ	Typical higher visuospatial performance scores than verbal scores	More even
Grand mal seizures	4–32%	Low incidence

overlap with some ASD features. The main differentiating features between ASD and intellectual disability are that children with intellectual disability syndromes generally display similar levels of global impairments in both verbal and nonverbal areas. In contrast, children with ASD are noticeably weaker in social interactions compared to other areas of performance and often have odd language usage. Children with intellectual disability generally relate verbally and socially to adults and peers in ways that are reminiscent of their mental age, not their chronologic age, but they exhibit a relatively even profile of limitations across various skills and domains.

Language Disorder

Some children with language disorders also have ASD features, which may present a diagnostic challenge. Table 5-3 summarizes the significant differences between ASD and language disorders.

Congenital Deafness or Hearing Impairment

Because children with ASD may appear mute or lack language development, we should rule out hearing impairment or congenital deafness. Differentiating factors include

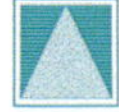

Table 5-3.
Autism Spectrum Disorder versus Language Disorder

Criteria	Autism Spectrum Disorder	Language Disorder
Incidence	1%	5 of 10,000
Sex ratio (M:F)	4:1	Equal or almost equal sex ratio
Family history of speech delay or language problems	<25% cases	<25% cases
Associated deafness	Very infrequent	Not infrequent
Nonverbal communication (e.g., gestures)	Impaired	Actively utilized
Language abnormalities (e.g., echolalia, stereotyped phrases out of context)	Present in a subset	Uncommon
Articulation problems	Infrequent	Frequent
Intellectual level	Impaired in a subset (about 30%)	Uncommon, less frequently severe
Patterns of intelligence quotient (IQ) tests	Typically lower on verbal scores than performance scores	Often verbal scores lower than performance scores
Impaired social communication, restricted and repetitive behaviors	Present	Absent or, if present, mild
Imaginative play	Often impaired	Usually intact

the following: infants with ASD may babble only infrequently, whereas deaf infants often have a history of relatively normal babbling that then gradually tapers off and may stop at 6 months to 1 year of age. Deaf children generally respond only to loud sounds, whereas children with ASD may ignore loud or normal sounds and respond to soft or low sounds. Most importantly, an audiogram or auditory-evoked potentials indicate a significant hearing loss in deaf children. Deaf children usually seek out nonverbal social communication with regularity and seek social interactions with peers and family members more consistently than children with ASD.

Psychosocial Deprivation

Severe neglect, maltreatment, and lack of parental care can lead to a child displaying apathy and withdrawn mood and behavior. Children who have endured early periods of maltreatment may have delayed language and motor skills. Children with language and motor delay that is not attributable to other causes such as in utero exposure to substances, intellectual disability, or medical illness generally improve when placed in favorable and enriched psychosocial environments. Some children with aberrant social behaviors are attributable to ASD may not improve significantly in enriched environments; however, most children with ASD develop some greater social skills and increased verbal abilities over time when provided with therapeutic interventions.

COURSE AND PROGNOSIS

ASD is typically a lifelong disorder with highly variable severity which impacts degree of learned improvements over time and overall prognosis. Children with ASD and IQs above 70 and with average adaptive skills, who develop communicative language by ages 5 to 7 years, have the best prognoses. A longitudinal study comparing symptoms in children with high-IQ ASD at the age of 5 years, and again at 13 years and older found that a small proportion no longer met criteria for ASD over time. Most of these youth demonstrated positive changes in communication and social skills over time. Early intensive behavioral interventions (BIs) can provide a profound positive impact on children with ASD, and in occasional cases, even lead to recovery and function within the average range.

The symptoms that do not seem to improve substantively over time with early BIs are often related to ritualistic and repetitive behaviors. There is some evidence base for supporting BIs such as ABA to reduce some repetitive behaviors in children with ASD; however, more research is still needed. The prognosis of a given child with ASD is generally when the home environment is supportive.

TREATMENT

The goals of treatment for children with ASD are to improve social interactions and communication, broaden strategies to integrate into schools, develop meaningful peer relationships, and increase long-term skills in independent living. Psychosocial treatment interventions aim to help children with ASD to develop skills in social conventions, increase socially acceptable and prosocial behavior with peers, and decrease odd behavioral symptoms. In many cases, a child may require language and academic remediation. Treatment goals include providing interventions for associated behaviors such as irritable and disruptive behaviors that may emerge in school and at home and may exacerbate during transitions. Children with intellectual disability require developmentally appropriate BIs to reinforce socially acceptable behaviors and encourage self-care skills. Parents of children with ASD often benefit from psychoeducation, support, and counseling in order to optimize their relationships and effectiveness with their children. Comprehensive treatment for ASD, including intensive behavioral programs like ABA, parent training, social skills groups, and academic/educational interventions, provides the most promising results. Components of treatment include expanding social skills, communication, and language, often through practicing imitation, joint attention, social reciprocity, and play in a directed but child-centered manner. Early intensive, comprehensive BIs targeting core features of ASD in children ranging in age from 2 to 5 years of age have shown increases in language acquisition, social interactions, and educational achievement at the end of the study period compared to control groups. The study periods ranged from 12 weeks to several years, and the settings were at home, in a clinic, or at school. The next section describes some comprehensive treatment models or adapted versions based on these studies.

Psychosocial Interventions

Early Intensive Behavioral and Developmental Interventions

UCLA/LOVAAS-BASED MODEL OF APPLIED BEHAVIOR ANALYSIS. This intensive and manualized intervention primarily utilizes techniques derived from ABA, given on a one-to-one basis for many hours per week. A therapist and a child will work on practicing specific social skills, language usage, and other target play skills, with reinforcement and rewards provided for accomplishments and mastery of skills.

EARLY START DENVER MODEL (ESDM). Interventions occur in naturalistic settings such as in daycare, at home, and during play with other children. Parents learn to be cotherapists and provide the training at home while educational settings also provide the interventions. The focus of the interventions is on developing basic play skills and relationship skills and integrating ABA into the interventions. This approach is focused on training for very young children and occurs within the context of the child's daily routine.

PARENT TRAINING APPROACHES. This includes Pivotal Response Training, in which parents learn to facilitate social and communication development within the home and during activities by targeting gateway or pivotal social behaviors for mastery by the child, with the expectation that once they master these central social skills, a natural generalizing of social behaviors would follow. The approach integrates extensive parent and family components into this type of intervention. Once parents learn the interventions, they gradually increase the frequency until they occur throughout the day with the child. Another example of a parent training approach is the Hanen More Than Words Program.

Social Skills Approaches

SOCIAL SKILLS TRAINING. Typically provided by therapeutic leaders to children of various ages in a group setting with peers, children are given guided practice in initiating social conversation and greetings, initiating games, and joint attention. The approach includes emotion identification and regulation in practice with recognizing and learning how to label emotions in given social situations, learning to attribute appropriate emotional reactions in others, and social problem-solving techniques. The goals are that, with practice in the group setting, the child will be able to use the techniques in less-structured settings and internalize strategies to interact positively with peers.

Behavioral Interventions (BIs) and Cognitive-Behavioral Therapy (CBT) for Repetitive Behaviors and Associated Symptoms

BEHAVIORAL THERAPY. ABA is somewhat effective in reducing some repetitive behaviors in children and adolescents with ASD. Early intervention helps for repetitive self-injurious behaviors; BIs may need to be combined with pharmacologic treatments to manage the symptoms adequately.

COGNITIVE-BEHAVIORAL THERAPY. There is a significant evidence base from randomized clinical trials for the efficacy of CBT for symptoms of anxiety, depression, and obsessive-compulsive disorders (OCDs) in children. There are fewer controlled trials of this treatment in children with ASD, although there are at least two published studies in which CBT was used to treat repetitive behavior in individuals with ASD.

Interventions for Comorbid Symptoms in Autism Spectrum Disorder

NEUROFEEDBACK. The goal of neurofeedback is to modify and diminish symptoms of attention-deficit/hyperactivity disorder (ADHD) and anxiety and increase social interaction in children and adolescents with ASD by providing enjoyable activities such as computer games or other games which reinforce the desired behavior. The child wears electrodes during neurofeedback that monitor electrical activity in the brain. The aim is to influence brainwave activity to prolong or produce electrical activity present during the desired behaviors. Neurofeedback devices do not correct the core features of ASD, but may improve associated anxiety, inattention, and social withdrawal and promote prosocial behavior.

INSOMNIA. Insomnia is a prevalent problem for children and adolescents with ASD, and both behavioral and pharmacologic interventions may improve this condition. The most common BI for insomnia in children with ASD is based on improving "sleep hygiene," that is, decreasing and removing evening stimulation such as activating screen games in the evening and creating a calming routine which is consistent and promotes relaxation. In other words, removing reinforcement and attention for being awake, leading to gradual extinction of the "staying awake" behavior. Several studies using massage therapy before bedtime in children with ASD between the ages of 2 years and 13 years provided an improvement in falling asleep and a sense of relaxation.

Educational Interventions for Children with Autism Spectrum Disorder

TREATMENT AND EDUCATION OF AUTISTIC AND RELATED COMMUNICATION-HANDICAPPED CHILDREN (TEACCH). Originally developed at the University of North Carolina at Chapel Hill in the 1970s, TEACCH involves structured teaching based on the notion that children with ASD have difficulty with perception. This teaching method incorporates many visual supports and a picture schedule to aid in teaching academic subjects as well as socially appropriate responses. Caregivers arrange the physical environment to support visual learning, and the day is structured to promote autonomy and social relatedness.

BROAD-BASED APPROACHES. These educational plans include a blend of teaching strategies that use behavioral analysis and also focus on language remediation. Behavioral reinforcement is provided for socially acceptable behaviors while teaching academic subjects. TEACCH can be part of a broader special educational program for ASD.

COMPUTER-BASED APPROACHES AND VIRTUAL REALITY. Computer-based and virtual reality approaches use computer programs to teach language acquisition and reading skills. This approach provides the child with a sense of mastery. It also delivers behaviorally based instruction in a modality that is appealing to the child. The Let's Face It! program is a computerized game that helps to teach children with ASD to recognize faces. It consists of seven interactive computer games that target changes in facial expression, attention to the eye region of the face, holistic face recognition, and identifying emotional expression. An randomized controlled trial (RCT) of this program with children with ASD provided evidence that after 20 hours of face training with Let's Face It!, compared to the control group, the trained children demonstrated improvement in their ability to focus on the eye region of a face and improved their analytic and holistic face-processing skills. Several studies using virtual reality environments to teach children with ASD social skills and interaction have provided evidence of their value. In one study, a virtual café for children with ASD allowed the children to practice ordering and paying for drinks and food by navigating with the use of a computer mouse.

Psychopharmacological Interventions

Psychopharmacological interventions in ASD help ameliorate behavioral symptoms rather than core features of ASD. Target symptoms include irritability, broadly including aggression, temper tantrums, and self-injurious behaviors, hyperactivity, impulsivity, and inattention.

Irritability. Two second-generation antipsychotics, risperidone and aripiprazole, have been approved by the Food and Drug Administration (FDA) in the United States for treatment of irritability in individuals with ASD. Risperidone is approved for irritability in children with ASD from 5 years of age. Aripiprazole is approved for irritability in children and adolescents with ASD from 6 years of age.

Risperidone, a high-potency antipsychotic with combined dopamine (D_2) and serotonin ($5\text{-}HT_2$) receptor antagonist properties, has been shown to subdue aggressive or self-injurious behaviors in children with and without ASD. There have been seven RCTs, three reanalysis studies, and two add-on studies, which have converged to confirm risperidone as an efficacious pharmacologic treatment for irritability in children and adolescents with ASD. Typical doses range from 0.5 to 1.5 mg. Some of the children in this study were also receiving intensive behavioral treatments. Risperidone is considered the first line of medication treatment for children and adolescents with ASD who exhibit severe irritability. Despite its efficacy, risperidone's main side effects of weight gain and increased appetite, metabolic side effects such as hyperglycemia, prolactin elevation, and dyslipidemia, along with other common adverse effects such as fatigue, drowsiness, dizziness, and drooling, have limited its use in some individuals. Risperidone should be used with caution in individuals with underlying cardiac abnormalities or hypotension, since risperidone may contribute to orthostatic hypotension. In further continuation studies of risperidone in the treatment of irritability in ASD, persistent efficacy, and tolerability were found over 6 months, with a rapid return of symptoms in good responders when discontinuing the risperidone. Other drugs studied in the treatment of irritability in ASD include aripiprazole and olanzapine.

Two extensive studies utilizing aripiprazole in the treatment of tantrums, aggression, and self-injury in children and adolescents with ASD found that aripiprazole was both efficacious and safe. Doses ranged from 5 to 15 mg/day. The main side effects included sedation, dizziness, insomnia, akathisia, nausea, and vomiting. Although weight gain was not as pronounced as with risperidone, it was still considered a moderate adverse event, with approximately 1.3 to 1.5 kg gained during an 8-week study period. The weight gain was similar at the lower and higher doses. Olanzapine, which blocks $5\text{-}HT_{2A}$ and D_2 receptors and blocks muscarinic receptors, has been studied in children and adolescents with ASD for the treatment of irritability with a trend toward a positive response; however, significant weight gain of approximately 3.5 kg occurred. The main side effect was sedation.

Hyperactivity, Impulsivity, and Inattention. Randomized placebo-controlled trials of methylphenidate for the treatment of hyperactivity, impulsivity, and inattention in children and adolescents with ASD have provided evidence of efficacy, although not as robust evidence as this medication has in children with ADHD symptoms without ASD. The Research Units of Pediatric Psychopharmacology found methylphenidate to be at least moderately efficacious at doses of 0.25 to 0.5 mg/kg for youth with ASD and ADHD symptoms. The efficacy of methylphenidate in this population was less effective than in children with ADHD without ASD, and children with ASD developed more frequent side effects, including increased irritability, compared to ADHD children. A study of methylphenidate in the treatment of hyperactivity and inattention in preschoolers with ASD found the stimulant safe and relatively efficacious; half of the preschoolers developed side effects including increased stereotypies, gastrointestinal upset, sleep problems, and emotional lability. Among nonstimulants, one double-blind placebo-controlled study of hyperactivity, impulsivity, and inattention using atomoxetine in children with ASD found that it was significantly more effective than placebo. Side effects included sedation, irritability, constipation, and nausea. Clonidine, an α-agonist, has also been studied in children with ASD for the treatment of hyperactivity with mixed results. Guanfacine may also help in some cases.

Repetitive and Stereotypic Behavior. Antidepressants and mood stabilizers have been studied for the treatment of these core symptoms of ASD without robust positive results. One study with fluoxetine found the medication group only slightly better and not significantly better than the placebo group regarding the target symptoms, and another trial with escitalopram found no difference between groups. Risperidone, however, was found to be effective in targeting irritability, and restrictive and repetitive behaviors were improved in some children. A recent systematic review and meta-analysis of randomized clinical trials for the treatment of restrictive and repetitive behaviors in ASD found no significant difference between agents including risperidone, fluoxetine, citalopram, and fluvoxamine, and placebo, respectively.

Agents Administered for Behavioral Impairment in Autism Spectrum Disorder Based on Open Trials. Quetiapine is an antipsychotic with more potent 5-HT_{2A} than D_2 receptor-blocking properties. Although there are only open-label trials with this agent, some experts use this when risperidone and olanzapine fail or are intolerable. Doses range from 50 to 200 mg/day. Adverse effects include drowsiness, tachycardia, agitation, and weight gain.

Clozapine has a heterocyclic chemical structure that is related to certain first-generation antipsychotics, such as loxapine, although clozapine carries a lower risk of extrapyramidal symptoms. It is not generally used in the treatment of aggression and self-injurious behavior unless those behaviors coexist with psychotic symptoms. The most severe adverse effect is agranulocytosis, which necessitates monitoring white blood cell count weekly during clozapine use. Its use is generally limited to treatment-resistant psychotic patients. According to a meta-analysis of published retrospective chart reviews by Rotharemel and colleagues in 2018, of open trials of clozapine in the treatment of severe disruptive behaviors in patients with ASD over 11 years, Clozapine could be efficacious in patients with ASD who do not response to other antipsychotics over time.

Ziprasidone has receptor-blocking properties at the 5-HT_{2A} and D_2 receptor sites and carries little risk of extrapyramidal and antihistaminic effects. No guidelines exist for its use in autistic children with aggressive and self-injurious behaviors; clinicians sometimes use it to treat these behaviors in treatment-resistant children. In studies of its use in adults with schizophrenia, dose ranges of 40 to 160 mg were effective. Adverse effects include sedation, dizziness, and lightheadedness. Before using this medication, the clinician should check an electrocardiogram. Open trials of ziprasidone have shown trends toward efficacy for extreme aggressive and self-injurious behavior in patients with ASD.

Lithium is efficacious in children with aggression without ASD, and it is used clinically in the treatment of aggressive or self-injurious behaviors in ASD when antipsychotic medications are not helpful. Open trials of lithium in the management of irritability and aggressive behaviors in patients with ASD have indicated that lithium could be efficacious in the treatment of these symptoms in ASD.

Agents Used for Behavioral Impairment in Autism Spectrum Disorder without Evidence of Efficacy. A double-blind study investigated the efficacy of amantadine, which blocks *N*-methyl-D-aspartate (NMDA) receptors, in the treatment of behavioral disturbance, such as irritability, aggression, and hyperactivity, in children with autism. Some researchers have suggested that abnormalities of the glutamatergic system may contribute to the emergence of ASDs. High glutamate levels occur in children with the formerly labeled Rett syndrome. In the amantadine study, 47% of children on amantadine were "improved" per their parents, and 37% of children on placebo were rated "improved" by parents in irritability and hyperactivity, although this difference was not statistically significant. Investigators rated the children on amantadine "significantly improved" for hyperactivity. A double-blind, placebo-controlled study of the efficacy of the anticonvulsant lamotrigine on hyperactivity in children with autism showed high rates of placebo improvement in ratings of hyperactivity, which were similar to response on the medication.

Clomipramine is sometimes used but lacks RCTs to provide evidence of positive results. Fenfluramine, which reduces blood serotonin levels, has also been used but appears to be ineffective. Improvement does not seem to be associated with a reduction in blood serotonin levels. Naltrexone, an opioid receptor antagonist, has been investigated without much success, based on the notion that blocking endogenous opioids would reduce autistic symptoms.

Tetrahydrobiopterin, a coenzyme that enhances the action of enzymes, was studied. However, the results were not significant. Post hoc analysis of the three core symptoms of autism—social interaction, communication, and stereotyped behaviors—revealed a significant improvement in social interaction score after 6 months of active treatment. There was a positive correlation between social response and IQ. These results suggest that there is a possible effect of tetrahydrobiopterin on the social functioning of children with autism.

A case report suggested that low-dose venlafaxine was efficacious in three adolescents and young adults with autistic disorder with self-injurious behavior and hyperactivity. The dose of venlafaxine used was 18.75 mg/day, and the efficacy continued over 6 months.

Complementary and Alternative Medicine (CAM) Approaches to Autism Spectrum Disorder

CAM is a group of nontraditional treatments used in conjunction with conventional treatments. Safe interventions that target both core and associated behavioral features of ASD with unknown efficacy include the following: music therapy, to promote communication and expression, and yoga, to promote attention and decrease activity level. A biologically based practice that appears to be safe and efficacious is melatonin, which reduces sleep-onset latency in children. Other biologic practices that appear to be safe but with unknown efficacy include vitamin C, multivitamins, essential fatty acids, and the amino acids carnosine and carnitine. Secretin is ineffective in RCTs in the treatment of ASD.

EPIDEMIOLOGY

Prevalence

Currently, 1 in 54 children in the United States is diagnosed with ASD, almost 2%, based on DSM-5 criteria. The diagnostic rate for ASDs has increased over the last two decades. Autistic disorder, based on DSM-IV-TR criteria, is believed to occur at a rate of about 8 cases per 10,000 children (0.08%). By definition, the onset of ASD is in the early developmental period; however, children with mild symptoms may go undetected until they are much older. Due to the delay between onset and diagnosis, the prevalence rates increase with age in young children.

Sex Distribution

ASD is diagnosed four times more often in boys than in girls. In clinical samples, girls with ASD more often exhibit intellectual disability than boys. One potential explanation for this is that girls with ASD without an intellectual disability may be less likely to be identified, referred clinically, and diagnosed.

ETIOLOGY AND PATHOGENESIS

Genetic Factors

Family and twin studies suggest that ASD has a complex heritable contribution; this contribution does not appear to be fully penetrant. Only 15% of cases of ASD appear to be associated with a known genetic mutation, in the vast majority of cases, its expression is dependent on multiple genes. Family studies have demonstrated increased rates of ASD in siblings of an index child, as high as 50% in some families with two or more children with ASD. Siblings of a child with ASD are also at increased risk for a variety of developmental impairments in communication and social skills, even when they do not meet the criteria for ASD.

The concordance rate of autistic disorder in two extensive twin studies was 36% in monozygotic pairs versus 0% in dizygotic pairs in one study and about 96% in monozygotic pairs versus about 27% in dizygotic pairs in the second study. High rates of cognitive impairments, in the nonautistic twin in monozygotic twins with perinatal complications, suggest that contributions of perinatal environmental factors interact with genetic vulnerability differentially in ASD.

The heterogeneity in the expression of symptoms in families with ASD suggests that there are multiple patterns of genetic transmission. Studies indicate that both an increase and decrease in specific genetic patterns may be risk factors for ASD. In addition to specific genetic factors, gender plays a substantial role in the expression of ASD. Genetic studies have identified two biologic systems involved in ASD: the consistent finding of elevated platelet serotonin (5-HT) and the mTOR, that is, mammalian target of rapamycin–linked synaptic plasticity mechanisms, which is disrupted in ASD. These will be discussed further in the next section.

Several genetic disorders cause ASD symptoms as part of a broader phenotype. The most common of these inherited disorders is fragile X syndrome, an X-linked recessive disorder that is present in 2% to 3% of individuals with ASD. Fragile X syndrome exhibits a nucleotide repeat in the 5′ untranslated region of the *FMNR1* gene, resulting in symptoms of ASD. Children with fragile X syndrome characteristically exhibit intellectual disability, gross and fine motor impairments, an unusual facies, macroorchidism, and significantly diminished expressive language ability. Tuberous sclerosis, another genetic disorder characterized by multiple benign tumors, inherited by autosomal dominant transmission, is found with higher frequency among children with ASD. Up to 2% of children with ASD also have tuberous sclerosis.

Researchers who screened the DNA of more than 150 pairs of siblings with ASD found evidence of two regions on chromosomes 2 and 7 containing genes that may contribute to ASD. Additional genes hypothesized to be involved in ASD are on chromosomes 16 and 17.

Biomarkers in Autism Spectrum Disorder

ASD is associated with several biomarkers, potentially resulting from interactions of genes and environmental factors, which then influence neuronal function, dendrite development, and contribute to altered neuronal information processing. Researchers have identified several biomarkers of abnormal signaling in the 5-HT system, the mTOR-linked synaptic plasticity mechanisms, and alterations of the γ-aminobutyric acid (GABA) inhibitory system.

The first biomarker identified in ASD was elevated serotonin in whole blood, almost exclusively in the platelets. Platelets acquire 5-HT through the process of SERT (serotonin transporter), known to be hereditary, as they pass through the intestinal circulation. The genes that mediate SERT (*SLC64A*), and the 5-HT receptor 5-HT$_{2A}$ gene (*HTR2A*) are known to be more heritable than ASD and encode the same protein in the platelets and the brain. Because 5-HT is known to be involved in brain development, the changes in 5-HT regulation may lead to alterations in neuronal migration and growth in the brain.

Both structural and functional neuroimaging studies have suggested specific biomarkers associated with ASD. Several studies found increased total brain volume in children younger than 4 years of age with ASD, whose neonatal head circumferences were within normal limits or slightly below. By about age 5 years, however, 15% to 20% of children with ASD developed macrocephaly. Additional studies found confirmatory data in samples of infants who later had ASD, who exhibited normal head circumferences at birth; by 4 years, 90% had larger brain volumes than controls, with 37% of the disordered group meeting criteria for macrocephaly. In contrast, structural magnetic resonance imaging (sMRI) studies of children with ASD ranging from 5 to 16 years did not find mean values of total brain volume increased. One study followed the size of the amygdala in youth with ASD in the first few years of life, and similarly, found an increased size in the first few years of life, followed by a decrease in size over time. Several studies have found enlarged striatum in young children with ASD, with a positive correlation of striatal size with the frequency of repetitive behaviors. The dynamic process of the atypical and changing total brain volume observed in children with ASD lends support for the overarching hypothesis that there are sensitive periods or "critical periods" within the brain's plasticity, which when disrupted, may contribute to the emergence of ASD.

Functional MRI (fMRI) studies have focused on identifying biomarkers; that is, the functional brain correlates of various observed core symptoms in ASD. fMRI studies of children, adolescents, and adults with ASD have employed tasks including face perception, neutral face tasks, "theory of mind" deficits, language and communication impairments, working memory, and repetitive behaviors. fMRI studies have provided evidence that individuals with ASD tend to scan faces differently than controls, in that they focus more on the mouth region of the face rather than on the eye region and rather than scanning the entire face multiple times, individuals with ASD focus more on individual features of the face. In response to socially relevant stimuli, researchers have concluded that individuals with ASD have greater amygdala hyperarousal. In terms of "theory of mind," that is, the ability to attribute emotional states to others, and to oneself, fMRI studies find differences in activation in brain regions such as the right temporal lobe and other areas of the brain known to become activated in controls during tasks involving the theory of mind. This difference has been hypothesized by some researchers to represent dysfunction of the mirror neuron system (MNS). Atypical patterns of frontal lobe activation have been found in multiple studies of ASD during face processing tasks, suggesting that this area of the brain may be critical in social perception and emotional reasoning. Decreased activation in individuals with ASD in the left frontal regions of the brain during memory and language-based tasks led researchers to hypothesize that individuals with ASD utilized more visual strategies during language processing than controls did.

Both sMRI and fMRI research have contributed to demonstrating brain correlates of core impairments observed in individuals with ASD.

Immunologic Factors

There is some evidence that immunologic incompatibility (i.e., maternal antibodies directed at the fetus) may contribute to ASD in some cases. The lymphocytes of some children with ASD react with maternal antibodies, which raise the possibility that embryonic neural tissues damage during gestation. These reports usually reflect single cases rather than controlled studies, and this hypothesis is still under investigation.

Prenatal and Perinatal Factors

A higher-than-expected incidence of prenatal and perinatal complications seems to occur in infants who are diagnosed with ASD in childhood. Prenatal factors that have been found to be associated with ASD in offspring are advanced maternal and paternal age at birth, maternal gestational bleeding, and gestational diabetes. Perinatal risk factors for ASD include umbilical cord complications, birth trauma, fetal distress, small for gestational age, low birth weight, low 5-minute Apgar score, congenital malformation, ABO blood group system or Rh factor incompatibility, and hyperbilirubinemia. Many of the obstetrical complications that are associated with risk for ASD are also risk factors for hypoxia, which may be an underlying risk factor itself. There is no sufficient evidence to implicate any one single perinatal or prenatal factor in ASD etiology, and a genetic predisposition to ASD may be interacting with perinatal factors.

Comorbid Neurologic Disorders

EEG abnormalities and seizure disorders occur with higher-than-expected frequency in individuals with ASD. Four percent to 32% of individuals with ASD have grand mal seizures at some time, and about 20% to 25% show ventricular enlargement on computed tomography (CT) scans. Various EEG abnormalities occur in 10% to 83% of children with the previously defined autistic disorder, and although no EEG finding is specific to autistic disorder, there is some indication of failed cerebral lateralization. The current consensus is that ASD is a set of behavioral syndromes caused by a multitude of factors acting on the CNS.

Psychosocial Theories

Psychosocial theories such as the idea that parental emotional factors contribute to the development of ASD have been debunked. Studies comparing parents of children with ASD with parents of typical children have shown no significant differences in child-rearing skills.

Further Readings

Aishworiya R, Valica T, Hagerman R, Restrepo B. An update on pharmacologic treatment of autism spectrum disorder. *Neurotherapeutics*. 2022;19(1):248–262.

Aman MG, Arnold LE, McDougle CJ, et al. Acute and long-term safety and tolerability of risperidone in children with autism. *J Child Adolesc Psychopharmacol*. 2005;15:869–884.

Boyd BA, McDonough SG, Bodfish JW. Evidence-based behavioral interventions for repetitive behaviors in autism. *J Autism Dev Disord*. 2012;42(6):1236–1248.

Buckley AW, Hirtz D, Oskoui M, et al. Practice guideline: Treatment for insomnia and disrupted sleep behavior in children and adolescents with autism spectrum disorder: Report of the Guideline Development,

Dissemination, and Implementation Subcommittee of the American Academy of Neurology. *Neurology.* 2020;94(9):392–404.
Dal Pai J, Wolff CG, Aranchipe CS, et al. COVID-19 pandemic and autism spectrum disorder, consequences to children and adolescents-a systematic review. *Rev J Autism Dev Disord.* 2022:1–26.
DeVane CL, Charles JM, Abramson RK, et al. Pharmacotherapy of autism spectrum disorder: results from the randomized BAART clinical trial. *Pharmacotherapy.* 2019;39(6):626–635.
Gardener H, Spiegelman D, Buka SL. Perinatal and neonatal risk factors for autism: a comprehensive meta-analysis. *Pediatrics.* 2011;128:344–355.
Genovese A, Butler MG. The autism spectrum: behavioral, psychiatric and genetic associations. *Genes (Basel).* 2023;14(3):677.
Hazlett HC, Poe M, Gerig G, et al. Magnetic resonance imaging and head circumference study of brain size in autism: birth through age 2 years. *Arch Gen Psychiatry.* 2005;62:1366–1376.
Kasari C, Sturm A, Shih W. SMARTer approach to personalizing intervention for children with autism spectrum disorder. *J Speech Lang Hear Res.* 2018;61(11):2629–2640.
Ke JY, Chen CL, Chen YJ, Chen CH, Lee LF, Chiang TM. Features of developmental functions and autistic profiles in children with fragile X syndrome. *Chang Gung Med J.* 2005;28:551–558.
Kirst S, Bögl K, Gross VL, Diehm R, Poustka L, Dziobek I. Subtypes of aggressive behavior in children with autism in the context of emotion recognition, hostile attribution bias, and dysfunctional emotion regulation. *J Autism Dev Disord.* 2022;52(12):5367–5382.
Lord C, Elsabbagh M, Baird G, Veenstra-Vanderweele J. Autism spectrum disorder. *Lancet.* 2018;392(10146):508–520.
Maniram J, Karrim SBS, Oosthuizen F, Wiafe E. Pharmacological management of core symptoms and comorbidities of autism spectrum disorder in children and adolescents: a systematic review. *Neuropsychiatr Dis Treat.* 2022;18:1629–1644.
Miano S, Ferri R. Epidemiology and management of insomnia in children with autistic spectrum disorders. *Pediatr Drugs.* 2010;12:75–84.
Miller LE, Dai YG, Fein DA, Robins DL. Characteristics of toddlers with early versus later diagnosis of autism spectrum disorder. *Autism.* 2021;25(2):416–428.
Nazeer A. Psychopharmacology of autistic spectrum disorders in children and adolescents. *Pediatr Clin N Am.* 2011;58:85–97.
Research Units on Pediatric Psychopharmacology Autism Network. Risperidone treatment of autistic disorder: longer-term benefits and blinded discontinuation after 6 months. *Am J Psychiatry.* 2005; 162:1361–1369.
Research Units on Pediatric Psychopharmacology Autism Network. Randomized, controlled crossover trial of methylphenidate in pervasive developmental disorders with hyperactivity. *Arch Gen Psychiatry.* 2005;62:1266–1274.
Robinson EB, Koenen KC, McCormick MC, et al. Evidence that autistic traits show the same etiology in the general population and at the quantitative extremes (5%, 2.5%, and 1%). *Arch Gen Psychiatry.* 2011; 68:1113–1121.
Rogers SJ, Vismara LA. Evidence-based comprehensive treatments for early autism. *J Clin Child Adolesc Psychol.* 2008;37:8–38.
Ronald A, Hoekstra RA. Autism spectrum disorders and autistic traits: a decade of new twin studies. *Am J Med Genet Part B.* 2011;156:255–274.
Rotharmel M, Szymoniak F, Pollet C, et al. Eleven years of clozapine experience in autism spectrum disorder: efficacy and tolerance. *J Clin Psychopharmacol.* 2018;38:577–581.
Salazar de Pablo G, Pastor Jordá C, Vaquerizo-Serrano J, et al. Systematic review and meta-analysis: efficacy of pharmacological interventions for irritability and emotional dysregulation in autism spectrum disorder and predictors of response. *J Am Acad Child Adolesc Psychiatry.* 2023;62(2):151–168.
Salehinejad MA, Ghanavati E, Glinski B, Hallajian AH, Azarkolah A. A systematic review of randomized controlled trials on efficacy and safety of transcranial direct current stimulation in major neurodevelopmental disorders: ADHD, autism, and dyslexia. *Brain Behav.* 2022;12(9):e2724.
Sikich L, Kolevzon A, King BH, et al. Intranasal oxytocin in children and adolescents with autism spectrum disorder. *N Engl J Med.* 2021;385(16):1462–1473.
Stigler KA, McDonald BC, Anand A, Saykin AJ, McDougle CJ. Structural and functional magnetic resonance imaging of autism spectrum disorders. *Brain Res.* 2011;1380:146–161.
Sugie Y, Sugie H, Fukuda T, Ito M. Neonatal factors in infants with autistic disorder and typically developing infants. *Autism.* 2005;9(5):487–494.
Tanaka JW, Wolf JM, Klaiman C, et al. Using computerized games to teach face recognition skills to children with autism spectrum disorder: the Let's Face it! Program. *J Child Psychol Psychiatry.* 2010;51:944–952.
Vanderbuilt Evidence-Based Practice Center, Nashville TN. Therapies for children with autism spectrum disorders. *Comparative Effectiveness Review.* 2011;26:1–13.
Veenstra-VanderWeele J, Blakely RD. Networking in autism: leveraging genetic, biomarker and model system findings in the search for new treatments. *Neuropsychopharmacology.* 2012;37:196–212.
Wang M, Reid D. Virtual reality in pediatric neurorehabilitation: attention deficit hyperactivity disorder, autism and cerebral palsy. *Neuroepidemiology.* 2011;36:2–18.
Wink LK, Erickson CA, McDougle CJ. Pharmacologic treatment of behavioral symptoms associated with autism and other pervasive developmental disorders. *Curr Treat Options Neurol.* 2010;12:529–538.
Yu Y, Chaulagain A, Pedersen SA, et al. Pharmacotherapy of restricted/repetitive behavior in autism spectrum disorder: a systematic review and meta-analysis. *BioMed Central (BMC) Psychiatry.* 2020;20:121.
Zuddas A, Zanni R, Usala T. Second generation antipsychotics (SGAs) for nonpsychotic disorders in children and adolescents: a review of the randomized controlled studies. *Eur Neuropsychopharmacol.* 2011;21:600–620.

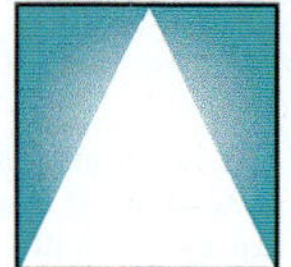

6 Attention-Deficit/ Hyperactivity Disorder

Attention-deficit/hyperactivity disorder (ADHD) is a neuropsychiatric condition affecting preschoolers, children, adolescents, and adults around the world, characterized by a pattern of diminished sustained attention, and increased impulsivity or hyperactivity. Based on family history, genotyping, and neuroimaging studies, there is clear evidence to support a biologic basis for ADHD. Although multiple regions of the brain and several neurotransmitters contribute to the emergence of symptoms, dopamine continues to be a focus of investigation regarding ADHD symptoms. The prefrontal cortex of the brain is a focus of interest because of its high utilization of dopamine and its reciprocal connections with other brain regions involved in attention, inhibition, decision-making, response inhibition, working memory, and vigilance. ADHD affects up to 5% to 8% of school-age children, with 60% to 85% of those diagnosed as children continuing to meet criteria for the disorder in adolescence, and up to 60% continuing to be symptomatic into adulthood. Children, adolescents, and adults with ADHD often have significant impairment in academic functioning as well as in social and interpersonal situations. ADHD is frequently associated with comorbid disorders, including learning disorders, anxiety disorders, mood disorders, and disruptive behavior disorders.

The DSM-5-TR includes the following criteria: "several inattentive or hyperactive-impulsive symptoms" must be present by age 12 years. Previous to the DSM-5 version, there were two subtypes: Inattentive and Hyperactive/Impulsive type. In DSM-5-TR, the subtypes have been replaced by the following three specifiers, which largely denote the same groups: (1) combined presentation, (2) predominantly inattentive presentation, and (3) predominantly hyperactive/impulsive presentation. Additional criteria DSM-5-TR include permitting comorbid ADHD and autism spectrum disorder diagnoses. In DSM-5-TR, for adolescents 17 years and older, only five symptoms, rather than six symptoms of either inattention or hyperactivity and impulsivity, are required. DSM-5-TR criteria include symptoms to reflect different presentations across the life span. To confirm a diagnosis of ADHD, impairment from inattention or hyperactivity and impulsivity must be present in at least two settings and interfere with developmentally appropriate social or academic functioning.

ADHD has historically been described in the literature using different terminology. In the early 1900s, impulsive, disinhibited, and hyperactive children—many of whom also had neurologic damage due to encephalitis—were grouped under the label *hyperactive syndrome.* In the 1960s, a heterogeneous group of children with poor coordination, learning disabilities, and emotional lability, but without specific neurologic disorders, were described as having "minimal brain damage"; however, over time, it became clear that this was an inappropriate term. There are many explanations for ADHD symptoms, including theories of abnormal arousal and reduced ability to modulate emotions. This theory was initially supported by the observation that stimulant medications increased sustained attention and improved focus. ADHD is one of the most well-researched childhood psychiatric disorders with several evidence-based treatments.

CLINICAL FEATURES

ADHD can have its onset in infancy, although it is rarely diagnosed until a child is at least toddler age. More commonly, infants with ADHD are active in the crib, sleep little, and cry a great deal.

In school, children with ADHD may attack a test rapidly but may answer only the first two questions. They may be unable to wait to be called on in school and may respond before everyone else. At home, caregivers cannot put them off for even a minute. Impulsiveness and an inability to delay gratification are characteristic. Children with ADHD are often susceptible to accidents.

The most cited characteristics of children with ADHD, in order of frequency, are hyperactivity, attention deficit (short attention span, distractibility, perseveration, failure to finish tasks, inattention, poor concentration), impulsivity (action before thought, abrupt shifts in activity, lack of organization, jumping up in class), memory and thinking deficits, specific learning disabilities, and speech and hearing deficits. Associated features often include perceptual-motor impairment, emotional lability, and developmental coordination disorder. A significant percentage of children with ADHD show behavioral symptoms of aggression and defiance. School difficulties, both learning and behavioral, commonly exist with ADHD. Comorbid communication disorders or learning disorders that hamper the acquisition, retention, and display of knowledge complicate the course of ADHD.

Andrew, an 8-year-old boy, was taken for an evaluation with a child and adolescent psychiatrist by his adoptive parents after his third grade teacher informed them that Andrew was on the verge of being suspended from school. Andrew's teacher reported that Andrew was unmanageable in the classroom due to his inability to sit in his seat, his disruptive impulsive behaviors, and recurrent aggressive behaviors toward his peers and his teacher in the classroom. Andrew's adoptive parents were surprised because Andrew was already receiving two resource room periods each day in which he received help with reading and math as well as speech therapy once a week. Andrew's adoptive parents knew very little about his biologic family other than that his biologic father had psychiatric problems and his biologic mother may have used drugs while she was pregnant. Andrew's parents provided foster care for Andrew since he was an infant and adopted Andrew when he was 2 years old. Andrew's foster parents knew that Andrew was a very active child, but they found him endearing and cute and believed that he would grow out of it. Since kindergarten, Andrew's teachers had complained that Andrew did not seem to listen and was unable to stay in his seat. Because Andrew was an engaging and cute child, his teachers in kindergarten and first grade made accommodations for him in their classrooms despite their concerns. When Andrew entered the second grade, however, it became clear to his teachers that, in addition to being hyperactive, Andrew was struggling with learning to read words and forming letters to write his name. Andrew's classroom contained 25 students, and his teacher complained that she did not have enough time to focus on his problems so the school initiated an Individualized Educational Plan (IEP) evaluation. Andrew was provided with resource room periods for academic remediation but continued to have problems getting along with his peers during lunch and at recess. Andrew was bossy and often argued with peers, who complained that he was not playing by the rules of their games. When he was challenged, Andrew became angry and would often impulsively push his classmates, which resulted in a physical altercation. At home, Andrew's adoptive parents became increasingly frustrated with Andrew because he was unable to complete a few math problems and or write a paragraph without continued nagging. Andrew was easily annoyed when frustrated and would often run around the house in a silly and disruptive manner. In school, Andrew was a good-hearted child who seemed to get along best with younger children. Andrew was not well-like by his classmates, and the teachers indicated that Andrew's peers avoided him because he was too rough during play, and he did not follow the rules of games. Andrew had difficulty waiting his turn, and when limits were set, he became easily provoked. Andrew became an outcast among his classmates and was often bullied by his classmates. Andrew was aware that he was not able to keep up with his classwork, and he told his adoptive parents that he was just "stupid." Andrew's adoptive parents began to notice that, despite his high activity level, Andrew seemed sad. One day after an altercation with several classmates, he told his adoptive parents that he wished he was dead. At this point, Andrew's parents became worried and decided that Andrew's teacher was right and took him for a psychiatric evaluation. During the initial psychiatric evaluation with a child and adolescent psychiatrist, Andrew presented as a well-developed, cute, and active child, who appeared distracted and fidgety and somewhat sad. When asked about school, Andrew said that he wanted to do "better" in school but that nobody liked him, he was too dumb to do his schoolwork, and he did not like doing homework. He denied suicidal thoughts and reported that he had only said that to his parents because he was angry at his peers. Andrew admitted that it was tough for him to understand his schoolwork and impossible to complete his assignments. The evaluation included several parent and teacher rating scales to be filled out by his adoptive parents and teacher. These included The Child Behavior Checklist and the SNAP Rating Scale. At the psychiatrist's follow-up appointment, Andrew's teacher and parents strongly endorsed similar symptoms, including poor organization, inability to follow directions, being forgetful in daily activities, and perpetual impulsivity, with several episodes of running into the street without looking, blurting things out in the classroom without raising his hand, and recurrent fights with peers. Andrew looked dejected in school when he was excluded from play activities by peers, and sullen or angry at home when his parents asked him to read or do homework. Based on the clinical history, the rating scales, and the teacher's report, a diagnosis of attention-deficit/hyperactivity disorder, with the DSM-5–specifier of combined presentation, was made. Andrew had displayed a depressed mood which did not meet full criteria for a depressive disorder. The treatment plan included a behavioral plan allowing Andrew to receive rewards for effort on his homework along with a trial of stimulant medication for his ADHD. A medical history and recent physical examination revealed a healthy boy without any systemic illnesses. Since Andrew did not have any history or symptoms of cardiac abnormalities, an EKG was not necessary for his current treatment. The psychiatrist started Andrew on a trial dose of a short-acting stimulant, methylphenidate at 10 mg, to determine if he could tolerate a stimulant without any unexpected sensitivities. Andrew had no adverse effects and was soon switched to a long-acting formulation (Concerta), 36 mg, which would last between 10 and 12 hours. Andrew displayed a partial response to this dose and became less restless and more focused, and his teacher reported that he was not getting out of his seat as often. Andrew continued to blurt out in class inappropriately, and he continued to have difficulty following directions. Since Andrew had no adverse effects but was still displaying

ADHD symptoms, his psychiatrist increased his Concerta to 54 mg/day. At this dose, Andrew was better at sitting and finishing his classwork and homework. However, Andrew's parents began to notice that he had insomnia—it was taking him several hours to fall asleep, and he was becoming fatigued from lack of adequate sleep. Andrew's treating psychiatrist believed that part of Andrew's new insomnia might be related to a rebound effect when the Concerta wore off. Since the Concerta at 54 mg was extremely effective, it was decided to maintain this dose of medication and address the insomnia. The psychiatrist discussed two sequential options with Andrew's parents to address insomnia. The first option was to initiate a 2-week trial of melatonin, 3 mg, to be taken after dinner to help with falling asleep and remaining asleep throughout the night. If melatonin was found to be ineffective, the second option was to initiate a trial of Intuniv, long-acting guanfacine to be administered at bedtime, which can also be effective for sleep. Andrew followed up with his psychiatrist after the 2-week trial of melatonin, and both Andrew and his parents agreed that it was not effective and so they were instructed to increase the melatonin dose to 5 mg after dinner for another 2-week trial and then evaluate its efficacy. When Andrew and his family returned to the psychiatrist in another 2 weeks, it was determined that even at this dose, melatonin was not helpful. At this point, a trial of Intuniv (long-acting guanfacine) 1 mg was initiated at bedtime. Within a few days, it became evident to Andrew and his family that Andrew became calmer after taking the 1 mg of Intuniv and was falling asleep within about 30 minutes. Over the next few months, Andrew's improvement was clear in that his grades were improved and he was less irritable and oppositional at home. However, Andrew still had social skills difficulties with peers and was still ostracized by peers for acting in a bossy manner. Andrew's parents discussed this with his treating psychiatrist and his teacher, and they both agreed that a weekly social skills therapy group would be helpful and his psychiatrist suggested a local psychologist who ran social skills groups especially for children with ADHD. A parent training group for parents of children with ADHD was also recommended for his parents to attend, which they did. At first, Andrew resisted attending these sessions, but after a going for a few weeks, Andrew received praise for demonstrating social skills he was taught in the group, and he also liked the snacks that he received at the end of each group. Over time, Andrew's parents got to know the parents of other children in the group and began to arrange play-dates for Andrew with these peers. Andrew and his new peers practiced their improved social behaviors with some parental supervision at first, and gradually they were able to play congenially in a more independent way. The combination of stimulant medication in the day time, Intuniv at night, his social skills group, and his parents improved parenting skills resulted in a significant improvement in Andrew's ADHD symptoms as well as his social interactions. Andrew demonstrated improvement in the quality of his relationships with peers in school and from his group, as well as in his family. (Adapted from Boland JB, Verduin ML, Ruiz P, eds. *Kaplan & Sadock's Synopsis of Psychiatry*. 12th ed. Wolters Kluwer; 2022.)

DIAGNOSIS

We can elicit the principal signs of inattention, impulsivity, and hyperactivity from a detailed history of a child's early developmental patterns along with direct observation of the child, especially in situations that require sustained attention. Hyperactivity may be more severe in some situations (e.g., school) and less marked in others (e.g., one-on-one interviews), and may be less evident in active outdoor sports and in stimulating or favorite video games. The diagnosis of ADHD requires persistent, impairing symptoms of either hyperactivity/impulsivity or inattention in at least two different settings. For example, most children with ADHD have symptoms in school and at home. Table 6-1 outlines the diagnostic criteria for ADHD.

Distinguishing features of ADHD are short attention span and high levels of distractibility for chronologic age and developmental level. In school, children with ADHD often exhibit difficulties following instructions and require increased individualized attention from teachers. At home, children with ADHD frequently have difficulty complying with their parents' directions and may need to be asked multiple times to complete relatively simple tasks. Children with ADHD typically act impulsively, are emotionally labile, explosive, lack focus, and are irritable.

Children for whom hyperactivity is a predominant feature are more likely to be referred for treatment earlier than are children whose primary symptoms are attention deficit. Children with the combined inattentive and hyperactive-impulsive symptoms of ADHD, or predominantly hyperactive-impulsive symptoms of ADHD, are more apt to have a stable diagnosis over time and to exhibit comorbid psychiatric disorders including disruptive behavior disorders, depressive disorders, and disruptive mood dysregulation disorder. Specific learning disorders in the areas of reading, arithmetic, language, and writing frequently occur in association with ADHD. We should assess global development to rule out other sources of inattention.

School history and teachers' reports are critical in evaluating whether a child's difficulties in learning and school behavior are caused primarily by inattention or compromised understanding of the academic material due to specific learning disorders. In addition to intellectual limitations, poor performance in school may result from developmental delays, social rejection, mood disorders, anxiety, or poor self-esteem. Assessment of social relationships with siblings, peers, and adults and engagement in free and structured activities may yield valuable diagnostic clues to the presence of ADHD. Children with ADHD who are well aware of their impairment may become demoralized or display a depressed mood. Even children who are not well aware of their ADHD diagnosis will not typically display a thought disorder or impaired reality testing. A child with ADHD may exhibit distractibility and perseveration and signs of visual-perceptual, auditory-perceptual, or language-based learning disorders.

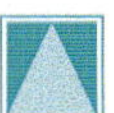

Table 6-1.
Attention-Deficit/Hyperactivity Disorder

	DSM-5-TR	ICD-10	ICD-11
Diagnostic name	Attention-Deficit/Hyperactivity Disorder	Hyperkinetic Disorders Disturbance of activity and attention	Attention deficit hyperactivity disorder
Duration	6 mo or longer		Persistent for ≥6 mo, begins before age 12 (usually)
Symptoms	A persistent pattern of either or both of Inattention, as evidenced by: • Failure to give attention to details or making frequent mistakes • Difficulty maintaining attention or focus • Not seeming to listen when spoken to • Failing to follow through with tasks or instructions • Difficulty organizing tasks • Avoiding or delaying tasks that require sustained mental effort or attention • Frequently losing or misplacing items • Easily distracted • Forgetfulness Hyperactivity/impulsivity, as evidenced by: • Fidgeting or restlessness • Inability to remain in a seat • Running around or climbing in inappropriate social situations • Inability to engage in quiet play or activities • Difficulty remaining still or inactive • Talking excessively • Blurting out answers without waiting for their turn • Difficulty waiting for one's turn • Frequently interrupting others Symptoms present before the age of 12, with symptoms present in ≥2 settings	Early onset (usually before the age of 5) of inability to engage in activities requiring prolonged attention, in addition to disorganization of task completion and excessive activity. There may also be associated impulsivity, recklessness, and social disinhibition.	• Inattention symptoms and/or a combination of hyperactivity and impulsivity symptoms • Outside the limits of normal variation expected for age and level of intellectual development • Symptoms vary according to chronologic age and disorder severity • Occur in a variety of settings Inattention • Difficulty sustaining attention • Easily distracted • Loses things • Hyperactivity • Excess motor activity • Difficulty engaging in activities quietly • Blurts out answers in school • Inappropriately acts out in response to stimuli
Required number of symptoms	≥6 symptoms of inattention (≥5 for adolescents/adults) and/or ≥6 of hyperactivity-impulsivity (≥5 for adolescents/adults)		
Psychosocial Consequences	Impairment in functioning		Impairment in functioning
Exclusions	Result of: • Other mental illness		Another mental disorder Substance or medication
Symptoms Specifiers	**Combined presentation** **Predominantly inattentive presentation** **Predominantly hyperactive/impulsive presentation**		Combined presentation Predominantly inattentive presentation Predominantly hyperactive/ impulsive presentation
Course specifiers	**In partial remission** (full/all criteria not met for prior 6 mo, though symptoms still causing significant impairment)		
Severity specifiers	**Mild** (few symptoms in excess of the minimum required for diagnosis, in addition to only minor impairment at most in functioning) **Moderate** (intermediate severity/ impairment) **Severe** (several symptoms of high severity and resulting in marked impairment)		

(continued)

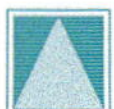

Table 6-1.
Attention-Deficit/Hyperactivity Disorder (Continued)

	DSM-5-TR	ICD-10	ICD-11
	Other Specified Attention-Deficit/ Hyperactivity Disorder Reserved for cases where above symptoms cause distress or impairment but do not meet full criteria for a diagnosis. **Unspecified Attention-Deficit Hyperactivity** Disorder is reserved for cases in which symptoms do not meet full criteria, and clinician chooses not to specify reasons for the disorder, or there is insufficient information.	Hyperkinetic conduct disorder—referring to symptoms present in the context of conduct disorder	**Other Specified Attention-Deficit/ Hyperactivity Disorder** **Unspecified Attention-Deficit Hyperactivity**

A neurologic examination may reveal visual, motor, perceptual, or auditory discriminatory immaturity or impairments without overt signs of visual or auditory disorders. Children with ADHD often have problems with motor coordination and difficulty copying age-appropriate figures, rapid alternating movements, right–left discrimination, ambidexterity, reflex asymmetries, and a variety of subtle nonfocal neurologic signs (soft signs).

If there are indications of possible absence spells, clinicians should obtain a neurologic consultation and an EEG to rule out a complex seizure disorder. A child with an unrecognized temporal lobe seizure focus may have behavior disturbances that can resemble those of ADHD.

Pathology and Laboratory Examination

Evaluation for ADHD includes a comprehensive psychiatric and medical history. This history includes prenatal, perinatal, and toddler information. Complications during the mother's pregnancy are also informative. Medical problems that may produce symptoms overlapping with ADHD include petit mal epilepsy, hearing and visual impairments, thyroid abnormalities, and hypoglycemia. A thorough cardiac history should be taken, including an investigation of the life history of syncope, family history of sudden death, and a cardiac examination of the child. If any cardiac risk factors are present, a cardiology consultation and examination are warranted, and an EKG and cardiac ultrasound may be obtained. No specific laboratory measures are pathognomonic of ADHD.

Children with ADHD typically have impairments in impulsivity and attention. A continuous performance task (CPT) is a computerized task in which a child presses a button each time a particular sequence of letters or numbers flashes on a screen. Children with ADHD often reveal difficulty with errors of commission, indicating impulsivity (pressing the button when the sequence has not emerged) or errors of omission, indicating impaired attention (failing to press the button when the sequence has been displayed). Although not a diagnostic tool for ADHD, a CPT can be useful in comparing a child with ADHD's performance before and on medication treatment, particularly at different doses.

DIFFERENTIAL DIAGNOSIS

There is a range within typical children of temperamental traits of high activity level and short attention span which does not cause impairment and is within the normal range for the child's age. Differentiating temperamental characteristics which do not cause impairment from the cardinal symptoms of ADHD before the age of 3 years is difficult because very young children typically have short attention spans and high levels of impulsivity. It is important to consider whether anxiety is a contributing factor in a child being evaluated for ADHD. Anxiety may accompany ADHD as a symptom or comorbid disorder, and anxiety can manifest with overactivity and easy distractibility.

It is not uncommon for a child with ADHD to become demoralized or, in some cases, to develop depressive symptoms in reaction to persistent frustration with academic and social difficulties and resulting in low self-esteem. Mania and ADHD share many core features, such as excessive verbalization, motoric hyperactivity, and high levels of distractibility. Although extremely rare in prepubertal children, mania in childhood typically presents with irritability rather than euphoria. Mania and ADHD can coexist, however, children and adolescents with bipolar I disorder exhibit more waxing and waning of mood cycles rather than the persistent hyperactivity and impulsivity of ADHD. Follow-up data of children who met the criteria for ADHD in childhood and subsequently developed bipolar disorder as adolescents or young adults suggest that certain clinical features in ADHD may predict future mania. Children with ADHD who had developed bipolar I disorder at 4-year follow-up had a higher number of comorbid disorders and a higher family history of bipolar disorders and other mood disorders than children without bipolar disorder.

We must also distinguish specific learning disorders from ADHD; a child may be unable to read or do mathematics because of a learning disorder rather than because of inattention. ADHD often coexists with one or more learning problems, including deficits in reading, mathematics, or written expression.

The DSM-5 includes Unspecified ADHD as a category for disturbances of inattention or hyperactivity that cause impairment but do not meet the full criteria for ADHD.

COURSE AND PROGNOSIS

The course of ADHD is variable. Symptoms persist into adolescence in 60% to 85% of cases and into adult life in approximately 60% of cases. The remaining 40% of cases may remit at puberty or in early adulthood. In some cases, the hyperactivity may disappear, but the decreased attention span and impulse-control problems persist. Overactivity is usually the first symptom to remit, and distractibility is the last. ADHD does not usually remit during middle childhood. A family history of the disorder predicts persistence, as do adverse life events and comorbidity with conduct symptoms, depression, and anxiety disorders. When remission occurs, it is usually between the ages of 12 and 20. After remission, with or without treatment, the child or adolescent can go on to have a productive adolescence and adult life, satisfying interpersonal relationships, and few significant sequelae. Even many teens and young adults with a persistent ADHD diagnosis can learn to manage their symptoms and lead productive lives. Most patients with ADHD achieve partial remission and have some increased risk for substance use disorders and mood disorders. Learning problems often continue throughout life.

In about 60% of cases, some symptoms persist into adulthood. Those who persist with the disorder may show diminished hyperactivity but remain impulsive and accident-prone. Although the educational attainments of people with ADHD as a group are lower than those of people without ADHD, early employment histories do not differ from those of people with similar educations.

Many children with ADHD have social skills difficulties. Socially impaired children with ADHD have significantly higher rates of comorbid psychiatric disorders and experience more problems with behavior in school as well as with peers and family members. Overall, the outcome of ADHD in childhood seems to be related to the degree of persistent comorbid psychopathology, including mood disorders, substance use disorders, chaotic family factors, and adverse childhood events. For optimal outcomes, it is essential to ameliorate children's social functioning, diminish aggression, and improve family functioning as early as possible.

TREATMENT

Pharmacotherapy

Pharmacologic treatment is considered the first line of treatment for ADHD. CNS stimulants are the first choice of agents in that they have the highest efficacy with generally mild, tolerable side effects. Children, adolescents, and adults with known cardiac risks and abnormalities require an evaluation by a cardiologist and clearance for the safe use of stimulants. In healthy youths, both short- and sustained-release preparations have excellent safety records. The newer preparations aim to maximize the target effects and minimize the adverse effects in individuals with ADHD who obtain a partial response from methylphenidate or whose dose was limited by side effects.

Current strategies favor once-a-day sustained-release stimulant preparations for their convenience and diminished rebound side effects. The advantages of the sustained-release preparations are that a single dose will sustain the effects all day, and the medication is sustained at an approximately even level in the body throughout the day. In general, the immediate-release preparations are expected to last 1 to 4 hours, and extended-release preparations are expected to last up to 8 hours, with exceptions for the transdermal patch, which lasts an hour after it is removed.

Nonstimulant medications approved by the FDA in the treatment of ADHD include atomoxetine, a norepinephrine uptake inhibitor. Unlike stimulants, atomoxetine carries with it a black-box warning for potential increases in suicidal thoughts or behaviors and requires children with ADHD to be monitored for these symptoms, similar to children taking antidepressants. α-agonists, including clonidine and guanfacine, are also useful in treating ADHD. The FDA has approved the extended-release form of clonidine and the extended-release form of guanfacine for the treatment of ADHD in children 6 years and older. Antidepressants, such as bupropion, have been used with variable success in the treatment of ADHD. Table 6-2 indicates FDA-approved ages for ADHD medications.

Stimulant Medications. Methylphenidate and amphetamine preparations are dopamine agonists; however, the precise mechanism of the stimulant's central action remains unknown. Methylphenidate preparations are highly effective in up to three-fourths of children with ADHD, with relatively few adverse effects. Concerta, the 10- to 12-hour extended-release OROS (osmotic controlled-release extended delivery system) form of methylphenidate, is administered once daily in the morning and is useful during school hours as well as after school during the afternoon and early evening. Both shorter forms of methylphenidate and Concerta have similar common adverse effects, including headaches, stomachaches, nausea, and insomnia. Some children experience a rebound effect, in which they become mildly irritable and appear to be slightly hyperactive for a brief period when the medication wears off. In children with a history of motor tics, we should observe them as, in some cases, methylphenidate can exacerbate the tics, whereas, in other children, the tics are unaffected or even improved. Because tics wax and wane, it is essential to observe their patterns over some time. Another common concern about

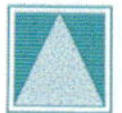

Table 6-2.
FDA Approval for ADHD Medications

Medication	Generic Name	FDA Approval Age (yr)
Methylphenidate		
Concerta	Methylphenidate (OROS long-acting)	6 and older
Ritalin	Methylphenidate	6 and older
Ritalin LA	Methylphenidate (long-acting)	6 and older
Metadate ER	Methylphenidate (extended-release)	6 and older
Metadate CD	Methylphenidate (extended-release)	6 and older
Methylin	Methylphenidate (oral solution and chewable tablet)	6 and older
Daytrana	Methylphenidate (patch)	6 and older
Adhansia XR	Methylphenidate (extended-release)	6 and older
Aptensio XR	Methylphenidate (extended-release)	6 and older
Cotempla XR-ODT	Methylphenidate (extended-release orally disintegrating tablet)	6–17
Jornay PM	Methylphenidate (extended-release)	6 and older
Quillichew	Methylphenidate (extended-release chewable)	6 and older
Quillivant ER	Methylphenidate (extended-release suspension)	6 and older
Dexmethylphenidate		
Focalin	Dexmethylphenidate	6 and older
Focalin XR	Dexmethylphenidate (extended-release)	6 and older
Dextroamphetamine		
Dexedrine	Dextroamphetamine	3 and older
Amphetamine		
Adzenys ER	Amphetamine (extended-release suspension)	6–12
Adzenys XR-ODT	Amphetamine (extended-release orally disintegrating tablet)	6–17
Dynavel XR	Amphetamine (extended-release suspension)	6 and older
Evekeo	Amphetamine	3 and older
Evekeo ODT	Amphetamine (orally disintegrating tablet)	6–17
Dextroamphetamine/amphetamine		
Adderall	Dextroamphetamine/amphetamine	3 and older
Adderall XR	Dextroamphetamine/amphetamine (extended-release)	6 and older
Mydayis	Dextroamphetamine/amphetamine (extended-release)	13 and older
Lisdexamfetamine		
Vyvanse	Lisdexamfetamine	6 and older
Nonstimulants		
Strattera	Atomoxetine	6 and older
α Agonists		
Kapvay	Clonidine (extended-release)	6–17
Intuniv	Guanfacine (extended-release)	6–17

the use of methylphenidate preparations over long periods is potential growth suppression. During periods of use, methylphenidate may cause slightly decreased rates of growth, and if used over many years continuously without any drug holidays, experts have noted a growth suppression of about several centimeters. When given "drug holidays" on weekends or summers, children tend to eat more and also make up the growth. The methylphenidate products can improve ADHD children's scores on tasks of vigilance, such as on math calculation tests, the CPT, and paired associations. Transdermal methylphenidate is available for children and adolescents. Advantages of this preparation include an alternative for children who have difficulties swallowing pills, and that the patch can individualize how many hours per day a given child with ADHD receives the medication. This option is useful because a child with ADHD who needs the medication in the late afternoons to do homework but develops insomnia if the medication is still present after dinner can remove the patch at the desired time. Thus, individualized delivery time may be provided for each child by how many hours they wear the patch.

In contrast, oral sustained-release forms of methylphenidate are those in which the release time continues for 12 hours after swallowing the pill. A double-blind, randomized study in children with ADHD who wore the methylphenidate patch for 12 hours at a time showed the efficacy of the patch preparation doses ranging from patches delivering 0.45 to 1.8 mg/hr of methylphenidate. A delay in the onset of the transdermal medication effect was approximately an hour. Side effects were similar to oral preparations of methylphenidate. Approximately half of the children exhibited at least minor erythematous reactions to the patch; however, these side effects are usually well tolerated by children on the patch. Dextroamphetamine and dextroamphetamine/amphetamine salt combinations are usually the second drugs of choice when methylphenidate fails.

CNS STIMULANT SIDE EFFECTS. CNS stimulants are generally well-tolerated, and the current expert consensus is that long-acting, once-a-day dosing is preferable for convenience and to minimize rebound side effects. Long-term tolerability of once-daily mixed amphetamine salts has shown mild side effects, most commonly decreased appetite, insomnia, and headache. There are a variety of strategies for children or adolescents with ADHD who respond favorably to methylphenidate but for whom insomnia has become a significant problem. Clinical strategies to manage insomnia include the use of melatonin, up to 10 mg/day, and α-adrenergic agents such as guanfacine, long-acting guanfacine (Intuniv), or clonidine. When ineffective, short-term use of diphenhydramine (25 to 75 mg) or low-dose trazodone (25 to 50 mg) can be used. In some cases, insomnia may attenuate on its own after several months of treatment.

Nonstimulant Medications. Atomoxetine is a norepinephrine uptake inhibitor approved by the FDA for the treatment of ADHD in children age 6 years and older. The mechanism of action is not well understood but likely involves selective inhibition of the presynaptic norepinephrine transporter. Atomoxetine absorbs well in the gastrointestinal tract, and it reaches maximal plasma levels in 1 to 2 hours after ingestion. It is useful for inattention as well as impulsivity in children and adults with ADHD. Its half-life is approximately 5 hours, and it is given twice daily in most cases. The most common side effects include diminished appetite, abdominal discomfort, dizziness, and irritability. In some cases, there were increases in blood pressure and heart rate. Atomoxetine is metabolized by the cytochrome P450 (CYP) 2D6 hepatic enzyme system. A small fraction of the population are poor metabolizers of CYP 2D6–metabolized drugs, and, for those individuals, plasma concentrations of the drug may increase as much as fivefold for a given dose of medication. Drugs that inhibit CYP 2D6, including fluoxetine, paroxetine, and quinidine, may lead to increased plasma levels of this medication. Despite its short half-life, research suggests that atomoxetine can reduce symptoms of ADHD in children during the school day when administered once daily. Another recent study of a combination of atomoxetine alone and combined with fluoxetine in the treatment of 127 children with ADHD and symptoms of anxiety or depression suggested that atomoxetine alone can lead to improvements in mood and anxiety. Children who received combined atomoxetine and fluoxetine experienced more significant increases in blood pressure and pulse than those taking atomoxetine only.

α-Agonists, both short-acting and the extended-release forms of clonidine hydrochloride and guanfacine, are FDA-approved for the treatment of ADHD in children and adolescents from 6 to 7 years of age. Clonidine, a centrally acting α_2-adrenergic receptor agonist, likely exerts its effect on the prefrontal cortex, although the mechanism of action is unknown. It is available in 0.1-mg and 0.2-mg tablets and is generally used twice daily, once in the morning and once at night, to provide an around-the-clock effect. Clonidine is initiated at 0.1 mg at bedtime, with incremental weekly increases of 0.1 mg. The maximum dose recommended is 0.2 mg twice daily. The extended-release formulation is not interchangeable with the short-acting clonidine. Because it is also an antihypertensive agent, it causes a decrease in blood pressure and heart rate. We should monitor vital signs in patients, especially during initiation and titration of the dose. Common side effects include somnolence, headache, upper abdominal pain, and fatigue. When tapering the drug, the rate should be no more than 0.1 mg every 3 to 7 days.

Extended-release guanfacine (Intuniv) is a once-a-day medication for children between 6 and 17 years of age, available in 1-mg, 2-mg, 3-mg, and 4-mg tabs. It is swallowed whole with liquids, and the patient should not take it with a high-fat meal. It is initiated as a 1-mg tab daily and titrated by 1 mg/day at 1-week intervals. The maximum dose approved is 4 mg/day. As a monotherapy, improvement in ADHD symptoms occur at 0.05 to 0.08 mg/kg once daily. As an adjunctive treatment, optimal doses are reported to range from 0.05 to 0.12 mg/kg/day. Common side effects include somnolence, sedation, fatigue, nausea, hypotension, insomnia, and dizziness. We should monitor the heart rate and blood pressure. When discontinuing the drug, one should use a gradual taper, decreasing by 1 mg every 3 to 7 days.

α-Adrenergic agents, including the short- and extended-release preparations of guanfacine and clonidine, are sometimes preferred treatments in children with ADHD and comorbid tic disorders when stimulants exacerbate the tics. Bupropion is somewhat useful for some children and adolescents in the treatment of ADHD. One multisite, double-blind, placebo-controlled study found a positive result regarding the efficacy of bupropion. No further studies have compared bupropion with other stimulants. There is a higher risk of seizures at doses of 400 mg/day or more.

Few data confirm the efficacy of SSRIs in the treatment of ADHD, but due to the frequency of comorbid depression and anxiety with ADHD, in cases of comorbidity, the SSRIs may be considered in conjunction with a stimulant.

Tricyclic drugs for ADHD are not generally recommended due to potential cardiac arrhythmia effects. The reports of sudden death in at least four children with ADHD using desipramine have made tricyclic antidepressants an unlikely choice. Antipsychotics are not recommended for the treatment of ADHD. However, in cases of intractable hyperactivity, usually in comorbid cases, antipsychotics may be considered for adolescents whose hyperactivity is causing potential harm to the patient and others. Antipsychotics are generally not chosen in the treatment of ADHD due to the risks of tardive dyskinesia, withdrawal dyskinesia, neuroleptic malignant syndrome, weight gain, and metabolic dysfunction.

Modafinil, another type of CNS stimulant, a narcolepsy treatment, may help treat adults with ADHD. Only one randomized, double-blind, placebo-controlled study of the efficacy and safety of modafinil film-coated tablets in approximately 250 adolescents with ADHD showed that 48% of those on active treatment were rated as "much" or "very much" improved compared with 17% of patients receiving placebo. The dosage range was from 170 to 425 mg, administered once daily and titrated to optimal doses based on efficacy and tolerability. Modafinil failed to receive FDA approval based on a Stevens–Johnson skin rash that occurred in a patient during the trial. The most common side effects included insomnia, headache, and decreased appetite.

Some clinicians use venlafaxine, especially for children and adolescents, with combinations of ADHD and depression or anxiety features. No clear empirical evidence supports the use of venlafaxine in the treatment of ADHD.

One open-label report of reboxetine, a selective norepinephrine reuptake inhibitor that is not available in the United States, in 31 children and adolescents with ADHD who were resistant to methylphenidate treatment suggested that this agent may have efficacy. In this open trial, reboxetine was initiated and maintained at 4 mg/day. The most common side effects included drowsiness, sedation, and gastrointestinal symptoms. Reboxetine and other new agents in this class await controlled studies.

Monitoring Pharmacologic Treatment

STIMULANTS. Stimulant medications have adrenergic effects and cause moderate increases in blood pressure and pulse rate. At baseline, the most recent American Academy of Child and Adolescent Psychiatry (AACAP) practice parameters recommend the following workup before starting the use of stimulant medications: physical examination, blood pressure, pulse, weight, and height. Screening electrocardiograms are not generally recommended prior to initiating stimulant medications unless there is a family history or risk factors for cardiac disease.

Children and adolescents using stimulants should have their height, weight, blood pressure, and pulse checked quarterly and have a physical examination annually. Monitoring starts with the initiation of medication. Because school performance is most markedly affected, we should give individual attention and effort to establishing and maintaining a close collaborative working relationship with a child's school personnel. In most patients, stimulants reduce overactivity, distractibility, impulsiveness, explosiveness, and irritability. No evidence indicates that medications directly improve any existing impairments in learning, although when the attention deficits diminish, children can learn more effectively. Stimulant medication has been shown to decrease aggressive behaviors in children with ADHD and can improve self-esteem when children are no longer constantly reprimanded for their behavior. Children treated with medications should be taught the purpose of the medication and encouraged to describe any side effects that they may be experiencing.

Psychosocial Interventions

Psychosocial interventions for children with ADHD include psychoeducation, academic organization skills remediation, parent training, behavior modification in the classroom and at home, CBT, and social skills training. These psychosocial interventions are not aimed at treating the core symptoms of ADHD; rather, they target ways to teach the child and parents strategies for managing their residual symptoms. There are various studies of social skills groups, behavioral training for parents of children with ADHD, and behavioral interventions at school and home, alone and in combination with medication management for ADHD. Evaluation and treatment of coexisting learning disorders or additional psychiatric disorders are essential.

Psychosocial interventions are not aimed at the core symptoms of ADHD. Rather, when we help children structure their environment, their anxiety and oppositional behaviors diminish. Parents and teachers should work together to develop concrete expectations for the child and a system of rewards when the child meets these expectations.

A common goal of therapy is to help parents of children with ADHD recognize and promote the notion that, although the child may not "voluntarily" exhibit symptoms of ADHD, they are still capable of being responsible for trying to meet reasonable expectations. We should also help parents recognize that, despite their child's difficulties, every child faces the usual tasks of maturation, including the significant building of self-esteem when they develop a sense of mastery. Therefore, children with ADHD do not benefit from being exempted from the majority of requirements, expectations, and planning applicable to other children. Parent training is an integral part of the psychotherapeutic interventions for ADHD. Most parental training helps parents develop usable behavioral interventions with positive reinforcement that target both social and academic behaviors.

Group therapy aimed at both refining social skills and increasing self-esteem and a sense of success may be beneficial for children with ADHD who have great difficulty functioning in group settings, especially in school. A recent year-long group therapy intervention in a clinical setting for boys with the disorder described the goals as helping the boys improve skills in game-playing and feeling a sense of mastery with peers. The researchers asked the boys to do a fun task in pairs, and then they were gradually asked to do projects in a group. The researchers directed them on how to follow instructions, wait, and pay attention and praised them for successful cooperation.

Multimodal Treatment Study of Children with ADHD (MTA Study)

The National Institute of Mental Health (NIMH)–supported Multimodal Treatment Study of Children with ADHD (The MTA Cooperative Group, 1999) was a 14-month–long randomized clinical trial involving six clinical sites comparing four treatment strategies. More than 500 children diagnosed with DSM-IV ADHD, combined type, were randomly assigned to: (1) systematic medication management utilizing an initial placebo-controlled titration and three times per day dosing 7 days per week and monthly 30-minute clinic visits; (2) behavior therapy consisting of 27 sessions of group parent training, eight individual parent sessions, an 8-week summer treatment program, 12 weeks of classroom administered behavior therapy with a half-time aide, and 10 teacher consultation sessions; (3) a combination of medication and behavior therapy; or (4) usual community care. All groups showed improvement over baseline; however, a combination of medication management and behavior therapy led to a greater reduction in symptoms in children with ADHD alone or ADHD and oppositional defiant disorder than in behavior therapy alone or community care. The combination treatment had significantly better outcomes for those children with ADHD and anxiety or mood disorders compared to behavioral treatment and community care. Combined treatment but not medication management was superior for improvement in oppositional and aggressive symptoms, anxiety and mood symptoms, teacher-rated social skills, parent–child relationships, and reading achievement. Furthermore, the mean dose of medication per day was less in the combination group than in the medication-only management group.

A follow-up of the MTA sample at 6 and 8 years revealed that the clinical presentation of the disorder, including the severity of ADHD, comorbid conduct disturbance, and intellect, were more reliable predictors of later functioning than the type of treatment received in childhood during the 14-month study period. The children maintained the improvements as long as they continued treatment, but 3 years after treatment, there was no difference between groups.

Overall, the evidence suggests that medication and psychosocial interventions for the combined type of ADHD in childhood provide the broadest benefit in functioning for this population. This recommendation is especially pertinent given the comorbidity of learning disorders, anxiety, mood disorders, and other disruptive behavior disorders that occur in children with ADHD.

EPIDEMIOLOGY

Rates of ADHD are 7% to 8% in prepubertal elementary school children in the United States. Epidemiologic studies suggest that ADHD occurs in about 5% of youth, including children and adolescents, and about 2.5% of adults. The rate of ADHD in parents and siblings of children with ADHD is two to eight times greater than in the general population. ADHD is more prevalent in boys than in girls, with the ratio ranging from 2:1 to as high as 9:1. First-degree biologic relatives (e.g., siblings of probands with ADHD) are at high risk for developing ADHD as well as other psychiatric disorders, including disruptive behavior disorders, anxiety disorders, and depressive disorders. Siblings of children with ADHD are also at higher risk than the general population for learning disorders and academic difficulties. The parents of children with ADHD show an increased incidence of substance use disorders. Symptoms of ADHD are often present by age 3 years, but unless they are very severe, the diagnosis is frequently not made until the child is in kindergarten or elementary school when teacher information is available comparing the index child to peers of the same age.

ETIOLOGY

Data suggest that the etiology of ADHD is mainly genetic, with a heritability of approximately 75%. ADHD symptoms are the product of complex interactions of neuroanatomical and neurochemical systems evidenced by data from twin and adoption family genetic studies, dopamine transport gene studies, neuroimaging studies, and neurotransmitter data. Most children with ADHD have no evidence of gross structural damage in the CNS. In some cases, contributory factors for ADHD may include prenatal toxic exposures, prematurity, and prenatal mechanical insult to the fetal nervous system. Some have suggested that food additives, colorings, preservatives, and sugar are possible contributing causes of hyperactive behavior; however, studies have not confirmed these theories. No research has established artificial food coloring or sugar as causes of ADHD. There is no clear evidence that omega-3 fatty acids are beneficial in the treatment of ADHD.

Genetic Factors

Evidence for a significant genetic contribution to ADHD has emerged from family studies, which reveal an increased concordance in monozygotic compared to dizygotic twins, as well as a marked increased risk of two to eight times for siblings as well as parents of an ADHD child, compared to the general population. Clinically, one sibling may have impulsivity/hyperactivity symptoms predominantly, and others may have predominantly inattention symptoms. Up to 70% of children with ADHD meet the criteria for a comorbid psychiatric disorder, including learning disorders, anxiety disorders, mood disorders, conduct disorders, and substance use disorders. Several hypotheses regarding the mode of transmission of ADHD have been proposed, including a sex-linked hypothesis, which would explain the significantly increased rates of ADHD in males. Other theories have focused on a model of the interaction of multiple genes that produces the various symptoms of ADHD. Numerous investigations continue to identify specific genes involved in ADHD. Cook and colleagues have found an association of the dopamine transporter gene (DAT1) with ADHD, although data from other research groups have not confirmed that result. Family studies and population-based studies have found an association between the dopamine four receptor seven-repeat allele (DRD4) gene and ADHD. Most molecular research on ADHD has focused on genes that influence the metabolism or action of dopamine. Continued investigation is necessary to clarify the complex relationships between multiple interactive genes and the emergence of ADHD.

Neurochemical Factors

Many neurotransmitters are likely associated with ADHD symptoms; however, dopamine is a primary focus of clinical investigation, and the prefrontal cortex has been implicated based on its role in attention and regulation of impulse control. Animal studies have shown that other brain regions, such as locus ceruleus, which consists predominantly of noradrenergic neurons, also play a significant role in attention. The noradrenergic system includes the central system (originating in the locus ceruleus) and the peripheral sympathetic system. Dysfunction in peripheral epinephrine, which causes the hormone to accumulate peripherally, may potentially feedback to the central system and "reset" the locus ceruleus to a lower level. In part, hypotheses regarding the neurochemistry of ADHD have arisen from the predictable effect of medications. Stimulants, known to be the most effective medications in the treatment of ADHD, affect both dopamine and norepinephrine, leading to neurotransmitter hypotheses that may include dysfunction in both the adrenergic and dopaminergic systems. Stimulants increase catecholamine concentrations by promoting their release and blocking their uptake.

Neurophysiologic Factors

EEG studies in ADHD children and adolescents over the last several decades have found evidence of increased theta activity, especially in the frontal regions. Further studies of youth with ADHD have provided data showing elevated beta activity in their EEG studies. Clarke and colleagues, studying EEG findings in children and adolescents over the last two decades, found that those ADHD children with the combined type of ADHD were the ones who showed significantly elevated beta activity on EEG, and further studies indicate that these youth also tend to show increased mood lability and temper tantrums. The current investigation of EEG in youth with ADHD has identified behavioral symptom clusters among children with similar EEG profiles.

Neuroanatomical Aspects

Researchers have hypothesized networks within the brain for promoting components of attention, including focusing, sustaining attention, and shifting attention. They describe neuroanatomical correlations for the superior and temporal cortices with focusing attention; external parietal and corpus striatal regions with motor executive functions; the hippocampus with encoding of memory traces; and the prefrontal cortex with shifting from one stimulus to another. Further hypotheses suggest that the brainstem, which contains the reticular thalamic nuclei function, is involved in sustained attention. A review of MRI, positron emission tomography (PET), and single-photon emission computerized tomography (SPECT) suggests that populations of children with ADHD show evidence of both decreased volume and decreased activity in prefrontal regions, anterior cingulate, globus pallidus, caudate, thalamus, and cerebellum. PET scans have also shown that female adolescents with ADHD have globally lower glucose metabolism than both control female and male adolescents without ADHD. One theory postulates that the frontal lobes in children with ADHD do not adequately inhibit lower brain structures, an effect leading to disinhibition.

Developmental Factors

Higher rates of ADHD are present in children who were born prematurely and whose mothers had infections during pregnancy. Perinatal insult to the brain during early infancy caused by infection, inflammation, and trauma may, in some cases, be contributing factors in the emergence of ADHD symptoms. Children with ADHD exhibit nonfocal (soft) neurologic signs at higher rates than those in the general population. Reports in the literature indicate that September is a peak month for births of children with ADHD with and without comorbid learning disorders. The implication is that prenatal exposure to winter infections during the first trimester may contribute to the emergence of ADHD symptoms in some susceptible children.

Psychosocial Factors

In utero, drug and alcohol exposure, severe chronic abuse, maltreatment, and neglect are associated with behavioral symptoms that overlap with ADHD, including poor attention and poor impulse control. Predisposing factors may include the child's temperament and genetic–familial factors.

Further Readings

American Psychiatric Association. *Diagnostic and Statistical Manual of Mental Disorders*. 5th ed, text revision. American Psychiatric Association; 2022.

Andrade BF, Courtney D, Duda S, et al. A systematic review and evaluation of clinical practice guidelines for children and youth with disruptive behavior: rigor of development and recommendations for use. *Clin Child Fam Psychol Rev*. 2019;22(4):527–548.

Barbaresi WJ, Campbell L, Diekroger EA, et al. Society for Developmental and Behavioral Pediatrics Clinical Practice Guideline for the assessment and treatment of children and adolescents with complex attention-deficit/hyperactivity disorder. *J Dev Behav Pediatr*. 2020; 41(Suppl 2S):S35–S57.

Becker SP. Systematic review: assessment of sluggish cognitive tempo over the past decade. *J Am Acad Child Adolesc Psychiatry*. 2021; 60:690–709.

Catalá-López F, Hutton B, Núñez-Beltrán A, et al. The pharmacological and non-pharmacological treatment of attention deficit hyperactivity disorder in children and adolescents: a systematic review with network meta-analyses of randomised trials. *PLoS One*. 2017;12(7):e0180355.

Chen Q, Brikell I, Lichtenstein P, et al. Familial aggregation of attention-deficit/hyperactivity disorder. *J Child Psychol Psychiatry*. 2017; 58(3):231–239.

Cortese S, Adamo N, Del Giovane C, et al. Comparative efficacy and tolerability of medications for attention-deficit hyperactivity disorder in children, adolescents, and adults: a systematic review and network meta-analysis. *Lancet Psychiatry*. 2018;5(9):727–738.

Cothros N, Medina A, Pringsheim T. Current pharmacotherapy for tic disorders. *Expert Opin Pharmacother*. 2020;21(5):567–580.

Coughlin CG, Cohen SC, Mulqueen JM, et al. Meta-analysis: reduced risk of anxiety with psychostimulant treatment in children with attention-deficit/hyperactivity disorder. *J Child Adolesc Psychopharmacol*. 2015;25(8):611–617.

Daley D, Van der Oord S, Ferrin M, et al; European ADHD Guidelines Group. Behavioral interventions in attention-deficit/hyperactivity disorder: a meta-analysis of randomized controlled trials across multiple outcome domains. *J Am Acad Child Adolesc Psychiatry*. 2014;53(8):835–847, 847.e1–e5.

Danielson ML, Bitsko RH, Ghandour RM, Holbrook JR, Kogan MD, Blumberg SJ. Prevalence of parent-reported ADHD diagnosis and associated treatment among US children and adolescents, 2016. *J Clinical Child & Adolescent Psychology*. 2018;47(2);199–212.

Demontis D, Walters RK, Martin J, et al; ADHD Working Group of the Psychiatric Genomics Consortium (PGC); Early Lifecourse & Genetic Epidemiology (EAGLE) Consortium; 23andMe Research Team. Discovery of the first genome-wide significant risk loci for attention deficit/hyperactivity disorder. *Nat Genet*. 2019;51(1):63–75.

Faraone SV, Banaschewski T, Coghill D, et al. The World Federation of ADHD International Consensus Statement: 208 evidence-based conclusions about the disorder. *Neurosci Biobehav Rev*. 2021;128:789–818.

Faraone SV, Larsson H. Genetics of attention deficit hyperactivity disorder. *Mol Psychiatry*. 2019;24(4):562–575.

Greenhill LL, Swanson JM, Hechtman L, et al. Trajectories of growth associated with long-term stimulant medication in the multimodal treatment study of attention-deficit/hyperactivity disorder. *J Am Acad Child Adolesc Psychiatry*. 2020;59(8):978–989.

Hoogman M, Muetzel R, Guimaraes JP, et al. Brain imaging of the cortex in adhd: a coordinated analysis of large-scale clinical and population-based samples. *Am J Psychiatry*. 2019;176(7):531–542.

Joshi G, Wilens T, Firmin ES, Hoskova B, Biederman J. Pharmacotherapy of attention deficit/hyperactivity disorder in individuals with autism spectrum disorder: a systematic review of the literature. *J Psychopharmacol*. 2021;35(3):203–210.

Kooij JJS, Bijlenga D, Salerno L, et al. Updated European Consensus Statement on diagnosis and treatment of adult ADHD. *Eur Psychiatry*. 2019;56:14–34.

The MTA Cooperative Group. A 14-month randomized clinical trial of treatment strategies for attention-deficit/hyperactivity disorder. Multimodal treatment study of children with ADHD. *Arch Gen Psychiatry*. 1999;56:1073–1086.

The MTA Cooperative Group. Moderators and mediators of treatment response for children with attention-deficit/hyperactivity disorder: the multimodal treatment study of children with attention-deficit/hyperactivity disorder. *Arch Gen Psychiatry*. 1999;56(12):1088–1096.

Nakao T, Radua J, Rubia K, Mataix-Cols D. Gray matter volume abnormalities in ADHD: voxel-based meta-analysis exploring the effects of age and stimulant medication. *Am J Psychiatry*. 2011;168(11):1154–1163.

Nigg JT, Lewis K, Edinger T, Falk M. Meta-analysis of attention-deficit/hyperactivity disorder or attention-deficit/hyperactivity disorder symptoms, restriction diet, and synthetic food color additives. *J Am Acad Child Adolesc Psychiatry*. 2012;51(1):86–97.e8.

Pereira-Sanchez V, Castellanos FX. Neuroimaging in attention-deficit/hyperactivity disorder. *Curr Opin Psychiatry*. 2021;34(2):105–111.

Pettersson E, Lichtenstein P, Larsson H, et al. Genetic influences on eight psychiatric disorders based on family data of 4,408,646 full and half-siblings, and genetic data of 333,748 cases and controls. *Psychol Med*. 2019;49(7):1166–1173.

Pliszka SR, Greenhill LL, Crismon LM, et al. The Texas Children's Medication Algorithm Project: report of the Texas Consensus Conference Panel on medication treatment of childhood attention-deficit/hyperactivity disorder. Part II: tactics. *J Am Acad Child Adolesc Psychiatry*. 2000;39(7):920–927.

Stevens LJ, Kuczek T, Burgess JR, Hurt E, Arnold LE. Dietary sensitivities and ADHD symptoms: thirty-five years of research. *Clin Pediatr (Phila)*. 2011;50:279–293.

Vitiello B, Lazzaretto D, Yershova K, et al. Pharmacotherapy of the preschool ADHD treatment study (PATS) children growing up. *J Am Acad Child Adolesc Psychiatry*. 2015;57(7):550–556.

Willcutt EG. The prevalence of DSM-IV attention-deficit/hyperactivity disorder: a meta-analytic review. *Neurotherapeutics*. 2012;9(3):490–499.

Wolraich ML, Hagan JF, Allan C, et al; Subcommittee on Children and Adolescents with Attention-Deficit/Hyperactive Disorder. Clinical practice guideline for the diagnosis, evaluation, and treatment of attention-deficit/hyperactivity disorder in children and adolescents. *Pediatrics*. 2019;144:e20192528.

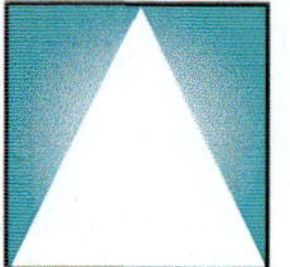

7 Specific Learning Disorder

Specific learning disorder in youth is a neurodevelopmental disorder produced by the interactions of heritable and environmental factors that influence the brain's ability to perceive or process verbal and nonverbal information efficiently. Children with the disorder have persistent difficulty learning academic skills in reading, written expression, or mathematics, beginning in early childhood, which is inconsistent with the overall intellectual ability of a child. Children with specific learning disorders often find it challenging to keep up with their peers in specific academic subjects, whereas they may excel in others. Academic skills may be compromised in specific learning disorders, including reading single words and sentences fluently, writing expression and spelling, and calculating and solving mathematical problems. Specific learning disorder results in unexpected underachievement based on the child's potential. Specific learning disorder in reading, spelling, and mathematics appears to aggregate in families. There is an increased risk of four to eight times in first-degree relatives for reading deficits and about five to ten times for mathematics deficits, compared to the general population. Specific learning disorder occurs two to three times more often in males than females. Learning problems in a child or adolescent identified in this manner can establish eligibility for academic services through the public school system.

The American Psychiatric Association's DSM-5-TR combines the DSM-IV diagnoses of reading disorder, mathematics disorder, and disorder of written expression, and learning disorder not otherwise specified into a single diagnosis: specific learning disorder. Learning deficits in reading, written expression, and mathematics in the DSM-5-TR are designated using specifiers. ICD-10 continues to separate the disorders. ICD-11 calls the disorder developmental learning disorder and follows criteria that are similar to DSM-5-TR.

DSM-5-TR notes that *dyslexia* is an equivalent term describing a pattern of learning difficulties, including deficits in accurate or fluent word recognition, poor decoding, and poor spelling. *Dyscalculia* is an alternative term referring to a pattern of deficits related to learning arithmetic facts, processing numerical information, and performing accurate calculations. Table 7-1 lists the approaches to diagnosing specific learning disorder.

Specific learning disorders of all types affect approximately 10% of youth. This disorder represents approximately half of all public school children who receive special education services in the United States. In 1975, Public Law 94–142 (the Education for All Handicapped Children Act, now known as the Individuals with Disabilities Education Act [IDEA]) mandated that all states provide all children with free and appropriate educational services. Since that time, the number of children identified with learning disorders has increased, and a variety of definitions of learning disabilities have arisen. For this diagnosis, a child's achievement must be significantly lower than expected in one or more of the following: reading skills, comprehension, spelling, written expression, calculation, mathematical reasoning, or the learning problems that interfere with academic achievement or activities of daily living. It is common for specific learning disorder to include more than one area of skill deficits.

Children with specific learning disorder in the area of reading can be identified by poor word recognition, slow reading rate, and impaired comprehension compared with most children of the same age. Current data suggest that most children with reading difficulties have speech sound processing skills deficits, regardless of their IQ. In DSM-5-TR, there is no longer a diagnostic criterion for specific learning disorder comparing the specific deficit to overall IQ. The current consensus is that children with reading impairment have trouble with word recognition and "sounding out" words because they cannot efficiently process and use phonemes (the smaller bits of words associated with particular sounds). An epidemiologic study found four profiles, including (1) weak reading, (2) weak language, (3) weak math, or (4) combined weak math and reading, accounting for 70% of children with specific learning impairments. Low scores in short-term memory for speech sounds characterized the profile with weak language, whereas low speech sound awareness was associated with the weak reading group but not the weak language group. Finally, another study found that the weak math group did not show speech sound deficits.

Severe specific learning disorder may make it agonizing for a child to succeed in school, often leading to demoralization, low self-esteem, chronic frustration, and

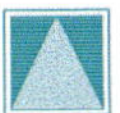

Table 7-1.
Specific Learning Disorder

	DSM-5-TR	ICD-10	ICD-11
Diagnostic name	Specific Learning Disorder	Specific Developmental Disorders of Scholastic Skills Specific Reading Disorder Specific Spelling Disorder Specific Disorder of Arithmetical Skills Mixed Disorder of Scholastic Skills	Developmental Learning Disorder
Duration	≥6 mo		Onset in early school years
Symptoms	Difficulties with learning or academics, below what would be expected per individual's age or school level, as evidenced by: • Inaccuracy or slowness with reading • Difficulty understanding or comprehending what is being read • Trouble with spelling • Difficulty with written expression • Difficulties with numbers or calculation • Difficulties with mathematical reasoning Symptoms begin during school-age years (but may become obvious during the later part of academic career)		The presence of significant limitations in learning academic skills of reading, writing, or arithmetic, resulting in a skill level markedly below what would be expected for age
Psychosocial Consequences	Impairment in functioning		Significant impairment to academic, occupational, or other areas of functioning
Exclusions	Result of: • Intellectual disability • Visual or auditory impairment • Another mental disorder • Another medical disorder • Psychosocial adversity • Result of inadequate educational instruction		External factors (economic, environmental disadvantage, lack of access to educational opportunities) Disorders of intellectual development, other neurodevelopmental disorders, and motor or sensory disorders
Symptoms Specifiers	***With impairment in reading*** ***With impairment in written expression*** ***With impairment in mathematics***		Impairment in reading Impairment in written expression Impairment in mathematics
Course specifiers			
Severity specifiers	**Mild** (minimal accommodations or support needed during school) **Moderate** (some accommodations needed) **Severe** (intensive individualized and specialized teaching needed for most of the schooling)		
Comments			Other specified impairments in learning Developmental Learning Disorder, Unspecified

compromised peer relationships. Specific learning disorder is associated with an increased risk of comorbid disorders, including attention-deficit/hyperactivity disorder (ADHD), communication disorders, conduct disorders, and depressive disorders. Adolescents with specific learning disorder are at least 1.5 times more likely to drop out of school, approximating rates of 40%. Adults with specific learning disorder are at increased risk for difficulties in employment and social adjustment. Specific learning disorder often extends to skills deficits in reading, writing, and mathematics.

Moderate to high heritability contributes to specific learning disorder, and many cognitive traits appear polygenic. Also, there is pleiotropy; the same genes may affect the skills necessary for diverse learning tasks. Factors such as perinatal injury and specific neurologic conditions may contribute to the development of specific learning disorder. Conditions such as lead poisoning, fetal alcohol syndrome, and in utero drug exposure are also associated with increased rates of specific learning disorder.

SPECIFIC LEARNING DISORDER WITH IMPAIRMENT IN READING

Reading impairment is present in up to 75% of children and adolescents with a specific learning disorder. Students with learning problems in other academic areas most commonly experience difficulties with reading as well.

Reading impairment is characterized by difficulty recognizing words, slow and inaccurate reading, poor comprehension, and difficulties with spelling. Reading impairment is often comorbid with other disorders in children, particularly ADHD. The historical term *developmental alexia* defines a developmental deficit in recognizing printed symbols. The term was simplified to *dyslexia* in the 1960s. Dyslexia was used extensively for many years to describe a reading disability syndrome that often included speech and language deficits and right–left confusion. Reading impairment is frequently accompanied by disabilities in other academic skills, and dyslexia remains an alternate term for a pattern of reading and spelling difficulties.

Clinical Features

We can usually identify children with reading disabilities by the age of 7 years (second grade). Reading difficulty may be apparent among classroom students who expect reading skills earlier. Children can sometimes compensate for reading disorders in the early elementary grades by using memory and inference, particularly in children with high intelligence. In such instances, the disorder may not be apparent until age 9 (fourth grade) or later. Children with reading impairment make many errors in their oral reading. The errors include omissions, additions, and distortions of words. Such children have difficulty distinguishing between printed letter characters and sizes, especially those that differ only in spatial orientation and length of a line. The problems in managing printed or written language can pertain to individual letters, sentences, and even a page. The child's reading speed is slow, often with minimal comprehension. Most children with reading disability have an age-appropriate ability to copy from a written or printed text, but nearly all spell poorly.

Associated problems include language difficulties, discrimination, and difficulty properly sequencing words. A patient might start with a word that occurs midway or at the end of a written sentence. Most children with reading disorder dislike and avoid reading and writing. They become anxious when confronted with demands that involve printed language. Many children with specific learning disorders who do not receive remedial education have a sense of shame and humiliation because of their continuing failure and subsequent frustration. The intensity of these feelings grows over time. Older children tend to be angry and depressed and exhibit poor self-esteem.

Jason, a 10-year-old boy, was referred for evaluation for failing to complete in-class assignments and homework and failing tests in reading, spelling, and arithmetic. For the past 2 years (grades 5 and 6), he attended a particular education class every morning in the local community school based on an assessment from the second grade. A subsequent psychoeducational assessment by a clinical psychologist confirmed reading problems. Jason was eligible for a full-day special education class, after which he started attending a program with eight other students ranging from 6 to 12.

A clinical interview with his parents revealed that Jason had a history of language delay. In preschool and kindergarten, Jason struggled with rhyming games, lacked interest in books, and preferred playing with construction toys. In the first grade, Jackson had more difficulty learning to read than other boys in his class and continued to have problems pronouncing multisyllabic words (e.g., he said "aminals" for "animals" and "sblanation" for "explanation"). Jason's father disclosed a history of personal reading problems, and Jason's older brother, 15 years of age, had ADHD, for which he took stimulant medication. Jason's parents were concerned about his poor focus in school and wondered whether he had ADHD. In the clinical interview with Jason, he rarely made eye contact, mumbled a lot, and struggled to find the right words (e.g., he manifested many false starts, hesitations, and nonspecific terms, such as "the thing that you draw ... um ... pencil—no ... um ... lines with"). He admitted to disliking school, adding, "Reading is boring and stupid—I'd rather be skateboarding." Jason complained about how much reading he was given—even in math—and commented, "Reading takes so much time. By the time I figure out a word, I can't remember what I just read, and so have to reread the stuff."

Psychoeducational assessment included the Wechsler Intelligence Scale for Children-IV, Clinical Evaluation of Language Fundamentals-IV (CELF-IV), the Wechsler

Individual Achievement Test-II, and self-ratings of anxiety, depression, and self-esteem. Results indicated low-average verbal and above-average performance IQ, poor word attack and word identification skills (below 12th percentile), poor comprehension (below ninth percentile), poor spelling (below sixth percentile), weak comprehension of oral language (below 16th percentile), elevated but subthreshold scores on the Children's Depression Inventory, and low self-esteem. Although Jason manifested symptoms of inattention, restlessness, and oppositional behavior (mainly at school), he did not meet the criteria for ADHD. Jason met DSM-5-TR criteria for a specific learning disorder, with deficits in reading and written expression. Recommendations included continuation in special education plus attendance at a summer camp specializing in children with reading disorder, as well as ongoing monitoring of self-esteem and depressive traits.

At 1-year follow-up, Jason and his parents reported striking improvements in his reading, overall school performance, mood, and self-esteem. Both Jackson and his family felt that the specialized instruction provided during the summer camp was beneficial. The program provided one-on-one focused and explicit instruction for 1 hour a day for 70 hours. Jason explained that he had been taught "like a game plan" to read and challenged the clinician to give him a "really tough long word to read." He demonstrated strategies that he had learned to read the word "unconditionally" and also explained what it meant. To boost his reading and comprehension fluency, he was given assignments to read along with audio-taped versions of books, the use of graphic organizers to facilitate reading comprehension, and continued participation in the summer camp reading program. (Adapted from Rosemary Tannock, Ph.D.)

Diagnosis

Reading impairment is diagnosed when a child's reading achievement is significantly below that expected of a child of the same age. Characteristic diagnostic features include difficulty recalling, evoking, and sequencing printed letters and words, processing sophisticated grammatical constructions, and making inferences. School failure and ensuing poor self-esteem can exacerbate the problems as a child becomes more consumed with a sense of failure and spends less time focusing on academic work. Students with reading impairment are entitled to an educational evaluation through the school district to determine eligibility for special education services. Special education classification, however, is not uniform across states or regions, and students with identical reading difficulties may be eligible for services in one region but ineligible in another.

Pathology and Laboratory Examination. No specific physical signs or laboratory measures are helpful in the diagnosis of reading deficits. Psychoeducational testing, however, is critical in determining these deficits. The diagnostic battery generally includes a standardized spelling test, written composition, processing and using oral language, design copying, and judgment of the adequacy of pencil use. The Woodcock–Johnson Psycho-Educational Battery–Revised reading subtests and the *Peabody Individual Achievement Test-Revised* help identify reading disability. A screening projective battery may include human-figure drawings, picture-story tests, and sentence completion. The evaluation should also include systematic observation of behavioral variables.

Differential Diagnosis

Comorbid disorders, such as language disorder, disability in written expression, and ADHD, often accompany reading deficits. Data indicate that children with reading disability consistently present difficulties with linguistic skills, whereas children with ADHD only do not. Children with reading disability without ADHD, however, may have some overlapping deficits in cognitive inhibition. For example, they perform impulsively on continuous performance tasks. Deficits in expressive language and speech discrimination, along with reading disorder, may lead to a comorbid diagnosis of language disorder. We should differentiate reading impairment from intellectual disability syndromes in which reading, along with most other skills, are below the achievement expected for a child's chronologic age. Intellectual testing helps to differentiate global deficits from more specific reading difficulties.

We can detect poor reading skills from inadequate schooling by comparing a child's achievement with a student's reading performance on standardized tests. We should rule out hearing and visual impairments with screening tests.

Comorbidity

Children with reading difficulties are at high risk for additional learning deficits, including mathematics and written expression. The DSM-5-TR Language disorder, also known as specific language impairment, has traditionally been viewed as distinct from dyslexia and dyscalculia. Children with language disorder have poor word knowledge, limited ability to form accurate sentence structure, and impaired ability to combine words to produce clear explanations. Children with language disorder may have delayed language acquisition and difficulties with grammar and syntactic knowledge. Specific learning disorder in the areas of reading and mathematics frequently occur comorbidly with language disorder. In one study, 19% to 63% of reading disorder patients also had language impairment.

Conversely, reading impairment occurs in 12.5% to 85% of individuals with language disorder. In twin studies, reading impairments are significantly higher in those children with specific learning impairment and family members of children with the disorder. There are also high rates of comorbidity between reading impairment and mathematics impairment; in some studies, the comorbidity is as high as 60%. It appears that children with both reading and math impairment may perform more poorly in mathematics; however, the reading skills of the comorbid children were no different from children with only reading disorder and not math disorder.

Comorbid psychiatric disorders are also frequent, such as ADHD, oppositional defiant disorder, conduct disorders, and depressive disorders, especially in adolescents. Data suggest that up to 25% of children with reading impairment may have comorbid ADHD. Alternately, between 15% and 30% of children diagnosed with ADHD have specific learning disorder. Family studies suggest that ADHD and reading impairment may share some degree of heritability. That is, some genetic factors contribute to both reading impairment and attentional syndromes. Youth with reading impairments have higher than average rates of depression on self-report measures and experience higher levels of anxiety symptoms than children without specific learning disorder. Furthermore, children with reading impairment are at increased risk for poor peer relationships and exhibit less skill in responding to subtle social cues.

Course and Prognosis

Children with a reading disability may gain knowledge of printed language during their first 2 years in grade school without remedial assistance. By the end of the first grade, many children with reading problems have learned to read a few words; however, by the third grade, keeping up with classmates is exceedingly difficult without remedial educational intervention. When remediation is instituted early, in milder cases, it may not be necessary after the first or second grade. In severe cases and depending on the pattern of deficits and strengths, remediation may continue into the middle and high school years.

Treatment

Remediation strategies for children with reading impairments focus on direct instruction that leads a child's attention to the connections between speech sounds and spelling. Effective remediation programs begin by teaching the child to make accurate associations between letters and sounds. This approach relies on the theory that the core deficits in reading impairments are related to difficulty recognizing and remembering the associations between letters and sounds. After mastering individual letter–sound associations, remediation can target more significant components of reading, such as syllables and words. We can determine the exact focus of any reading program only after accurately assessing a child's specific deficits and weaknesses. Positive strategies include small, structured reading groups that offer individual attention and make it easier for a child to ask for help.

Children and adolescents with reading difficulties are entitled to an individual education program (IEP) the public school system provides. However, for high school students with persistent reading disorders and ongoing difficulties with decoding and word identification, IEP services may not be sufficient to remediate their problems. A study of students with reading disorders in 54 schools indicated that specific high school–level goals are not adequately met solely through school remediation. High schoolers with persisting reading difficulties may benefit more from individualized reading remediation.

Reading instruction programs such as the Orton Gillingham and Direct Instructional System for Teaching and Remediation (DISTAR) approach begin by concentrating on individual letters and sounds, advance to the mastery of simple phonetic units, and then blend these units into words and sentences. Thus, if children learn to cope with graphemes, they will learn to read. Other reading remediation programs, such as the Merrill program and the *Science Research Associates, Inc. (SRA) Basic Reading Program,* begin by introducing whole words and then teach children how to break them down and recognize the sounds of the syllables and the individual letters in the word. Another approach teaches children with reading disorders to recognize whole words through visual aids, bypassing the sounding-out process. One such program is called the *Bridge Reading Program.* The Fernald method uses a multisensory approach that combines teaching whole words with a tracing technique so that the child has kinesthetic stimulation while learning to read the words.

Epidemiology

An estimated 4% to 8% of youth in the United States have been identified with dyslexia, encompassing a variety of reading, spelling, and comprehension deficits. Three to four times as many boys as girls have reading impairments in clinically referred samples. In epidemiologic samples, however, rates of reading impairments are much closer among boys and girls. Boys with reading impairment are referred for psychiatric evaluation more often than girls due to comorbid ADHD and disruptive behavior problems. There is no apparent gender differential among adults who report reading difficulties.

Etiology

Data from cognitive, neuroimaging, and genetic studies suggest that reading impairment is a neurobiologic disorder with a significant genetic contribution. It reflects a deficiency in processing sounds of speech sounds and, thus, spoken language. Children who struggle with reading most likely also have a deficit in speech sound processing skills. Children with this deficit cannot adequately identify the parts of words that denote specific sounds, leading to difficulty recognizing and "sounding out" words. Youths with reading impairment are slower than peers in naming letters and numbers. The core deficits for children with reading impairment include poor processing of speech sounds and deficits in comprehension, spelling, and sounding out words.

Because reading impairment typically includes a language deficit, we believe the left brain is the anatomical site of this dysfunction. Several studies using MRI have suggested that the planum temporale in the left brain shows less asymmetry than the same site in the right brain in children with both language disorders and specific learning disorder. PET studies have led some researchers to conclude that left temporal blood flow patterns during language tasks differ between children with and without learning disorders. Cell analysis studies suggest that, in reading-impaired individuals, the visual magnocellular system (typically containing large cells) contains more disorganized and smaller cell bodies than expected. Studies indicate that 35% to 40% of first-degree relatives of children with reading deficits also have a reading disability. Several studies have suggested that chromosome 6 maps to phonologic awareness (i.e., the ability to decode sounds and sound out words).

Furthermore, the ability to identify single words maps to chromosome 15. Impairment in reading and spelling likely links to susceptibility loci on multiple chromosomes. Although a recent research study identified a locus on chromosome 18 strongly influencing single-word reading and phoneme awareness, generalist genes are likely responsible for learning disorders. Many genes associated with specific learning disorder may also influence normal variation in learning abilities. Also, genes that affect reading abilities, for example, are hypothesized to affect written expression and mathematics skills.

Several historical hypotheses about the origin of reading deficits are now known to be untrue. The first myth is that visual–motor problems cause reading impairments, sometimes called *scotopic sensitivity syndrome.* There is no evidence that children with reading impairment have visual problems or difficulties with their visual–motor system. The second false theory is that allergies can cause or contribute to reading disability. Finally, unsubstantiated theories have implicated the cerebellar–vestibular system as the source of reading disabilities.

Research in cognitive neuroscience and neuropsychology supports the hypothesis that encoding processes and working memory, rather than attention or long-term memory, are areas of weakness for children with reading impairment. One study found an association between dyslexia and birth in May, June, and July, suggesting that prenatal exposure to maternal infectious illness, such as influenza, in the winter months may contribute to reading disabilities. Complications during pregnancy and prenatal and perinatal difficulties are common in the histories of children with reading disabilities. Meager birth weight and severely premature children are at higher risk for specific learning disorder. Children born very preterm are at increased risk for minor motor, behavioral, and specific learning disorder.

An increased incidence of reading impairment occurs in intellectually average children with cerebral palsy and epilepsy. Children with postnatal brain lesions in the left occipital lobe, resulting in right visual-field blindness, experience reading impairments. Similarly, youths with lesions in the splenium of the corpus callosum that block the transmission of visual information from the intact right hemisphere to the language areas of the left hemisphere experience reading impairments.

Children malnourished for long periods during early childhood are at increased risk of compromised performance cognition, including reading.

SPECIFIC LEARNING DISORDER WITH IMPAIRMENT IN MATHEMATICS

Children with mathematics difficulties have difficulty learning and remembering numerals, cannot remember basic facts about numbers, and are slow and inaccurate in computation. There are four groups of skills for which children with this disorder have poor achievement: linguistic skills (those related to understanding mathematical terms and converting written problems into mathematical symbols), perceptual skills (the ability to recognize and understand symbols and order clusters of numbers), mathematical skills (basic addition, subtraction, multiplication, division, and following the sequencing of basic operations), and attentional skills (copying figures correctly and observing operational symbols correctly). There are a variety of terms used over the years to denote various difficulties with math skills, including *dyscalculia, congenital arithmetic disorder, acalculia, Gerstmann syndrome,* and *developmental arithmetic disorder;* these terms have been used to denote the difficulties present in mathematics disorder. Core deficits in dyscalculia are in processing numbers, and good language abilities are needed to count, calculate, and understand mathematical principles accurately.

Mathematics deficits can, however, occur in isolation or conjunction with language and reading impairments. According to the DSM-5-TR, the diagnosis of specific learning disorder with impairment in mathematics consists of deficits in arithmetic counting and calculations, difficulty remembering mathematics facts, and potentially counting on fingers instead. Additional deficits include difficulty with mathematical concepts and reasoning, leading to difficulties applying procedures to solve quantitative problems. As documented by standardized academic achievement testing, these deficits lead to skills substantially below what is typical for the child's age and cause significant interference in academic success.

Clinical Features

Common features of mathematics deficit include difficulty learning number names, remembering the signs for addition and subtraction, learning multiplication tables, translating word problems into computations, and performing calculations at the expected pace. We can detect most children with mathematics deficits during the second and third grades of elementary school. A child with poor mathematics abilities typically has problems with concepts, such as counting and adding even one-digit numbers, compared with classmates of the same age. During the first 2 or 3 years of elementary school, a child with poor mathematics skills may get by in mathematics by relying on rote memory. However, soon, as mathematics problems require discrimination and manipulation of spatial and numerical relations, a child with mathematics difficulties is overwhelmed.

Some investigators have classified mathematics deficiencies into the following categories: difficulty learning to count meaningfully, difficulty mastering cardinal and ordinal systems, difficulty performing arithmetic operations, and difficulty envisioning clusters of objects as groups. Children with mathematics difficulty have trouble associating auditory and visual symbols, understanding the conservation of quantity, remembering sequences of arithmetic steps, and choosing principles for problem-solving activities. Children with these problems are presumed to have good auditory and verbal abilities; however, in many cases, mathematics deficits may occur with reading, writing, and language problems. In these cases, the other deficiencies may compound the impairment of poor mathematics skills.

Mathematics difficulty, in fact, often coexists with other disorders affecting reading, expressive writing, coordination, and language. Spelling problems, deficits in memory or attention, and emotional or behavioral problems may be present. Young grade-school children may exhibit specific learning problems in reading and writing, and we should evaluate these children for mathematics deficits. The exact relationship between mathematics deficits and the deficits in language and dyslexia is not clear. Although children with language disorder do not necessarily experience mathematics deficiencies, these conditions often coexist, and both are associated with impairments in decoding and encoding processes.

Sophia, an 8-year-old girl, was referred for evaluation of impairing problems in attention and academic achievement, which were first noted in kindergarten but were now causing difficulty at home and school. Sophia attended a regular third-grade class in a local public school, which she had been attending since midway through kindergarten.

Sophia's history included a mild delay in speech acquisition (e.g., first words at approximately 18 months of age and short sentences at approximately 3 years). However, she had no major developmental problems until kindergarten, when her teacher raised concerns about inattentiveness, difficulty following instructions, and difficulty mastering basic number concepts (e.g., inaccurate counting of sets of objects). A speech, language, and hearing assessment completed at the end of kindergarten revealed mild language problems that did not warrant specific intervention. School reports from grades 1 and 2 noted ongoing concerns about inattention, poor reading skills, difficulty mastering simple arithmetic facts, and "careless mistakes in copying numbers from the board and doing addition and subtraction." These problems continued through grade 2, despite some in-school accommodations (e.g., moving Sophia's seat closer to the teacher) and modifications (e.g., providing her with printed sheets of arithmetic problems so she did not need to copy them herself). Sophia's parents reported a 3-year history of losing things, fidgeting at the dinner table, having difficulty concentrating on games and homework, and forgetting to bring notes to and from school. The psychological assessment included the Wechsler Intelligence Scale for Children-III, Clinical Evaluation of Language Fundamentals-IV, Comprehensive Test of Phonological Processing, and the Woodcock–Johnson Psycho-Educational Battery–III. Results indicated average intelligence, with relatively weaker performance on tests of perceptual organization, weak phonologic (speech sound) awareness, mild deficits in receptive and expressive language, and reading and arithmetic abilities that were well below grade level. Parent and teacher ratings on a standardized behavior questionnaire (Conners' Rating Scales–Long Form) were above the clinical threshold for ADHD.

Sophia was given a diagnosis of ADHD, predominantly inattentive type, and specific learning disorder with impairment in reading, based on the history, school achievement, and standardized assessment. She did not meet the criteria for communication disorder, and her doctors thought that her mathematics problems did not cause impairment like her reading disorder and ADHD did. Recommendations included the following: family psychoeducation clarifying the ADHD and specific learning disorder, remedial interventions for reading, and treatment of her ADHD with a long-acting stimulant agent.

At 1-year follow-up, Sophia and her parents reported noticeable improvement with inattention but ongoing problems with reading and more significant math deficits. Her clinicians added mathematics remediation to her weekly schedule. Two years later, when Sophia was 11 years of age, her parents called for an "urgent reevaluation" due to a sudden worsening of her difficulties at home and school. Clinical evaluation revealed adequate stimulant treatment response to her ADHD, more marked deficits in reading speed accuracy compared to others her age, and significant deficits in mathematics. Sophia's parents reported that she had started lying about having mathematics homework or refused to do it, was suspended from mathematics class twice in the past 3 months because of oppositional behavior and had failed sixth-grade mathematics. Sophia acknowledged disliking and worrying about math: "Whenever the teacher starts asking questions and looks in my direction, my mind just goes blank, and I feel sort of shaky—it's so bad in tests that I have to leave class to get myself together."

At this point, her team noted an additional component of anxiety to be contributing to her school impairments. Added recommendations included increased specific educational remediation for mathematics. At follow-up, Sophia reported that the resource teacher had taught her some helpful strategies to address her mathematics anxiety, classify word problems, and differentiate critical information from irrelevant information. She continued to be a robust responder to long-acting stimulants for her ADHD and had only minimal difficulties concentrating on homework after school. (Adapted from Rosemary Tannock, Ph.D.)

Diagnosis

We diagnose a specific learning disorder in mathematics when a child's mathematical reasoning or calculation skill remains significantly below that expected for that child's age for at least 6 months, even when administering remedial interventions. Many different skills contribute to mathematics proficiency. These include linguistic skills, conceptual skills, and computational skills. Linguistic skills involve understanding mathematical terms and word problems and translating them into the proper mathematical process. Conceptual skills involve the recognition of mathematical symbols and being able to use mathematical signs correctly. Computational skills include correctly lining up numbers and following the "rules" of the mathematical operation.

Pathology and Laboratory Examination. No physical signs or symptoms indicate mathematics disorder, but educational testing and standardized measurement of intellectual function are necessary to make this diagnosis. The *Keymath Diagnostic Arithmetic Test* measures several areas of mathematics, including knowledge of mathematical content, function, and computation. It assesses the ability in mathematics of children in grades 1 to 6.

Course and Prognosis

A child with a specific learning disorder in mathematics is usually identifiable by the age of 8 years (third grade). The disorder is apparent in some children as early as 6 years (first grade); in others, it may not be apparent until age 10 (fifth grade) or later. Too few data are currently available from longitudinal studies to predict developmental and academic progress patterns of children classified as having mathematics disorder in early school grades. On the other hand, children with a moderate mathematics disorder who do not receive intervention may have complications, including continuing academic difficulties, shame, poor self-concept, frustration, and depression. These complications can lead to reluctance to attend school and demoralization about academic success.

Differential Diagnosis

We should differentiate mathematics deficits from global causes of impaired functioning, such as intellectual disability. Inadequate schooling can affect a child's arithmetic performance. Conduct disorder or ADHD can occur comorbidly with specific learning disorder in mathematics, and in these cases, we would make both diagnoses.

Comorbidity

Mathematics deficits are comorbid with deficits in both reading and written expression. Children with mathematics difficulties may also be at higher risk for expressive language problems and developmental coordination disorder.

Treatment

It is best to treat mathematics difficulties for children with early interventions that lead to improved skills in basic computation. Specific learning disorder in reading and mathematics difficulties can impede progress; however, children are responsive to early grade school remediation. Children with indications of mathematics disorder as early as kindergarten require help understanding which digit in a pair is larger, counting abilities, identifying numbers, and remembering sequences. Flashcards, workbooks, and computer games can be a viable part of this treatment. One study indicated that mathematics instruction is most helpful when focusing on problem-solving activities, including word problems, rather than only computation. *Project MATH,* a multimedia self-instructional or group-instructional in-service training program, has been successful for some children with mathematics disorder. Computer programs can be helpful and can increase compliance with remediation efforts.

Social skills deficits can contribute to a child's hesitation in asking for help, so a child with a mathematics disorder may benefit from gaining positive problem-solving skills in the social arena and mathematics.

Epidemiology

Mathematics disability alone is estimated to occur in about 1% of school-age children, which is about one of every five children with specific learning disorder. Epidemiologic studies have indicated that up to 6% of school-age children have some difficulty with mathematics, with a prevalence of 3.5 to 6.5 for impairing forms of dyscalculia. Although specific learning disorders occur two to three times more often in males overall, mathematics deficits may be more frequent in girls than in reading. Many studies of learning disorders in children have grouped reading, writing, and mathematics disability, which makes it more difficult to ascertain the precise prevalence of mathematics disability.

Etiology

As with other areas of specific learning disorder, mathematics deficiency has a significant genetic contribution. Comorbidity with reading deficits is common and ranges from 17% to 60%. One theory proposed a neurologic deficit in the right cerebral hemisphere, particularly in the occipital lobe areas. These regions are responsible for processing visual–spatial stimuli that, in turn, are responsible for mathematical skills. This theory, however, has received little support in subsequent neuropsychiatric studies.

The causes of deficits in mathematics are multifactorial, including genetic, maturational, cognitive, emotional, educational, and socioeconomic factors. Prematurity and low birth weights are risk factors for specific learning disorder, including mathematics. Compared with reading abilities, arithmetic abilities seem to depend more on the amount and quality of instruction.

SPECIFIC LEARNING DISORDER WITH IMPAIRMENT IN WRITTEN EXPRESSION

Written expression is the most complex skill for understanding language and expressing thoughts and ideas. Writing skills correlate highly with reading for most children; however, for some youth, reading comprehension may far surpass their ability to express complex thoughts. In some cases, written expression is a sensitive index of more subtle language usage deficits typically not detected by standardized reading and language tests.

Deficits in written expression include writing skills significantly below the expected level for a child's age and education. Such deficits impair the child's academic performance and writing in everyday life. Components of writing disorder include poor spelling, errors in grammar and punctuation, and poor handwriting. Spelling errors are among the most common difficulties for a child with a writing disorder. Spelling mistakes are often phonetic errors or erroneous spelling that sounds correct. Common spelling errors include *fone* for phone or *beleeve* for believe.

Historically, experts considered dysgraphia (i.e., poor writing skills) a reading disorder; however, written expression impairment can occur independently. The terms previously used to describe writing disability include *spelling disorder* and *spelling dyslexia.* Writing disabilities are often associated with other forms of specific learning disorders; however, impaired writing ability may be identified later than other forms because it is generally acquired later than verbal language and reading.

In contrast with the DSM-5-TR, which includes specific learning disorder in written expression, ICD-10 includes a separate specific spelling disorder.

Clinical Features

Youth with impairments in written expression struggle early in grade school with spelling words and expressing their thoughts according to age-appropriate grammatical norms. Their spoken and written sentences contain an unusually large number of grammatical errors and poor paragraph organization. Affected children commonly make simple grammatical errors, even when writing a short sentence. For example, despite constant reminders, affected youth frequently fail to capitalize the first letter of the first word and end the sentence with a period. Typical features of impaired written expression include spelling errors, grammatical errors, punctuation errors, poor paragraph organization, and poor handwriting.

In higher grades in school, affected youth's written sentences become more conspicuously primitive, odd, and inaccurate compared to typical students at their grade level. For youth with impaired written expression, word choices are often erroneous and inappropriate, paragraphs are disorganized and not in proper sequence, and spelling accuracy becomes increasingly difficult as their vocabulary becomes more extensive and abstract. Associated features of writing impairments may include reluctance to go to school, refusal to do assigned written homework, and concurrent academic difficulties in other areas.

Many children with impaired written expression understandably become frustrated and angry and harbor feelings of shame and inadequacy regarding poor academic achievement. In some cases, depressive disorders can result from a growing sense of isolation, estrangement, and despair. Young adults with impaired written expression who do not receive remedial intervention continue to have writing skills deficits and a persistent sense of incompetence and inferiority.

Oliver, an 11-year-old boy, was referred for evaluation of increasing problems in school over 2 years, including failure to complete assigned schoolwork and homework, inattention and oppositional behavior, and deteriorating grades and test scores. At the time of assessment, he was in a regular fifth-grade class in a public school, which he had been attending since grade 1.

A clinical interview with parents revealed that Oliver had a twin brother (monozygotic) with a history of language problems for which he had received speech-language therapy in the preschool years and remedial reading in the primary grades. However, according to parental reports and scores on standardized oral language tests administered in the preschool years, Oliver had not exhibited speech or language development difficulty. His current and previous school reports indicate that Oliver participated well in class discussions and had no difficulty reading or doing mathematics; however, his written work was far below grade level. In each of the last 2 years, his teachers had expressed increasing concerns about Oliver's refusal to complete written work, failure to hand in homework, daydreaming and fidgeting in class, and withdrawal from class activities. Oliver admitted to an increasing dislike of school, especially writing assignments. He explained, "It's writing all day long—even in math and science. I know how to do the problems and the experiments, but I hate having to write it all down—my mind just goes blank." Oliver complained, "My teacher is always on me, telling me that I'm lazy and haven't done enough and that my writing is atrocious. He tells me I've got a bad attitude—so why would I want to go to school?" Oliver and his parents reported that he has been down over the past year, increasingly frustrated with school, and has refused to do homework. They all agree that Oliver had experienced a few brief episodes of depressed mood.

Testing by a clinical psychologist revealed average to high-average scores on the verbal and performance scales of the Wechsler Intelligence Scale for Children-III and average scores on the reading and arithmetic subtests of the Wide Range Achievement Test-3 (WRAT-3). However, the WRAT-3 spelling subtest scores were below the 9th percentile, significantly below age and ability expectations. Examination of his spelling errors revealed that his spelling was typically phonologically accurate (i.e., could plausibly be pronounced to sound like the target word). However, he used letter sequences that did not resemble English, regardless of pronunciation (e.g., "houses" was written as "howssis," "phones" was written as "fones," and "exact" was "egszakt"). Moreover, his performance was well below age and grade on standardized tests of written expression (TOWL-3), as well as on a brief (5-minute) informal assessment of expository text generation on a favorite topic (e.g., a newspaper article on a recent sports event). During the 5-minute writing activity, he frequently stared out the window, shifted positions, and chewed on his pencil. He would often get up to sharpen his pencil and sigh when he put pencil to paper, writing slowly and laboriously. At the end of 5 minutes, he had produced three short sentences without any punctuation or capitalization that were barely legible, containing several misspellings and grammatical errors that were not linked semantically. By contrast, later in the assessment, he described the sporting event with detail and enthusiasm. A speech-language evaluation revealed average scores on standard tests of oral language (Clinical Evaluation of Language Fundamentals-IV). However, in a nonword repetition test, he omitted sounds or syllables in a multisyllabic word, which was sensitive to mild residual and written language impairments.

The clinical team diagnosed a specific learning disorder with impairment in written expression based on Oliver's inability to compose written text, poor spelling, and grammatical errors, without problems in reading or mathematics or a history of language impairments. He did not meet the full diagnostic criteria for any other DSM-5-TR disorder, including oppositional defiant disorder, ADHD, or mood disorder. Recommendations included the following: psychoeducation, the need for educational accommodations (e.g., provision of additional time for test-taking and written assignments, specific educational intervention to facilitate written expression and to teach note-taking, and use of specific computer software to support written composition and spelling), and counseling should his depressed mood continue or worsen. (Adapted from Rosemary Tannock, Ph.D.)

Diagnosis

The DSM-5-TR diagnosis of specific learning disorder with impairment in written expression depends on a child's poor ability to use punctuation and grammar accurately in sentences and inability to organize paragraphs or to articulate ideas in writing. Compared to others of the same age, poor performance in composing written text may also include poor handwriting and impaired ability to spell and place words sequentially in coherent sentences. In addition to spelling mistakes, youth with impaired written expression make grammatical mistakes, such as using incorrect tenses, forgetting words in sentences, and placing words incorrectly. Punctuation may be incorrect, and the child may be unable to remember which words begin with capital letters. Additional symptoms of impaired written expression include the formation of illegible, inverted letters and mixtures of capital and lowercase letters in a given word. Other features of writing disorders include poor organization of written stories, which lack critical elements such as "where," "when," and "who," or clear expression of the plot.

Pathology and Laboratory Examination. Whereas no physical signs of a writing disorder exist, educational testing helps diagnose writing disorder. Diagnosis depends on a child's writing performance being markedly below expected production for his age, as confirmed by an individually administered standardized expressive writing test. Currently available tests of written language include the Test of Written Language (TOWL), the Diagnostic Evaluation of Writing Skills (DEWS), and the Test of Early Written Language (TEWL). We should also evaluate for impaired vision and hearing.

When there are impairments in written expression, we should administer a standardized intelligence test, such as The Wechsler Intelligence Scale for Children-Fifth Edition (WISC-V), to determine the child's overall intellectual capacity.

Course and Prognosis

Specific learning disorder with impairment in writing, reading, and mathematics often coexist, and additional language disorder may be present as well. A child with all of the above disabilities will likely be diagnosed with language disorder first and impaired written expression last. In severe cases, an impaired written expression is apparent by age 7 (second grade); in less severe cases, the disorder may not be apparent until age 10 (fifth grade) or later. Youth with mild and moderate impairment in written expression fare well if they receive timely remedial education early in grade school. Severely impaired written expression requires continual, extensive remedial treatment through the late part of high school and even into college.

The prognosis depends on the severity of the disorder, the age or grade when starting the remedial intervention, the length and continuity of treatment, and the presence or absence of associated or secondary emotional or behavioral problems.

Differential Diagnosis

It is crucial to determine whether disorders such as ADHD or major depression are interfering with a child's focus and thereby preventing the production of adequate writing in the absence of a specific writing impairment. If true, treatment for the other disorder should improve a child's writing performance. Common comorbid disorders with writing disability are language disorder, mathematics disorder, developmental coordination disorder, disruptive behavior disorders, and ADHD.

Comorbidity

Children with impaired writing ability are significantly more likely to have language disorder and impairments in reading and mathematics compared to the general population of youth. ADHD occurs with higher frequency in children with writing disability than in the general population. Youth with specific learning disorder, including writing disability, are at higher risk for social skills difficulties, and some develop poor self-esteem and depressive symptoms.

Treatment

Remedial treatment for writing disability includes direct practice in spelling and sentence writing and reviewing grammatical rules. Intensive and continuous administration of individually tailored, one-on-one expressive and creative writing therapy appears to influence a favorable outcome. Teachers in some special schools devote as much as 2 hours a day to such writing instruction. This intervention largely depends on the relationship between the child and the writing specialist. Success or failure in sustaining the patient's motivation affects the treatment's long-term efficacy. Associated secondary emotional and behavioral problems should be given prompt attention, with appropriate psychiatric treatment and parental counseling.

Epidemiology

The prevalence of specific learning disorder with impairment in written expression occurs in 5% to 15% of school-age children. Over time, specific learning disorder remits in many youths, leading to a persistent rate of specific learning disorder of 4% in adults. The gender ratio in writing deficits is two to three to one in boys compared with girls. Impaired written expression often occurs along with deficits in reading, but not always.

Etiology

The causes of writing disability are likely similar to reading disorder, that is, underlying deficits in using language components related to letter sounds. Genetic factors are a significant factor in the development of writing disability. Writing difficulties often accompany language disorder, leading an affected child to struggle with understanding grammatical rules, finding words, and expressing ideas clearly. According to one hypothesis, impairment in written expression may result from the combined effects of language disorder and reading disorder. Most youths with impaired written expression have first-degree relatives with similar difficulties. Children with limited attention spans and high levels of distractibility may find writing an arduous task.

Further Readings

Archibald LMD, Cardy JO, Joanisse MF, Ansari D. Language, reading, and math learning profiles in an epidemiological sample of school age children. *PLoS One*. 2013;8(10):e77463.

Bernstein S, Atkinson AR, Martimianakis MA. Diagnosing the learner in difficulty. *Pediatrics*. 2013;132(2):210–212.

Boxer O. Specific learning disorder. In: Boland RJ, Verduin ML, eds. *Kaplan & Sadock's Comprehensive Textbook of Clinical Psychiatry*. 11th edition. Wolters Kluwer; 2025.

Büber A, Başay Ö, Şenol H. The prevalence and comorbidity rates of specific learning disorder among primary school children in Turkey. *Nord J Psychiatry*. 2020;74(6):453–460.

Butterworth B, Kovas Y. Understanding neurocognitive developmental disorders can improve education for all. *Science*. 2013;340(6130):300–305.

Callaway E. Dyscalculia: number games. *Nature*. 2013;493(7431):150–153.

de Zeeuw EL, de Geus EJC, Boomsma DI. Meta-analysis of twin studies highlights the importance of genetic variation in primary school educational achievement. *Trends Neurosci Educ*. 2015;4(3):69–76.

Hedges JH, Adolph KE, Amso D, et al. Play, attention, and learning: how do play and timing shape the development of attention and influence classroom learning? *Ann N Y Acad Sci*. 2013;1292(1):1–20.

Klatte M, Bergstrom KM, Lachmann T. Does noise affect learning? A short review on noise effects on cognitive performance in children. *Front Psychol*. 2013;4:578.

Locke R, Scallan S, Mann R, Alexander G. Clinicians with dyslexia: a systematic review of effects and strategies. *Clin Teach*. 2015;12(6):394–398.

Peterson RL, Pennington BF. Developmental dyslexia. *Annu Rev Clin Psychol*. 2015;11:283–307.

Swanson E, Vaughn S. Learning disabilities: academic and mental health needs. In: Holt MK, Grills AE, eds. *Critical Issues in School-based Mental Health: Evidence-Based Research, Practice, and Interventions*. Routledge; 2015.

Tannock R. Provision of evidence-based intervention is not part of the DSM-5 diagnostic criteria for specific learning disorder. *Eur Child Adolesc Psychiatry*. 2016;25(2):209–210.

Tannock R. Specific learning disabilities in DSM-5: are the changes for better or worse? *Int J Res Learn Disabil*. 2013;1(2):2–30.

8 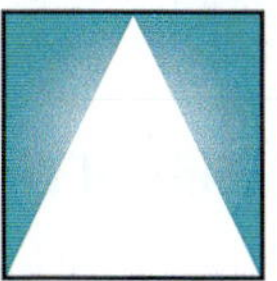

Motor Disorders: Developmental Coordination Disorder, Stereotypic Movement Disorder

DEVELOPMENTAL COORDINATION DISORDER

Developmental coordination disorder is a neurodevelopmental disorder in which a child's fine or gross motor coordination is slower, less accurate, and more variable than in peers of the same age. Affecting about 5% to 6% of school-age children, 50% of children with developmental coordination disorder also have comorbid attention-deficit/hyperactivity disorder (ADHD) or dyslexia. A meta-analysis of recent research on developmental coordination disorder concluded that three general areas of deficits contribute to the disorder: (1) poor predictive control of motor movements, (2) deficits in rhythmic coordination and timing, and (3) deficits in executive functions, including working memory, inhibition, and attention.

Children with developmental coordination disorder struggle to perform the motor activities of daily life, such as jumping, hopping, running, or catching a ball. Children with coordination problems may also agonize over using utensils, tying their shoelaces, or writing. A child with developmental coordination disorder may exhibit delays in achieving motor milestones, such as sitting, crawling, and walking, because of clumsiness, yet they may excel at verbal skills.

Thus, Developmental coordination disorder may be characterized by either clumsy gross or fine motor skills, resulting in poor performance in sports and academic achievement because of poor writing skills. A child with developmental coordination disorder may bump into things more often than siblings or drop things. In the 1930s, the term *clumsy child syndrome* began to be used in the literature to denote a condition of awkward motor behaviors not due to any specific neurologic disorder or damage. This term continues to identify children's imprecise or delayed gross and fine motor behavior, resulting in subtle motor inabilities but often significant social rejection. Gross and fine motor impairment in developmental coordination disorder is not from a medical condition, such as cerebral palsy, muscular dystrophy, or a neuromuscular disorder. Currently, specific indications are that perinatal problems, such as prematurity, low birth weight, and hypoxia, may contribute to the emergence of developmental coordination disorders. Children with developmental coordination disorder are at higher risk for language and learning disorders. A strong association exists between speech and language problems and coordination problems, as well as an association of coordination difficulties with hyperactivity, impulsivity, and reduced attention span.

Children with developmental coordination disorder may resemble younger children because of their inability to master motor activities typical for their age group. For example, elementary school children with developmental coordination disorder may not be adept at bicycle riding, skateboarding, running, skipping, or hopping. In middle school, children with this disorder may have trouble in team sports, such as soccer, baseball, or basketball. In the preschool-age group, fine motor skill manifestations of developmental coordination disorder typically include clumsiness using utensils and difficulty with buttons and zippers. In older children, using scissors and more complex grooming skills, such as styling hair or putting on makeup, is difficult. Peers often ostracize children with developmental coordination disorder because of their poor skills in many sports, and they often have longstanding difficulties with peer relationships. DSM-5-TR categorizes developmental coordination disorder as a motor disorder, along with stereotypic movement disorder and tic disorders.

Clinical Features

The clinical signs suggesting the existence of developmental coordination disorder are evident as early as infancy and, in some cases, when a child begins to attempt tasks requiring motor coordination. The essential clinical feature is significantly impaired performance in motor coordination. The difficulties in motor coordination may vary with a child's age and developmental stage (Table 8-1).

In infancy and early childhood, the disorder may manifest in delays in developmental motor milestones, such as turning over, crawling, sitting, standing, walking, buttoning shirts, and zipping up pants. Between 2 and 4 years of age, clumsiness appears in almost all activities requiring motor coordination. Affected children cannot hold objects and drop them easily, their gait may be unsteady, they often trip over their feet, and they may bump into other children while attempting to go around them. Older children may display impaired motor coordination in table games, such as putting together puzzles or building blocks, and in any ball game. Although no specific features are pathognomonic of developmental coordination disorder, there is a delay in developmental milestones. Many children with the disorder also have speech and language difficulties. Older children may have secondary problems, including academic difficulties, as well as poor peer relationships based on social rejection. Children with motor coordination problems are more likely to have problems understanding subtle social cues, and their peers often reject them. A recent study indicated that children with motor difficulties perform more poorly on scales that measure the recognition of static and changing facial expressions of emotion. This finding likely correlates with the clinical observations that children with motor coordination have difficulties in social behavior and peer relationships.

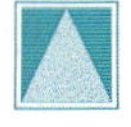

Table 8-1. Manifestations of Developmental Coordination Disorder

Gross Motor Manifestations

Preschool age

Delays in reaching motor milestones, such as sitting, crawling, and walking

Balance problems: falling, getting bruised frequently, and poor toddling

Abnormal gait

Knocking over objects, bumping into things, and destructiveness

Primary-school age

Difficulty with riding bikes, skipping, hopping, running, jumping, and doing somersaults

Awkward or abnormal gait

Older

Poor at sports, throwing, catching, kicking, and hitting a ball

Fine Motor Manifestations

Preschool age

Difficulty learning dressing skills (tying, fastening, zipping, and buttoning)

Difficulty learning feeding skills (handling knife, fork, or spoon)

Primary-school age

Difficulty assembling jigsaw pieces, using scissors, building with blocks, drawing, or tracing

Older

Difficulty with grooming (putting on makeup, blow-drying hair, and doing nails)

Messy or illegible writing

Difficulty using hand tools, sewing, and playing piano

Jimmy was referred for evaluation to determine his need for adaptive physical education (PE), age 9 years. Jimmy was failing PE, was unable to run a mile, and he could not throw or catch the ball, and was generally slow motorically. His classmates laughed because he looked so "funny" while running, and he always seemed to be getting hit with the ball instead of catching it. Jimmy was always picked last for team sports games and was beginning to be bullied by his classmates for his poor physical skills. Jimmy already had an accommodation for more time on tests due to his previously diagnosed ADHD. He was being treated with Vyvanse, which was working well. A developmental history revealed that Jimmy was born prematurely at 31 weeks, and his motor milestones were all delayed, although speech milestones were right on time. Currently, Jimmy was unable to tie his shoes correctly, and he struggled to handwrite letters correctly, but his parents were hoping that he would outgrow those problems. Upon questioning Jimmy's current motor skills, it became apparent that not only was he having coordination problems but that he was now being rejected by peers and had become quite socially isolated. At home, Jimmy's parents had accepted the fact that he was just a clumsy boy and noted that Jimmy constantly spilled his drinks and was awkward when he used a fork. His food often fell off a fork or spoon before it reached his mouth, and he had great difficulty using a knife and a fork. A comprehensive assessment of fine and gross motor skills yielded the following results: Jimmy was able to hop, but he could not skip without briefly stopping after each step. He could stand with both feet together but could not stand on tiptoe. Jimmy held a ball bounced to him at chest level, and he could not catch a ball bounced to him on the ground from a distance of 15 ft. Jimmy's agility and coordination were measured with the Bruininks–Oseretsky Test of Motor Proficiency (BOTMP), which revealed functioning levels commensurate with those of an average 7-year-old child.

Jimmy was referred to a neurologist for a comprehensive evaluation to rule out neurologic disorders. On neurologic examination, Jimmy was found to have no signs of a specific neurologic disorder. Neurologic examination was negative for conditions that could account for his poor motor skills. Based on the history and findings on the BOTMP, Jimmy was given a diagnosis of DCD. Jimmy's symptoms included gross and fine motor impairments, poor balance, and mild hypotonia. Based on an individualized educational plan (IEP) meeting with his school, it became evident that Jimmy required an adaptive PE program for DCD and had other specific learning disorders. In addition to his known ADHD, Jimmy was found to have a writing disability. A treatment plan was developed that included twice weekly with an occupational therapist who used perceptual-motor exercises to improve his fine motor skills, particularly targeting writing and the use of utensils. Jimmy was also enrolled in a treatment program using motor imagery training to improve clumsiness and was also referred to a social skills group to help him deal more effectively with his peers.

Jimmy was relieved to be receiving help, especially for his handwriting and PE class, which he had been close to failing. Over a period of 4 months of treatment, Jimmy showed some improvement in the legibility of his handwriting, although he remained a slow writer. He was responsive to the stimulant medication, and his academic achievement improved as his attention span increased. Jimmy was receiving more praise from his teachers than ever before, and his classmates were teasing him less. As he began to feel better about himself, he began to try to play sports informally with his peers, although not competitively. He was given a modified PE program in school, and he was not required to play on teams, but he practiced throwing and catching a ball and was allowed to walk his mile at a slower time. Jimmy continued to exhibit some impairment in fine motor skills over the year, and he was cooperative with the therapeutic interventions, showed some continual improvement, and demonstrated improved peer relationships. (Courtesy of Caroly Pataki, M.D. and Sarah Spence, M.D.)

Diagnosis

The diagnosis of developmental coordination disorder depends on poor performance in activities requiring coordination for a child's age and intellectual level. The diagnosis is based on a history of the child's delay in achieving early motor milestones and on direct observation of current deficits in coordination. An informal screen for developmental coordination disorder involves asking the child to perform tasks involving gross motor coordination (e.g., hopping, jumping, and standing on one foot); fine motor coordination (e.g., finger-tapping and shoelace tying); and hand-eye coordination (e.g., catching a ball and copying letters). We should consider what is expected of a child of a certain age to judge possible poor performance. A mildly clumsy child with unimpaired functioning does not qualify for a diagnosis of developmental coordination disorder. Table 8-2 compares the diagnostic approaches to developmental coordination disorder.

The diagnosis may be associated with below-normal scores on performance subtests of standardized intelligence tests and normal or above-normal scores on verbal subtests. Specialized motor coordination tests such as the Bender Visual Motor Gestalt Test, the Frostig Movement Skills Test Battery, and the Bruininks–Oseretsky Test of Motor Development can be helpful. We should consider the child's age and ensure that there is no better

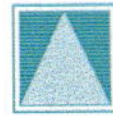

Table 8-2.
Developmental Coordination Disorder

	DSM-5-TR	ICD-10	ICD-11
Diagnostic name	Developmental Coordination Disorder	Specific Developmental Disorder of Motor Function	Developmental Motor Coordination Disorder
Duration	Onset in the early developmental period		Onset in the early developmental period
Symptoms	The development of coordinated motor skills is far behind what would be expected for an individual's chronologic age	Significant impairment in motor coordination	Significant delay in the acquisition of gross or fine motor skills and impairment in the execution of coordinated motor skills May manifest as: Clumsiness Slowness Inaccuracy of motor performance Coordinated motor skills are markedly below that expected on the basis of age
Psychosocial consequences	Resulting in impaired ability to play, perform self-care, and function		Limitations in activities of daily living, school work, vocation, leisure activities, or other important areas of functioning
Exclusions		General intellectual retardation Any specific congenital or neurologic disorder	Disease of the nervous system Disease of the musculoskeletal system Connective tissue disease Sensory impairment Disorder of intellectual development
Symptom specifiers	Result of: *Another neurologic condition* *Intellectual disability* *Visual impairment*		

explanation, such as a neurologic or neuromuscular condition. Examination, however, may occasionally reveal slight reflex abnormalities and other soft neurologic signs.

Differential Diagnosis

The differential diagnosis includes medical conditions that produce coordination difficulties (e.g., cerebral palsy and muscular dystrophy). In autism spectrum disorder (ASD) and intellectual disability, coordination usually does not stand out as a significant deficit compared with other skills. Children with neuromuscular disorders may exhibit more global muscle impairment than clumsiness and delayed motor milestones. Neurologic examination and workup usually reveal more extensive deficits in neurologic conditions than developmental coordination disorder. Extremely hyperactive and impulsive children may be physically careless because of their high levels of motor activity. Clumsy gross and fine motor behavior and ADHD, as well as reading difficulties, are highly associated.

Comorbidity

Developmental coordination disorder is strongly associated with ADHD, specific learning disorder, particularly in reading, as well as language disorder. Children with coordination difficulties have higher-than-expected rates of language disorder, and studies of children with language disorder report very high rates of "clumsiness." Developmental coordination disorder is also associated, but less strongly, with specific learning disorder with impairment in mathematics and written expression. A study of children with developmental coordination disorder reported that, although motor coordination is critical for accuracy in tasks that require speed, poor motor coordination does not correlate with the degree of inattention. Thus, in children comorbid for ADHD and developmental coordination disorder, children with the most severe ADHD do not necessarily have the worst developmental coordination disorder. Functional neuroimaging, pharmacologic, and neuroanatomical studies suggest that motor coordination depends on the integration of sensory input and an action response, not purely through sensorimotor function and higher-level thinking. Investigations of comorbid developmental coordination disorder and ADHD are trying to ascertain whether this comorbidity is due to overlapping genetic factors.

Peer relationship problems are common among children with developmental coordination disorders because of rejection that often occurs along with their poor performance in sports and games that require good motor skill. Adolescents with coordination problems often exhibit poor self-esteem and academic difficulties. Recent studies underscore the importance of attention to both the victimization of children and adolescents with developmental motor coordination by peers and the potential resulting damage to self-worth. Children and adolescents with developmental coordination disorder often are victims of bullying and have higher rates of poor self-esteem that often deserves clinical attention.

Course and Prognosis

Historically, experts believed that developmental coordination spontaneously typically improved over time. However, longitudinal studies have shown that motor coordination problems can persist into adolescence and adulthood. When mild to moderate clumsiness is persistent, some children can compensate by developing an interest in other skills. Some studies suggest a more favorable outcome for children with average or above-average intellectual capacity in that they develop strategies to develop friendships that do not depend on physical activities. Clumsiness typically persists into adolescence and adult life. One study following a group of children with developmental coordination problems over a decade found that the clumsy children remained less dexterous, showed poor balance, and continued to be physically awkward. The affected children were also more likely to have both academic problems and poor self-esteem. Children with developmental coordination disorder have also been shown to be at higher risk for obesity, have difficulties with running, and are at greater risk of future cardiovascular diseases.

Treatment

Interventions for children with developmental coordination disorder utilize multiple modalities, including visual, auditory, and tactile materials targeting perceptual-motor training for specific motor tasks. Two broad categories of interventions are the following: (1) deficit-oriented approaches, including sensory integration therapy, sensorimotor-oriented treatment, and process-oriented treatment, and (2) task-specific interventions, including neuromotor task training and cognitive orientation to daily occupational performance (CO-OP). More recently, therapists have incorporated motor imagery into treatment. These approaches involve visual imagery exercises using a computer; they have a broad range of foci, including predictive timing for motor tasks, relaxation, mental preparation, visual modeling of fundamental motor skills, and mental rehearsal of various tasks. This type of intervention derives from the notion that improved internal representation of a movement task will improve a child's motor behavior.

The treatment of developmental coordination disorder generally includes versions of sensory integration programs and modified physical education. Sensory integration programs, usually administered by occupational therapists, consist of physical activities that increase motor and sensory function awareness. For example, a child who bumps into objects often might be tasked with trying to balance on a scooter, under supervision, to improve balance and body awareness. Therapists often give tasks to children with difficulty writing letters to increase their awareness of hand movements. School-based occupational therapies for motor coordination problems in writing include utilizing mechanisms that provide resistance or vibration during writing exercises to improve grip and practicing vertical writing on a chalkboard to increase arm strength and stability while writing. These programs improve the legibility of students' writing, but not speed, because students learn to write with greater accuracy and deliberate letter formation. Many schools also allow and may even encourage children with coordination difficulties that affect writing to use computers to write reports and long papers.

Adaptive physical education programs help children enjoy exercise and physical activities without the pressures of team sports. These programs generally incorporate certain sports actions, such as kicking a soccer ball or throwing a basketball. Children with coordination disorder may also benefit from social skills groups and other prosocial interventions. The Montessori technique may promote motor skill development, especially with preschool children, because this educational program emphasizes the development of motor skills. Small studies have suggested that exercise in rhythmic coordination, practicing motor movements, and learning to use word-processing keyboards may be beneficial. Parental counseling may help reduce parents' anxiety and guilt about their child's impairment, increase their awareness, and facilitate their confidence to cope with the child.

An investigation of children with developmental coordination disorder showed positive results using a computer game designed to improve the ability to catch a ball. These children improved their game scores by practicing virtual catching without specific instructions on utilizing the visual cues. This finding has implications for treatment in that the practice of specific motor tasks, even without overt instructions, can positively influence certain types of motor task coordination.

Epidemiology

The prevalence of developmental coordination disorder is about 5% to 6% of school-age children. The male-to-female ratio in referred populations tends to show increased rates of the disorder in males, but schools refer boys more often for testing and special education evaluations. About two males out of every female are affected.

Etiology

The causes of developmental coordination disorder are multifactorial and likely include genetic and developmental factors. Risk factors postulated to contribute to this disorder include prematurity, hypoxia, perinatal malnutrition, and low birth weight. Prenatal exposure to alcohol, cocaine, and nicotine likely contributes to both low birth weight and cognitive and behavioral abnormalities. Children born prematurely have developmental coordination disorder rates of up to 50%. Researchers have proposed that the cerebellum may be the neurologic substrate for comorbid cases of developmental coordination disorder and ADHD. Neurochemical abnormalities and parietal lobe lesions may contribute to coordination deficits. Studies of postural control, the ability to regain balance after being in motion, indicate that children with developmental coordination disorder who have adequate balance when standing still cannot accurately correct for movement, resulting in impaired balance compared with other children. A study concluded that neural signals from the brain to particular muscles involved in balance are neither being optimally sent nor received in children with developmental coordination disorder. These findings have also implicated the cerebellum as a potential anatomical site for the dysfunction of developmental coordination disorder. There are several theories regarding the mechanisms of developmental coordination disorder. One example called the automatization deficit hypothesis, suggests that, similar to dyslexia, children with developmental coordination disorder have difficulty developing automatic motor skills. Another popular suggestion is the internal modeling deficit hypothesis, which suggests that children with developmental coordination disorder cannot perform the typical internal cognitive models that predict the sensory consequences of motor commands. The cerebellum is vital in motor coordination and developmental coordination disorder in both scenarios.

STEREOTYPIC MOVEMENT DISORDER

Stereotypic movements include a diverse range of repetitive behaviors that usually emerge in the early developmental period, appear to lack a clear function, and sometimes cause an interruption in daily life. These movements are typically rhythmic, such as hand flapping, body rocking, hand waving, hair twirling, lip-licking, skin picking, or self-hitting. Stereotypic movements often appear self-soothing or self-stimulating; however, they can sometimes result in self-injury. Stereotypic movements appear to be involuntary; however, they frequently can be suppressed with a concentrated effort. Stereotypic movement disorder occurs with increased frequency in children with ASD and intellectual disability, but it also exists in typically developing children. Stereotypic movements (head-banging, face slapping, eye-poking, or hand-biting) can cause significant self-harm. Nail-biting, thumb-sucking, and nose-picking are often not included as symptoms of stereotypic movement disorder because they rarely cause impairment. When impairment occurs, however, they can be included in stereotypic movement disorder. Stereotypic movements share several features with tics, including the repetitive, seemingly involuntary, and characteristically identical nature of the movements each time they are displayed. However, distinguishing features of stereotypical movements compared to tics include a younger age of onset, lack of changing anatomical locations, lack of premonitory "urge," and decreased response to medication management.

According to DSM-5-TR, stereotypic movement disorder includes repetitive, seemingly driven, and purposeless motor behavior that interferes with social, academic, or other activities and may result in self-harm.

Diagnosis and Clinical Features

The presence of multiple repetitive, stereotyped symptoms tends to occur frequently among children with ASD and intellectual disability, particularly when the intellectual disability is severe. Patients with multiple stereotyped movements frequently have other significant mental disorders, including disruptive behavior disorders or neurologic conditions. In extreme cases, severe mutilation and life-threatening injuries can result from self-inflicted trauma. Table 8-3 compares the diagnostic approaches to diagnosing stereotypic movement disorder.

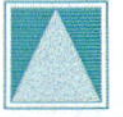

Table 8-3.
Stereotypic Movement Disorder

	DSM-5-TR	ICD-10	ICD-11
Diagnostic name	Stereotypic Movement Disorder	Stereotyped Movement Disorders	Stereotyped Movement Disorder
Duration			Onset in the early developmental period. Persists ≥ several months
Symptoms	Repetitive and seemingly purposeless movements with onset during the developmental period	The presence of voluntary, repetitive, stereotyped, and seemingly purposeless movements outside of any other psychiatric or neurologic condition; may include such things as repeatedly rocking, hand-flapping, or biting	Voluntary, repetitive, stereotyped, apparently purposeless, and often rhythmic movements
Psychosocial consequences	Marked interference in activities and functioning		Marked interference in activities and functioning or result in self-inflicted injury
Exclusions	Other medical condition Substance or medication induced, including withdrawal Other mental disorder	Tic disorder Trichotillomania Stereotypies that are part of a broader psychiatric condition Nail-biting Nose-picking Movement disorders of organic origin	
Symptom specifiers	With self-injurious behavior Without self-injurious behavior Associate with a known medical or genetic condition, neurodevelopmental disorder, or environmental factor		With self-injury Without self-injury
Course specifiers			
Severity specifiers	**Mild** (symptoms easily suppressed by sensory stimulus or distraction) **Moderate** (significant behavioral modification needed to control symptoms) **Severe** (continuous measures taken to prevent harm or injury)		
Comments			Stereotyped Movement Disorder, Unspecified

Head-Banging. Head-banging exemplifies a stereotypic movement disorder that can result in functional impairment. Typically, head-banging begins during infancy, between 6 and 12 months. Infants strike their heads with a definite rhythmic and monotonous continuity against the crib or another hard surface. They seem absorbed in the activity, persisting until they become exhausted and fall asleep. Head-banging is often transitory but sometimes persists into middle childhood. Head-banging, a component of temper tantrums, differs from stereotypic head-banging and ceases after the tantrums, controlling their secondary gains.

Nail-Biting. Nail-biting begins as early as 1 year and increases incidence until age 12. Most cases are not sufficiently severe to meet the DSM-5-TR diagnostic criteria for stereotypic movement disorder. In rare cases, children cause physical damage to the fingers themselves, usually by associated biting of the cuticles, which leads to secondary infections of the fingers and nail beds. Nail-biting seems to occur or increase in intensity when a child is either anxious or stressed. Some of the most severe nail biting occurs in children with severe or profound intellectual disability. However, many nail-biters have no noticeable emotional disturbance.

Pathology and Laboratory Examination. No specific laboratory measures are helpful in the diagnosis of stereotypic movement disorder.

Differential Diagnosis

The differential diagnosis of stereotypic movement disorder includes obsessive-compulsive disorder (OCD) and tic disorders, both of which are exclusionary criteria in DSM-5-TR. Although stereotypic movements can often be voluntarily suppressed and are not spasmodic, it is difficult to differentiate these features from tics in all cases. A study of stereotyped movements compared with tics found that stereotyped movements tended to be longer in duration and displayed more rhythmic qualities than tics. Tics seemed to occur more when a child was in an "alone" condition than when the child was in a play condition, whereas stereotypic movements occurred with the same frequency in these two different conditions. Stereotypic movements seem self-soothing, whereas tics are often associated with distress.

Differentiating dyskinetic movements from stereotypic movements can be difficult. Because antipsychotic medications can sometimes suppress stereotypic movements, clinicians should note any stereotypic movements before initiating treatment with an antipsychotic agent. Stereotypic movement disorder may be diagnosed concurrently with substance-related disorders (e.g., amphetamine use disorders), severe sensory impairments, central nervous system (CNS) and degenerative disorders (e.g., Lesch–Nyhan syndrome), and severe schizophrenia.

Course and Prognosis

The duration and course of stereotypic movement disorder vary, and the symptoms may wax and wane. Up to 60% to 80% of normal toddlers show transient rhythmic activities that seem purposeful and comforting and tend to disappear by 4 years of age. When stereotypic movements emerge more severely later in childhood, they typically range from brief episodes occurring under stress to an ongoing pattern in the context of a chronic condition, such as ASD or intellectual disability. Even in chronic conditions, stereotypic behaviors may come and go. Stereotypic movements are often prominent in early childhood and diminish as the child ages.

The severity of the dysfunction caused by stereotypic movements varies with the frequency, amount, and degree of associated self-injury. Children who exhibit frequent, severe, self-injurious stereotypic behaviors have the poorest prognosis. Repetitive episodes of head-banging, self-biting, and eye-poking can be challenging to control without physical restraints. Most nail-biting is benign and often does not meet the diagnostic criteria for stereotypic movement disorder. Bacterial and fungal infections can occur in severe cases where the child repetitively damages their nail beds. Although chronic stereotypic movement disorders can severely impair daily functioning, several treatments help control the symptoms.

Treatment

When stereotypic movements occur in the absence of any other symptoms or disorders, they may not warrant pharmacologic treatment. Treatment modalities yielding the most promising effects include behavioral techniques, such as habit reversal and differential reinforcement of other behaviors, as well as pharmacologic interventions. A recent report on utilizing habit reversal (in which the therapist trains the child to replace the undesired repetitive behavior with a more acceptable behavior) and reinforcement for reducing the unwanted behavior indicated that these treatments had efficacy among 12 typically developing children between 6 and 14 years. One case report detailed a successful habit reversal treatment of a 3-year-old with severe stereotypic movements, which was implemented mainly at home by her parents.

Pharmacologic interventions have been used in clinical practice to minimize self-injury in children whose stereotyped movements caused significant harm to their bodies. Small open-label studies have reported some benefits from atypical antipsychotics, and case reports have indicated the use of selective serotonin retuptake inhibitors (SSRIs) in the management of self-injurious stereotypies. The dopamine receptor antagonists are often used to treat stereotypical movements and self-injurious behavior. The SSRI agents may be influential in diminishing stereotypies; however, this is still under investigation. Open trials suggest that both clomipramine and fluoxetine may decrease self-injurious behaviors and other stereotypic movements in some patients.

Epidemiology

Repetitive movements are common in infants and young children, with greater than 60% of parents of children between the ages of 2 and 4 years reporting transient emergence of these behaviors. The most frequent age of onset is in the second year of life. Epidemiologic surveys estimate that up to 7% of otherwise typically developing children exhibit stereotypic behaviors. A prevalence of about 15% to 20% in children younger than the age of 6 years has been reported for displaying stereotypic behavior, with diminishing rates over time. The prevalence of self-injurious behaviors, however, is in the range of 2% to 3% among children and adolescents with intellectual disability. Stereotypic movements appear to occur in about twice as many boys as girls. Determining which cases are sufficiently severe to confirm a diagnosis of stereotypic movement disorder may be difficult. Stereotypic behaviors occur in 10% to 20% of children with intellectual disability, with increased rates being proportional to the level of severity. Self-injurious behaviors frequently occur in genetic syndromes, such as Lesch–Nyhan syndrome, and children with sensory impairments, such as blindness and deafness.

Etiology

The etiology of stereotypic movement disorder includes environmental, genetic, and neurobiologic factors. Although the neurobiologic mechanisms of stereotypic movement disorder have yet to be proven, given their similarity to other involuntary movements, stereotypic movement disorder likely originates from the basal ganglia. Dopamine and serotonin are likely to be involved in their emergence. Dopamine agonists tend to induce or increase stereotypic behaviors, whereas dopamine antagonists sometimes decrease them. One study found that 17% of typically developing children with stereotypic movement disorder had a first-degree relative with the disorder, and 25% had a first- or second-degree relative with stereotypic movement disorder. Transient stereotypic behaviors in very young children can be considered a normal developmental phenomenon. Genetic factors likely play a role in some stereotypic movements, such as the X-linked recessive deficiency of enzymes leading to Lesch–Nyhan syndrome, which has predictable features including intellectual disability, hyperuricemia, spasticity, and self-injurious behaviors. Other minimal stereotypic movements that do not usually cause impairment (e.g., nail-biting) also appear to run in families. Some stereotypic behaviors seem to emerge or become exaggerated in situations of neglect or deprivation; such behaviors as head-banging correlate with psychosocial deprivation.

Further Readings

Anderson KE, Stamler D, Davis MD, et al. Deutetrabenazine for the treatment of involuntary movements in patients with tardive dyskinesia (AIM-TD): a double-blind, randomized, placebo-controlled, phase 3 trial. *Lancet Psychiatry*. 2017;4(8):595–604.

Bhidayasiri R, Jitkritsadakul O, Friedman JH, Fahn S. Updating the recommendations for treatment of tardive syndromes: a systematic review of new evidence and practical treatment algorithm. *J Neurol Sci*. 2018;389:67–75.

Blank R, Smits-Engelsman B, Polatajko H, Wilson P; European Academy for Childhood Disability. European Academy for Childhood Disability: recommendations on the definition, diagnosis and intervention of developmental coordination disorder (long version). *Dev Med Child Neurol*. 2012;54(1):54–93.

Doyle RL. Stereotypic movement disorders in children. In: Boland RJ, Verduin ML, eds. *Kaplan & Sadock's Comprehensive Textbook of Psychiatry*. 11th ed. Wolters Kluwer; 2024.

Ferguson GD, Jelsma D, Jelsma J, Smits-Engelsman BCM. The efficacy of two task-oriented interventions for children with developmental coordination disorder: neuromotor task training and Nintendo Wii Fit training. *Res Dev Disabil*. 2013;34(9):2449–2461.

Fernandez HH, Factor SA, Hauser RA, et al. Randomized controlled trial of deutetrabenazine for tardive dyskinesia: the ARM-TD study. *Neurology*. 2017;88(21):2003–2010.

Smits-Engelsman BCM, Blank R, van der Kaay AC, et al. Efficacy of interventions to improve motor performance in children with developmental coordination disorder: a combined systematic review and meta-analysis. *Dev Med Child Neurol*. 2013;55(3):229–237.

Vishwanath V, Mitchell W. Developmental coordination disorder. In: Boland RJ, Verduin ML, eds. *Kaplan & Sadock's Comprehensive Textbook of Psychiatry*. Eleventh edition. Wolters Kluwer; 2024.

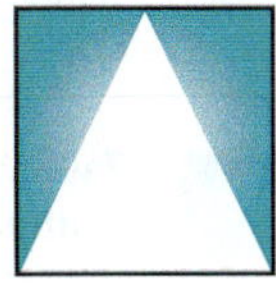

9 Feeding and Eating Disorders of Infants, Children and Adolescents: Pica, Rumination Disorder, Anorexia Nervosa; and Bulimia Nervosa

Feeding and eating disorders of infancy and childhood are persistent disturbances in eating or eating-related behaviors that can lead to significant impairments in physical health and psychosocial functioning. The DSM-5-TR category *Feeding and Eating Disorders* includes pica, rumination disorder, avoidant/restrictive food intake disorder (ARFID), anorexia nervosa, bulimia nervosa, and binge eating disorders. The first three (pica, rumination disorder, and ARFID) are usually, but not always, associated with infancy and childhood, whereas the latter three (anorexia nervosa, bulimia nervosa, and binge eating disorders) typically occur in adolescence or early adulthood. Anorexia nervosa typically begins in mid to late adolescence (14 to 18 years), with about 20% reporting symptoms by age 14 years and about 60% reporting onset by the age of 18 years.

PICA

Pica is persistent ingestion of nonnutritive substances over a period of at least 1 month. Typically, no specific biologic conditions account for pica, and the eating behavior is not part of a culturally normative practice, or normative development. In some cases, however, pica may be associated with nutritional deficiencies including iron-deficiency anemia, calcium deficiency, or zinc deficiency. In many cases, the disorder is only recognized when medical problems emerge, such as intestinal obstruction, intestinal infections, or poisonings, such as lead poisoning due to eating lead-containing paint chips. Pica is more frequent in the context of autism spectrum disorder or intellectual disability; it is only diagnosed as pica when it is severe and persistent enough to warrant clinical attention. Pica can emerge in young children, adolescents, or adults; however, childhood onset is most commonly reported. Pica occurs in both males and females. Among adults, certain forms of pica, including geophagia (clay eating) and amylophagia (starch eating), have been reported in pregnant women.

Diagnosis and Clinical Features

Eating nonedible substances repeatedly after 18 months of age is not typical; however, DSM-5-TR suggests a minimum age of 2 years when making a diagnosis of pica to exclude developmentally expected mouthing of objects which results in ingestion. Pica behaviors, however, may begin in infants 12 to 24 months of age. Specific substances ingested vary with their accessibility, and they increase with a child's mastery of locomotion and the resultant increased independence and decreased parental supervision. Typically, infants may ingest paint, plaster, string, hair, and cloth, whereas older toddlers and young children with pica may ingest dirt, animal feces, small stones, and paper. The clinical implications can be benign or life-threatening, depending on the objects ingested. Among the most severe complications are lead poisoning (usually from lead-based paint), intestinal parasites after ingestion of soil or feces, anemia and zinc deficiency after ingestion of clay, severe iron deficiency after ingestion of large quantities of starch, and

Table 9-1.
Comparative Diagnostic Criteria for Pica

	DSM-5-TR	ICD-10	ICD-11
Diagnostic name	Pica	Pica in Infancy and Childhood Pica in Adults	Pica
Duration	≥1 month	Persistent	Persistent, but can be episodic or variable, or chronic and continuous
Symptoms	Eating substances that are not foods and not nutritional Behavior is inappropriate for development level	Eating nonnutritive substances	Consuming nonnutritive substances Severe enough to require clinical attention Inappropriate for age
Psychosocial consequences			Risks to health/functional impairment
Exclusions	Other medical condition Other mental illness		Other medical conditions, such as a nutritional deficiency
Course specifiers			It can be episodic or variable, or chronic and continuous
Severity specifiers	In remission		

intestinal obstruction from the ingestion of hairballs, stones, or gravel. Except in autism spectrum disorder and intellectual disability, pica often remits by adolescence. Pica associated with pregnancy is usually limited to the pregnancy itself. Table 9-1 provides comparative diagnostic criteria for pica according to DSM-5-TR, ICD-10, and ICD-11.

Clara was 2½ years of age when her mother urgently brought her to the emergency room due to severe abdominal pain and lack of appetite. Clara's mother reported that she was still mouthing many objects but refused to eat regular food. The emergency room physician observed Clara to be pale, thin, and listless. Clara sucked her thumb and quietly looked down while her mother reported that Clara often chewed on her clothing and from chips that came off the wall.

Clara was admitted to the pediatric unit and a comprehensive blood panel revealed that Clara was anemic and suffered from lead poisoning. While on the pediatric inpatient unit, a child psychiatric consultation revealed that Clara's mother was overwhelmed, caring for her five young children, and often left Clara to play by herself for hours in her crib. During these times, Clara played quietly and did not call out for her mother. Clara's mother was a single mother, living with her five children and four other family members in a three-bedroom apartment. Her 7-year-old daughter had behavior problems, and her 6- and 4-year-old sons were impulsive and hyperactive, requiring constant supervision. Clara's 18-month-old sister was an engaging and active little girl, whereas Clara was withdrawn and would sit quietly, rocking herself, sucking her thumb, or chewing on her shirt.

A report was made to child protective services based on Clara's mother's suspected neglect and inability to protect her children from danger. After a full evaluation by child protective services, it was determined that Clara's mother was not neglectful but overwhelmed, and that she was very appreciative to accept help from social services. The treatment plan included increased support for Clara's mother by other relatives living in the home, the removal of any lead paint from the walls in their current apartment, and a plan to seek better living arrangements for the family and provide a safe environment for the children. Clara's mother received guidance in enrolling Clara in a preschool program, and her older sister and two brothers in an after-school program that provided structure and stimulation, and some respite time for the mother. Clara's mother eagerly agreed to participate in a parent management training program. Family therapy was started to help Clara's mother to better understand Clara's developmental needs and to practice these proposed interactions in the sessions with Clara. Once Clara's mother felt more supported and less overwhelmed, she was able to become more empathic and warmer toward Clara. When Clara began chewing on her shirt, her mother learned to instead engage her in a play activity rather than ignoring her. Clara and her mother continued in therapy for a year, during which their relationship gradually became more interactive and warmer, while Clara's chewing and eating of nonnutritive substances significantly decreased.

Pathology and Laboratory Examination. No single laboratory test confirms or rules out a diagnosis of pica, but several laboratory tests are useful because abnormal levels of lead are sometimes associated. Levels of iron and zinc in serum should be determined and corrected if low. In rare cases, when a paucity of iron or zinc is found, administering oral iron and zinc may ameliorate the pica. A hemoglobin level should be determined to rule out anemia.

Differential Diagnosis

The differential diagnosis of pica includes avoidance of food, anorexia, or rarely iron and zinc deficiencies. Pica may occur in conjunction with failure to thrive and can be comorbid with schizophrenia, autism spectrum disorder, and Kleine–Levin syndrome. In psychosocial dwarfism, a dramatic but reversible endocrinologic and behavioral form of failure to thrive, children often show bizarre behaviors, including ingesting toilet water, garbage, and other nonnutritive substances. Lead intoxication may be associated with pica. In children who have pica that warrants clinical intervention as well as a known medical disorder, both disorders should be diagnosed.

Course and Prognosis

The prognosis for pica is usually good, and typically in children with normal intellectual function, pica generally remits spontaneously within several months. In childhood, pica usually resolves with increasing age; in pregnant women, pica resolves after delivery. In some adolescents with pica, particularly in those with autism spectrum disorder and intellectual disability, pica can continue for years.

Treatment

The first step in determining the appropriate treatment of pica is to investigate the specific environmental and psychosocial situation in which the behaviors emerged. When pica occurs in the context of child neglect or maltreatment, those circumstances must be immediately corrected. Exposure to toxic substances, such as lead, must also be eliminated. No definitive treatment exists for pica per se beyond education and behavior modification. Treatments emphasize psychosocial, environmental, behavioral, and family guidance approaches. It is essential to address significant psychosocial stressors. When lead is present in the surroundings, it must be eliminated or rendered inaccessible, or the child and their family should move.

When pica persists in the absence of any toxic manifestations, behavioral techniques are typically employed. Techniques include positive reinforcement, modeling, behavioral shaping, and overcorrection treatment. Increasing parental attention, stimulation, and emotional nurturance may yield positive results. A study found that pica occurred most frequently in impoverished environments, and in some patients, correcting an iron or zinc deficiency has eliminated pica. Medical complications (e.g., lead poisoning) that develop secondarily to the pica also require treatment.

Epidemiology

The prevalence of pica is unclear. A survey of a large clinic population reported that 75% of 12-month-old infants and 15% of 2- to 3-year-old toddlers placed nonnutritive substances in their mouth; however, this behavior is developmentally appropriate and typically does not result in ingestion. Pica is more common among children and adolescents with autism spectrum disorder and intellectual disability. Up to 15% of persons with severe intellectual disability reportedly have engaged in pica. Pica appears to affect both sexes equally.

Etiology

Pica is most often a transient disorder that typically lasts for several months and then remits. In younger children, those with delays of speech and social development are more likely to have it. Among adolescents with pica, a substantial number of them exhibited depressive symptoms and use of illicit drugs. Nutritional deficiencies in minerals such as zinc or iron (found in, e.g., dirt or ice) may rarely be a cause. In some cases of pica, we also find severe child maltreatment in the form of parental neglect and deprivation. Lack of supervision and general neglect, as well as inadequate feeding of infants and toddlers, may increase the risk of pica.

RUMINATION DISORDER

Rumination is an effortless and painless regurgitation of partially digested food into the mouth soon after a meal, which is either swallowed or spit out. Rumination is a developmentally normative behavior in infants under a year, who initiate regurgitation by putting their thumb or hand in the mouth, sucking their tongue rhythmically, and arching their back. Persistent rumination behavior is more likely to occur in infants who receive inadequate emotional interaction and have learned to soothe and may stimulate themselves through rumination. However, rumination syndromes also occur in children and adolescents, in which case rumination is a functional gastrointestinal disorder. According to DSM-5-TR, rumination disorder is diagnosed when rumination behaviors occur repeatedly for at least one month after a period of normal functioning and are not better accounted for by gastrointestinal illness or another psychiatric or medical condition.

The pathophysiology of rumination is not well understood; however, it often involves a rise in intragastric pressure generated by either voluntary or unintentional contraction of the abdominal wall muscles causing movement of gastric contents back up into the esophagus. The onset of the disorder can occur in infancy, childhood, or adolescence. In infants, it typically occurs between 3 and 12 months of age, and once the regurgitation occurs, the food may be swallowed or spit out. Infants who ruminate strain with their backs arched and head back to bring the food back into their mouths and appear to find the experience pleasurable. Infants who are "experienced" ruminators can bring up the food through tongue movements and may not spit out the

Table 9-2.
Comparative Diagnostic Criteria for Rumination Disorder

	DSM-5-TR	ICD-10	ICD-11
Diagnostic name	Rumination Disorder	Feeding Disorder of Infancy and Childhood: Rumination Disorder of Infancy	Rumination–Regurgitation Disorder
Duration	≥1 month		≥ several times per week Sustained for several weeks
Symptoms	Repeated regurgitation of food		Intentional regurgitation of food
Psychosocial consequences			Risks to health/functional impairment
Exclusions	Other eating disorder Other mental illness Other medical conditions, including gastrointestinal disorders		Age <2 Other medical condition Adult rumination syndrome Nausea or vomiting
Severity specifiers	In remission		

food at all, but rather hold it in their mouths and reswallow it. The disorder is not common in older children, adolescents, and adults. It varies in severity and is sometimes associated with medical conditions, such as hiatal hernia, leading to esophageal reflux. In its most severe form, the disorder can cause malnutrition and be fatal.

Rumination disorder can be diagnosed even if an infant maintains a healthy weight. Failure to thrive, therefore, is not a criterion of this disorder, but it is sometimes a sequela. An awareness of the disorder is essential to avoid misdiagnosis and unwarranted tests and treatment.

Diagnosis and Clinical Features

The DSM-5-TR notes that the essential feature of the disorder is repeated regurgitation and rechewing of food for at least 1 month after a period of normal functioning. Patients bring partially digested food into their mouth without nausea, retching, or disgust; on the contrary, it may appear to be pleasurable. This activity may be distinguished from vomiting by its purposeful movements which are observable in some infants who induce it. The food is then ejected from the mouth or swallowed.

Initially, rumination may be challenging to distinguish from the regurgitation that frequently occurs in healthy infants. In infants with persistent and frequent rumination behaviors, however, the differences are apparent. Although spontaneous remissions are common, secondary complications can develop, such as progressive malnutrition, dehydration, and lowered resistance to disease. Failure to thrive, with the absence of growth and developmental delays in all areas, can occur in the most severe cases. Additional complications may occur if the primary caregiver of a given infant with rumination becomes tense or discouraged by the persistent symptoms, viewing it as her feeding failure, as this may lead to more tension and more rumination after feedings. Table 9-2 provides the comparative diagnostic criteria according to the DSM-5-TR, ICD-10, and ICD-11 for rumination disorder.

Pablo was 9 months old when his mother brought him to his pediatrician for evaluation of persistent, repetitive ruination behaviors which had been occurring for the past month. After a pediatric evaluation, Pablo was then evaluated by a gastroenterologist, who found that all of Pablo's medical tests were normal. Finally, Pablo was evaluated by a child and adolescent psychiatrist who specialized in feeding disorders of infancy. Pablo was born full-term and had developed typically until 8 weeks of age when he began to regurgitate large amounts of milk just after feedings. Initially, his pediatrician diagnosed him with gastroesophageal reflux and recommended thickening his feedings. Pablo responded well to the thickened formula, his regurgitation diminished, and he gained weight adequately. Pablo continued to do well, and his mother decided to go back to work when Pablo was 8 months old. He was cared for by a young nanny, who spent all day with Pablo until his mother returned from work. Pablo and his nanny seemed to have a warm rapport with each other; however, he started again to regurgitate his meals soon after his mother left for work each morning. The regurgitation seemed to increase in frequency and intensity within the first 2 weeks of the mother's return to work. At this point, Pablo regurgitated after almost every meal, and he began to lose weight. A gastroenterologist evaluated Pablo with a barium swallow and noted that, during the test, Pablo put his hand in his mouth, which seemed to induce the regurgitation. Pablo did not seem to be distressed during regurgitation; in fact, he seemed to be enjoying it.

Pablo's mother reported that even when she fed him at home in the evenings, as soon as Pablo finished feeding, he purposefully placed his hand in his mouth and induced regurgitation. When his mother restricted his hand, Pablo was able to move his tongue back and forth in a rhythmic manner until he regurgitated again. Pablo continued this rhythmic tongue movement repeatedly, even when he could not bring up any more of his feeding, and appeared to be enjoying this behavior.

Due to Pablo's weight loss and slight dehydration, Pablo was hospitalized and began to receive nasojejunal tube feedings. During feedings, a private duty nurse or his parents played with him and distracted him during attempts to put his hand in his mouth or thrust his tongue rhythmically. Pablo became increasingly engaged in this playful activity, and his ruminative activity decreased accordingly. After 2 weeks in the hospital, they started small feedings by mouth, some of which he would bring up with his tongue. The nursing staff and his mother continued the "distracting" intervention in order to interrupt his rumination during meals. Pablo's mother slowly increased his feedings while playing with him during and after, and she was able to interest him in other activities so that he would not ruminate. Pablo's mother decided not to return to work at this time. After 4 weeks of slow incremental increases in his feedings, Pablo was able to take all his feedings by mouth without ruminating, and his nasojejunal tube was removed. Pablo and his mother continued to use stimulating and distracting activities during and just after meals, which Pablo became very engaged in, and over time, his ruminating behavior extinguished completely.

Pathology and Laboratory Examination. No specific laboratory examination is pathognomonic of rumination disorder; however, rumination disorder is not uncommonly associated with gastrointestinal abnormalities. Clinicians should evaluate other physical causes of vomiting, such as pyloric stenosis and hiatal hernia, before making the diagnosis of rumination disorder. Rumination disorder can lead to states of malnutrition and dehydration. In very severe cases, laboratory measures of endocrinologic function, serum electrolytes, and a hematologic workup may determine the need for medical intervention.

Differential Diagnosis

To make the diagnosis of rumination disorder, clinicians must rule out primary gastrointestinal congenital anomalies, infections, and other medical illnesses that could account for frequent regurgitation. Pyloric stenosis is usually associated with projectile vomiting and is generally evident before 3 months of age when rumination has its onset. Rumination may occur with autism spectrum disorder and intellectual disability, in which stereotypic behaviors and eating disturbances are not uncommon. Rumination behavior may occur comorbidly in youth with severe anxiety disorders, as well. Rumination disorder may also occur in patients with other eating disorders, such as anorexia nervosa and bulimia nervosa.

Course and Prognosis

Rumination disorder has a high rate of spontaneous remission. Indeed, many cases of rumination disorder may develop and remit without ever being diagnosed. Limited data are available about the prognosis of rumination disorder in adolescents and adults. Behavioral interventions using habit-reversal techniques may significantly lead to improved prognosis.

Treatment

The treatment of rumination disorder is often a combination of education and behavioral techniques. Sometimes, an evaluation of the mother–child relationship reveals deficits that can be influenced by offering guidance to the mother. Behavioral interventions, such as habit-reversal, can reinforce an alternate behavior that becomes more compelling than the behaviors leading to regurgitation. Aversive behavioral interventions, such as squirting lemon juice into the infant's mouth whenever rumination occurs, have been used in the past to diminish rumination behavior. Aversive interventions are not currently recommended, and current consensus supports the use of habit-reversal techniques.

Medication is not a standard part of the treatment of rumination. Case reports, however, cite a variety of medications, including metoclopramide, cimetidine, and even antipsychotics such as haloperidol, as helpful. The treatment of adolescents with rumination disorder is often complicated and includes a multidisciplinary approach consisting of individual psychotherapy, nutritional intervention, and pharmacologic treatment for frequent comorbid anxiety and depressive symptoms.

Epidemiology

Rumination is a rare disorder. It seems to be more common among male infants and emerges between 3 months and 1 year of age. It persists more frequently among children, adolescents, and adults with intellectual disability. Adults with rumination are usually of normal weight.

Etiology

Rumination is associated with high intragastric pressure and the ability to contract the abdominal wall to cause retrograde movement of the gastric contents into the esophagus. Several studies have elucidated other gastrointestinal symptoms, such as gastroesophageal reflux, that may accompany rumination. Although rumination disorder most typically occurs in infants, there are some reports in which older children and adolescents with gastrointestinal conditions or other symptoms exhibit rumination as well. For example:

In a study of 2,163 children in Sri Lanka between the ages of 10 and 16 years, it was found that rumination behaviors were present in 5.1% of boys and 5.0% of girls. In 94.5% of youth who ruminated, the regurgitation occurred in the first hour after the meal, and 73.6% reported reswallowing the regurgitated food, whereas the rest spit it out. Only 8.2% of this sample reported daily episodes of regurgitation, whereas 62.7% experienced weekly symptoms. Associated gastrointestinal symptoms reported in this sample included abdominal pain, bloating, and weight loss. Approximately 20% of youth with rumination in this sample also experienced other gastrointestinal symptoms. Another survey of 147 patients from 5 to 20 years of age found the mean age of onset of rumination was 15 years, and these patients were symptomatic after each meal; 16% of this sample met criteria for a psychiatric disorder, 3.4% had anorexia or bulimia nervosa, and 11% had a surgical procedure. Additional gastrointestinal symptoms in this sample included abdominal pain in 38%, constipation in 21%, nausea in 17%, and diarrhea in 8%. In some cases, vomiting secondary to gastroesophageal reflux or an acute illness precedes a pattern of rumination that lasts for several months. In many cases, children classified as ruminators have gastroesophageal reflux or hiatal hernia.

It appears, for some infants, that the rumination behavior is self-soothing or produces a sense of relief, leading to a continuation of behaviors to bring it about. In youth with autism spectrum disorder or intellectual disability, rumination may serve as a self-stimulatory behavior. Overstimulation and tension are contributing factors in rumination. Behaviorists attribute persistent rumination to the positive reinforcement of pleasurable self-stimulation and to the attention a baby receives from others as a consequence of the disorder.

AVOIDANT/RESTRICTIVE FOOD INTAKE DISORDER

ARFID, formerly known as feeding disorder of infancy or early childhood, is characterized by a lack of interest in food, or its avoidance based on the sensory features of the food or the perceived consequences of eating. According to the DSM-5-TR, ARFID is manifested by a persistent failure to meet nutritional or energy needs, as evidenced by one or more of the following: significant weight loss or failure to achieve expected weight, nutritional deficiency, dependence on enteral feedings or nutritional supplements, or marked interference with psychosocial functioning. It may take the form of outright food refusal, food selectivity, eating too little, food avoidance, and delayed self-feeding. We should not make the diagnosis in the context of anorexia nervosa or bulimia nervosa, or if caused by a medical condition, by another mental disorder, or by a genuine lack of available food.

Infants and children with ARFID may be withdrawn, irritable, apathetic, or anxious. Due to the infant's avoidant behavior during feeding, there is less touching and holding between caregivers and infants during the feeding process compared with other infants. Some reports suggest that food avoidance or restriction may be relatively longstanding; however, in most cases, typical eating behavior is achieved by adolescence. Table 9-3 provides comparative diagnostic criteria for avoidant/

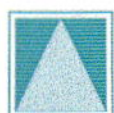

Table 9-3.
Comparative Diagnostic Criteria for Avoidant/Restrictive Food Intake Disorder

	DSM-5-TR	ICD-10	ICD-11
Diagnostic name	Avoidant/Restrictive Food Intake Disorder (ARFID)	Other Eating Disorder	ARFID
Symptoms	Eating/Feeding disturbance associated with: • Significant weight loss/lack of expected weight gain • Significant nutritional deficiency • Needing enteral feeding or oral supplements		Avoidance or restriction of food intake • Insufficient intake for nutritional needs • Nutritional deficiencies • Dependence on supplements or tube feeding • Other negative effects on health
Required number of symptoms			Any of the above or functional impairment
Psychosocial consequences	Functional impairment		Functional impairment
Exclusions	Food insecurity Culturally sanctioned practice Other eating disorder Other medical condition		Food insecurity Other medical condition Substance or medication, including withdrawal Other mental illness
Course specifiers	In remission		

restrictive food intake according to DSM-5-TR, ICD-10, and ICD-11.

Differential Diagnosis

When it emerges in infants, ARFID must be differentiated from structural problems with an infant's gastrointestinal tract that may be contributing to discomfort during the feeding process. Because feeding disorders and organic causes of swallowing difficulties often coexist, it is essential to rule out medical reasons for feeding difficulties. A study of video fluoroscopic evaluation of children with feeding and swallowing problems revealed that clinical evaluation was 92% accurate in identifying those children at increased risk of aspiration. This type of evaluation is necessary before psychotherapeutic interventions in cases where a medical contribution to feeding problems is suspected.

Course and Prognosis

Most infants identified with feeding disorder within the first year of life and who receive treatment do not go on to develop malnutrition, growth delay, or failure to thrive. When feeding disorders have their onset later, in children 2 to 3 years of age, growth and development can be affected when the disorder lasts for several months. In older children or adolescents, the feeding disorder typically interferes with social functioning until treated. About 70% of infants who persistently refuse food in the first year of life continue to have some eating problems during childhood.

Tina was 6 months old when her parents became concerned that she was having increasing feeding difficulties. Tina's parents consulted with their pediatrician to determine whether she had developed a medical illness accounting for her an exacerbation of feeding difficulties, irritability, and poor weight gain since birth. On examination by the pediatrician, Tina was small and slight, but she did not appear to be lethargic or malnourished. Tina had exhibited feeding difficulties since she was an infant. She was full-term and weighed 7 lb at birth; however, she had been unable to breastfeed due to turning away and not ingesting enough breast milk. When she was 4 weeks old, Tina's mother had reluctantly switched her to bottle feedings in the hope of promoting weight gain because she was losing weight. Tina's intake improved somewhat on bottle feedings, she gained weight very slowly, and she was still less than 8 lb at 3 months of age. Since then, she has gained a minimal amount each month to maintain a low but adequate weight. Tina's mother appeared exhausted and described that Tina would drink only up to about 6 oz at a time, or two bites of baby food, and then wiggle, cry, and refuse to continue with the feeding. However, after an hour or two she would often cry again as if she were hungry. Tina and her mother could not settle her into a good rhythm of feeding, and continued attempts by her mother to feed her would lead her to cry inconsolably. Tina's mother reported approximately 10 to 15 attempts at feeding her both liquids and solids in 24 hours. Tina was described as an irritable and fussy baby who cried multiple times during the day and at night. Tina was still unable to sleep through the night at 6 months old and woke her family several times each night with her crying. Tina's developmental milestones, such as sitting up, tracking, and making sounds, were as expected for her age. Tina's pediatrician did not find any medical reasons to account for Tina's feeding problems. The pediatrician referred Tina and her family to a child and adolescent psychiatrist who specialized in infant feeding disorders. The psychiatrist's observation of Tina and her mother's interactions during feeding and play revealed that Tina was a very alert and wiggly baby who had difficulty sitting still. While drinking from the bottle, Tina would kick her feet and move around, and if the bottle slipped out of her mouth, she did not try to find it to continue feeding. When Tina's mother attempted to feed Tina baby foods, she seemed disinterested, and her mother had to coax her to open her mouth. The more that her mother tried to feed her, the more upset Tina would become, and this process usually ended in her crying. Tina's mother reported that she was always anxious during meals, and she would try to convince Tina to take small spoonful of baby food while sitting in her highchair. Tina wriggled during these sessions and tried to get out of her highchair. After repeated unsuccessful attempts of adequate feeding, Tina and her mother both became frustrated and tired and would take a break. The psychiatrist noted that Tina was a very active and excitable baby who had difficulty keeping calm during feedings. After reviewing the videotape with the mother, the psychiatrist explored ways in which the mother could facilitate calming Tina before and during meals. Using a quiet corner in the house and singing to Tina gently before feeding resulted in Tina becoming calmer during meals. As she became calmer, she was able to drink more substantial amounts of milk, eat more solid foods, and wait longer between meals. This improvement, in turn, relieved her mother's anxiety and helped both to have calmer and more successful interactions.

Treatment

Most interventions for feeding disorders aim to optimize the interaction between the mother and infant during feedings and identify any factors that can be changed to promote better ingestion. The psychiatrist helps the mother to become more aware of the infant's stamina for the length of individual feedings, the infant's biologic regulation patterns, and the infant's fatigue level to increase the level of engagement between mother and infant during feeding.

Some experts have proposed a transactional model of intervention for infants who exhibit the "difficult" temperamental traits of emotional intensity, stubbornness, lack of hunger cues, and irregular eating and sleeping patterns. The treatment includes education for the parents regarding the temperamental traits of the infant, exploration of the parents' anxieties about the infant's nutrition, and training for the parents regarding changing their behaviors to promote internal regulation of eating in the infant. Parents are encouraged to feed the infant regularly at 3- to 4-hour intervals and offer only water between meals. The parents learn to deliver praise to the infant for any self-feeding efforts, regardless of the amount of food ingested. Furthermore, parents learn to limit any distracting stimulation during meals and give attention and praise to positive eating behaviors rather than intense negative attention to inappropriate behavior during meals. This training process for parents is intense even though brief. Many parents can facilitate improved eating patterns in the infant as a result. In extreme cases, if an infant tires before ingesting an adequate amount of nutrition, it may be necessary to begin treatment with the placement of a nasogastric tube for supplemental oral feedings.

Medication is not a standard component of treatment for feeding disorders. In the extreme cases in which an older child or preadolescent develops failure-to-thrive and is also comorbid for anxiety and mood symptoms, parenteral nutrition interventions may be necessary. Anecdotal reports in extreme cases describe the introduction of risperidone to aid with weight gain.

Epidemiology

Reported rates of transient feeding difficulties have ranged from 15% to 35% of infants and young children. A study of restrictive eating difficulties in Swedish 9- and 12-year-olds found that restrictive eating problems were present in 0.6% of their sample. However, another study of avoidant eating patterns in young children in Germany found that some degree of avoidance was present in up to 53% of children. Thus, we should separate avoidant eating behaviors without impairment of nutritional state or psychosocial functioning from restricted eating disturbances leading to significant functional impairment. A survey of feeding problems in nursery school children revealed a prevalence of 4.8% with equal gender distribution. In that study, children with feeding problems exhibited more somatic complaints and mothers of affected infants exhibited an increased risk of anxiety symptoms. Data from community samples estimate a prevalence of failure-to-thrive syndromes in approximately 3% of infants, with approximately half of those infants exhibiting feeding disorders.

ANOREXIA NERVOSA

Anorexia nervosa is a severe disorder that typically emerges in adolescence or young adulthood. According to the DSM-5-TR, anorexia nervosa is characterized by three essential criteria, restriction of nutritional intake leading to a significantly low body weight, intense fear of gaining weight or becoming fat, and a disturbance of the way that one's body weight or shape is experienced.

Two subtypes of anorexia nervosa exist: restricting type and binge-eating/purging type. The theme in both anorexia nervosa subtypes is the relentless drive to remain thin as a vital source of self-esteem, with persistent behavior that interferes with weight gain.

Young adolescents with anorexia nervosa generally lose weight by drastically reducing their total food intake. In older adolescents and young adults, some not only diet but will also regularly engage in binge eating, followed by purging behaviors. Some patients routinely purge after eating small amounts of food. Anorexia nervosa is much more prevalent in females than in males, accounting for more than 90% of those persons with the diagnosis. Hypotheses of underlying psychological disturbances in adolescents with the disorder include conflicts surrounding the transition from girlhood to womanhood and difficulty establishing a sense of autonomy. Bulimic symptoms can occur as part of anorexia nervosa or as a separate disorder. Persons with either subtype of anorexia nervosa and/or those with bulimia nervosa are excessively preoccupied with weight, food, and body shape. The outcome of anorexia nervosa varies from spontaneous recovery to a waxing and waning course to death.

Diagnosis and Clinical Features

The onset of anorexia nervosa usually occurs during adolescence or young adulthood. The restricting subtype is associated with an earlier age of onset, a better prognosis, and increased risk of switching to the binging/purging subtype. In the United States, the lifetime prevalence of anorexia nervosa is approximately 0.80%. A switch from the restricting type of anorexia nervosa to the binging/purging type generally indicates that the clinical impairment has worsened. Comparative diagnostic criteria for anorexia nervosa according to DSM-5-TR, ICD-10, and ICD 11 are shown in Table 9-4.

Intense fear of gaining weight and becoming obese is present in all patients with the disorder and undoubtedly contributes to their even resistance to therapy. Most intense efforts to lose weight and maintain an underweight status occur secretly. Patients with anorexia nervosa usually refuse to eat with their families or friends in private or in public places. They lose weight by drastically reducing their total food intake, with a strong aversion to any food that contains fat or carbohydrates.

The term anorexia is a misnomer because the loss of appetite is usually rare until late in the disorder. Evidence that patients are frequently obsessing about food is their passion for collecting recipes and for preparing elaborate meals for others. Some patients cannot continuously control their voluntary restriction of food intake, and so have eating binges. These binges usually occur secretly, often

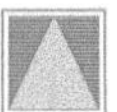

Table 9-4.
Comparative Diagnostic Criteria for Anorexia Nervosa

	DSM-5-TR	ICD-10	ICD-11
Diagnostic name	Anorexia Nervosa	Anorexia Nervosa	Anorexia Nervosa
Symptoms	Food restriction leading to abnormally low weight Fear of gaining weight and behaviors to prevent weight gain Distorted body image • Misperceiving weight or shape • Self-evaluation based on thinness, lack of recognition of the seriousness of one's weight	Deliberate weight loss induced by the patient Fear of being fat or flabby Associated physiologic disturbances due to low weight Specific Behaviors: • Restricted diet • Excess exercise • Binging behavior • Use of appetite suppressants and diuretics	Low body weight Typically BMI <18.5 kg/m^2 in adults, and under 5th percentile in children and adolescents Pattern or restrictive eating or other behavior for maintaining a low weight Usually associated with fear of weight gain Excess preoccupation with body weight or shape
Required number of symptoms	All		
Exclusions		Loss of appetite (physical or psychological)	Other medical condition Food insecurity
Symptom specifiers	Restricting type: Primary behaviors are dieting, fasting, and exercise for the last 3 mo Binge eating type: Binging and purging behavior for the last 3 mo This can include the use of laxatives or other substances to aid in purging		
Course specifiers	Partial remission: symptoms present but no longer an abnormally low weight Full remission: No symptoms for a sustained period		
Severity specifiers	Severity is measured by BMI level Mild: BMI ≥17 kg/m^2 Moderate: BMI ≥16, <17 kg/m^2 Severe: BMI ≥15, <16 kg/m^2 Extreme: BMI <15 kg/m^2		
Comments		If lacking core symptoms, the diagnosis of "Atypical Anorexia Nervosa" is made	

at night, and are frequently followed by self-induced vomiting. Patients abuse laxatives and diuretics to lose weight and engage in ritualistic exercising, which can include extensive cycling, walking, jogging, and running long distances each day.

Adolescents with anorexia nervosa often display peculiar behavior surrounding food. While eating meals, they often try to dispose of food surreptitiously in their napkins or hide it in their pockets. They cut their food into tiny pieces and spend a great deal of time rearranging these pieces on their plates. If someone confronts the patient about the behavior, the adolescent often denies that it is unusual or flatly refuses to discuss it.

Obsessive-compulsive behavior, depression, and anxiety are other psychiatric symptoms of anorexia nervosa most frequently noted clinically. Patients tend to be rigid and perfectionistic, often leading to excellent performance in school and sports activities. Many adolescent patients with anorexia nervosa have delayed social development and do not engage in social or romantic relationships typical for their age group.

Adolescents with anorexia nervosa come to medical attention when their weight loss becomes apparent to parents, teachers, or coaches of sports teams. As the weight loss becomes profound, physical signs such as hypothermia (as low as 35 °C), dependent edema, bradycardia, hypotension, and lanugo (the appearance of neonatal-like hair) appear, and patients show a variety of metabolic changes. Medical complications of anorexia nervosa are listed in Table 9-5.

Table 9-5.
Medical Complications of Anorexia Nervosa

Disorder and System Affected	Consequence
Anorexia Nervosa—Restricting Type	
Vital signs	Bradycardia, hypotension with marked orthostatic changes, hypothermia, poikilothermia
General	Muscle atrophy, loss of body fat
Central nervous system	Generalized brain atrophy with enlarged ventricles, decreased cortical mass, seizures, abnormal electroencephalogram
Cardiovascular	Peripheral (starvation) edema, decreased cardiac diameter, narrowed left ventricular wall, decreased response to exercise demand, superior mesenteric artery syndrome
Renal	Prerenal azotemia
Hematologic	Anemia of starvation, leukopenia, hypocellular bone marrow
Gastrointestinal	Delayed gastric emptying, gastric dilatation, decreased intestinal lipase and lactase
Metabolic	Hypercholesterolemia, nonsymptomatic hypoglycemia, elevated liver enzymes, decreased bone mineral density
Endocrine	Low luteinizing hormone, low follicle-stimulating hormone, low estrogen or testosterone, low/normal thyroxine, low triiodothyronine, increased reverse triiodothyronine, elevated cortisol, elevated growth hormone, partial diabetes insipidus, increased prolactin
Anorexia Nervosa—Binging and Purging Type	
Metabolic	Hypokalemic alkalosis or acidosis, hypochloremia, dehydration
Renal	Prerenal azotemia, acute and chronic renal failure
Cardiovascular	Arrhythmias, myocardial toxicity from emetine (ipecac)
Dental	Lingual surface enamel loss, multiple caries
Gastrointestinal	Swollen parotid glands, elevated serum amylase levels, gastric distention, irritable bowel syndrome, melanosis coli from laxative abuse
Musculoskeletal	Cramps, tetany

Subtypes. Anorexia nervosa has two clinical subtypes: food restricting and purging. In the food-restricting category, more commonly occurring in younger adolescents than adults, food intake is highly restricted (with attempts to consume fewer than 300 to 500 calories per day and no grams of fat). The adolescent may be relentlessly and compulsively over exercising, even with overuse athletic injuries. In the binging/purging subtype, adolescents alternate attempts at rigorous dieting with intermittent binge or purge episodes. Purging represents a secondary compensation for the unwanted calories, most often accomplished by self-induced vomiting, frequently by laxative abuse, less frequently by diuretics, and occasionally with emetics. Sometimes, repetitive purging occurs without prior binge eating, after ingesting only relatively few calories. Both types may become socially isolated and exhibit anxiety and depressive symptoms. Over exercising and perfectionistic traits are also common in both subtypes of anorexia nervosa.

Those who practice binge eating and purging share many features with people who have bulimia nervosa without anorexia nervosa. Adolescents with binging and purging are more likely to be associated with substance abuse and impulse control disorders. Adolescents with restricting anorexia nervosa typically have obsessive-compulsive traits concerning food and other matters. Some adolescents with anorexia nervosa may purge but not binge.

Patients with anorexia nervosa are often secretive, deny their symptoms, and resist treatment. In almost all cases, relatives or friends must confirm a patient's history. The mental status examination usually shows an adolescent who is alert and knowledgeable on the subject of nutrition and who is excessively preoccupied with food and weight.

Sometimes anorexia nervosa is triggered in an adolescent who started out with average weight after learning about "health" in school, or after joining a dance team or track team in which an optimal weight is identified by the coach. Once triggered, an adolescent might start training for hours a day, more than her teammates, begin to perceive herself as fat, and believe that her performance would be enhanced if she lost weight. After persistently dieting, however, once an adolescent's body mass index falls below about 17.5, her performance may actually decline. Adolescents with anorexia nervosa may push themselves in sports when they feel that their performance has declined, until the coach disallows them from participating in team activities. With the loss of a sporting activity and the continued intense fear of becoming fat, an adolescent may further restrict food intake. At the extreme, an adolescent may stop eating any food containing fat, and may subsist on salad, vegetables, and occasional fruits such as apples or oranges. At this point, an adolescent generally becomes amenorrheic, and her hair may be thinning. Some adolescents at the peak of their weight loss do not appear to be fully alert in conversation and are often in need of a partial hospital program or inpatient eating disorder program.

Pathology and Laboratory Examination. Adolescents with anorexia nervosa must have a thorough general physical and neurologic examination. If the patient is vomiting, hypokalemic alkalosis may be present. Because most patients are dehydrated, serum electrolyte levels must be determined initially and periodically. Hospitalization may be necessary to deal with medical complications.

A complete blood count often reveals leukopenia with relative lymphocytosis in emaciated patients with anorexia nervosa. If binge eating and purging are present, serum electrolyte determination reveals hypokalemic alkalosis. Fasting serum glucose concentrations are often low during the emaciated phase, and serum salivary amylase concentrations may increase if the patient is vomiting.

Electrocardiographic (ECG) changes, such as T-wave flattening or inversion, ST segment depression, and lengthening of the QT interval, have been noted in the emaciated stage of anorexia nervosa. The ST segment and T-wave changes are usually secondary to electrolyte disturbances; emaciated patients have hypotension and bradycardia. ECG changes may also result from potassium loss, which can lead to death. Young girls may have a high serum cholesterol level. All these values revert to normal with nutritional rehabilitation and cessation of purging behaviors. Endocrine changes related to being underweight may occur. These can include amenorrhea, mild hypothyroidism, and hypersecretion of corticotrophin-releasing hormone, which revert to normal with weight gain.

Differential Diagnosis

The differential diagnosis of anorexia nervosa is complicated, as patients often deny symptoms, are secretive about their eating habits, and resist seeking treatment. Thus, it may be difficult to identify the mechanism of weight loss and the patient's associated ruminative thoughts about distortions of body image.

We should differentiate eating disorders from one another. Attention to specific criteria, including whether the patient is of average weight, is essential. However, the two conditions can coexist.

We must ascertain that a patient does not have a medical illness that can account for the weight loss (e.g., a brain tumor or cancer). Weight loss, peculiar eating behaviors, and vomiting can occur in several mental disorders. Depressive disorders and anorexia nervosa have several features in common, such as depressed feelings, crying spells, sleep disturbance, obsessive ruminations, and occasional suicidal thoughts. The two disorders, however, have several distinguishing features. In general, a patient with a depressive disorder has decreased appetite, whereas a patient with anorexia nervosa claims to have a normal appetite and to feel hungry; only in the severe stages of anorexia nervosa do patients have decreased appetite.

In contrast to ADHD or agitated depression, the over activity seen in anorexia nervosa is planned and ritualistic. The preoccupation with recipes, the caloric content of foods, and the preparation of gourmet feasts is typical of patients with anorexia nervosa but is absent in patients with a depressive disorder. In depressive disorders, patients have no intense fear of obesity or disturbance of body image.

Weight fluctuations, vomiting, and peculiar food handling may occur in somatization disorder. On rare occasions, a patient may have both a somatization disorder and anorexia nervosa, in which case we should diagnose both. In general, patients with somatization disorder have less weight loss than patients with anorexia nervosa and do not fear weight gain. Amenorrhea for 3 months or longer is unusual in somatization disorder.

Patients with schizophrenia that include delusions about food rarely are concerned with caloric content. More likely, they believe someone poisoned the food. Patients with schizophrenia are rarely preoccupied with a fear of becoming obese and do not have the hyperactivity seen with anorexia nervosa. Patients with schizophrenia have bizarre eating habits but not the entire syndrome of anorexia nervosa.

There are rare conditions of unknown etiology in which a hyperactive vagus nerve causes changes in eating patterns that are associated with weight loss, sometimes severe. In such cases, we may see bradycardia, hypotension, and other parasympathomimetic signs and symptoms. Because the vagus nerve relates to the enteric nervous system, eating may be associated with gastric distress such as nausea or bloating. Patients do not generally lose their appetite. Treatment is symptomatic. Anticholinergic drugs can reverse hypotension and bradycardia, which may be life-threatening.

Comorbidity

The suicide rate is higher in persons with the binge eating–purging type of anorexia nervosa than in those with the restricting type.

Binge eating–purging persons are likely to be associated with substance abuse, impulse control disorders, and personality disorders. Persons with restricting anorexia nervosa often have obsessive-compulsive traits concerning food and other matters. Some persons with anorexia nervosa may purge but not binge.

Course and Prognosis

The precise course of the illness varies substantially, although specific patterns have emerged in the literature. Follow-up studies of adolescents with anorexia nervosa reveal that, at the time of assessment, approximately 30% to 50% have achieved full recovery, and 10% to 20% remain chronically ill. The remainder improve but continue to struggle with certain disordered behaviors. The chronically ill group often requires multiple hospitalizations. Of note, anorexia nervosa has a mortality rate as high as that associated with any psychiatric illness. Compared to the general population, individuals with the illness are up to six times more likely to die. The majority of deaths are attributable to medical complications of low weight and malnourishment, but a smaller, yet significant, proportion of deaths (approximately 1 in 5) are due to suicide.

Although additional research is needed to identify predictors of outcome in anorexia nervosa, studies have found that adolescents with a shorter duration of illness tend to have a better prognosis, emphasizing the importance of early detection and intervention. Studies examining inpatients with anorexia nervosa just before and after discharge have also identified specific predictors of posttreatment outcomes. Individuals who achieve full weight-restoration on an inpatient unit and maintain their weight in the first month after discharge are, perhaps unsurprisingly, more likely to remain at a healthy weight up to a year after treatment. Lower BMI at discharge and weight loss in the first month after treatment, on the other hand, predict more unsatisfactory long-term outcomes. In addition, individuals who demonstrate an ability to consume a diet that is high in variety and energy density (i.e., a greater concentration of kcal/g) before discharge seem to do better after treatment.

Treatment Approach

Given the complicated psychological and medical implications of anorexia nervosa, a comprehensive treatment plan, including hospitalization when necessary and both individual and family therapy, is recommended. It is important to consider behavioral, interpersonal, and cognitive approaches. In many cases, medication may also help.

Hospitalization. The first consideration in the treatment of anorexia nervosa is to restore patient's nutritional state; dehydration, starvation, and electrolyte imbalances can seriously compromise health and, in some cases, lead to death. When deciding whether to hospitalize a patient, we should consider the patient's medical condition and the amount of structure needed to ensure cooperation. In general, adolescents with anorexia nervosa who are about 20% below expected weight for their height and age require inpatient programs followed by intensive outpatient programs. Adolescents 30% below their expected weight require psychiatric hospitalization for up to 6 months.

Inpatient adolescent psychiatric programs for patients with anorexia nervosa generally use a combination of a behavioral management approach, individual psychotherapy, family education and therapy, and, in some cases, psychotropic medications. Staff members maintain a firm yet supportive approach to patients, often through a combination of positive reinforcers (praise) and negative reinforcers (restriction of exercise). The program must have some flexibility for individualizing treatment to meet patient's needs and cognitive abilities.

Most adolescents with anorexia nervosa deny symptoms and resist treatment until they are pressured by family members and medical teams. Adolescents rarely accept the recommendation of hospitalization without arguing and criticizing the proposed program. Family support and confidence in the physicians and treatment team are essential for reinforcing the firm recommendations made on the unit. Adolescents may make many dramatic pleas to their families to obtain release from the hospital program. Compulsory admission or commitment is only possible when the risk of death from the complications of malnutrition is imminent. In less severe cases, an adolescent may gain the specified amount of weight by the time of each outpatient visit, but such behavior is uncommon, and a period of inpatient care is usually necessary.

HOSPITAL MANAGEMENT. The following considerations apply to the general management of adolescents with anorexia nervosa during a hospitalized treatment program. Adolescents should be weighed on a regular basis, twice weekly in some programs. Some adolescents attempt to drink large amounts of water (water loading) prior to being weighed to increase their weight, so observation is needed prior to being weighed. If vomiting is occurring despite being monitored, hospital staff members must monitor serum electrolyte levels regularly and watch for the development of hypokalemia. Because adolescents with anorexia nervosa may try to regurgitate food after meals, direct observation by staff for a period of time is typically built in the milieu. Many adolescents complain of constipation during their hospital stay which normalizes over time. Adolescents with constipation are often prescribed stool softeners, but never laxatives. Due to the serious risk of refeeding syndrome when patients immediately start eating an enormous number of calories, which can result in large electrolyte shifts that potentially cause seizures, heart failure, and coma, slow refeeding is necessary. In some inpatient eating disorder programs, adolescents start with 300 calorie meals three times per day. Increases in calories per meal and meal frequency typically leads to three meals plus two or three snacks. Liquid food supplementation is typically only recommended when a patient does not finish their solid meal or snack. After discharge from the hospital, adolescents are recommended to step down to an intensive outpatient program until they are ready to continue in outpatient treatment. Once they leave the hospital for home, most adolescents who have just been discharged from inpatient programs will require supervision while eating meals by their families.

Psychotherapy

FAMILY-BASED THERAPY. Family-based therapy (FBT) is an effective component of treatment for anorexia nervosa for patients who do not require inpatient treatment, particularly in patients under the age of 18. FBT generally consists of three phases of treatment. In phase one, treatment focuses on the restoration of the patient's physical health, with decisions about what or when the adolescent will eat largely made by the parents. Once the patient has begun to gain weight and shown improvement in symptoms of anorexia nervosa, FBT moves on to phase two. In this phase, the patient gradually begins to take responsibility for decisions about eating. In phase three, the focus shifts to the patient's psychological growth and development.

COGNITIVE-BEHAVIORAL THERAPY. Cognitive and behavioral therapy principles are utilized in both inpatient and outpatient settings and have been found to be helpful within these settings to manage weight gain. Monitoring is an essential component of cognitive-behavioral therapy (CBT). Therapists help patients to monitor their food intake, their feelings and emotions, and their meal programs. Therapists work on cognitive restructuring to identify negative automatic thoughts and to challenge distorted core beliefs. Problem-solving is a specific method whereby patients learn how to think through and devise strategies to cope with their food-related and social problems.

DYNAMIC PSYCHOTHERAPY. Dynamic expressive-supportive psychotherapy can be helpful in the treatment of adolescents with anorexia nervosa, but the process is often difficult and painstaking. Adolescents with anorexia nervosa view their symptoms as constituting the core of their specialness, and therapists may rely on other members of a treatment team, such as nutritionists or dieticians, to monitor and manage specific food choices and eating behaviors. In the opening phase of the psychotherapy, the goal is to build a therapeutic alliance. Adolescents may experience a therapist's "interpretations" as though someone else was telling them what they feel and thereby minimizing and invalidating their own experiences. Therapists who empathize with patients' points of view and take an active interest in what their patients think and feel, however, convey to patients that their autonomy is respected. Psychotherapists must be flexible, persistent, and durable in the face of adolescents who are rigidly attached to their maladaptive cognitions and behaviors.

Pharmacotherapy. Pharmacologic studies have not yet identified any medication that yields a definitive improvement of the core symptoms of anorexia nervosa. Some studies have reported on the use of atypical antipsychotics, particularly olanzapine, for weight gain, or to manage extreme states of anxiety, although larger studies or meta-analyses have not supported this. When using atypical antipsychotics, the metabolic and cardiac risks associated with these medications, particularly in a population already at risk for cardiac complications, require close monitoring. Antidepressants, including selective serotonin reuptake inhibitors (SSRIs), have been prescribed to adolescent patients with anorexia nervosa without consistent results, though typically antidepressants are not helpful while patients are in an undernourished state. In patients with anorexia nervosa and coexisting depressive disorders, pharmacologic treatment is recommended for the depressive condition. In some patients, depression improves or resolves with weight gain and normalized nutritional status.

Epidemiology

Various studies have documented a significant increase in incidence rates (the number of new cases in the population over a set time) in 15- to 19-year-old females in recent years. It remains unclear if this increase signifies an earlier age of illness onset or more rapid recognition and intervention. The point prevalence estimate of DSM-5-TR diagnoses of anorexia nervosa is between 0.6% and 0.8%. The lifetime prevalence rates of anorexia nervosa have been reported to be up to 4% among females and 0.3% among males.

Although epidemiologic studies indicate that it may occur as many as 10 times more frequently in females, anorexia nervosa does affect males. Research suggests that anorexia nervosa, which occurs much more commonly in females, occurs in men and boys more frequently than previously believed. It may go unrecognized in men for a variety of reasons. Males may be reluctant to seek treatment out of shame, and clinicians may be less likely to recognize the syndrome in male versus female patients. Anorexia nervosa is a world-wide disorder and impacts individuals of all racial and socioeconomic backgrounds.

Etiology

Genetic and Biologic Factors. A specific gene in anorexia nervosa has not yet been identified; however, several lines of evidence suggest that genetic vulnerability plays an important role in the development of the illness. Family studies have provided useful information about genetic susceptibility, demonstrating that individuals with a family history of anorexia nervosa are much more likely than those with no family history to receive a diagnosis during their lifetime. The risk of developing the illness is up to 11 times greater in individuals with a first-degree relative who has experienced the illness. A relative with a history of a different eating disorder also increases this risk. Twin studies have demonstrated that concordance rates of anorexia nervosa are substantially higher in monozygotic twins compared to dizygotic twins, suggesting that something more than the family environment is at play in increasing the odds of illness development. Studies of the serotonin transporter gene provide some evidence that this gene may interact with environmental influences to play a role in the development of anorexia nervosa. Once anorexia nervosa emerges, both the biologic and psychological changes to the body that occur in the starvation state, including depression and obsessionality, may contribute to maintaining the disorder.

Developmental Factors. Anorexia nervosa typically develops during adolescence, suggesting that developmental factors increase the risk for the emergence of this disorder. Adolescence represents a time of increased biologic, psychological, and social maturation. The experience of going through puberty and experiencing changes to body shape or weight may serve as a major stressor for some, triggering or worsening body dissatisfaction and low self-esteem. In addition, major social and psychological transitions which occur throughout adolescence, including identity and role formation, increasing independence from parents, and the initiation of romantic relationships, may result in extreme stress for some adolescents. These developmental stressors may work to catalyze the eating disorder.

Psychological Factors. Several psychological factors appear to confer added risk for developing anorexia nervosa. Certain personality traits, including high levels of perfectionism, self-discipline, harm avoidance, and self-criticism, are common in adolescents with the disorder. Individuals with the restricting subtype, in particular, exhibit low impulsivity and are much more likely to delay rewards than individuals without the illness. Cognitive inflexibility is usually prominent, as well. In a subset of individuals, mood and anxiety disorders or symptoms precede the development of anorexia nervosa. Obsessive-compulsive disorder (OCD) and obsessive-compulsive personality traits also appear to serve as vulnerability factors.

Environmental and Social Factors. Environmental and social factors, experienced in the family or school setting to cultural ideals, may play a role in the development of anorexia nervosa. The influence of family functioning style as a potential predisposing factor remains controversial. No specific family functioning style appears to be either a necessary or sufficient requirement for developing an eating disorder. As in most psychiatric disorders, various family dysfunctional styles appear to act as nonspecific vulnerability factors and hamper recovery.

Activities that emphasize weight may increase the probability of developing anorexia nervosa or another eating disorder during adolescence. Ballet, gymnastics, modeling, and weight-restricted sports like wrestling or light-weight rowing may lead to preoccupation with body form and unhealthy attempts to control weight. As many of these activities likely select for individuals who are higher in perfectionism, another risk factor for anorexia nervosa, they may be even more likely to contribute to illness onset.

Concerns that social media plays a role in the development of anorexia nervosa may be true for vulnerable adolescents. The cultural ideal of thinness, which is certainly perpetuated by all kinds of media, may fuel the overvaluation of shape and weight that marks both anorexia nervosa and bulimia nervosa in adolescents. Nonetheless, classic anorexia nervosa remains rare, and research indicates that neither social media nor other media exposure alone is likely to cause an eating disorder.

BULIMIA NERVOSA

Adolescents with bulimia nervosa have episodes of binge eating combined with compensatory ways of preventing weight gain. Bulimia nervosa, according to an epidemiologic report, has a peak incidence between 15 and 19 years of age. Bulimia nervosa has been reported to have a lifetime prevalence rate of about 3% in females and about 1% in males. A typical binge may continue until physical discomfort, such as abdominal pain or nausea, terminates it. Adolescents often have feelings of guilt, depression, or self-disgust after an episode of binge eating. Unlike adolescents with anorexia nervosa, those with bulimia nervosa typically maintain average body weight.

For some adolescents, bulimia nervosa may represent a rebound reaction to an attempt to become very thin but failing to sustain prolonged semi starvation or severe hunger. Eating binges may represent "breakthrough eating" episodes of giving in to hunger pangs generated by efforts to limit eating to maintain a socially desirable level of thinness. For some adolescents, binge eating is a means of self-soothing during times of emotional distress. In all of the above situations, eating binges lead to a sense of guilt, shame, and panic as individuals feel that their eating behaviors are more and more out of control. The undesired but irresistible binges lead to subsequent attempts to prevent the feared weight gain by a variety of compensatory behaviors, such as purging or excessive exercise.

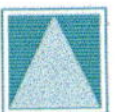

Table 9-6.
Comparative Diagnostic Criteria for Bulimia Nervosa

	DSM-5-TR	ICD-10	ICD-11
Diagnostic name	Bulimia Nervosa	Bulimia Nervosa	Bulimia Nervosa
Duration	Occurs ≥1/wk for 3 mo		Usually ≥1/wk for 1 mo

Symptoms	Repeated binge-eating episodes
	• Occurring within 2-hr period
	• Loss of control during the episode
	• Compensatory behaviors to prevent weight gain, such as
	  • Purging
	  • Laxatives
	  • Diuretics, other substances
	  • Excessive exercise
	  • Fasting
	• Self-evaluation based on weight and shape
		Binging
		Preoccupation with weight control
		Preoccupation with body shape and weight
		Associated physiologic disturbances due to repeated vomiting
		Specific compensatory behaviors:
		• Vomiting
		• Use of purgatives
			Frequent episodes of binge eating
			Compensatory behaviors to prevent weight gain, most commonly purging
			Excess preoccupation with body weight or shape

Required number of symptoms	All	Not specified	
Psychosocial consequences			Distress or functional impairment
Exclusions	Does not occur only during episodes of anorexia nervosa		Anorexia nervosa
Course specifiers	Partial remission: Full symptoms no longer met for a sustained time Full remission: No symptoms for a sustained period		
Severity specifiers	Severity is measured by the average number of compensatory behaviors in a week's time Mild: 1–3 Moderate: 4–7 Severe: 8–13 Extreme: 14+		

Diagnosis and Clinical Features

Adolescents with bulimia nervosa have binge episodes with compensatory behaviors. Like adolescents with anorexia nervosa, they fear becoming fat; however, they are not severely thin. The comparative diagnostic criteria for bulimia nervosa in DSM-5-TR, ICD-10, and ICD-11 are shown in Table 9-6.

When making a diagnosis of bulimia nervosa, clinicians should explore the possibility that the adolescent has experienced a brief or prolonged prior bout of anorexia nervosa, which is present in approximately half of those with bulimia nervosa. In adolescents with bulimia nervosa, approximately 40% report purging by vomiting, use of laxatives, or diuretics, while the others use excessive exercise or fasting to control their weight. According to DMS-5-TR, in order to meet diagnostic criteria for bulimia nervosa, binge eating with inappropriate compensatory behaviors must occur on average at least once per week for at least 3 months.

Vomiting is frequent and is often induced by sticking a finger down the throat. Some patients can vomit at will. Vomiting decreases abdominal pain and the feeling of being bloated and allows patients to continue eating without fear of gaining weight. The acid content of vomitus can damage tooth enamel, a not uncommon finding in patients with the disorder. Depression, sometimes called postbinge anguish, often follows an episode of binge eating. During binges, patients eat a variety of foods, often food that is sweet, high in calories, and generally soft or smooth textured, such as peanut butter, or cakes and pastry. Some patients prefer bulky foods without regard to taste. The food is eaten secretly and rapidly and is sometimes not even chewed.

Most patients with bulimia nervosa are within their normal weight range, but some may be underweight or overweight.

Sophia was a 17-year-old teen who was admitted to an adolescent eating disorders inpatient program after her parents found out that she was failing in school and absent from classes due to increasingly frequent episodes of binging during the school day. Sophia had always been an outgoing, gregarious girl who was considered a "people person" by her family, teachers, and peers. Sophia's parents noticed a change in her over the past 3 months. She had become more isolated, often skipped family meals, and seemed sad and listless in the evenings. Sophia was a junior in high school and she had previously been an active participant in school, both socially and academically. She had stopped talking to her friends in the evenings and preferred to be alone in her room. Sophia had always felt that she was too "chunky" and often tried to diet by skipping meals during the day, and she would tend to eat too much "junk food" in the evening. When she felt she had eaten too much, Sophia would induce vomiting by sticking her finger down her throat. Sophia had been able to maintain a normal body weight and many active friendships during high school until now. Sophia's eating pattern changed over the past few months. She would quietly leave school after a few periods in the morning and secretly purchase large amounts of food, such as a jar of peanut butter, a large bag of potato chips, and a bag of chocolate chip cookies. Sophia began to hide in the alleys near her school and binge on the foods she had purchased for about an hour. Sophia felt that she couldn't control her binging behavior, although she felt shame and self-loathing after she finished. One the binge was over, Sophia would feel uncomfortable mentally and physically and knew that she had to make herself vomit. Lately, Sophia's daytime binge eating occurred daily and seemed to be taking over her life. Sophia realized that she was failing in school due to her binges and felt powerless to control them. Sophia also used laxatives daily since she feared that she would gain weight and that vomiting was not enough. Sophia had always been active and ran for at least an hour a day. Sophia's goal was to lose weight, but instead she feared that her binges would surely cause weight gain. Although Sophia went to great lengths to hide her binging and purging, she was so depressed and disgusted with herself, she felt some relief when she disclosed her binging to her parents and accepted admission to an eating disorder program. Sophia had gotten to the point where she did not even have to stick her finger down her throat to induce vomiting, and she sometime vomited small amounts when she was not trying to vomit. On examination, she was still at normal weight with a BMI of 23. Sophia's dentition showed signs of enamel erosion, and her cheeks seemed slightly puffy. There were superficial scratches on her wrist from when she cut herself several weeks ago in despair. Sophia had normal electrolytes on laboratory evaluation.

During her stay in the adolescent eating disorders program, Sophia had nutritional counseling and ate regularly scheduled meals, during and after which she had to be observed for 30 minutes. After meals, she could use the bathroom but was instructed not to flush the toilet. On her 3rd day in the program, a staff member found a small plastic bag of partially digested food in a trash can in the hospital courtyard where she was allowed to jog for a period of 30 minutes after meals. After this incident, her treatment plan was modified so that staff would observe her for an hour after meals. Sophia's courtyard jogging was restricted for the next period, as well. One evening, a staff member observed her doing calisthenics in her room in the middle of the night. Sophia's treatment consisted of a behavioral meal plan, therapeutic sessions with her parents, and individual therapy sessions which focused on her difficulties with self-esteem and interpersonal interactions. Sophia reported that she still had strong urges to binge, and that she had persistent depressive symptoms without suicidal thoughts. Sophia's inpatient psychiatrist prescribed fluoxetine 20 mg/ day, and gradually titrated it up to 40 mg/day. Sophia reported after several weeks that both her depressive symptoms and her urges to binge had decreased moderately. Sophia's attempts at purging also significantly diminished. After 6 weeks in the inpatient unit, Sophia was considered appropriate to step down to the intensive outpatient program and continue her meal management and therapy as an outpatient. Sophia continued to struggle with some urges to binge and purge but was able to control her eating and was able to return to school successfully.

Pathology and Laboratory Examination. Bulimia nervosa can result in electrolyte abnormalities and various degrees of starvation, although it may not be as apparent as in low-weight patients with anorexia nervosa. Thus, even normal-weight patients with bulimia nervosa should have laboratory studies of electrolytes and metabolism. In general, thyroid function remains intact in bulimia nervosa, but patients may show no suppression on a dexamethasone-suppression test. Dehydration and electrolyte disturbances are likely to occur in patients with bulimia nervosa who purge regularly. These patients commonly exhibit hypomagnesemia and hyperamylasemia. Although not a core diagnostic feature, many patients with bulimia nervosa have menstrual disturbances. Hypotension and bradycardia occur in some patients.

Differential Diagnosis

A diagnosis of bulimia nervosa is not made if the binge-eating and purging behaviors occur exclusively during episodes of anorexia nervosa. In such cases, the diagnosis is anorexia nervosa, binge eating–purging type. In addition, bulimia nervosa should be distinguished from binge-eating disorder, which typically includes binge-eating behaviors but no compensatory or purging behaviors.

Some patients with bulimia nervosa have multiple comorbid impulsive behaviors, including substance abuse, and lack of ability to control themselves in such diverse areas as money management (resulting in impulse buying and compulsive shopping) and sexual relationships (often resulting in a short, passionate attachment and promiscuity). They may exhibit self-mutilation, chaotic emotions, and chaotic sleeping patterns. They may exhibit traits of or the full diagnosis of bipolar II disorder. When bulimia nervosa co-occurs with bipolar II disorder, both disorders are diagnosed.

Comorbidity

Bulimia nervosa occurs in individuals with high rates of mood disorders and impulse control disorders. Bulimia nervosa also co-occurs with substance use disorders, particularly alcohol. Patients with bulimia nervosa also have increased rates of anxiety disorders, bipolar I and II disorders, dissociative disorders, and histories of sexual abuse. Individuals with bulimia nervosa who purge may be at risk for certain medical complications, such as hypokalemia from vomiting or laxative abuse and hypochloremic alkalosis. Those who vomit repeatedly are at risk for gastric and esophageal tears, although these complications are rare.

Lists comorbid psychiatric conditions associated with anorexia nervosa and bulimia nervosa. The lifetime rate of depression in adolescents and adults with anorexia nervosa is about 50%, and the lifetime rate of social phobia (social anxiety disorder) is more than 20%. Obsessive-compulsive features, both related to and unrelated to food, are often present in anorexia nervosa. When obsessions and compulsions are severe and not related to food, body shape, and weight, a concurrent diagnosis of obsessive-compulsive disorder may be made.

Course and Prognosis

Bulimia nervosa is characterized by higher rates of partial and full recovery compared with anorexia nervosa. Those receiving treatment fare much better than those who are untreated. Untreated patients tend to remain chronic or may show small, but generally unimpressive, degrees of improvement with time. Research has yet to identify any clear predictors of outcome in bulimia nervosa. Studies have examined a variety of potential prognostic factors, including duration of illness, age of onset, illness severity, comorbid diagnoses, and personality characteristics, with mixed results. In individuals who receive treatment for bulimia nervosa, studies have found that rapid symptom reduction predicts better treatment outcomes.

Treatment Approach

Most patients with uncomplicated bulimia nervosa do not require hospitalization. In general, patients with bulimia nervosa are not as secretive about their symptoms as patients with anorexia nervosa. Therefore, outpatient treatment is usually not difficult, but psychotherapy is frequently stormy and prolonged. In some cases—when eating binges are out of control, outpatient treatment does not work, or a patient exhibits such additional psychiatric symptoms as suicidality and substance abuse—hospitalization may become necessary. Also, electrolyte and metabolic disturbances resulting from severe purging may necessitate hospitalization.

Psychotherapy

COGNITIVE-BEHAVIORAL THERAPY. CBT should be considered the benchmark, first-line treatment for bulimia nervosa. The data supporting the efficacy of CBT are based on strict adherence to rigorously implemented, highly detailed, manual-guided treatments that include about 18 to 20 sessions over 5 to 6 months. CBT implements several cognitive and behavioral procedures to (1) interrupt the self-maintaining behavioral cycle of binging and dieting and (2) alter the individual's dysfunctional cognitions, specifically beliefs about food, weight, body image, and overall self-concept.

OTHER MODALITIES. Given its effectiveness in anorexia nervosa, clinicians have also used family-based treatment (FBT) for bulimia nervosa in adolescents. In addition, controlled trials have shown that a variety of novel ways of administering and facilitating CBT are effective for bulimia nervosa. These include "stepped-care" programs and internet-based platforms, computer-facilitated programs, email-enhanced programs, and administration of CBT via telemedicine to remote areas. Finally, emerging evidence suggests that dialectical behavior therapy may be effective.

Pharmacotherapy. Antidepressant medications help treat bulimia nervosa, particularly the SSRI fluoxetine. Fluoxetine can reduce binge eating and purging, independent of the presence of a mood disorder. Dosages of fluoxetine that are effective in decreasing binge eating, however, may be higher (60 to 80 mg a day) than those used for depressive disorders. Other antidepressants that may be helpful include other SSRIs (although concerns about prolonged QT intervals with higher doses limit the utility of citalopram in this population). Tricyclic antidepressants (TCAs; particularly amitriptyline and desipramine), trazodone, and monoamine oxidase inhibitors (MAOIs) are not typically recommended in this population. Bupropion is relatively contraindicated due to an increased risk of seizure in this population. In general, most of the antidepressants other than fluoxetine have been effective at dosages usually given in the treatment of depressive disorders. Medication is helpful in patients with comorbid depressive disorders and in diminishing urges to binge in bulimia nervosa. Topiramate may have some efficacy in reducing binge episodes in bulimia nervosa, as may lisdexamfetamine, especially for adolescents with comorbid ADHD. Evidence indicates that CBT and medications (particularly fluoxetine) are the most effective combination.

Epidemiology

As with anorexia nervosa, rates of bulimia nervosa have increased with changes to diagnostic criteria. However, before the recent modifications appearing in DSM-5 and

DSM-5-TR, studies suggested that the incidence of the illness had decreased in recent years. Using DSM-5-TR criteria, the lifetime prevalence of bulimia nervosa in women is approximately 3%, and point prevalence is close to 0.6%. The average age of onset also seems to have decreased, although this finding may be an artifact of earlier detection. Like anorexia nervosa, the disorder is more common in women than in men, although approximately 1% of males suffer from this disorder during their lifetime.

Etiology

Genetic and Biologic Factors. As in anorexia nervosa, genetics likely play a role in the development of bulimia nervosa, as evidenced by twin and family studies. Individuals with a family history of bulimia nervosa, mood disorder, substance use disorder, or obesity are at higher risk for developing the syndrome.

Neurobiologic disturbances are also present in individuals with bulimia nervosa and may increase the probability of binge eating. In particular, individuals with the disorder tend to display delayed gastric emptying, increased stomach capacity, and reduced secretion of cholecystokinin (CCK), a peptide hormone released by the small intestine that helps to signal satiety during food consumption. Together, disruptions to these neurobiologic processes may put individuals at elevated risk for overeating.

Developmental Factors. The same psychological and social stressors of puberty and adolescence that put individuals at risk for anorexia nervosa also confer risk for bulimia nervosa. Developmental transition periods involving increasing social demands and individuation are typical contributing factors in the emergence of both anorexia nervosa and bulimia nervosa.

Psychological Factors. Unlike individuals with anorexia nervosa, those with bulimia nervosa tend to exhibit high levels of novelty seeking and impulsivity. They also tend to display elevated levels of harm-avoidance, negative emotionality, and stress reactivity. Afflicted individuals are more likely than others to experience a comorbid substance use disorder and engage in self-harm, leading to speculation that a subset of individuals with bulimia nervosa may have a propensity toward impulsivity across a range of problematic behaviors. Mood and anxiety disturbances appear to serve as risk factors for bulimia nervosa, as well.

Just as the starvation state works to maintain anorexia nervosa, the cycle of binge eating and purging often becomes self-sustaining in bulimia nervosa. Individuals with bulimia nervosa tend to restrict their food intake outside of binge episodes, which puts them at increased risk for episodes of overeating. In turn, after experiencing a binge episode and the resulting compensatory behaviors, individuals often renew their commitment to restrictive eating in an attempt to avoid future overeating episodes. Thus, this cycle tends to become self-perpetuating and works to maintain the disorder.

Environmental and Social Factors. Individuals with bulimia nervosa are likely affected by similar environmental and social stressors as those with anorexia nervosa; however, their symptoms may or may not overlap.

Further Readings

Agras WS, Bohon C. Cognitive behavioral therapy for the eating disorders. *Annu Rev Clin Psychol*. 2021;17:417–438.

Baudinet J, Eisler I, Dawson L, Simic M, Schmidt U. Multi-family therapy for eating disorders: a systematic scoping review of the quantitative and qualitative findings. *Int J Eat Disord*. 2021;54(12):2095–2120.

Bills E, Greene D, Stackpole R, Egan SJ. Perfectionism and eating disorders in children and adolescents: a systematic review and meta-analysis. *Appetite*. 2023;187:106586.

Brennan C, Illingworth S, Cini E, Bhakta D. Medical instability in typical and atypical adolescent anorexia nervosa: a systematic review and meta-analysis. *J Eat Disord*. 2023;11(1):58.

Cass K, McGuire C, Bjork I, Sobotka N, Walsh K, Mehler PS. Medical complications of anorexia nervosa. *Psychosomatics*. 2020;61(6):625–631.

Castillo M, Weiselberg E. Bulimia nervosa/purging disorder. *Curr Probl Pediatr Adolesc Health Care*. 2017;47(4):85–94.

Charrat JP, Massoubre C, Germain N, Gay A, Galusca B. Systematic review of prospective studies assessing risk factors to predict anorexia nervosa onset. *J Eat Disord*. 2023;11(1):163.

Couturier J, Isserlin L, Norris M, et al. Canadian practice guidelines for the treatment of children and adolescents with eating disorders. *J Eat Disord*. 2020;8:4.

Crow SJ. Pharmacologic treatment of eating disorders. *Psychiatr Clin N Am*. 2019;42(2):253–262.

Cucinotta U, Romano C, Dipasquale V. A systematic review to manage avoidant/restrictive food intake disorders in pediatric gastroenterological practice. *Healthcare (Basel)*. 2023;11(16):2245.

Di Cara M, Rizzo C, Corallo F, et al. Avoidant restrictive food intake disorder: a narrative review of types and characteristics of therapeutic interventions. *Children (Basel)*. 2023;10(8):1297.

Frank GKW, Shott ME, DeGuzman MC. The neurobiology of eating disorders. *Child Adolesc Psychiatr Clin N Am*. 2019;28(4):629–640.

Friars D, Walsh O, McNicholas F. Assessment and management of cardiovascular complications in eating disorders. *J Eat Disord*. 2023;11(1):13.

Gorrell S, Loeb KL, Le Grange D. Family-based treatment of eating disorders: a narrative review. *Psychiatr Clin North Am*. 2019;42(2):193–204.

Guerdjikova AI, Mori N, Casuto LS, McElroy SL. Update on binge eating disorder. *Med Clin N Am*. 2019;103(4):669–680.

Hagan KE, Walsh BT. State of the art: the therapeutic approaches to bulimia nervosa. *Clin Ther*. 2021;43(1):40–49.

Kishi T, Kafantaris V, Sunday S, Sheridan EM, Correll CU. Are antipsychotics effective for the treatment of anorexia nervosa? Results from a systematic review and meta-analysis. *J Clin Psychiatry*. 2012;73(6):e757–e766.

Milano W, De Rosa M, Milano L, Capasso A. Night eating syndrome: an overview. *J Pharm Pharmacol*. 2012;64(1):2–10.

Monteleone AM, Pellegrino F, Croatto G, et al. Treatment of eating disorders: a systematic meta-review of meta-analyses and network meta-analyses. *Neurosci Biobehav Rev*. 2022;142:104857.

Muratore AF, Attia E. Psychopharmacologic management of eating disorders. *Curr Psychiatry Rep*. 2022;24(7):345–351.

Perez M, Warren CS. The relationship between quality of life, binge-eating disorder, and obesity status in an ethnically diverse sample. *Obesity (Silver Spring)*. 2012;20(4):879–885.

Poulsen S, Lunn S, Daniel SIF, et al. A randomized controlled trial of psychoanalytic psychotherapy or cognitive-behavioral therapy for bulimia nervosa. *Am J Psychiatry*. 2014;171(1):109–116.

Rajindrajith S, Devanarayana NM, Perera BJC. Rumination syndrome in children and adolescents: a school survey assessing prevalence and symptomatology. *BMC Gastroenterol*. 2012;12:163–169.

Reinecke RD. Family-based treatment of eating disorders in adolescents: current insights. *Adolesc Health Med Ther*. 2017;8:69–79.

Tack J, Blondeau K, Boecxstaens V, Rommel N. Review article: the pathophysiology, differential diagnosis and management of rumination syndrome. *Ailment Pharmacol Ther*. 2011;33(7):782–788.

Uniacke B, Walsh BT. Eating disorders. *Ann Intern Med*. 2022;175(8): ITC113–ITC128.

van Eeden AE, van Hoeken D, Hoek HW. Incidence, prevalence and mortality of anorexia nervosa and bulimia nervosa. *Curr Opin Psychiatry*. 2021;34(6):515–524.

Vander Wal JS. Night eating syndrome: a critical review of the literature. *Clin Psychol Rev*. 2012;32(1):49–59.

Volpe U, Tortorella A, Manchia M, Monteleone AM, Albert U, Monteleone P. Eating disorders: what age at onset? *Psychiatry Res*. 2016;238:225–227.

Williams DE, McAdam D. Assessment, behavioral treatment, and prevention of pica: clinical guidelines and recommendations for practitioners. *Res Develop Disab*. 2012;33(6):2050–2057.

Yamamiya Y, Desjardins CD, Stice E. Sequencing of symptom emergence in anorexia nervosa, bulimia nervosa, binge eating disorder, and purging disorder in adolescent girls and relations of prodromal symptoms to future onset of these eating disorders. *Psychol Med*. 2023;53(10):4657–4665.

Zipfel S, Wild B, Groß G, et al; ANTOP study group. Focal psychodynamic therapy, cognitive behaviour therapy, and optimised treatment as usual in outpatients with anorexia nervosa (ANTOP study): randomised controlled trial. *Lancet*. 2014;383(9912):127–137.

10

Trauma- and Stressor-Related Disorders in Children

This section includes disorders in which a traumatic or significantly stressful event is a necessary diagnostic criterion, according to the DSM-5-TR. Included here are reactive attachment disorder, disinhibited social engagement disorder, and posttraumatic stress disorder (PTSD).

Both reactive attachment disorder and disinhibited social engagement disorder are comprised of inappropriate attachment behavior; however, in DSM-5-TR, reactive attachment disorder is characterized by withdrawn/inhibited behaviors, and disinhibited social engagement disorder is characterized by disinhibited attachment behaviors.

POSTTRAUMATIC STRESS DISORDER OF INFANCY, CHILDHOOD, AND ADOLESCENCE

PTSD, formerly grouped with anxiety disorders, is now categorized under Trauma- and Stressor-Related Disorders in DSM-5-TR. along with other disorders caused by trauma or stress.

In the United States, the rates of children and adolescents exposed to violence and traumatic events are extremely high. In a nationally representative sample of children and adolescents, exposure to at least one traumatic event was up to 60%, with a lifetime rate ranging from 80% to 90%. Traumatic events can include physical or sexual abuse, domestic violence, motor vehicle accidents, severe medical illnesses, or natural or human-created disasters. A significant number of children and adolescents who experience traumatic events will develop PTSD. In children younger than the age of 6 years, spontaneous and intrusive memories may be expressed in their play or occur in frightening dreams, even when it may be challenging to connect the dreams or intrusive thoughts to a traumatic event. The child may also display inexplicable agitation, fear, or disorganization.

Diagnosis and Clinical Features

PTSD requires an exposure to a traumatic event consisting of either direct personal experience or witnessing an event involving the threat of death, serious injury, or severe harm. The most common traumatic exposures for children and adolescents include physical or sexual abuse, emotional abuse, exposure to violence, and severe neglect. Additional adverse events for children include school or community violence. Less common, albeit equally traumatic, are being kidnapped; exposure to terrorist attacks; motor vehicle or household accidents. In addition, natural or man-made disasters, such as floods, hurricanes, tornadoes, fires, explosions, or airplane crashes are traumatic events. A child with PTSD experiences either intrusive memories of the event, recurrent frightening dreams, dissociative reactions including flashbacks in which the child feels as if the traumatic event is recurring, or intense psychological distress when exposed to reminders of the trauma. Table 10-1 compares the diagnostic criteria for PTSD.

To meet the DSM-5-TR criteria for PTSD in children or adolescents, one or more symptoms in the following categories are present following exposure to the adverse event:

- Intrusive thoughts: One or more symptom of intrusive and distressing thoughts
- Avoidance: One or more symptom of persistent avoidance of stimuli associated with the traumatic event
- Negative mood and thoughts: Two symptoms of negative changes in thoughts and mood associated with the traumatic event
- Changes in arousal: Marked changes in arousal and reactivity as evidenced by at least two symptoms

Symptoms of PTSD include *reexperiencing* traumatic events in at least one of the following ways. Children may have intrusive thoughts, memories, or images that spontaneously recur, or body sensations that remind them of the event. In very young children, it is common to observe play that includes elements of the traumatic event, or inappropriate behaviors (e.g., sexual behaviors). Children may experience periods during which they either act or feel as though the event is taking place presently; this is a dissociative event usually described by adults as a "flashback."

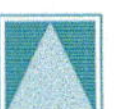

Table 10-1.
Comparison of Diagnostic Criteria for Posttraumatic Stress Disorder

	DSM-5-TR	ICD-10	ICD-11
Diagnostic name	Posttraumatic Stress Disorder	Posttraumatic Stress Disorder	Posttraumatic Stress Disorder
Duration	≥1 mo	Symptoms arise in weeks to months following the traumatic event	
Symptoms	History of exposure to (directly experiencing, repeated exposure, witnessing in person, learning of occurrence in close acquaintance) actual threatened death, severe injury, or sexual trauma Intrusive symptoms • Involuntary intrusive memories • In children <6 yr may see a reenactment of the event through play • Recurrent nightmares/dreams of the event • In children <6 yr, frightening dreams without identifiable content may be present • Dissociative responses or reliving of prior experience (i.e., flashbacks) • Psychological distress related to exposure to stimuli that are reminders of prior trauma • Presence of physiologic response to stimuli that are reminders of prior trauma • Avoidance of stimuli associated with prior experience of trauma • Avoidance of memories related to trauma • Avoidance of external reminders of the trauma • Negative mood or cognitions related to trauma • Impairment in memories related to the event • Negative perceptions of self and others • Cognitive distortions related to the event • Excessive guilt, anger, or fear • Diminished interest and social withdrawal • Subjective detachment from others • Difficulty experiencing positive feelings in response to previously pleasurable stimuli • Altered level of arousal • Irritability and/or anger • Risk taking • Hypervigilance • Increased startle response • Difficulties with concentration • Sleep disturbances	Symptoms arise as a delayed or prolonged response to a single or recurrent stressful experience that is life-threatening or catastrophic in severity The traumatic event would cause distress in most individuals Symptoms may include • Flashbacks • Dreams/nightmares • Emotional blunting and subjective numbness • Social withdrawal/ detachment • Anhedonia • Avoidance • Hyperarousal/ hypervigilance • Sleep disturbance May or may not be associated with co-occurring anxiety and/or depression	Exposure to an extremely threatening or horrifying event. Following the event develops symptoms in all three of the following categories: • Reexperiencing the trauma • Avoiding reminders of the trauma • Persistent perception of heightened threat (e.g., hypervigilance)
Required number of symptoms	In addition to a history of exposure to trauma, they must have • ≥1 symptom of intrusion • ≥1 symptom of avoidance • ≥2 symptoms of negative mood/cognition • ≥2 symptoms of arousal alterations	Any of the above	
Psychosocial consequences	Marked distress and impairment in functioning		Impairment in functioning
Exclusions	Exposure through media, electronics, movies, or photo Related to substance use Related to another medical condition		Acute stress reaction Complex posttraumatic stress disorder

(continued)

Table 10-1.
Comparison of Diagnostic Criteria for Posttraumatic Stress Disorder (Continued)

	DSM-5-TR	ICD-10	ICD-11
Symptoms specifiers	**With dissociative symptoms:** • **Depersonalization:** perception of feeling outside one's own body • **Derealization:** perception of the surrounding environment being unreal or distorted		
Course specifiers	With delayed expression • All diagnostic criteria are not met until ≥6 mo after an initial traumatic event		

Another critical symptom cluster of PTSD is *avoidance,* in which children may make active physical efforts to avoid the places, people, or situations that would present traumatic reminders of the event. The third cluster of diagnostic criteria for PTSD is *negative alterations in cognition and mood* following the trauma. In children 6 years or younger, according to DSM-5-TR, negative alterations in cognition may take the form of socially withdrawn behavior, reduction of expressing positive emotions, diminished interest in play, and feelings of shame, fear, and confusion. In children older than 6 years of age, these may take the form of an inability to remember parts of a traumatic event, that is, psychological amnesia or persistent negative feelings about oneself, including horror, anger, guilt, or shame. After a traumatic event, children may experience a sense of detachment from their usual play activities ("psychological numbing") or a diminished capacity to feel emotions. Older adolescents may express a fear that they expect to die young (sense of foreshortened future).

The final category of symptoms involves *changes in arousal* that were not present before the traumatic exposure, such as difficulty falling asleep or staying asleep, hypervigilance regarding safety, and increased checking that doors are locked or exaggerated startle reaction. In some children, hyperarousal can present as a generalized inability to relax with increased irritability, outbursts, and impaired ability to concentrate.

To meet the diagnostic criteria for PTSD, according to the DSM-5-TR, the symptoms must be present for more than 1 month and cause distress and impairment in critical functional areas of life. When the diagnostic symptoms of PTSD are met following the traumatic event, persist for at least 3 days, but resolve within 1 month, a diagnosis of Acute Stress Disorder is made. In some cases, the PTSD symptoms increase over time, and it is not until more than 6 months have elapsed after the exposure to the trauma that the whole syndrome emerges; in that case, the diagnosis is PTSD, delayed onset.

It is not uncommon for children and adolescents with PTSD to experience feelings of guilt, mainly if they have survived the trauma and others in the situation did not. They may blame themselves for the demise of the others and may go on to develop a comorbid depressive episode. Childhood PTSD is also associated with increased rates of other anxiety disorders, depressive episodes, substance use disorders, and attentional difficulties. DSM-5-TR includes a specifier *With dissociative symptoms,* which can present as either *Depersonalization,* in which there are recurrent experiences of feeling detached, as if outside of one's own body, or *Derealization,* in which the world feels unreal, dreamlike, and distant. A final specifier, *With delayed expression,* indicates that the full diagnostic criteria were not met until 6 months after the traumatic event, although some symptoms may present earlier.

Pathology and Laboratory Examination. Although reports indicate some alterations in both neurophysiologic and neuroimaging studies of children and adolescents with PTSD, no current laboratory tests can help in making this diagnosis.

Differential Diagnosis

Several overlapping symptoms exist between childhood PTSD and presentations of childhood anxiety disorders, such as separation anxiety disorder, obsessive-compulsive disorder (OCD), or social anxiety disorder, in which recurrent intrusive thoughts or avoidant behaviors occur. Children with depressive disorders often exhibit withdrawal and a sense of isolation from peers as well as guilt about life events over which they have no control. Irritability, poor concentration, sleep disturbance, and decreased interest in usual activities occur in both PTSD and major depressive disorder.

Children who have lost a loved one in a traumatic event may go on to experience both PTSD and a major depressive disorder when bereavement persists beyond its expected course. Children with PTSD may also be confused with children who have disruptive behavior disorders because they often show poor concentration, inattention, and irritability. It is critical to elicit a history of traumatic exposure and evaluate the chronology of the trauma and the onset of the symptoms to make an accurate diagnosis of PTSD.

Lina was a 15-year-old high school sophomore who was outgoing, bubbly, and highly popular with her friends and her teachers. She was a good student and participated in many after school activities including drama club, and she was on the track team. Lina had many friends, but she had two best friends who she walked to and from school with because they all lived in the same apartment complex. Lina was walking with her two friends as usual, when suddenly a car ran a stop sign and hit one of them. The injured teen fell to the ground unconscious while the other two screamed and called 911. An ambulance came quickly and transported the injured teen to the hospital. The injured teen had sustained a concussion and was kept in the hospital overnight for observation but was otherwise not hurt. Lina and her friend stayed with their injured friend for the afternoon and evening, but later went to their respective homes. Lina kept replaying the accident over and over again in her mind and started to have thoughts that it was probably her fault because she was walking farthest from the street on the sidewalk, while her friend was closest to the street. Lina tried to sleep but was unable to stay asleep all night. After her friend was discharged from the hospital and returned to school, Lina worried constantly about her safety and didn't want to be separated from her all day. Lina felt that she had to watch over her friend so that another terrible accident wouldn't happen. Lina became withdrawn and no longer wanted to walk to school, and she convinced her older brother to drive her and her friends to and from school. Lina closed her eyes tight each time they passed the spot where the accident had taken place. Lina stopped participating in after school activities, because she felt she had to stay with her friend to watch over her. Lina became so distracted with fears of being separated with her friend and replaying the scene of the accident over and over that she was unable to do her homework and her grades began to fall. She found herself tearful multiple times per day without realizing why. Lina's parents and her friends noticed that she was no longer the outgoing, fun-loving teen she used to be, and she seemed to have turned most of her energy inward. She looked sad and seemed on edge all of the time. She jumped when someone approached her and began to spend more time alone. Lina's friends finally told her parents that Lina was not acting like herself and that she told them that she was always sad and anxious, worried constantly, and was internally distracted by intrusive thoughts of the accident. Lina's parents sought help for Lina, and she was diagnosed with PTSD. Lina began trauma-focused cognitive-behavioral therapy (CBT) and seemed to be benefitting from it.

Course and Prognosis

For some children and adolescents with milder forms of PTSD, symptoms may persist for 1 to 2 years, after which they diminish and attenuate. In more severe circumstances, however, PTSD syndromes persist for many years or decades in children and adolescents, with spontaneous remission in only a portion of them.

The prognosis of untreated PTSD has become an issue of growing concern for researchers and clinicians who have documented a variety of severe comorbidities and psychobiological abnormalities associated with PTSD. In one study, children and adolescents with severe PTSD were at risk for decreased intracranial volume, diminished corpus callosum area, and lower IQs compared to children without PTSD. Children and adolescents with histories of physical and sexual abuse have higher rates of depression and suicidality themselves and in their offspring as well. This risk highlights the importance of early recognition and treatment of PTSD that may significantly improve the long-term outcome among youth.

Treatment

Trauma-Focused Cognitive-Behavioral Therapy. Randomized clinical trials have provided evidence for the efficacy of trauma-focused cognitive-behavioral therapy (TF-CBT) in the treatment of PTSD in children and adolescents. This treatment is generally administered over 10 to 16 treatment sessions. The treatment includes nine components itemized in the acronym PRACTICE. TF-CBT entails the inclusion of gradual exposure to feared stimuli as a critical element. Such stimuli encompass places, people, sounds, and situations. The first component of TF-CBT is *Psychoeducation* regarding the nature of typical emotional and physiologic reactions to traumatic events and PTSD. Next, *Parenting Skills* involve sessions focused on guiding parents on providing praise, administering a time out, contingency reinforcement programs, and troubleshooting for specific symptoms in a given child. Component 3 is *Relaxation,* in which children learn to utilize muscle relaxation, focused breathing, affective modulation, thought-stopping, and other cognitive techniques to diminish feelings of helplessness and distress. Component 4 is *Affective Expression and Modulation,* geared to help children and their parents to identify their feelings, interrupt disturbing thoughts with positive imagery, and teach positive self-talk and social skills building. Component 5 is *Cognitive Coping and Processing,* which deals specifically with reviewing the Cognitive Triangle, in which the therapist and child explore the relationship between thoughts, feelings, and behaviors. The child learns to challenge unhelpful thoughts with practice. In Component 6, *Trauma Narrative,* the story of the traumatic event and its sequelae are developed over time by the child, with the therapist's support, using a depiction of words, art, or another creative form. Eventually, they share this with the parent. Component 7, *In Vivo Exposure and Mastery of Trauma Reminders,* is a session that reviews with the child how to deal with situations that are a reminder of the trauma and how to maintain control over distressing feelings associated with it. Component 8 is *Conjoint Child–Parent Sessions*; this component may involve several sessions in which the child and parent share their understanding of the process of the therapy and the gains that they have made. Finally, Component 10, *Enhancing Future Safety,* involves sessions that focus on the changes made in the family to ensure the safety of the child. These final sessions also promote healthy communication between the child and the parents.

A variant of TF-CBT for PTSD is called *eye movement desensitization and reprocessing* (EMDR), in which the therapist combines exposure and cognitive reprocessing interventions with directed eye movements. This technique is not as well accepted as the more extensive TF-CBT detailed above.

Cognitive-Behavioral Intervention for Trauma in Schools. Cognitive-behavioral intervention for trauma in schools (CBITS) is an intervention that administers treatment in the school setting for children who screen positive for PTSD and whose parents agree to treatment in school. It consists of 10 weekly group sessions, one to three individual imaginal exposure sessions, two to four optional sessions with parents, and one parent education session. Similar to TF-CBT, CBITS incorporates psychoeducation, relaxation training, cognitive coping skills, gradual exposure to traumatic memories through a narrative, in vivo exposure, and affect modulation, cognitive restructuring, and social problem-solving. In one randomized controlled trial (RCT), 86% of students in the CBITS group reported significantly decreased PTSD symptoms compared to the waitlist controls. Students who received CBITS also reported lower depression scores. Among parents whose children received CBITS treatment, 78% reported decreased psychosocial problems in their children. After CBITS treatment, the children sustained improvements in both the PTSD and depression symptoms at 6 months.

Structured Psychotherapy for Adolescents Responding to Chronic Stress. Structured psychotherapy for adolescents responding to chronic stress (SPARCS) consists of a group intervention, generally administered in 16 sessions, with a focus on the needs of adolescents between the ages of 12 and 19 years who have lived with chronic trauma and may also carry a diagnosis of PTSD. Investigators have tested SPARCS in a trial of multicultural teens and young adults with moderate or severe trauma exposure. Most of the participants were female and comprised multiple ethnic groups: 67% African American; 12% Latino; 21% Caucasian. SPARCS demonstrated efficacy in reducing traumatic stress symptoms, mainly in the largest group, the African American group. SPARCS utilizes cognitive-behavioral techniques and also incorporates many of the components of TF-CBT. Also, SPARCS includes mindfulness techniques and relaxation.

Trauma Affect Regulation: Guide for Education and Therapy. Trauma affect regulation: guide for education and therapy (TARGET), an affect regulation therapy, combines CBT components, such as cognitive processing, with affect modulation. We would usually consider this for adolescents between the ages of 13 and 19 who experience maltreatment or chronic traumatic exposure to such things as community violence or domestic violence. It usually requires 12 sessions which focus on past or current situations. As with SPARCS treatment, gradual exposure may occur in the context of recounting past trauma but is not a core component of the treatment. A randomized trial with 59 delinquent girls aged 13 to 17 years who met full or partial criteria for PTSD found that TARGET reduced anxiety, anger, depression, and PTSD cognitions. TARGET is a promising treatment for girls with histories of delinquency, especially to reduce anger and to enhance optimism and self-efficacy.

Psychopharmacological Treatment. Although there is data to suggest that pharmacologic agents such as selective serotonin reuptake inhibitor (SSRI) antidepressants may be effective to treat PTSD in adults, there is little evidence base for pharmacologic treatments for PTSD in children and adolescents. Clinicians have used several pharmacologic agents to treat symptoms in children and adolescents with PTSD, often focused on diminishing intrusive thoughts, hyperarousal, and avoidance, with some success and mixed results. Given the frequent comorbidity of depressive disorder, anxiety disorders, and behavioral problems associated with PTSD, psychopharmacological agents for these disorders and symptoms are often utilized.

Sertraline and paroxetine are approved by the FDA in the treatment of PTSD in adults; however, there is scant evidence to support their efficacy for the core symptoms of PTSD in youth. An RCT of TF-CBT plus sertraline compared to TF-CBT plus placebo in 24 children with PTSD found that both groups had a significant reduction in PTSD symptoms, with no significant difference between the groups. One multicenter placebo-controlled study of 131 children aged 6 to 17 years with PTSD evaluated sertraline over 10 weeks. Results showed sertraline to be a safe treatment; however, it was not effective when compared to placebo. An RCT using citalopram did not show the superiority of citalopram over placebo in the treatment of core PTSD symptoms. There is, however, evidence suggesting that the use of SSRIs in traumatized children with burns may be preventive regarding the development of PTSD. Published literature demonstrates that up to 50% of children with moderate to severe burns develop PTSD. Thus, preventive strategies are essential. A randomized controlled study of sertraline to prevent PTSD found that children who received sertraline, flexibly dosed between 25 and 150 mg/day, had a decrease in parent-reported symptoms of PTSD over 8 weeks compared to a placebo group. Among the child-reported symptoms, however, there was no significant difference between the two groups.

Psychiatrists sometimes use antiadrenergic agents to treat dysregulation of the noradrenergic system in adults and youth with PTSD. α_2-agonists such as clonidine and guanfacine, for example, have been used to decrease norepinephrine release, whereas centrally acting β-antagonists such as propranolol and α_1-antagonists such as prazosin are hypothesized to improve hyperarousal and intrusive thoughts through attenuation of norepinephrine postsynaptically. Although there are some data in adults with PTSD to support the use of these agents, there are mainly case reports for youths. There is a suggestion that guanfacine may reduce nightmares in children with PTSD and that clonidine may diminish symptoms of reenactment of traumatic events in children. One report of propranolol treatment in 11 pediatric patients, with a mean age of 8.5 years, who had PTSD from sexual or physical abuse and exhibited agitation and hyperarousal indicated some decrease in symptoms in 8 of the 11 children studied. Another open study of transdermal clonidine treatment of preschoolers with PTSD suggests that clonidine may be efficacious in this population in decreasing activation and hyperarousal. An additional open trial of oral clonidine with dosage ranges of 0.05 to 0.1 mg twice daily similarly suggests that this medication may provide some relief for the symptoms of hyperarousal, impulsivity, and agitation in young children with PTSD.

Second-generation antipsychotics such as risperidone, olanzapine, quetiapine, ziprasidone, and aripiprazole have been studied in adults with PTSD with mixed results. Risperidone and aripiprazole both have FDA approval for use in children and adolescents with aggression, severe behavioral dyscontrol, and severe psychiatric disorders; however, there are no controlled trials with children with PTSD. For example, there is one case series of three preschool-age children who exhibited symptoms of acute stress disorder and who had severe thermal burns and improved after being treated with risperidone.

In children and adolescents with PTSD, there is one open-label trial of carbamazepine and one trial of sodium valproate. In the carbamazepine trial, all 28 improved at blood levels of 10 to 11.5 μg/mL. In the sodium valproate trial, there was some improvement at higher doses of the drug. These agents have not been shown to be efficacious in the treatment of PTSD in youth.

Given that many children and adolescents with PTSD have comorbid depressive and anxiety disorders, we would recommend SSRIs as a first-line pharmacologic option for children with PTSD and those disorders.

Epidemiology

Epidemiologic studies of children 9 to 17 years of age have found 3-month prevalence rates of PTSD ranging from 0.5% to 4%. An epidemiologic survey of preschoolers aged 4 to 5 years found a rate of PTSD of 1.3%.

Children exposed chronically to trauma, such as child abuse, or traumas resulting in a broader disruption of entire communities, such as war, have the highest risk of developing PTSD. In addition to the staggering rate of the full-blown disorder of PTSD among youth, several studies indicate that most children exposed to severe or chronic trauma develop PTSD symptoms sufficiently severe to disrupt functioning, even in the absence of the full diagnosis.

Etiology

Biologic Factors. Risk factors in children for developing PTSD include preexisting anxiety disorders and depressive disorders. A prospective study found that, among children exposed to traumatic events, those with anxiety disorders and teacher ratings of externalizing behavior problems by the age of 6 years were at increased risk for PTSD. Furthermore, children with an IQ higher than 115 at age 6 years were at lower risk for developing PTSD. Also, among children exposed to trauma, those who developed PTSD were at higher risk of developing comorbid disorders such as depression. This comorbidity suggests that a genetic predisposition for anxiety disorders, as well as a family history indicating an increased risk of depressive disorders, may predispose a trauma-exposed child to develop PTSD. Children with PTSD exhibit increased excretion of adrenergic and dopaminergic metabolites, smaller intracranial volume and corpus callosum, memory deficits, and lower IQs compared with age-matched controls. Adults with PTSD have been found to have an overactive amygdala and decreased hippocampal volume. Whether the above findings are sequelae of PTSD or markers of vulnerability to the disorder remains a focus of investigation.

Psychological Factors. Although the exposure to trauma is the initial etiologic factor in the development of PTSD, the enduring symptoms typical of PTSD, such as avoidance of the place where the trauma occurred, can be conceptualized, in part, as the result of both classical and operant conditioning. Extreme physiologic responses may accompany the fear of a given traumatic event, such as an adolescent who was terrorized by an attack by a group of students near a school, who then develops an extreme adverse physiologic reaction each time they are near the school. This reaction is an example of classical conditioning in that a neutral cue (the school) has become paired with an intensely fearful past event. Operant conditioning occurs when a child learns to avoid traumatic reminders to prevent distressing feelings from arising. For example, if a child was in a motor vehicle accident, the child may then refuse to ride in cars altogether to prevent adverse physiologic reactions and fear from occurring.

Another mechanism in developing and maintaining symptoms of PTSD is through modeling, which is a form of learning. For example, when parents and children experience traumatic events, such as natural disasters, children may emulate parental responses, such as avoidance, withdrawal, or extreme expressions of fear, and "learn" to respond to their memories of the traumatic event in the same manner.

Social Factors. Family support and reactions to traumatic events in children may play a significant role in the development of PTSD in that adverse parental emotional reactions to a child's abuse may increase that child's risk of developing PTSD. Lack of parental support and psychopathology among parents—especially maternal depression—have been identified as risk factors in the development of PTSD after a child experiences a traumatic event.

REACTIVE ATTACHMENT DISORDER AND DISINHIBITED SOCIAL ENGAGEMENT DISORDER

Reactive attachment disorder and disinhibited social engagement disorder are clinical disorders characterized by aberrant social and attachment behaviors in a child that reflect grossly negligent parenting and maltreatment that disrupted the development of normal attachment behavior. A diagnosis of either reactive attachment disorder or disinhibited social engagement disorder rests on the presumption that the cause is caregiving deprivation. This fundamental relationship is the product of a young child's need for protection, nurturance, and comfort, and the interaction of the parents and child in fulfilling these needs.

Based on observations of a young child and parents during a brief separation and reunion, designated the "strange situation procedure" and pioneered by Mary Ainsworth and colleagues, researchers have designated a child's basic pattern of attachment to be characterized as secure, insecure, or disorganized. Children who exhibit secure attachment behavior experience their caregivers as emotionally available and appear to be more exploratory and well-adjusted than children who exhibit insecure or disorganized attachment behavior. Insecure attachment results from a young child's perception and experience of the primary caregiver not being consistently available. In contrast, disorganized attachment behavior in a child results from experiencing both the need for proximity to the caregiver and apprehension in approaching the caregiver. These early patterns of attachment influence a child's future capacities for affect regulation, self-soothing, and relationship building. According to the DSM-5-TR, reactive attachment disorder is characterized by a consistent pattern of emotionally withdrawn responses toward adult caregivers, limited positive affect, sadness, and minimal social responsiveness to others, and concomitant neglect, deprivation, and lack of appropriate nurturance from caregivers. Reactive attachment disorder is, presumably, due to grossly pathologic caregiving received by the child. The pattern of caregiver care may take the form of disregard for a child's emotional or physical needs or repeated changes of caregivers, as when a child is frequently relocated during foster care. The symptoms are not due to autism spectrum disorder, and the child must have a developmental age of at least 9 months.

Pathologic caretaking can result in two distinct attachment disorders: reactive attachment disorder, in which the disturbance takes the form of the child failing to initiate and respond to nurturing in most social interactions in a developmentally typical way; and disinhibited social engagement disorder, in which the disturbance takes the form of undifferentiated, unselective, and inappropriate social behaviors with familiar and unfamiliar adults.

In disinhibited social engagement disorder, according to DSM-5-TR, a child actively approaches and interacts with unfamiliar adults in an overly familiar way, either verbally or physically. They check for or seek out their caregiver less often and are willing to go with unfamiliar adults without hesitation. These behaviors in disinhibited social engagement disorder are not accounted for by impulsivity, although socially disinhibited behavior is predominant. These patterns of disinhibited, developmentally inappropriate behaviors are presumed to be caused by pathogenic caregiving. Thus, for both reactive attachment disorder and disinhibited social engagement disorder, aberrant caretaking is presumed to be the predominant cause of the child's inappropriate behaviors.

These disorders may also result in a picture of failure to thrive, in which an infant may show physical signs of malnourishment and does not exhibit the expected developmental motor and verbal milestones.

Diagnosis and Clinical Features

Children with reactive attachment disorder and/or disinhibited social engagement disorder may initially be identified by a preschool teacher or by a pediatrician based on direct observation of the child's inappropriate social responses. These diagnoses rely at least partially on documented evidence of pervasive disturbance of attachment leading to inappropriate social behaviors present before the age of 5 years. The clinical picture varies greatly, depending on a child's chronologic and mental ages, but expected social behavior is not evident. Often, a child with an attachment disorder may not be progressing developmentally or is frankly malnourished. Perhaps the most common clinical picture of an infant with severe reactive attachment disorder is the nonorganic failure to thrive. Such infants usually exhibit hypokinesis, dullness, listlessness, and apathy, with poverty of spontaneous activity. Infants look sad, joyless, and miserable. Some infants also appear frightened and watchful, with a radar-like gaze. Table 10-2 compares the diagnostic approaches to reactive attachment disorder and Table 10-3 compares them for disinhibited social engagement disorder.

Infants with attachment disorders exhibit delayed responsiveness to a stimulus that would elicit fright or

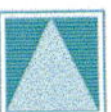

Table 10-2.
Comparison of Diagnostic Criteria for Reactive Attachment Disorder

	DSM-5-TR	ICD-10	ICD-11
Diagnostic name	Reactive Attachment Disorder	Reactive Attachment Disorder of Childhood	Reactive Attachment Disorder
Symptoms	Behavioral pattern characterized by emotional withdrawal • Not seeking or not responding to emotional comforting • A pattern of social/emotional disturbance • Lack of mood reactivity or positive affective response to stimuli • Inappropriate mood lability/irritability/sadness • History of exposure to severely insufficient caregiving • Severe neglect • Unstable caregiving environment with frequent changes in caregivers • Being raised in unusual care settings • Evidence for the disorder after the developmental age of 9 mo and before age 5 yr	A pattern of abnormal social relationships involving emotional disturbance and behavioral changes • i.e., fear, hypervigilance, poor socialization, aggression toward self and others, delayed growth in some instances Symptoms present before 5 yr of age Likely occur as a direct result of neglect, abuse, or maltreatment during rearing	History of grossly insufficient care • Disregard for the child's physical and emotional needs • Frequent changes in primary caregivers • Rearing in unusual settings • Maltreatment Abnormal attachment behaviors • Minimal seeking of comfort when distressed • Minimal response to comfort when offered Insufficient care is presumed to be responsible for the child's behaviors Evidence for the disorder after the developmental age of 9 mo and before age 5 yr
Required number of symptoms	All of the above categories, with behavioral symptoms, felt to be the direct result of exposure to inadequate caregiving or rearing environment		
Psychosocial consequences	Significant disturbance of behavior		
Exclusions	Autism spectrum disorder	Asperger syndrome Disinhibited attachment disorder of childhood Maltreatment syndromes Normal variation in the pattern of selective attachment Sexual or physical abuse in childhood, resulting in psychosocial problems	Autism spectrum disorder Not confined to one relationship
Symptom specifiers		Specifiers for: Failure to thrive [R62.51] Growth retardation	
Course specifiers	**Persistent** (>12 mo)		
Severity specifiers	**Severe:** All symptom criteria met, with symptoms presenting at a high level of severity as well		

withdrawal from a healthy infant. Infants with failure to thrive and reactive attachment disorder appear significantly malnourished, and many have protruding abdomens. Infants with attachment disorders may exhibit weight that is below the third percentile and markedly below the appropriate weight for their height. If serial weights are available, the weight percentiles may have decreased progressively because of an actual weight loss or a failure to gain weight as height increases. Head circumference is usually average for the infant's age. Muscle tone may be weak. The skin may be colder and paler or more mottled than the skin of a healthy child. Laboratory findings may indicate coincident malnutrition, dehydration, or concurrent illness. Bone age is usually retarded. Growth hormone levels are usually normal or elevated, a finding suggesting that growth failure in these children is secondary to caloric deprivation and malnutrition. Cortisol secretion in children with reactive attachment disorder or disinhibited social engagement disorder is lower than in typically developing children. For children with

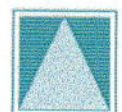

Table 10-3.
Comparison of Diagnostic Criteria for Disinhibited Social Engagement Disorder

	DSM-5-TR	ICD-10	ICD-11
Diagnostic name	Disinhibited Social Engagement Disorder	Disinhibited Attachment Disorder of Childhood	Disinhibited Social Engagement Disorder
Symptoms	Childhood pattern of approaching unfamiliar adults • Lack of inhibition in approaching unfamiliar adults • Overly familiar behavior toward unfamiliar adults • Reduced frequency of checking in with known adult/caregiver figure • Minimal or no hesitation to venture forth with an unfamiliar adult History of exposure to insufficient care • History of neglectful rearing environment • A pattern of instability and frequent changes in caregiver • Raised in an unusual setting for child rearing • The developmental age of ≥9 mo and before age 5 yr	A pattern of nonselective attachment, attention-seeking, indiscriminate behaviors with peers and strangers Abnormal social interaction patterns arise before the age of 5 yr It may or may not be associated with emotional or behavioral disturbance	History of grossly insufficient care • Disregard for the child's physical and emotional needs • Frequent changes in primary caregivers • Rearing in unusual settings • Maltreatment Abnormal attachment behaviors • Overly familiar behaviors with adult strangers • Decreased checking back with caregiver • Willing to go off with unfamiliar adults with little hesitation • Evidence for the disorder after age 1 yr or developmental age of 9 mo and before age 5 yr
Required number of symptoms	Two symptoms of disinhibited behavior with an unfamiliar adult, in addition to a history of exposure to an abnormal child rearing environment as above, are related to the development of abnormal behavior		
Psychosocial consequences	Significant disturbance of behavior resulting in impaired safety and/or functioning		
Exclusions	Symptoms limited to impulsivity without socially disinhibited behavior	Asperger syndrome Hospitalism in children Hyperkinetic disorders Reactive attachment disorder of childhood	Asperger syndrome Adjustment disorder Attention deficit hyperactivity disorder Reactive attachment disorder of childhood
Course specifiers	**Persistent** Present for ≥12 mo		
Severity specifiers	**Severe:** Child exhibiting all symptoms, with all symptoms at relatively high levels		

failure to thrive, improvement physically and weight gain generally rapidly occurs after hospitalization.

Socially, the infants with reactive attachment disorder usually show little spontaneous activity and a marked diminution of both initiative toward others and reciprocity in response to the caregiving adult or examiner. Both mother and infant may be indifferent to separation on hospitalization or to termination of subsequent hospital visits. The infants frequently show none of the normal upset, fretting, or protest about hospitalization. Older infants usually show little interest in their environment. They may not play with toys, even if encouraged; however, they rapidly or gradually take an interest in and relate to their caregivers in the hospital.

Children with disinhibited social engagement disorder appear to be overly friendly and familiar with little fear.

Adoptive parents brought their 7-year-old boy, Kim, for evaluation because of his hyperactivity, as well as inappropriate social behavior with peers at school as reported by his teacher. Kim was adopted at 4 years of age, having spent most of his life in an orphanage in China where he received care from a rotating shift of caregivers. Although he had been below the fifth percentile for height and weight at the time he was adopted, he quickly approached the 15th percentile in his new home. Kim's adoptive parents were frustrated by his inability to show a specific bond with affection toward them, even when they were affectionate toward him. Kim's parents had initially worried about an intellectual problem, although testing and his capacity to engage, albeit not normally, with many adults and many children suggested otherwise. Kim's parents thought he was indiscriminately too friendly, talking to anyone and often following strangers without hesitation. He showed little empathy when others were hurt, although he would sit on the laps of teachers and students without asking. Kim often sustained minor injuries because of seemingly reckless behavior, although he had an extremely high pain tolerance. His parents focused on problem behaviors at home to decrease his impulsive behavior, which improved with much prompting; however, he remained oddly overfriendly at home and in school. The psychiatrist diagnosed the child with disinhibited social engagement disorder. (Adapted from Neil W. Boris, M.D. and Charles H. Zeanah Jr., M.D.)

Pathology and Laboratory Examination. Although no single specific laboratory test can make a diagnosis, many children with reactive attachment disorder have disturbances of growth and development. Thus, establishing a growth curve and examining the progression of developmental milestones may help determine whether associated phenomena, such as failure to thrive, are present.

Differential Diagnosis

The differential diagnosis of reactive attachment disorder and disinhibited social engagement disorder must take into account that many other psychiatric disorders may arise in conjunction with maltreatment, including depressive disorders, anxiety disorders, and PTSD. Psychiatric disorders to consider in the differential diagnosis include language disorders, autism spectrum disorder, intellectual disability, and metabolic syndromes. Children with autism spectrum disorder are typically well nourished and of age-appropriate size and weight, and are generally alert and active, despite their impairments in reciprocal social interactions. Significant intellectual disability is often present in children with an autism spectrum disorder, whereas when intellectual disability occurs with reactive attachment disorder or disinhibited social engagement disorder, it is generally relatively mild. Children with disinhibited social engagement disorder often show comorbid Attention-Deficit/Hyperactivity Disorder (ADHD), PTSD, and language disorder or delay. Furthermore, children with disinhibited social engagement disorder symptoms may have complex neuropsychiatric problems.

Course and Prognosis

Most of the historical data available on the natural course of children with reactive attachment disorder and disinhibited social engagement disorder come from follow-up studies of children in residential facilities with histories of severe neglect. Findings from these studies suggest that children with reactive attachment disorder who are later adopted into caring environments improve in their attachment behaviors and may normalize over time. Children with disinhibited social engagement disorder, however, appear to have more difficulty developing attachments to new caregivers. Children with disinhibited social engagement disorder who exhibit indiscriminate social behavior also tend to have poor peer relationships. The duration and severity of the neglect influence the prognosis for both disorders. The degree of resulting impairment does, as well. Constitutional and nutritional factors interact in children, who may either respond resiliently to treatment or continue to fail to thrive. The amount of treatment and rehabilitation that the family receives affects the child. Children who have multiple problems stemming from pathogenic caregiving may recover physically faster and more completely than they do emotionally.

Treatment

The first consideration in treating reactive attachment disorder or disinhibited social engagement disorder is a child's safety. Thus, the management of these disorders must begin with a comprehensive assessment of the current level of safety and adequate caregiving. When there is suspicion of maltreatment persisting in the home, usually, the first decision is whether to hospitalize the child or to attempt treatment while the child remains in the home. If we suspect neglect or emotional, physical, or sexual abuse, we must report it to the appropriate law enforcement and child protective services in the area. The therapeutic strategy depends on the child's physical and emotional state and the level of pathologic caregiving. It is important to determine the nutritional status of the child and the presence of ongoing physical abuse or threat. Hospitalization is necessary for children with malnourishment.

Along with an assessment of the child's physical well-being, an evaluation of the child's emotional condition is essential. Immediate intervention must address the parents' awareness and capacity to participate in altering the injurious patterns that have heretofore ensued. The treatment team must begin to improve the unsatisfactory relationship between caregiver and child. This intervention usually requires extensive and intensive therapy and education with the mother or with both parents when possible.

In one study, parents of 120 children between 11.7 and 31.9 months, identified as being at risk for neglect, were randomly assigned to an intervention for at-risk parents called Attachment and Biobehavioral Catch-up (ABC) or to a control intervention. The purpose of the ABC intervention was to decrease frightening behavior toward the infant by parents and to increase sensitive and nurturing interactions between parents and infants. The investigators manualized the intervention to guide the parents in how to provide those interactions with their infants. They evaluated the children after 10 sessions, and the 60 children who received the ABC intervention showed significantly lower rates of disorganized attachment (32%) and higher rates of secure attachment (52%) compared to those who received the control intervention (disorganized attachment 57%; secure attachment 33%).

The authors concluded that we could enhance parental nurturance and sensitivity through a comprehensive and explicit intervention such as the ABC intervention and can measure significant improvements in attachment behaviors in young children after 10 sessions.

The caregiver–child relationship is the basis of the assessment of reactive attachment disorder and disinhibited social engagement disorder symptoms and the substrate from which to modify attachment behaviors. Structured observations allow a clinician to determine the range of attachment behaviors established with various family members. We may work closely with the caregiver and the child to facilitate higher sensitivity in their interactions. Three primary psychotherapeutic modalities help promote bonds between children and caregivers. First, a clinician can target the caregiver to promote positive interaction with a child who does not yet have the repertoire to respond positively. Second, a clinician can work with the child and the caregiver together as a dyad to advocate for practicing appropriate positive reinforcement for each other. Through the use of videotapes, therapists can view parent–child interactions and suggest modifications to increase positive engagement. The third modality for clinical intervention is through individual work with the child. Working with the child and caregiver together is often more effective in producing more emotionally meaningful exchanges than working with the parent or child individually.

Psychosocial interventions for families in which a child has reactive attachment disorder or disinhibited social engagement disorder include (1) psychosocial support services, including hiring a homemaker, improving the physical condition of the apartment, or obtaining adequate housing, improving the family's financial status, and decreasing the family's isolation; (2) psychotherapeutic interventions, including individual psychotherapy, psychotropic medications, and family or marital therapy; (3) educational counseling services, including mother–infant or mother–toddler groups, and counseling to increase awareness and understanding of the child's needs and to develop parenting skills; and (4) provisions for close monitoring of the progression of the patient's emotional and physical well-being. Sometimes, separating a child from the stressful home environment temporarily, as in hospitalization, allows the child to break out of the accustomed pattern. A neutral setting, such as the hospital, is the best place to start with families who are genuinely available emotionally and physically for intervention. If interventions are not feasible or inadequate, or if they fail, we must consider placing the child with relatives or in foster care, adoption, or in a group home or residential treatment facility.

Epidemiology

Few data exist on the prevalence, sex ratio, or familial pattern of reactive attachment disorder and disinhibited social engagement disorder. Both disorders probably occur in less than 1% of the population. A study of 1,646 children aged 6 to 8 years old, living in a deprived sector of urban United Kingdom, found that the prevalence of reactive attachment disorder in this population was 1.4%. However, other studies of selected high-risk populations have estimated that about 10% of young children with documented neglectful and grossly pathologic caregiving exhibit reactive attachment disorder, and up to 20% of children in this situation exhibit disinhibited social engagement disorder. In a retrospective report of children in one county of the United States who were removed from their homes because of neglect or abuse before the age of 4 years, 38% exhibited signs of either reactive attachment disorder or disinhibited social engagement disorder. Another study established the reliability of the diagnosis by reviewing videotaped assessments of at-risk children interacting with caregivers, along with a structured interview with the caregivers. Given that pathogenic care, including maltreatment, occurs more frequently in the presence of general psychosocial risk factors, such as poverty, disrupted families, and mental illness among caregivers, these circumstances are likely to increase the risk of reactive attachment disorder and disinhibited social engagement disorder.

Etiology

The core features of reactive attachment disorder and disinhibited social engagement disorder are disturbances of normal attachment behaviors. These behaviors occur in the face of caregiver social neglect or deprivation due to a persistent absence of attention to basic needs for comfort, stimulation, and affection. The inability of a young child to develop normative social interactions that culminate in aberrant attachment behaviors in reactive attachment disorder is inherent in the disorder's definition. Reactive attachment disorder and disinhibited social engagement disorder are presumed to be due to maltreatment of the child, including emotional neglect, physical abuse, or both. Grossly pathogenic care of an infant or young child by the caregiver presumably causes the markedly disturbed social relatedness that is evident. The emphasis is on the unidirectional cause; that is, the caregiver does something inimical or neglects to do something essential for the infant or child. In evaluating a patient for whom such a diagnosis is appropriate, however, clinicians should consider the contributions of each member of the caregiver–child dyad and their interactions. Exacerbating factors may include the temperament of a child and severe caregiver mismatch. The likelihood of neglect increases with a parental psychiatric disorder, substance abuse, intellectual disability, the parent's harsh upbringing, social isolation, deprivation, and premature parenthood (i.e., adolescent). These factors compromise parental ability to attend to the needs of the child, as the parents focus primarily on their existence. Frequent changes of the primary caregivers, for example, from multiple foster care placements or repeated lengthy hospitalizations, may also lead to impaired attachment. In the general population, a study of 1,600 children found that those children with reactive attachment disorder/disinhibited social engagement disorder showed a constellation of symptoms characterized by early symptomatic syndromes eliciting neurodevelopmental clinical examinations (ESSENCE). Some of the associated symptoms in children with reactive attachment disorder/disinhibited social engagement disorder include a higher risk of failure to gain weight as neonates, feeding difficulty, and poor impulse control. These traits are likely to emerge because of both genetic and environmental factors. The authors found that children with reactive attachment disorder/disinhibited social engagement disorder were more likely to have multiple psychiatric comorbidities, lower IQs compared to the general population, and more behavioral problems. Thus, a broad assessment may be necessary to identify symptoms and disorders associated with reactive attachment disorder/disinhibited social engagement disorder.

Further Readings

Bernard K, Dozier M, Bick J, Lewis-Morrarty E, Lindheim O, Carlson E. Enhancing attachment organization among maltreated children: results of a randomized clinical trial. *Child Dev*. 2012;83(2):623–636.

Bohus M, Kleindienst N, Hahn C, et al. Dialectical behavior therapy for posttraumatic stress disorder (DBT-PTSD) compared with cognitive processing therapy (CPT) in complex presentations of PTSD in women survivors of childhood abuse: a randomized clinical trial. *JAMA Psychiatry*. 2020;77(12):1235–1245.

Brown EJ, Cohen JA, Mannarino AP. Trauma-focused cognitive-behavioral therapy: the role of caregivers. *J Affect Disord*. 2020;277:39–45.

Choi KR, Seng JS, Briggs EC, et al. The dissociative subtype of posttraumatic stress disorder (PTSD) among adolescents: co-occurring PTSD, depersonalization/derealization, and other dissociation symptoms. *J Am Acad Child Adolesc Psychiatry*. 2017;56(12):1062–1072.

Cohen JA, Mannarino AP. Trauma-focused cognitive behavioral therapy for children and families. *Child Adolesc Psychiatr Clin N Am*. 2022; 31(1):133–147.

Cohen JA, Mannarino AP. Trauma-focused cognitive behavioral therapy for childhood traumatic separation. *Child Abuse Negl*. 2019;92:179–195.

Cohen JA, Mannarino AP, Deblinger E. *Treating Trauma and Traumatic Grief in Children and Adolescents*. The Guilford Press; 2009.

Cohen JA, Mannarino AP, Perel JM, Staron V. A pilot randomized controlled trial of combined trauma-focused CBT and sertraline for childhood PTSD symptoms. *J Am Acad Child Adolesc Psychiatry*. 2007;46(7):811–819.

Dorsey S, Briggs EC, Woods BA. Cognitive behavioral treatment for posttraumatic stress disorder in children and adolescents. *Child Adolesc Psychiatr Clin N Am*. 2011;20(2):255–269.

Ford JD, Steinberg KL, Hawke J, Levine J, Xhang W. Randomized trial comparison of emotion regulation and relational psychotherapies for PTSD in girls involved in delinquency. *J Clin Child Adolesc Psychol*. 2012;41(1):27–37.

Gillies D, Maiocchi L, Bhandari AP, Taylor F, Gray C, O'Brien L. Psychological therapies for children and adolescents exposed to trauma. *Cochrane Database Syst Rev*. 2016;10(10):CD012371.

Herringa RJ. Trauma, PTSD, and the developing brain. *Curr Psychiatry Rep*. 2017;19(10):69.

Jaycox LH, Cohen JA, Mannarino AP, et al. Children's mental health care following Hurricane Katrina: a field trial of trauma-focused psychotherapies. *J Traum Stress*. 2010;23(2):223–231.

Karadag M, Gokcen C, Sarp AS. EMDR therapy in children and adolescents who have post-traumatic stress disorder: a six-week follow-up study. *Int J Psychiatry Clin Pract*. 2020;24(1):77–82.

Kay C, Green J. Reactive attachment disorder following early maltreatment: systematic evidence beyond the institution. *J Abnorm Child Psychol*. 2013;41(4):571–581.

Kočovská E, Puckering C, Follan M, et al. Neurodevelopmental problems in maltreated children referred with indiscriminate friendliness. *Res Dev Disabil*. 2012;33(5):1560–1565.

Kočovská E, Wilson P, Young D, et al. Cortisol secretion in children with symptoms of reactive attachment disorder. *Psychiatr Res*. 2013; 209(1):74–77.

Maercker A, Cloitre M, Bachem R, et al. Complex post-traumatic stress disorder. *Lancet*. 2022;400(10345):60–72.

Minnis H. Reactive attachment disorder in the general population: a hidden ESSENCE disorder. *Sci World J*. 2013;2013:818157.

Minnis H, Macmillan S, Pritchett R, et al. Prevalence of reactive attachment disorder in a deprived population. *Br J Psychiatry*. 2013;202(5): 342–346.

Moner N, Soubelet A, Barbieri L, Askenazy F. Assessment of PTSD and posttraumatic symptomatology in very young children: a systematic review. *J Child Adolesc Psychiatr Nurs*. 2022;35(1):7–23.

Peters W, Rice S, Cohen J, et al. Trauma-focused cognitive-behavioral therapy (TF-CBT) for interpersonal trauma in transitional-aged youth. *Psychol Trauma*. 2021;13(3):313–321.

Robb AS, Cueva JE, Sporn J, Yang R, Vanderberg DG. Sertraline treatment of children and adolescents with posttraumatic stress disorder: a double-blind placebo-controlled trial. *J Child Adolesc Psychopharmacol*. 2010;20(6):463–471.

Ross SL, Sharma-Patel K, Brown EJ, Huntt JS, Chaplin WF. Complex trauma and trauma-focused cognitive-behavioral therapy: how do trauma chronicity and PTSD presentation affect treatment outcome? *Child Abuse Negl*. 2021;111:104734.

Task Force on Research Diagnostic Criteria: Infancy Preschool. Research diagnostic criteria for infants and preschool children: the process and empirical support. *J Am Acad Child Adolesc Psychiatry*. 2003;42(12):1504–1512.

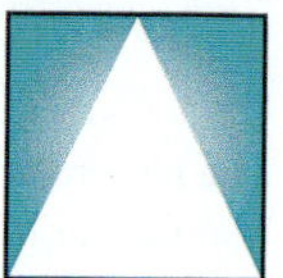

11 Depressive Disorders and Suicide in Children and Adolescents

Depressive disorders in youth represent a significant public health concern, because they are prevalent and result in long-term adverse effects on a youth's cognitive, social, and psychological development. Major depressive disorder, persistent depressive disorder, and disruptive mood dysregulation disorder (described in Chapter 13) all lead to an increased risk of long-term impairments in academics and relationships with family and peers. Depressive disorders affect approximately 2% to 3% of children and up to about 8% to 12% of adolescents. Earlier onset of major depression is associated with more lifetime depressive episodes and suicide attempts and poorer quality of life than later age onset of depression. Due to the long-term adverse outcome of depressive disorders in youth, the need for early identification and access to evidence-based interventions including cognitive-behavioral therapy (CBT) and antidepressant agents is extremely important.

Depressive disorders run in families, with the highest risk in children whose parents experienced early-onset depression; however, twin studies have demonstrated that major depression is only moderately heritable, with genetics accounting for approximately 40% to 50% of risk, emphasizing environmental stressors and adverse events as significant contributors.

The core features of major depression in children, adolescents, and adults are strikingly similar; however, the developmental level of the child or adolescent influences the clinical presentation. The DSM-5-TR uses the same criteria for major depressive disorder in youth as in adults, except that for children and adolescents, *irritable mood* may replace a *depressed mood* in the diagnostic criteria.

Most children and adolescents with depressive disorders do not attempt nor complete suicide; however, severely depressed youth often have suicidal ideation, and suicide remains the most severe risk of major depression. Conversely, many children and adolescents who engage in suicidal behavior do not have a depressive disorder. Epidemiologic data suggest that depressed youth with recurrent active suicidal ideation, including a plan, who have made prior attempts, are at higher risk to complete suicide.

Mood disorders in children and adolescents have been studied systematically in multisite randomized clinical trials (RCTs) over the last few decades, including the Treatment of Adolescent Depression Study (TADS), which provides evidence of the efficacy of both CBT as well as selective serotonin reuptake inhibitors (SSRIs). In more severe forms of major depression, combined CBT plus SSRIs appear to provide the highest treatment efficacy.

Increased recognition of depressive disorders in preschool populations has sparked clinicians and researchers to develop psychosocial interventions such as Parent–Child Interaction Therapy Emotion Development (PCIT-ED), which was developed specifically for this age group. The expression of depressed mood usually varies with the developmental stage. Very young children with major depression are often observed to be sad, listless, or apathetic, even though they may not articulate these feelings verbally. Perhaps surprisingly, mood-congruent auditory hallucinations occur in young children with major depression. Somatic complaints such as headaches and stomachaches, withdrawn and sad appearance, and poor self-esteem are more universal symptoms. In late adolescence, youth with more severe forms of depression often display pervasive anhedonia, severe psychomotor retardation, delusions, and a sense of hopelessness. Symptoms that emerge with the same frequency, regardless of age and developmental level, include suicidal ideation, depressed or irritable mood, insomnia, and diminished ability to concentrate.

Developmental factors influence the expression of depressive symptoms. Fortunately, depressed young children who exhibit recurrent suicidal ideation are rarely able to propose a realistic suicide plan or to carry out such a plan. Children's moods are especially vulnerable to the adverse influences of severe psychosocial stressors, such as chronic family discord, abuse and neglect, and academic failure. Young children with major depressive disorder have higher incidences of abuse and neglect. Children in families with significant psychosocial burdens, such as parental mental illness, domestic violence, substance abuse, or poverty, are at higher risk of developing a depressive disorder. Children who develop depressive disorders in response to acute toxic family stressors may have remission of depressive symptoms when the stressors diminish or when supported in a more nurturing family environment. Depressive disorders are typically episodic, albeit typically lasting 9 months to a year; however, their onset may be insidious and remain unidentified until clear indicators of impairment in peer relationships, poor academic function, or observable withdrawal from activities emerge.

Attention-deficit/hyperactivity disorder (ADHD), oppositional defiant disorder, and disruptive behavior disorders are not infrequently comorbid with a major depressive episode. In some cases, disruptive behaviors or disturbances of conduct, in the context of a major depressive episode, may resolve with treatment of the depression.

To make an accurate diagnosis, clinicians must clarify the chronology of the symptoms to identify whether a given behavior (e.g., poor concentration, defiance, or temper tantrums) was present before the depressive episode or is more likely a response to it.

DIAGNOSIS AND CLINICAL FEATURES

Major Depressive Disorder

It is easiest to diagnose major depressive disorder in children and adolescents when the disorder emerges acutely in a youth without a previous psychiatric disorder. In many cases, however, the onset is insidious, and the disorder occurs in a youth who has already experienced psychiatric symptoms such as an anxiety disorder, attentional problems, or intermittent depressive symptoms.

According to the DSM-5-TR, criteria for major depressive disorder in children and adolescents include either a depressed mood or loss of interest or pleasure which has been present for at least a 2-week period. For children, the depressed mood may be displayed as an irritable mood. In addition to one of the above pervasive symptoms, at least four of the following symptoms are required: weight loss or failure to make expected weight gain for children (a change of at least 5% of body weight in a month), or an increase or decrease in appetite; insomnia or hypersomnia nearly every day; psychomotor agitation or retardation; fatigue or loss of energy nearly every day; feelings of worthlessness or excessive or inappropriate guilt; diminished ability to think or concentrate, or indecisiveness; or recurrent thoughts of death, recurrent suicidal ideation, suicide attempt, or suicide plan. The symptoms must cause impairment in functioning or significant distress. Table 11-1 shows comparative diagnostic criteria for major depression.

A major depressive episode in a prepubertal child is more likely to include somatic complaints, psychomotor agitation, and potentially mood-congruent hallucinations. Anhedonia is also frequent, but anhedonia, as well as hopelessness, psychomotor retardation, and delusions, are more common in adolescent and adult major depressive episodes than in young children. Feelings of

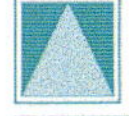

Table 11-1.
Comparative Diagnostic Criteria for Major Depressive Disorder

	DSM-5-TR	ICD-10	ICD-11
Diagnostic name	Major Depressive Disorder	Major Depressive Episode	Major Depressive Disorder
Duration	2-wk period	N/A	
Symptoms	Dysphoria/depressed mood Anhedonia Change in weight or appetite Change in sleep pattern Psychomotor disturbance: agitation or retardation Fatigue/decreased energy Depressive ruminations: worthlessness, guilt Poor concentration Recurrent thoughts of death, suicidal ideation, or a plan	Lowered mood Reduced energy Decreased activity Reduced capacity for enjoyment Reduced interest Reduced concentration Fatigue after even minimal effort Disturbed sleep/early morning awakening Disturbed appetite/weight loss Poor self-esteem Poor self-confidence Guilt or worthlessness Mood unreactive to circumstances Anhedonia Worse symptoms in the AM Psychomotor disturbance: agitation or retardation Loss of libido	**Affective Cluster** • Depressed mood • Anhedonia **Cognitive-behavioral cluster** • Poor concentration • Low self-worth or inappropriate guilt • Hopelessness • Recurrent thoughts of death, suicidal ideation, or a plan **Neurovegetative cluster** • Disrupted sleep • Change in appetite • Psychomotor agitation/retardation • Fatigue/decreased energy
Required number of symptoms	5 (one of these has to be symptom 1 or 2 listed above)	N/A	5 (≥1 from the affective cluster)

(continued)

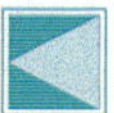

Table 11-1.
Comparative Diagnostic Criteria for Major Depressive Disorder (Continued)

	DSM-5-TR	ICD-10	ICD-11
Psychosocial consequences	Distress or impaired functioning (social, occupational, or other significant areas)	Depends on severity	Significant impairment in ≥1 domain
Exclusions	Other medical condition Substance or medication, including withdrawal Other mental illness History of: • manic episode • hypomanic episode	Adjustment disorder Conduct disorder Recurrent depressive disorder (which is considered a separate diagnosis)	Bereavement Mixed episode bipolar disorder Other medical consideration Effects of substance or medication

Symptoms specifiers	**With anxious distress**
	• 2+ symptoms of anxiety
	With mixed features
	• 3+ manic/hypomanic symptoms occurring during the depressive episode (if occur independently, diagnose bipolar disorder)
	With melancholic features
	• Loss of pleasure or reactivity to pleasure
	• 3+ of the following:
	  • Severe depression/despair
	  • Mood worse in AM
	  • Early morning awakening
	  • Psychomotor disturbance
	  • Anorexia/weight loss
	  • Guilt
	With atypical features
	• Mood reactivity
	• ≥2:
	  • Increased appetite/weight
	  • Hypersomnia
	  • Leaden Paralysis
	  • Rejection sensitivity
	  • With mood-congruent psychotic features
	  • With mood-incongruent psychotic features
	With psychotic features
	Symptoms occur only during a depressive episode. Also specify if delusions are mood congruent or incongruent.
	With catatonia
	• Must be present during most depressive episodes
	With peripartum onset
	With seasonal pattern
	• Usually occurs during a specific season
		Depressive reaction
		Psychogenic depression
		Reactive depression
			Mild
			Moderate
			Severe
			Unspecified
			With/without psychotic symptoms
			With prominent anxiety symptoms
			With panic attacks
			Current depressive episode persistent
			Current depressive episode with melancholia
			With seasonal pattern
			Associated with pregnancy, childbirth, or puerperium

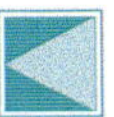

Table 11-1.
Comparative Diagnostic Criteria for Major Depressive Disorder (Continued)

	DSM-5-TR	ICD-10	ICD-11
Course specifiers	**In partial remission:** full criteria no longer met **In full remission:** no symptoms of an episode for the past 2 mo	**Recurrent Depressive Disorder** (Coded as a separate disorder) Repeated episodes of the above symptoms No mania	**In partial remission** **In full remission**
Severity specifiers	**Mild:** Minimum # symptoms **Moderate:** between mild and severe **Severe:** # of symptoms, the severity of symptoms, or dysfunction is much more than required for a diagnosis	**Mild** • 2–3 symptoms • Functions normally despite the distress **Moderate** • 4+ symptoms • Difficulty with functioning **Severe** • Several symptoms marked and distressing • Loss of self-esteem/feels worthless and guilty • Suicidal ideation/acts • Somatic symptoms of depression **Severe with psychotic symptoms** • As above but with psychosis • Other • Atypical depression • Single episodes of "masked depression" Unspecified	

restlessness, irritability, aggression, reluctance to cooperate in family ventures, withdrawal from social activities, and isolation from peers often occur in adolescents with major depression. School difficulties often occur in youth with major depression. Depressed adolescents may become less attentive to personal appearance and show increased sensitivity to rejection by peers and in romantic relationships.

School-age children can be reliable reporters about their emotions, relationships, and difficulties in psychosocial functions. Children may report depressive feelings in terms of anger or feeling "mad" rather than sad. Clinicians should assess the duration and frequency of the depressive mood to differentiate relatively universal, short-lived, and sometimes frequent periods of sadness, usually after a frustrating event, from a valid, persistent depressive mood. In very young children, estimates of duration of symptoms and mood may be unreliable.

Mood disorders are more often chronic when they begin in early childhood. Childhood-onset depressive disorders are often the most severe form of mood disorder and more likely to emerge in families with multiple first degree relatives with mood disorders. Functional impairment associated with a depressive disorder in childhood extends to practically all areas of a child's psychosocial world; school performance and behavior, peer relationships, and family relationships all suffer. Children with academic proficiency may be able to compensate for their mood disorder due to their academic skill. In many cases, however, school performance is impaired by a combination of difficulty concentrating, slowed thinking, lack of interest and motivation, fatigue, sleepiness, depressive ruminations, and preoccupations. Learning problems secondary to depression are typically corrected rapidly after a child's recovery from the depressive episode.

Children and adolescents, especially younger children with severe forms of major depressive disorder, may have auditory hallucinations or delusions. Typically, psychotic symptoms in youth with depression are consistent with the depressed mood and occur with the depressive episode. Depressive hallucinations usually consist of a single voice speaking to the person from outside their head, with derogatory or suicidal content. Depressive delusions center on themes of guilt, physical disease, death, nihilism, deserved punishment, personal inadequacy, and in some cases, persecution. These delusions are rare in prepuberty, probably because of cognitive immaturity, but are present in about half of psychotically depressed adolescents.

Persistent Depressive Disorder (Dysthymic Disorder)

In children and adolescents, persistent depressive disorder consists of a depressed or irritable mood for most of the day, more days than not, for at least 1 year. DSM-5-TR notes that in children and adolescents, irritable mood can replace the depressed mood criterion in place for adults, and that the duration criterion is 1 year (rather than 2 years as for adults). According to the DSM-5-TR diagnostic criteria, two or more of the following symptoms must accompany the depressed or irritable mood: low self-esteem, hopelessness, poor appetite or overeating, insomnia or hypersomnia, low energy or fatigue, or poor concentration or difficulty making decisions. During the year of the disturbance, these symptoms do not resolve for more than 2 months at a time. The diagnostic criteria for persistent depressive disorder specify that during the first year, no major depressive episode emerges. To meet the DSM-5-TR diagnostic criteria for persistent depressive disorder, a child or adolescent must not have a history of a manic or hypomanic episode. Persistent depressive disorder is not diagnosed if the symptoms occur exclusively during a chronic psychotic disorder or if they are the direct effects of a substance or a general medical condition. DSM-5-TR provides specifiers for early-onset (before 21 years of age) or late-onset (after 21 years of age). Table 11-2 provides comparative diagnostic criteria for Persistent Depressive Disorder (Dysthymic Disorder) in DSM-5-TR, ICD 10, and ICD 11.

A child or adolescent with persistent depressive disorder may have had a major depressive episode before developing persistent depressive disorder; however, it is much more common for a child with persistent depressive disorder for more than 1 year to develop a concurrent episode of major depressive disorder. In this case, both depressive diagnoses apply (double depression). Persistent depressive disorder in youth is known to have an average age of onset that is several years earlier than the typical onset of major depressive disorder. In some youth, all diagnostic criteria for persistent depressive disorder are met, except that the episode does not last for

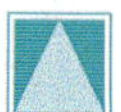

Table 11-2.
Comparative Diagnostic Criteria for Persistent Depressive Disorder/Dysthymic Disorder

	DSM-5-TR	ICD-10	ICD-11
Diagnostic name	Persistent Depressive Disorder	Dysthymia	Dysthymic Disorder
Duration	Symptoms continuously present for ≥2 yr No time during the affected period of no symptoms for >2 mo		≥2 yr
Symptoms	Depressed mood most of the time on a majority of days over a period of ≥2 yr (NOTE: In children, irritability may be present, and duration must be for a period of ≥1 yr) During the depressed period: • Abnormal appetite (↑ or ↓) • Abnormal sleep (↑ or ↓) • ↓ energy • ↓ self-esteem • ↓ concentration or ↑ indecisiveness • Hopelessness	Chronically depressed mood that does not meet criteria for a depressive episode, though criteria may have been met in the past	Persistent depressed mood Additional symptoms of depression. May include: • Anhedonia or decreased interest • Poor concentration • Low self-worth or inappropriate guilt • Hopelessness • Disturbed sleep • Change in appetite • Fatigue or low energy
Required number of symptoms	≥2 bulleted symptoms		
Psychosocial consequences	Marked distress and/or functional impairment		Marked distress and/or functional impairment
Exclusions	This cannot occur if a history of bipolar disorder Other medical condition Substance or medication, including withdrawal Other mental illness	Result of: • Anxiety • Depression • Bereavement • Schizophrenia	A depressive episode in the first 2 yr of the disorder History of manic, mixed, or hypomanic episodes Other medical condition Substance or medication, including withdrawal

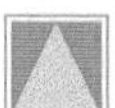

Table 11-2.
Comparative Diagnostic Criteria for Persistent Depressive Disorder/Dysthymic Disorder (Continued)

	DSM-5-TR	ICD-10	ICD-11
Symptoms specifiers	**With pure dysthymic syndrome:** Criteria for the depressive episode not met in the last 2 yr **With persistent major depressive episode:** Has met diagnostic criteria for a depressive episode for an entire 2-yr period **With intermittent major depressive episode, with current episode:** Though may currently meet criteria for major depressive disorder, has had a period of ≥8 wk during the prior 2-yr period during which symptoms were below the diagnostic threshold for a depressive episode **With intermittent major depressive episode, without current episode:** Does not currently meet criteria for a depressive episode, though has experienced ≥1 depressive episode over the course of the prior 2 yr. **With anxious distress:** Including ≥2 symptoms among feeling tense, restlessness, difficulty with concentration due to worrying, excessive fear without an identifiable cause, fear of loss of control **With mixed features:** Full criteria met for either depressive or manic/hypomanic episode, with additional symptoms of depressive or manic/hypomanic period without also meeting full criteria **With melancholic features:** Involving loss of pleasure, reduced reactivity with ≥3 of the following: • Depressed mood/despair • Depressive symptoms worse in the morning • Early morning awakening • Psychomotor changes • Loss of appetite/weight loss • Excessive guilt **With atypical features:** During most days, an individual is experiencing mood reactivity with ≥2 symptoms: • Weight gain or increased appetite • Excessive sleeping • Leaden paralysis • A pattern of heightened interpersonal rejection sensitivity **With mood-congruent psychotic features:** Mood-congruent delusions or hallucinations **With mood-incongruent psychotic features:** Mood-incongruent delusions or hallucinations		
Course specifiers	**With peripartum onset:** Full criteria for a mood episode are met during pregnancy or within 4 wk of delivery		
Severity specifiers	**Mild:** Few symptoms in excess of minimum diagnostic criteria, with no to minimal impairment and/or distress **Moderate:** Moderate symptomatology and impairment **Severe:** Symptoms in marked excess of minimum diagnostic requirement, with marked distress and impairment in functioning		

a whole year, or they experience remission from symptoms for more than 2 months. These mood presentations in youth may predict additional mood disorder episodes in the future. Current evidence suggests that the longer, more recurrent, and less directly related to social stress these episodes are, the higher the likelihood of future severe mood disorder. When minor depressive episodes follow a significant stressful life event by less than 3 months, it is more likely to meet criteria for an adjustment disorder.

Bereavement

Bereavement is a state of grief related to the death of a loved one. Bereavement often presents with symptoms which overlap with those of a major depressive episode such as sadness, insomnia, diminished appetite, and, in some cases, weight loss. Grieving children may become withdrawn and appear sad and avoid even their favorite activities.

In DSM-5-TR, bereavement is not a mental disorder; yet uncomplicated bereavement, that is, grief that is considered a typical response, is a condition that may be a focus of clinical attention. Children during a typical bereavement period may also meet the criteria for major depressive disorder. Symptoms indicating major depressive disorder exceeding typical bereavement include intense guilt related to issues beyond those surrounding the death of the loved one, preoccupation with death other than thoughts about being dead to be with the deceased person, morbid preoccupation with worthlessness, marked psychomotor retardation, prolonged severe functional impairment, and hallucinations other than transient perceptions of the voice of the deceased person.

Bereavement in a child may be characterized in the following way. For example, a child may feel devastated and abandoned if they must leave their home after the death of an only parent. Children who lose loved ones may feel a sense of guilt that death may have occurred because they were "bad" or did not perform as expected.

Prolonged Grief Disorder

Prolonged grief disorder in DSM-5-TR is defined by persistent grief for more than 1 year after the loss in adults, and more than 6 months after the loss in children and adolescents. This diagnosis is included in DSM-5-TR within the Trauma- and Stressor-Related Disorders section. Persistent grief is characterized by either intense yearning for the lost person or preoccupation with thoughts of the person, or both, every day. In children and adolescents, the persistent preoccupations may be about the cause or situation in which the death occurred. Three additional symptoms must be present daily or nearly every day. Prolonged grief disorder may include some symptoms overlapping with posttraumatic stress disorder (PTSD) such as avoidance of reminders of the person who was lost or emotional numbness. Other grief symptoms may include feeling that part of oneself has died, a strong sense of disbelief about the death, difficulties carrying on social relationships, feeling that life is now meaningless, and intense emotional pain and loneliness.

Rina was a 13-year-old eighth grader in middle school who was brought to the emergency room by police after walking into oncoming traffic at school. After school ended that day, Rina walked into the street across from the school when the light had just turned red. She didn't cross the street but just stood in the middle of it. The cars were driving slowly and stopped, since it was in a school zone. A parent of another student saw her and called 911. Two police stationed in their car across the street from the school responded. The police were about to issue Rina a citation for crossing against the red light; however, when they inquired as to why she was in the middle of the street, she informed them that she was trying to kill herself. The police placed Rina in the police car without a struggle and brought her to the local hospital's emergency room. Rina's mother was contacted and met Rina in the emergency room. Rina was not hurt physically, and a child and adolescent psychiatrist was called to evaluate her. When asked what had happened, Rina became tearful. She said she didn't want to live and was hoping she would be hit by a car and killed. Rina had a past history of ADHD and reported that numerous peers had bullied her the last 2 years because she was overweight and often blurted things out in class. Rina has a history of being an outcast and teased in school ever since she entered middle school in the sixth grade. Rina had been feeling sad and despondent ever since starting the eighth grade, and it just kept getting worse. She did not have friends in school and began to isolate herself from her family. Rina had been obsessing about death for several months and impulsively tried to kill herself today. Rina reported that on this day, a girl in her class had tried to trip her so she would fall down the stairs, and then started laughing at her with a few other girls. Rina reported that peers teased her and rejected her daily saying that they didn't want to be friends with someone who was "stupid and fat." Rina had made a few friends in the seventh grade who used to come defend her, but they had moved on to other friends in the eighth grade, excluding her from social activities. Rina disclosed that she had been sad for the last 2 years and thought about suicide recurrently over the last year. When Rina was asked by the child and adolescent psychiatrist whether she still felt suicidal, she replied, "Yes, I will try again to kill myself as soon as I get out of here."

Rina was an average student except that she needed more time than her classmates to finish assignments, especially ones that required a lot of writing. Rina was passing math, but this semester she was failing history. In a separate interview with Rina's mother, she reported that Rina had always had some difficulty making friends and had been treated for ADHD, but she was shocked to hear that Rina had reported sadness and suicidal thoughts for the past 2 years. Rina's mother felt that Rina was exaggerating her difficulties and wanted to take Rina home.

Rina had previously seen a counselor in school a few times last year due to her impulsive behavior, but the issues of depression or suicide did not come up. Rina has an older brother and a younger brother who are well adjusted;

however, her mother had experienced several episodes of significant depression. When interviewing Rina and her mother together, Rina was able, with some encouragement, to let her mother know how depressed, hopeless, and suicidal she felt, and why. Rina's mother burst into tears, and Rina tried to comfort her mother.

Rina was placed on a 72-hour hold for danger to self and referred to an adolescent psychiatric inpatient unit for further evaluation and treatment. The treatment team diagnosed major depression, started Rina on fluoxetine, and recommended CBT and psychoeducation for the family. After several weeks in the hospital, Rina was feeling better and was no longer actively suicidal. After she was discharged, Rina and her family followed up with the recommendations for CBT, and she continued on the fluoxetine.

Pathology and Laboratory Examination

No laboratory test is useful for diagnosis. If a child or adolescent also complains of symptoms of hypothyroidism, that is, dry skin, coldness, lethargy, for example, then a screening test for thyroid function may be indicated.

Rating scales for depressive symptoms administered to the child or adolescent and parent may be helpful in the evaluation of depressive disorders. The Patient Health Questionnaire-9 (PHQ-A) modified for youth is a frequently used self-report screening instrument for depression in youth aged 11 to 17 years. The scale has 9 depression symptom items rated on a 4-point scale from 0 (none) to 3 (nearly every day). Scores range from 0 to 27. A PHQ-A score ≥10 is typically the cut-off threshold to indicate the need for further evaluation to determine if all criteria are met for a diagnosis of major depression. This scale can be administered on an iPad. It may also be useful for monitoring treatment outcomes.

The Children's Depression Rating Scale—Revised (CDRS-R) is a 17-item instrument administered by the clinician separately to the parent and child or adolescent. The clinician scores a rating for each item using the information from both the parent and the child. The scale assesses affective, somatic, cognitive, and psychomotor symptoms. A cumulative score of 40 is a marker for moderate depression and a score of 45 or higher for significant depression.

DIFFERENTIAL DIAGNOSIS

There is much symptom overlap between major depressive disorder and many other child and adolescent psychiatric disorders, which can complicate the differential diagnosis. Irritability is often found in disruptive mood dysregulation disorder, persistent depressive disorder, bipolar disorder, PTSD disorder, and generalized anxiety disorder. Children with attention-deficit/hyperactivity disorder who are struggling in school and have difficulty with peer relationships may exhibit a depressed mood, low self-esteem, irritability, and behavioral outbursts. Anxiety symptoms and disorders in youth often coexist with depressive disorders. Anxiety disorders and oppositional defiant disorders may have some symptom features of depression and disruptive mood dysregulation disorder. Children with pervasive developmental disorder may present with depressive symptoms but not fulfill diagnostic criteria for a depressive disorder.

It is important for a clinician to consider bipolar disorders I and II in the differential diagnosis of a major depressive episode. The clinician should ask about a past or present history of manic or hypomanic symptoms. It is important to consider in the differential diagnosis the distinction between agitated depressive or manic episodes and ADHD, both of which may present with persistent excessive activity and restlessness.

Age is an important factor in interpreting diagnostic symptoms. Prepubertal children do not typically show symptoms of agitated depression, such as handwringing and pacing. Instead, an inability to sit still, irritability, and frequent temper tantrums are the most common symptoms. Sometimes an accurate diagnosis becomes evident only after remission of the depressive episode.

A substance-induced mood disorder may be challenging to differentiate from other mood disorders until detoxification occurs. Alcohol or drug use can complicate adolescent depression. One study found that up to 17% of adolescents with depressive disorder received an initial evaluation due to substance abuse.

COURSE AND PROGNOSIS

The course and prognosis of major depression in youths depend on the severity of illness. The mean length of an episode of major depression in children and adolescents is about 8 months. Recovery rates from a given episode of depression are high in youth, even without treatment, although treatment may shorten the length of the episode. More than 90% of moderately to severely depressed children and adolescents typically recover from an episode of major depression within 1 to 2 years. Important mediating factors include the rapidity of interventions and the degree of response to the interventions. The age of onset, severity, and the presence of comorbid disorders also influence course and prognosis.

In general, the younger the age of onset, the higher the recurrence of multiple episodes, and the increased likelihood of comorbid disorders which predict a poorer prognosis. The cumulative probability of another episode of major depression in youth is 20% to 60% within 2 years and 70% by 5 years. The most significant risk for relapse is in the 6 months to 1 year after discontinuing treatment. Depressed children who live in families with high levels of chronic conflict are more likely to have relapses. The relapse rate for childhood depression into adulthood is also high. In a community sample, 45% of adolescents with a history of major depression developed another episode of major depression in early adulthood.

Youth with major depression are at higher risk for the development of a future bipolar disorder compared to adults. Estimates of the incidence of children with an episode of major depression developing bipolar disorder range from 20% to 40%. Clinical characteristics of a depressive episode in youth suggesting the highest risk of developing bipolar I disorder include hallucinations and delusions, psychomotor retardation, and a family history of bipolar illness. In a longitudinal study of prepubertal children with major depression, 33% developed bipolar I disorder, whereas 48% went on to develop bipolar II or bipolar disorder not otherwise specified by early adulthood.

Depressive disorders are associated with short- and long-term peer relationship difficulties and complications, compromised academic achievement, and persistently low self-esteem. Persistent depressive disorder has an even more protracted recovery than major depressive disorder; the mean episode length is about 4 years. Early-onset persistent depressive disorder is associated with significant risks of comorbidity with major depressive disorder (70%), bipolar disorder (13%), and future substance abuse (15%). The risk of suicide, which accounts for about 12% of adolescent mortalities, is significant among adolescents with depressive disorders.

TREATMENT

The American Academy of Child and Adolescent Psychiatry (AACAP) practice parameters, AACAP's official Clinical Practice Guideline for the Assessment and Treatment of Children and Adolescents With Major and Persistent Depressive Disorders by Walter and colleagues (2023), as well as consensus reports of experts such as the Texas Children's Medication Algorithm Project (TMAP), provide evidence-based recommendations for the treatment of youth with depressive disorders. These include the following recommendations:

1. Psychoeducation and supportive interventions as a first intervention for youth with mild forms of depression.
2. Psychotherapeutic interventions for youth such as CBT and interpersonal therapy (IPT) as an initial intervention for youth with a moderate depressive episode.
3. For youth with moderate or severe or very severe depression, or recurrent episodes with significant impairment and with active suicidal thoughts or behaviors or psychosis, recommended interventions include initiation of combined pharmacotherapy and CBT. Pharmacotherapy typically includes a trial of an SSRI such as fluoxetine or another agent within the same class.

Psychiatric Hospitalization

When evaluating a youth for major depression, clinicians should assess for suicidal thoughts, behaviors, and a history of suicidal behavior. Safety is the most immediate and important consideration in assessing depression in youth; that is, a determination as to whether immediate psychiatric hospitalization is necessary. Depressed children and adolescents who express active suicidal thoughts or behaviors most often require some extended evaluation in the safety of the psychiatric hospital to protect them from immediate self-destructive impulses and behaviors.

Evidence-Based Treatment Studies

The Treatment for Adolescents With Depression Study (TADS) divided 439 adolescent subjects into four groups treated for 12 weeks with either fluoxetine alone (10 mg to 40 mg/day), fluoxetine in combination with cognitive-behavioral therapy (CBT), CBT alone, or placebo. Based on the Children's Depression Rating Scale (CDRS), combination treatment had significantly superior response rates compared with either treatment alone. Based on the Clinical Global Impressions (CGI) scale, at 12 weeks, scores of much or very much improved were 71% for the combined treatment group, 60.6% for the fluoxetine group, 43.2% for the CBT alone group, and 34.4% for the placebo group. At 12 weeks, combination treatment was the optimal strategy in the treatment of adolescent depression. By the end of 9 months of treatment, however, response rates for each group had converged, so that response for the combination group was 86%, fluoxetine group response was about 81%, and CBT-alone group response rate was 81%. The long-term effectiveness of treatments for adolescent depression demonstrates that for moderately ill adolescents, fluoxetine, CBT, or the combination is efficacious. However, the addition of CBT to fluoxetine decreased persistent suicidal ideation and potential treatment-related emergence of suicidal ideation.

A second large multicenter randomized placebo-controlled trial, Treatment of Resistant Depression in Adolescents (TORDIA), included adolescents with moderate to severe major depression who had not responded to a 2-month trial with an SSRI antidepressant. The investigators in this study randomly assigned 334 adolescents between 12 and 18 years of age to a different SSRI agent (either citalopram, paroxetine, citalopram, or another antidepressant class, venlafaxine) with or without concurrent CBT. The SSRI plus CBT group and the venlafaxine plus CBT group had higher response rates of improvement (54.8%) than the group on medications alone (40.5%). There were no differences found in the response rates between antidepressant agents.

Psychosocial Interventions

Cognitive-Behavioral Therapy. CBT is an efficacious intervention for the treatment of moderately severe depression in children and adolescents. CBT aims to challenge maladaptive beliefs and enhance problem-solving abilities and social competence. A review of controlled cognitive-behavioral studies in children and adolescents revealed that, as with adults, both children and adolescents showed consistent improvement with these methods. Other "active" treatments, including relaxation techniques, were also shown to be helpful as an adjunctive treatment for mild to moderate depression. Findings from one large, controlled study comparing cognitive-behavioral interventions with nondirective supportive psychotherapy and systemic behavioral family therapy showed that 70% of adolescents had some improvement with each of the interventions; cognitive-behavioral intervention had the most rapid effect. Another controlled study comparing a brief course of CBT with relaxation therapy favored cognitive-behavioral intervention. At a 3- to 6-month follow-up, however, no significant differences existed between the two treatment groups. This effect resulted from relapse in the cognitive-behavioral group, along with continued recovery in some patients in the relaxation group. Factors that seem to interfere with treatment responsiveness include the presence of comorbid anxiety disorder that probably was present before the depressive episode. Longer-term CBT is efficacious in the treatment of depression and has the advantage of mitigating suicidal ideation.

Interpersonal Psychotherapy

Interpersonal psychotherapy (IPT) focuses on improving depression through a focus on ways in which depression interferes with interpersonal relationships and overcoming these challenges. The four main areas of focus with IPT include loss, interpersonal disputes, role transition, and interpersonal deficits. A modification of IPT to more specifically address depression of adolescents (IPT-A) includes a focus on separation from parents, authority figures, peer pressures, and dyadic relationships. IPT-A has been studied on an outpatient basis as well as in a school-based clinic setting. A 12-week study of 48 adolescents with major depression randomly assigned to IPT-A or clinical monitoring found that the group receiving IPT-A showed decreased depressive symptoms, increased social functioning, and improved problem solving compared to the other group. In the school-based health clinic, depressed adolescents were randomly assigned to IPT-A or treatment as usual for 16 weeks. Trained clinic staff administered the treatment. At the end of 16 weeks, those adolescents receiving IPT-A had more significant symptom reduction and improved overall functioning; older and more severely depressed adolescents seemed to benefit most significantly.

Parent–Child Interaction Therapy

PCIT-ED for preschool depression, a modification of PCIT historically used in the treatment of disruptive disorders for children, was piloted in an RCT for 54 depressed preschoolers. Fifty-four depressed young children from ages 3 to 7 years received either PCIT-ED or psychoeducation with their caregivers. PCIT-ED was manualized and consisted of three modules conducted over 14 sessions in 12 weeks. The core modules of PCIT—Child-Directed Interaction (CDI) and Parent-Directed Interaction (PDI)—were utilized and limited to four sessions each. The focus of these modules is to strengthen the parent–child relationship by coaching parents in positive play techniques, giving effective directives to the child, and responding to disruptive behavior in firm but not punitive ways. The novel portion of the treatment targeting preschool depression consisted of a 6-week Emotion Development (ED) module, which focused on helping the parent to be a more effective emotion guide and affect regulator for the child. As part of the ED module, the parent learns to accurately recognize their emotions as well as the child's and serves to help regulate the child's emotions. The team developed a psychoeducation control condition, Developmental Education and Parenting Intervention (DEPI), for parents using small group sessions. The DEPI condition was designed to educate parents about child development and emphasized emotional and social development without individual coaching or practice with behavioral techniques as provided in the PCIT-ED group. Primary outcome measures included parent's report of the child's symptoms of depression using a structured instrument, the Preschool Age Psychiatric Assessment (PAPA), and the investigators measured depression severity pretreatment and posttreatment using parent ratings on the Preschool Reelings Checklist—Scale Version (PFC-S), a 20-item checklist. Results revealed that both groups showed significant improvement, with improvement in the PCIT-ED group concerning emotion recognition, child executive functioning, and parenting stress. This pilot study indicates that PCIT-ED is a promising novel intervention for preschool depression that deserves further investigation.

Pharmacotherapy

Fluoxetine and escitalopram have FDA approval in the treatment of major depression in adolescents (Table 11-3). The TADS of fluoxetine in depressed children and adolescents demonstrated the efficacy of fluoxetine. RCTs have demonstrated the efficacy of escitalopram. The common side effects of both of the above SSRIs are similar to those found for adults: headache, gastrointestinal symptoms, sedation, and insomnia.

Short-term RCTs have demonstrated the efficacy of citalopram and sertraline compared with placebo in the treatment of major depression in children and adolescents. Sertraline was efficacious in two multicenter, double-blind placebo-controlled trials of 376 children and adolescents. The doses of sertraline ranged from 50 to 200 mg a day. Nearly 70% of the subjects had a greater than 40% decrease in depression rating scale

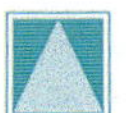

Table 11-3.
FDA-Approved Medications for Depressive Disorders in Youth

Medication	Class	Age Range	Mood Episode
Fluoxetine (Prozac)	Selective serotonin reuptake inhibitor (SSRI) antidepressant	8–17 yr	Unipolar major depression
Escitalopram (Lexapro)	SSRI antidepressant	12–17 yr	Unipolar major depression
Lurasidone (Latuda)	Second-generation antipsychotic	10–17 yr	Bipolar major depressive episode
Olanzapine-fluoxetine (OFC) (Zyprexa-Prozac)	Second-generation antipsychotic–SSRI antidepressant	10–17 yr	Bipolar depressive episode

scores (compared with 56% in the placebo group). The most common side effects are anorexia, vomiting, diarrhea, and agitation.

Citalopram has been demonstrated in one RCT in the United States to be efficacious in 174 children and adolescents treated with citalopram at doses of 20 to 40 mg a day for 8 weeks. Significantly more of the group on citalopram showed improvement compared with placebo on the depression rating scale (CDRS-R). A significantly increased response rate (response defined as less than 28 on CDRS-R) of 35% occurred in the citalopram group, compared with 24% of the placebo group. Common side effects that emerged included headache, nausea, insomnia, rhinitis, abdominal pain, dizziness, fatigue, and flulike symptoms.

RCTs to date that have not shown efficacy on primary outcome measures include those using mirtazapine and tricyclic antidepressants. A meta-analysis of SSRI trials in depressed children and adolescents found the efficacy of SSRIs compared to placebo with an average response rate of 60% for the SSRI compared to 49% for placebo.

Starting doses of SSRIs for prepubertal children are lower than doses recommended for adolescents or adults.

A potential side effect of SSRIs, especially in young depressed children, is behavioral activation or induction of hypomanic symptoms. If behavioral activation occurs, the medication should be discontinued to determine if the symptoms resolve. Activation due to SSRIs, however, does not necessarily predict a future diagnosis of bipolar disorder.

Venlafaxine was effective in the TORDIA study; however, adverse effects, including increased blood pressure, have made this agent a second-line choice compared to the SSRIs.

Tricyclic antidepressants lack evidence-based data and have significant cardiac risks, including arrhythmias, and they are not recommended as first or second line treatments for depression in youth.

About 60% of youth with major depression respond to adequate trials of an antidepressant agent and/or psychotherapy, which leaves about 40% resistant to evidence-based treatments. It is important to note that expected response to SSRI antidepressant agents varies with the age group of the depressed patients being treated. Young children and older adults, as a group, have less robust responses to SSRI agents in the treatment of major depression. Age-dependent group differences in response rates to SSRIs in the treatment of major depression may be related to environmental factors, such as influences of family and social factors. In addition, there may be neurobiologic differences between the emergence of early-onset major depression as compared to onset in adulthood.

Ketamine is being investigated for treatment-resistant depression in adolescents. In an open label study, 13 adolescents received intravenous ketamine infusion and 38% met criteria for clinical response. In a double-blind cross-over trial that included 17 adolescents with treatment resistant depression, single dose intravenous ketamine was shown to be significantly superior to midazolam on depression rating scores. Response rates were 76% for ketamine versus 35% for midazolam. Ketamine was associated with transient dissociative symptoms.

Transcranial magnetic stimulation (TMS) has been investigated in open studies which have suggested some effectiveness for treatment resistant depression in adolescents. However, a recent double-blind randomized sham-controlled trial did not demonstrate superiority of 10-Hz TMS compared to sham TMS for adolescents with treatment-resistant depression. Response rates were 41.7% for active TMS and 36.4% for sham treatment.

FDA Warning and Suicidality. In September 2004, the FDA received information from their Psychopharmacologic Drug and Pediatric Advisory Committee indicating an increased risk of suicidality in those children who were on active antidepressant medications, based on their review of reported suicidal thoughts and behavior among depressed children and adolescents who participated in RCTs with nine different antidepressants. Although there were no suicides, the rates of suicidal thinking and behaviors were 2% for patients on placebo, versus 4% among patients on antidepressant medications. The FDA, following the recommendation of their advisory committees, instituted a "black box" warning to the health professional label of all antidepressant medication indicating the increased risk of suicidal thoughts and behaviors in children and adolescents, and the need for close monitoring for these symptoms. Several reviews since 2004, however, concluded that the data do not indicate a significant increase in the risk of suicide or serious suicide attempts after starting treatment with antidepressant drugs.

Duration of Treatment. Based on available longitudinal data and the natural history of major depression in children and adolescents, current recommendations include maintaining antidepressant treatment for 1 year in a depressed child who has achieved a good response, and to then discontinue the medication at a time of relatively low stress for a medication-free period.

Pharmacologic Treatment Strategies for Resistant Depression. Pharmacologic recommendations for a depressed youth who does not respond to the first SSRI agent prescribed is to switch to another SSRI agent. This recommendation is based on the expert consensus well as the expert consensus and the results of the TORDIA. The TORDIA study protocol offered treatment with a second SSRI agent to youth who did not respond to their first SSRI medication. If a second SSRI was not effective, augmentation strategies or a trial of an antidepressant agent from another class of medications were offered.

Electroconvulsive Therapy

Electroconvulsive therapy (ECT) is rarely used for adolescents, although published case reports indicate its efficacy in adolescents with depression and mania. Currently, case reports suggest that ECT may be a relatively safe and useful treatment for adolescents who have persistent severe affective disorders, particularly with psychotic features, catatonic symptoms, or persistent suicidality.

EPIDEMIOLOGY

Depressive disorders increase in frequency with increasing age in the general population. Mood disorders among preschool-age children are estimated to occur in about 0.3% of community samples, and 0.9% in clinic settings. The prevalence of major depression in school-age children is 2% to 3%. Depression in referred samples of school-age children occurs at the same frequency in boys as in girls, with some surveys indicating a slightly increased rate among boys. In adolescents, the prevalence rate of major depression is from 8% to 12% and two to three times more likely in females than males. By age 18 years, the cumulative incidence of major depression is 20%. Children with a family history of major depression in a first-degree relative are about three times more likely to develop the disorder than those without family histories of affective disorders. The prevalence of persistent depressive disorder in children ranges from 0.6% to 4.6% and in adolescence increases to 1.6% to 8%. Children and adolescents with persistent depressive disorder have a high likelihood of developing major depressive disorder at some point after 1 year of persistent depressive disorder. The rate of developing a major depression on top of persistent depressive disorder (double depression) within 6 months of persistent depressive disorder is estimated to be about 9.9%.

Among psychiatrically hospitalized children and adolescents, the rates of major depressive disorder are close to 20% for children and 40% for adolescents.

ETIOLOGY

Considerable evidence indicates that the clinical features of major depression in youth are extremely similar to those in adults. However, given the less robust response to SSRI antidepressants in the treatment of early-onset major depression compared to that of adults 21 to 35 years of age, it is likely that the combined neurobiology of early-onset major depression as well as the environmental variables may contribute to these differences.

SUICIDE

In the United States, suicide is the second leading cause of death among children and adolescents aged 10 to 19 years, after accidental death. Throughout the world, suicide rarely occurs in children who have not reached puberty. In the last 15 years, the rates of both completed suicide and suicidal ideation have decreased among adolescents. This decrease appears to coincide with the increase in SSRI medications prescribed to adolescents with mood and behavioral disturbance.

Suicidal Ideation and Behavior

Suicidal thoughts or suicidal ideation may wax and wane and can vary in nature from passive thoughts of death (e.g., I would be better off dead, or I wish to die), to active suicidal ideation (e.g., I would like to kill myself, I would like to jump off a building), to suicidal ideation with a plan and intent (e.g., I plan to kill myself by hanging myself, I plan to kill myself by swallowing a bottle of pills).

Suicidal ideation, gestures, and attempts are frequently, but not necessarily, associated with depressive disorders. Reports indicate that as many as half of suicidal individuals express suicidal intentions to a friend or a relative within 24 hours before enacting suicidal behavior.

Suicidal ideation occurs in all age groups and with the highest frequency in children and adolescents with severe mood disorders. More than 12,000 children and adolescents are hospitalized in the United States each year because of suicidal threats or behavior, but completed suicide is rare in children younger than 12 years of age. A young child is rarely capable of designing and carrying out a realistic suicide plan. Cognitive immaturity seems to play a protective role in preventing even children who wish they were dead from committing suicide. Completed suicide occurs about five times more often in adolescent boys than in girls, although the rate of suicide attempts is at least three times higher among adolescent girls than among boys. Suicidal ideation is not a static phenomenon; it can wax and wane frequently with time.

The decision to engage in suicidal behavior may be made impulsively without much forethought, or the decision may be the culmination of prolonged rumination.

When assessing acute risk for suicide, factors that must be assessed urgently are those that increase distress and impulsivity and the availability and plan to use a lethal method. High levels of distress often accompany hopelessness, mixed and irritable bipolar states, agitation, psychosis, emotion dysregulation, anxiety and panic, and significant insomnia.

The method of the suicide attempt influences the morbidity and completion rates, independent of the severity of the intent to die at the time of the suicidal behavior. The most common method of completed suicide in children and adolescents is the use of firearms, which accounts for about two-thirds of all suicides in boys and almost one-half of suicides in girls. The second most common method of suicide in boys, occurring in about one-fourth of all cases, is hanging; in girls, about one-fourth commit suicide through the ingestion of toxic substances. Carbon monoxide poisoning is the next most common method of suicide in boys, but it occurs in less than 10%; suicide by hanging and carbon monoxide poisoning are equally frequent among girls and account for about 10% each. Additional risk factors in suicide include a family history of suicidal behavior, exposure to family violence, impulsivity, substance abuse, and availability of lethal methods. Gender differences in nonfatal suicidal behavior among ninth-grade adolescents in a survey of students in 100 high schools found that 19.8% of female students had serious suicidal thoughts, and 10.8% of females attempted suicide. In male students, 9.3% had a history of suicidal thoughts, and 4.9% attempted suicide. In this study, female students showed evidence of higher levels of mood and anxiety problems, whereas males had a slightly higher level of disruptive behavior problems. Female students reported higher levels of depression, anxiety, somatic complaints, and increased levels of emotional and behavioral problems than males. In young adolescents, even without meeting full criteria for psychiatric disorders, females report more psychopathology along with a higher likelihood of nonfatal suicidal behavior.

Diagnosis and Clinical Features of Suicidality

The characteristics of adolescents who attempt suicide and those who complete suicide are similar. Up to 40% of youth who report a plan to attempt suicide have made a previous attempt. Direct questioning of children and adolescents about suicidal thoughts is necessary because studies have consistently shown that caregivers are frequently unaware of these ideas in their children. Suicidal thoughts (i.e., children talking about wanting to harm themselves) and suicidal threats (e.g., children stating that they want to jump in front of a car) are more common than suicide completion.

Most older adolescents with suicidal behavior meet the criteria for one or more psychiatric disorders, often including major depressive disorder, bipolar disorder, and psychotic disorders. Youth with mood disorders in combination with substance abuse and a history of aggressive behavior are at particularly high risk for suicide. The most common precipitating factors in younger adolescent suicide completers appear to be impending disciplinary actions, impulsive behavioral histories, and access to loaded guns, particularly in the home. Adolescents without mood disorders with histories of disruptive and violent, aggressive, and impulsive behavior may be susceptible to suicide during family or peer conflicts. High levels of hopelessness, poor problem-solving skills, and a history of aggressive behavior are risk factors for suicide. A less common profile of an adolescent who completes suicide is one of high achievement and perfectionistic character traits facing a perceived failure, such an academically proficient adolescent humiliated by a poor grade on an examination.

Findings from a World Health Organization mental health survey revealed that a range of psychiatric disorders increases the risk of suicidal ideation across the lifespan. Youth with psychiatric disorders characterized by severe anxiety and poor impulse control are at higher risk to act on suicidal ideation. In psychiatrically disturbed and vulnerable adolescents, suicide behavior may represent impulsive responses to recent stressors. Typical precipitants of suicidal behavior include conflicts and arguments with family members and boyfriends or girlfriends. Alcohol and other substance use can further predispose an already vulnerable adolescent to suicidal behavior. In other cases, an adolescent attempts suicide in anticipation of punishment after being caught by the police or other authority figures for a forbidden behavior.

About 40% of youth who complete suicide had previous psychiatric treatment, and about 40% had made a previous suicide attempt. A child who has lost a parent by any means before age 13 is at higher risk for mood disorders and suicide. The precipitating factors include loss of face with peers, a broken romance, school difficulties, unemployment, bereavement, separation, and rejection. There are reports of clusters of suicides that occur among adolescents who know one another and go to the same school. Suicidal behavior can precipitate other such attempts within a peer group through identification—so-called copycat suicides. Some studies have found a transient increase in adolescent suicides after television programs in which the central theme was the suicide of a teenager.

In general, although imitation may play a role in the timing of suicide attempts by vulnerable adolescents, the overall suicide rate does not seem to increase over time when media exposure increases. Direct exposure to peer suicide increases the risk of depression and PTSD syndromes rather than suicide.

Treatment of Suicidality

The prognostic significance of suicidal ideation and behaviors in adolescents is complex and ranges from relatively low lethality to high risk for completion. One of the challenges in addressing suicide is to identify children and adolescents with suicidal ideation, and particularly those who have untreated psychiatric disorders, as the risk of completed suicide increases with age, as does the onset of an untreated psychiatric disorder. Clinicians should always evaluate adolescents who come to medical attention because of suicidal attempts to determine whether hospitalization is necessary. Pediatric patients who present to the emergency room with suicidal ideation benefit from an intervention that occurs in the emergency room to ensure that the patient is transitioned to outpatient care when hospitalization is not necessary. We should hospitalize youths who fall into high-risk groups until acute suicidality is no longer present. Adolescents at higher risk include those who have made previous suicide attempts, especially with a lethal method, males older than 12 years of age with histories of aggressive behavior or substance abuse, use of a lethal method, and severe major depressive disorder with social withdrawal, hopelessness, and persistent suicidal ideation.

Relatively few adolescents evaluated for suicidal behavior in a hospital emergency room subsequently receive ongoing psychiatric treatment. Factors that may increase the probability of psychiatric treatment include psychoeducation for the family in the emergency room, diffusing acute family conflict, and setting up an outpatient follow-up during the emergency room visit. Emergency room discharge plans often include providing an alternative if suicidal ideation recurs and a telephone hotline number for the adolescent and the family in case suicidal ideation reappears.

Scant data exist to evaluate the efficacy of various interventions in reducing suicidal behavior among adolescents. CBT alone and in combination with SSRIs decreased suicidal ideation in depressed adolescents over time in the TADS, a large multisite study; however, these interventions do not work immediately, so we should take safety precautions for high-risk situations. Dialectical behavior therapy (DBT), a long-term behavioral intervention useful for individuals or groups of patients, can reduce suicidal behavior in adults, but there are no significant studies in adolescents. Components of DBT include mindfulness training to improve self-acceptance, assertiveness training, instruction on avoiding situations that may trigger self-destructive behavior, and increasing the ability to tolerate psychological distress. This approach warrants investigation among adolescents.

Given the reduction in completed suicide among adolescents over the last decade, during the same period in which SSRI treatment in the adolescent population has markedly risen, SSRIs may have been instrumental in this effect. Given the risk of the increased rate of suicidal thoughts and behaviors among depressed children and adolescents (indicated in RCTs with antidepressant medications and leading to the "black box" warning for all antidepressants for depressed youth), we must closely monitor youths for increased suicidality while taking antidepressants.

Epidemiology of Suicidality

Deaths by suicide among youth are much rarer than suicidal behavior, they were reported to occur in 10.5/100,000 of adolescents aged 15 to 19 in 2019, and 2.57/100,000 of youth aged 10 to 14 in 2019. Suicide remains the second leading cause of death for children and youth aged 10 to 24. The reported rate of death by suicide in children aged 5 to 9 years is variable, with some reports indicating it to be 0.04/100,000 in children. The variability in reported rates may be in part because suicide deaths in this age range are often not listed by coroners or medical examiners as suicide, who may believe that children younger than 10 years old may not appreciate the seriousness of suicide, despite the evidence that children as young as 5 years old do die by suicide. Further, even in older children and adolescents, the cause of death by suicide is often misclassified as unintentional accident.

Etiology of Suicidality

Universal features in adolescents who resort to suicidal behaviors are the inability to find effective solutions to ongoing problems and the lack of coping strategies to deal with immediate crises. A sense of hopelessness and inability to improve their circumstances may contribute to a decision to act on suicidal thoughts.

Genetic Factors. Completed suicide and suicidal behavior are two to four times more likely to occur in individuals with a first-degree family member with similar behavior. Family suicide risk studies support a genetic contribution to suicidal behavior. There is also a higher concordance for suicide among monozygotic twins compared to dizygotic twins. Studies have investigated the possible contributions of the short allele of the serotonin transporter promoter polymorphism (5-HTTLPR) to suicidal behaviors, although, to date, the evidence has not been consistent. Current studies are seeking to investigate correlations between genetic vulnerability and environment and timing interactions as multiple variables that may interact to increase the risk of suicidal behavior.

Biologic Factors. Investigators have found a relationship between altered central serotonin with suicide as well as impulsive aggression. Studies document a reduction in the density of serotonin transporter receptors in the prefrontal cortex and serotonin receptors among individuals with suicidal behaviors. Postmortem studies in adolescents who have completed suicide show the most significant alterations in the prefrontal cortex and hippocampus, brain regions that are also associated with emotion regulation and problem-solving. These studies have found altered serotonin metabolites, alteration in 5-HT2A binding, and decreased activity of protein kinase A and C. Decreased levels of the serotonin metabolite 5-hydroxyindoleacetic acid (5-HIAA) are found in the cerebrospinal fluid (CSF) of depressed adults who attempted suicide by violent methods. Meta-analyses suggest an association between the short S-allele of the serotonin transporter promoter gene and depression as well as suicidal behavior, particularly when combined with adverse life events.

Psychosocial Factors. Although severe major depressive illness is the most significant risk factor for suicide, increasing its risk by 20%, many severely depressed individuals are not suicidal. A sense of hopelessness, impulsivity, recurrent substance use, a history of aggressive behavior, and access to a lethal method are associated with an increased risk of suicide. Exposure to violent and abusive homes results in a wide range of psychopathological symptoms. Aggressive, self-destructive, and suicidal behaviors seem to occur with the greatest frequency among youth who have endured chronically stressful family lives. The most significant family risk factor for suicidal behavior is maltreatment, including physical and sexual abuse and neglect. The single largest association is between sexual abuse and suicidal behavior. Large community studies have provided data suggesting that youth at risk for suicidal behavior include those who feel disconnected, isolated, or alienated from peers. Sexual orientation with peer and/or family rejection, isolation, and discrimination is a risk factor, with increased rates of suicidal behavior of two to six times among youth who identify themselves as gay, lesbian, bisexual, or transgender. Protective factors mitigating the risk of suicidal behavior are youth who have a secure connection to school, peers, and family even in the face of other risk factors.

Further Readings

Ayvaci ER, Croarkin PE. Special populations: treatment-resistant depression in children and adolescents. *Psychiatr Clin North Am.* 2023;46(2):359–370.

Bayer JK, Rapee RM, Hiscock H, Ukoumunne OC, Mihalopoulos C, Wake M. Translational research to prevent internalizing problems in early childhood. *Depress Anxiety.* 2011;28(1):50–57.

Brent D, Emslie G, Clarke G, et al. Switching to another SSRI or to venlafaxine with or without cognitive behavioral therapy for adolescents with SSRI-resistant depression: the TORIDA randomized controlled trial. *JAMA.* 2008:299(8):901–913.

Christiansen E, Larsen KJ. Young people's risk of suicide attempts after contact with a psychiatric department—a nested case-control design using Danish register data. *J Child Psychol Psychiatry.* 2011;52:102.

Correll CU, Kratocvil CJ, March JS. Developments in pediatric psychopharmacology: focus on stimulants, antidepressants, and antipsychotics. *J Clin Psychiatry.* 2011;72(5):655–670.

Daly M. Prevalence of depression among adolescents in the U.S. from 2009 to 2019: analysis of trends by sex, race/ethnicity, and income. *J Adolesc Health.* 2022;70(3):496–499.

Field T. Prenatal depression effects on early development: a review. *Infant Behav Dev.* 2011;34(1):1–14.

Frodl T, Reinhold E, Koutsoulieris N, et al. Childhood stress, serotonin transporter gene and brain structures in major depression. *Neuropsychopharmacology.* 2010;35(6):1383–1390.

Harro J, Kiive E. Droplets of black bile? Development of vulnerability and resilience to depression in young age. *Psychoneuroendocrinology.* 2011;36(3):380–392.

Hetrick SE, McKenzie JE, Bailey AP, et al. New generation antidepressants for depression in children and adolescents: a network meta-analysis. *Cochrane Database Syst Rev.* 2021;5(5):CD013674.

Hughes CW, Emslie GJ, Crimson ML, et al; The Texas Consensus Conference Panel on Medication Treatment of Childhood Major Depressive Disorder. Texas Children's Medication Algorithm Project: update from Texas Consensus Conference Panel on medication treatment of childhood major depressive disorder. *J Am Acad Child Adolesc Psychiatry.* 2007;46(6):667–686.

Kaess M, Parzer P, Haffner J, et al. Explaining gender differences in non-fatal suicidal behavior among adolescents: a population-based study. *BMC Public Health.* 2011;11:597–603.

Luby J, Lenze S, Tillman R. A novel early intervention for preschool depression: findings from a pilot randomized controlled trial. *J Child Psychol Psychiatry.* 2012;53(3):313–322.

March J, Silva S, Petrycki S, et al. The Treatment for Adolescents with Depression Study (TADS): long-term effectiveness and safety outcomes. *Arch Gen Psychiatry.* 2007;64(10):1132–1143.

Newton AS, Hamm MP, Bethell J, et al. Pediatric suicide-related presentations: a systematic review of mental health care in the emergency room department. *Ann Emerg Med.* 2010;56(6):649–659.

Nock MK, Hwang I, Sampson N, et al. Cross-national analysis of the associations among mental disorders and suicidal behavior: findings from the WHO World Mental Health Surveys. *PLoS Med.* 2009;6(8):1–13.

Olfson M, Shaffer D, Marcus SC, Greenberg T. Relationship between antidepressant medication treatment and suicide in adolescents. *Arch Gen Psychiatry.* 2003;60(10):978–982

Rosso IM, Cintron CM, Steingard RJ, Renshaw PF, Young AD, Yurgelun-Todd DA. Amygdala and hippocampus volumes in pediatric major depression. *Biol Psychiatry.* 2005;57(1):21–26

Singh MK, Gorelik AJ, Stave C, Gotlib IH. Genetics, epigenetics, and neurobiology of childhood-onset depression: an umbrella review. *Mol Psychiatry.* 2024;29(3):553–565.

Strawn JR, Mills JA, Suresh V, et al. The impact of age on antidepressant response: a mega-analysis of individuals with major depressive disorder. *J Psychiatr Res.* 2023;159:266–273.

Turecki G, Brent DA, Gunnell D, et al. Suicide and suicide risk. *Nature Reviews Disease Primers.* 2019;5(1):74.

von Knorring AL, Olsson GI, Thomsen PH, Lemming OM, Hulten A. A randomized, double-blind, placebo-controlled study of citalopram in adolescents with major depressive disorder. *J Clin Psychopharmacol.* 2006;26(3):311–315.

Wagner KD. Pharmacotherapy for major depression in children and adolescents. *Prog Neuropsychopharmacol Biol Psychiatry.* 2005;29(5):819–826.

Wagner KD. Depressive disorders and suicide in children and adolescents. In: Sadock BJ, Sadock VA, Ruiz P, eds. *Kaplan & Sadock's Comprehensive Textbook of Psychiatry.* 9th ed. Vol. 2. Wolters Kluwer Health/Lippincott Williams & Wilkins; 2009.

Walter HJ, Abright AR, Bukstein OG, et al. Clinical practice guideline for the assessment and treatment of children and adolescents with major and persistent depressive disorders. *J Am Acad Child Adolesc Psychiatry.* 2023;62(5):479–502.

Weigle PE, Shafi RMA. Social media and youth mental health. *Curr Psychiatry Rep.* 2024;26(1):1–8.

Whittington CJ, Kendall T, Fonagy P, Cottrell D, Cotgrove A, Boddington E. Selective serotonin reuptake inhibitors in childhood depression: systematic review of published versus unpublished data. *Lancet.* 2004;363(9418):1341–1345.

Wilson S, Dumornay NM. Rising rates of adolescent depression in the United States: challenges and opportunities in the 2020s. *J Adolesc Health.* 2022;70(3):354–355.

Zalsman G. Timing is critical: gene, environment and timing interactions in genetics of suicide in children and adolescents. *Eur Psychiatry.* 2010;25(5):284–286.

12

Early-Onset Bipolar Disorder

Early-onset bipolar disorder refers to children and adolescents who are diagnosed with bipolar disorder before the age of 18 years. Early-onset bipolar disorder has been studied in some epidemiologic and treatment studies in two subgroups: prepubertal children diagnosed by 12 years of age, and adolescents diagnosed at the age of 13 years or older. Bipolar disorder in prepubertal children 12 years and younger is a rare disorder, whereas it more frequently emerges in adolescents and resembles adult bipolar disorder more closely. Over the past two decades, there was a significant increase in the diagnosis of bipolar I disorder made in youth referred to psychiatric outpatient clinics and inpatient units. Questions and controversy emerged among clinicians and researchers regarding the phenotype of bipolar disorder, particularly in prepubertal youth, mainly due to bipolar disorder diagnoses made in children with persistent irritability and mood dysregulation and lack of discrete mood episodes. These "atypical" or wide definitions of bipolar symptoms among prepubertal children often include extreme mood dysregulation, severe temper tantrums, intermittent aggressive or explosive behavior, and high levels of distractibility and inattention. This constellation of mood and behavior disturbance in the majority of prepubertal children with a current diagnosis of bipolar disorder is nonepisodic, although fluctuation of irritability and temper outbursts occur. Follow-up studies of prepubertal children with nonepisodic severe mood dysregulation and irritability reveal that the majority of these children do not develop classic bipolar disorder, instead, as they grow older, symptoms of anxiety and depressive symptoms persisted. The high frequency of the chronic, severe irritability and temper outbursts in children who did not develop typical bipolar disorder led to the inclusion of a new mood disorder in youth, which was first included in DSM-5, and currently included in DSM-5-TR, named *Disruptive Mood Dysregulation Disorder*. (Please see Chapter 13 for more information about this disorder.) It was observed that many children with nonepisodic mood dysregulation and irritability have previous diagnoses of Attention-Deficit/Hyperactivity Disorder (ADHD). Family studies of children with ADHD have not revealed an increased rate of bipolar I disorder. Children with "atypical" bipolar disorders, however, are frequently severely impaired, are challenging to manage in school and at home, and may even require psychiatric hospitalization. In another study, investigators followed 84 children with "severe mood dysregulation" who also had at least three manic symptoms plus distractibility for approximately 2 years. The investigators found that only one child experienced a hypomanic or mixed episode. Although childhood severe mood dysregulation is common in community samples—one study reported a lifetime prevalence of 3.3% in youth 9 to 19 years of age—its relationship to future bipolar disorder remains questionable. A longitudinal community-based study that followed children and adolescents with nonepisodic irritability over 20 years found that these children were at higher risk for depressive disorders and generalized anxiety disorder than bipolar disorders.

Among adults and older adolescents with bipolar disorder who present with classic manic episodes, a major depressive episode typically precedes a manic episode. A classic manic episode in an adolescent, like in a young adult, typically emerges as a distinct departure from a preexisting state often characterized by grandiose and paranoid delusions and hallucinatory phenomena. According to DSM-5-TR, the criteria for a manic episode in children and adults are the same.

When mania emerges in an adolescent, there is a higher incidence of psychotic features, including delusions and hallucinations, which most typically involve grandiose notions about their power and worth, than in adults. Persecutory delusions and flight of ideas are not uncommon. Significant impairment of reality testing is common in adolescent manic episodes. In adolescents with major depressive disorder which precedes a manic episode and a diagnosis of bipolar I disorder, those at highest risk have family histories of bipolar I disorder and exhibit more acute, severe depressive episodes with higher incidence of psychosis, hypersomnia, and psychomotor retardation.

DIAGNOSIS AND CLINICAL FEATURES

Early-onset bipolar disorder uses the same diagnostic criteria in DSM-5-TR that is used in adults. Children diagnosed with early-onset bipolar disorder using a broader, nonepisodic set of symptoms than delineated in DSM-5-TR, may fit more accurately into the newer diagnosis of disruptive mood dysregulation disorder. This group of children displays severe mood dysregulation, irritability, and explosive outbursts. Irritability persists in between outbursts. It is rare for a prepubertal child to exhibit grandiose thoughts or euphoric mood; for the most part, children diagnosed with early-onset bipolar disorder are intensely emotional with a fluctuating but overriding negative mood. Current diagnostic criteria for bipolar disorders in children and adolescents in DSM-5-TR are the same as those used in adults. The clinical picture of early-onset bipolar disorder is complicated by the prevalence of comorbid psychiatric disorders including ADHD, anxiety, and disruptive behavior disorders. Tables 12-1 and 12-2 show the comparative diagnostic criteria for bipolar disorder type 1 and type 2, respectively, in the DSM-5-TR, ICD-10 and ICD-11.

Pathology and Laboratory Examination

No specific laboratory indices are currently helpful in making the diagnosis of bipolar disorders among children and adolescents.

DIFFERENTIAL DIAGNOSIS

The most critical clinical entities to distinguish from early-onset bipolar disorder are also the disorders with which it is most frequently comorbid. Included are

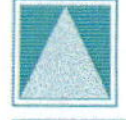

Table 12-1.
Comparative Diagnostic Criteria for Bipolar I Disorder

	DSM-5-TR	ICD-10	ICD-11
Diagnostic name	Bipolar I Disorder	Bipolar Affective Disorder **NOTE*: ICD-10 does not distinguish between bipolar I and II, requiring only a history of discrete episodes of mania, hypomania, and/or depression, with episodes demarcated by switches in mood/affect	Bipolar I Disorder
Duration	Manic episode: 1 wk+ Hypomanic episode: 4 days+ Major depressive episode: 2 wk+	Manic episode: 1 wk+ Hypomanic episode: 4 days+ Major depressive episode: 2 wk+	1 wk+
Symptoms	**Manic or hypomanic episodes** • Abnormally ↑ or irritable mood (required) • Grandiose thoughts • ↓ need for sleep • Pressured speech • Racing and expansive thoughts • Distractibility • Hyperactivity • Impulsivity/high-risk activities **Depressive episodes** Similar to that for major depressive disorder	History of episodes of mania, hypomania, and/or depression Switches in mood/affect **Mania** • Abnormally ↑ or irritable mood (required) • Abnormally elevated or irritable mood • ↑ activity • ↑ talkativeness • flight of ideas/racing thoughts • Social disinhibition • ↓ need for sleep • Grandiose thoughts • Distractibility • Impulsivity/recklessness • Hypersexuality **Hypomania** • Abnormally ↑ mood (required) • Psychomotor agitation • ↑ talkativeness • Poor concentration/distractibility • ↓ need for sleep • Hypersexuality • Impulsivity or ↑ spending • Overfamiliarity **Depressive Episode** • Depressed mood • Loss of interest or pleasure • Decreased energy	**Manic episode** • Extreme mood state (euphoria, irritability, or expansiveness) • ↑ activity • Talkativeness • Flight of ideas • ↑ self-esteem • ↓ need for sleep • Distractibility • Impulsivity • ↑ libido, sociability, or goal-directed activity **Mixed Episode** Several prominent manic and several prominent depressive symptoms

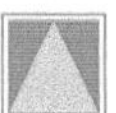

Table 12-1.
Comparative Diagnostic Criteria for Bipolar I Disorder (Continued)

	DSM-5-TR	ICD-10	ICD-11
		Additional symptoms: • Low self-esteem • Excessive guilt or shame • Recurrent thoughts of death or suicide • Poor concentration • Psychomotor changes • Sleep disturbance • Change in appetite and/or weight	
Required number of symptoms	≥1 manic episode Abnormally ↑ or irritable mood (requires 3 of the other symptoms [4 if irritable mood])	**Bipolar affective disorder, current episode hypomanic** Hypomania (elevated mood and ≥3 symptoms) History of a prior affective episode (manic, hypomanic, depressed, mixed) **Bipolar affective disorder, current episode manic** Mania (elevated or irritable mood and ≥3 symptoms [four if irritable mood]) History of prior affective episodes (manic, hypomanic, depressed, mixed) **Bipolar disorder, current episode mild/moderate/ severe depression** Depressive episode (2/3 of the first two symptoms and two more of the additional symptoms) History of prior affective episodes (manic, hypomanic, depressed, mixed) **Bipolar disorder, current episode mixed** A mixture or rapid alternation of hypomanic, manic, and/or depressive symptoms (defined above) History of prior affective episodes (manic, hypomanic, depressed, mixed)	≥1 manic or mixed episode consisting of first two symptoms listed above, plus several of the other symptoms listed
Exclusions	Other medical condition Substance or medication, including withdrawal Other mental illness	Psychoactive substance use Another mental disorder	Other medical condition Substance or medication, including withdrawal
Psychosocial consequences	Manic episode: impaired functioning or needing hospitalization Hypomanic episode: no impairment or need for hospitalization Depressive episode: marked distress and/ or psychosocial impairment		Impairment in ≥1 functional domain, or requiring intensive treatment (hospitalization), or includes hallucinations or delusion
Symptom specifiers	**Mild**—2 symptoms **Moderate**—3 symptoms **Moderate–Severe**—4–5 symptoms **Severe**—4–5 symptoms + motor agitation **With mixed features** Either a depressive or manic/hypomanic episode	**Current episode hypomanic** **Current episode manic without psychotic symptoms** **Current episode manic with psychotic symptoms** **Mood congruent** **Mood incongruent** **Current episode of depression** **Current episode mixed** **Currently in remission**—no symptoms; history of previous episodes	**Current/most recent episode:** Manic Hypomanic Depressive Mixed **With/without psychotic symptoms** **With prominent anxiety symptoms**

(continued)

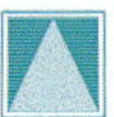

Table 12-1.
Comparative Diagnostic Criteria for Bipolar I Disorder (Continued)

	DSM-5-TR	ICD-10	ICD-11
	Additional symptoms of depressive or manic/hypomanic period (not full criteria) **With rapid cycling** ≥4 mood episodes in 1 yr ≥2-mo period of partial/full remission between episodes **With melancholic features** Similar to that for major depressive disorder **With atypical features** Similar to that for major depressive disorder **With anxious distress:** ≥2 symptoms among the following: • Feeling tense • Restlessness • Difficulty with concentration due to worrying • Excess fear without cause • Fear of loss of control	**With somatic syndrome** ≥4 of the following: • Loss of interest or pleasure • Lack of emotional reactivity • Early morning awakening • Depression gets worse in the mornings • Psychomotor changes • Loss of appetite • Weight loss • Loss of sexual drive	**With panic attacks** **With seasonal pattern** **With rapid cycling** **Associated with pregnancy, childbirth, or the puerperium**
Course specifiers	**With peripartum onset:** episode occurs during pregnancy or within 4 wk after delivery **With seasonal pattern:** pattern present for ≥2 yr		
Severity specifiers		**For the current episode of depression** **Mild:** 4 symptoms **Moderate:** 6 symptoms, including ≥2 among loss of pleasure, depressed mood, and low energy **Severe:** ≥8 symptoms, including all loss of pleasure, depressed mood, and low energy **Without psychotic symptoms** **With psychotic symptoms** **Mood congruent** **Mood incongruent**	**Mild** **Moderate** **Severe** **Unspecified severity**

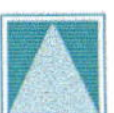

Table 12-2.
Comparative Diagnostic Criteria for Bipolar II Disorder

	DSM-5-TR	ICD-10	ICD-11
Diagnostic name	Bipolar II Disorder	Bipolar Affective Disorder **NOTE:* ICD-10 does not distinguish between Bipolar I and II, requiring only a history of discrete episodes of mania, hypomania, and/or depression, with episodes demarcated by switches in mood/affect.	Bipolar Type II Disorder
Duration	**Hypomanic episode:** lasting ≥4 days, with symptoms present most of the day for most days **Major depressive episode**: symptoms lasting ≥2 wk	Manic episode: lasting ≥1 wk Hypomanic episode: lasting ≥4 days Major depressive episode: symptoms lasting ≥2 wk	Several days
Symptoms	Hypomanic episodes involve abnormally elevated or irritable mood with: • Grandiosity • ↓ need for sleep • Pressured speech • Racing thoughts with expansiveness of thought • Distractibility • Goal-directed or non–goal-directed hyperactivity • Engagement in high-risk activity or ↑ impulsivity Depressive episode involving depressed mood and/or decreased interest/pleasure with: • Unintentional weight loss or change in appetite • Disruption of sleep • Psychomotor changes • Loss of energy • Difficulty with concentration and/or attention • Excessive feelings of worthlessness and/or guilt • Recurrent thoughts of death, including passive and/or active suicidal ideation	History of discrete episodes of mania, hypomania, and/or depression, with episodes demarcated by switches in mood/affect Episodes are defined as follows: **Mania:** abnormally elevated or irritable mood with ≥3 of the following (≥4 if mood irritable) • ↑ activity • ↑ talkativeness • Flight of ideas/racing thoughts • Social disinhibition • ↓ need for sleep • Grandiosity • Distractibility • ↑ recklessness and impulsivity • Hypersexuality **Hypomania:** abnormally elevated mood with ≥3 of the following: • Psychomotor agitation • ↑ talkativeness • Poor concentration or increased distractibility • ↓ need for sleep • Hypersexuality • Impulsivity or ↑ spending • Overfamiliarity Depressive episode: 4 total symptoms from among the following: ≥2: • Depressed mood • Loss of interest or pleasure • Decreased energy Additional symptoms: • Low self-esteem • Excessive guilt or shame • Recurrent thoughts of death or suicide • Poor concentration • Psychomotor changes • Sleep disturbance • Change in appetite and/or weight	**Hypomanic episode** Elevation of mood or irritability outside of the usual mood range Increased activity Talkativeness Flight of ideas ↑ self-esteem ↓ need for sleep Distractibility Impulsivity ↑ libido, sociability, or goal-directed activity **Depressive episode** *See depressive disorders*
Required number of symptoms	Lifetime history of a hypomanic episode involving elevated/irritable mood with ≥3 of the above symptoms (4 if mood irritable)	**Bipolar affective disorder, current episode hypomanic**—meets the above criteria for hypomania (elevated mood with ≥3 listed symptoms) and has a history of prior affective episodes (manic, hypomanic, depressed, mixed)	≥1 hypomanic episode ≥1 depressive episode

(*continued*)

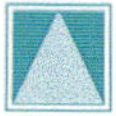

Table 12-2.
Comparative Diagnostic Criteria for Bipolar II Disorder (Continued)

	DSM-5-TR	ICD-10	ICD-11
	Lifetime history of a depressive episode with ≥5 of the above symptoms, which must include ≥1 of depressed mood or loss of pleasure	**Bipolar affective disorder, current episode manic**—meets above criteria for mania (elevated or irritable mood with ≥3–4 listed symptoms) and has a history of prior affective episodes (manic, hypomanic, depressed, mixed) **Bipolar disorder, current episode mixed**—mixture or rapid alteration in hypomanic, manic, and/or depressive symptoms, with symptoms present most of the time for ≥2 wk, in addition to having a history of prior affective episodes (manic, hypomanic, depressed, mixed) **Bipolar disorder, current episode mild/moderate/severe depression**—current symptoms meet criteria for a depressive episode, in addition to having a history of prior affective episodes (manic, hypomanic, depressed, mixed)	
Exclusions	Other medical condition Substance or medication, including withdrawal Other mental illness	Psychoactive substance use Another mental disorder	H/o manic episodes Other medical condition Effect of substance or medication
Psychosocial consequences	Hypomanic episode: NO marked impairment in functioning and NO hospitalization necessitated Depressive episode: marked distress and/or impairment in psychosocial functioning		Does not cause marked functional impairment
Symptom specifiers	**Current episode:** ***Depressed*** ***Hypomanic*** **Additional specifiers to be added to the above:** **With anxious distress:** including ≥2 symptoms among feeling tense, restlessness, difficulty with concentration due to worrying, excessive fear without an identifiable cause, fear of loss of control **With mixed features**—full criteria met for either depressive or manic/hypomanic episode, with additional symptoms of depressive or manic/hypomanic period without also meeting full criteria **With rapid cycling**—the presence of ≥4 mood episodes over the course of a 12-mo period, with ≥2-mo period of partial/full remission between mood episodes	**Current episode hypomanic** **Current episode manic without psychotic symptoms** **Current episode manic with psychotic symptoms** • ***With mood-congruent psychotic symptoms*** • ***With mood-incongruent psychotic symptoms*** **Current episode moderate or mild depression**—≥4 (mild) or 6 (moderate) symptoms present, including ≥2 among loss of pleasure, depressed mood, and low energy **With somatic syndrome**—≥4 of the following: • Loss of interest or pleasure • Lack of emotional reactivity • Early morning awakening • Depression gets worse in the mornings • Psychomotor changes • Loss of appetite • Weight loss • Loss of sexual drive **Without somatic syndrome** **Current episode severe depression without psychotic symptoms**—≥8 symptoms present, including all 3 of loss of pleasure, depressed mood, and low energy **Current episode severe depression with psychotic symptoms**—≥8 symptoms present, including all 3 of loss of pleasure, depressed mood, and low energy, occurring either • ***With mood-congruent psychotic symptoms*** • ***With mood-incongruent psychotic symptoms***	**Current/most recent episode** Hypomanic Depressive **With/without psychotic symptoms** **With prominent anxiety symptoms** **With panic attacks** **With seasonal pattern** **With rapid cycling** **Associated with pregnancy, childbirth, or the puerperium**

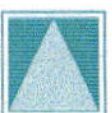

Table 12-2.
Comparative Diagnostic Criteria for Bipolar II Disorder (Continued)

	DSM-5-TR	ICD-10	ICD-11
	With melancholic features—involving loss of pleasure, reduced reactivity with ≥3 of the following: • Depressed mood/despair • Depressive symptoms worse in the morning • Early morning awakening • Psychomotor changes • Loss of appetite/weight loss • Excessive guilt **With atypical features:** during most days, an individual is experiencing mood reactivity with ≥2 symptoms of: • Weight gain or increased appetite • Excessive sleeping • Leaden paralysis • A pattern of heightened interpersonal rejection sensitivity **With mood-congruent psychotic features**—mood-congruent delusions or hallucinations **With mood-incongruent psychotic features**—mood-incongruent delusions or hallucinations **With catatonia**—catatonic features present during most of the mood episode	**Current episode mixed** **Currently in remission**—does not currently meet criteria for an affective episode despite a prior history of a manic or hypomanic episode	
Course specifiers	**With peripartum onset**—full criteria for a mood episode are met during pregnancy or within 4 wk of delivery **With seasonal pattern** (for ≥1 type of episode)—pattern present for ≥2 yr **In partial remission** **In full remission**		
Severity specifiers	**Mild**—few symptoms in excess of minimum diagnostic criteria, with no to minimal impairment and/or distress **Moderate**—moderate symptomatology and impairment **Severe**—symptoms in marked excess of minimum diagnostic requirement, with marked distress and impairment in functioning	See the above criteria for mild, moderate, and severe depression	Mild Moderate Severe
Comments	**Note**: A diagnosis of bipolar II cannot be made if there is a history of a manic episode, in which case a diagnosis of bipolar I disorder would be made.		

ADHD, oppositional defiant disorder, conduct disorder, anxiety disorders, and depressive disorders.

Although childhood ADHD tends to have its onset earlier than pediatric mania, current evidence from family studies supports the presence of ADHD and bipolar disorders as highly comorbid in children, and the concurrence is not because of the overlapping symptoms that the two disorders share. In a recent study of more than 300 children and adolescents who attended a psychopharmacology clinic and received a diagnosis of ADHD, bipolar disorder was also evident in almost one-third of those children with ADHD who had combined type and hyperactive type. It was less frequent (i.e., in less than 10%) in children with ADHD, inattentive type.

COMORBIDITY

ADHD is the most common comorbid condition among youth with early-onset bipolar disorder and occurs in up to 90% of prepubertal children and up to 50% of adolescents diagnosed with bipolar disorder. Comorbid ADHD creates a significant source of diagnostic confusion in children with early-onset bipolar disorder since the two disorders share many diagnostic criteria, including distractibility, hyperactivity, and talkativeness. Even when removing the overlapping symptoms from the diagnostic count, a significant percentage of children with bipolar disorder continued to meet the full criteria for ADHD. This implies that both disorders, with their distinct features, are present in many cases.

Children and adolescents with bipolar disorder have higher-than-expected rates of panic and other anxiety disorders. In youth with the narrow phenotype of bipolar disorders, up to 77% have been diagnosed with an anxiety disorder. The lifetime prevalence of panic disorder was 21% among subjects with the broader phenotype of bipolar disorder compared with 0.8% in those without mood disorders. Patients diagnosed with bipolar disorder who have comorbid high levels of anxiety symptoms are reported as adults to have higher risks of alcohol abuse and suicidal behavior. On the other hand, children who exhibit the broader phenotype of bipolar disorder are at higher risk of going on to have anxiety disorders as well as depressive disorders.

CASE 1—PREPUBERTAL PRESENTATION

Trina is a 9-year-old adopted child who was recently psychiatrically hospitalized after repeated aggressive and assaultive behavior toward her adoptive mother, leaving bruises on her arms and legs from Trina's kicks and punches. Trina has a long history of excessively severe tantrums, comprised of assaultive and self-injurious behavior, since before her parents adopted her at the age of 3 years. Trina was extremely hyperactive and impulsive in school and had been diagnosed and treated for ADHD when she was 6 years old. Trina's more recent psychiatric evaluation as an outpatient led to a diagnosis of early-onset bipolar disorder. Trina has always been irritable and explosive, with a short fuse. It was reported that she had been exposed to alcohol and methamphetamine in utero. Trina had become increasingly hard to manage at home, refused to go to school, yelled and screamed for hours on a daily basis, and often hit and repeatedly kicked her adoptive parents by the time she was 7 years old. During her psychiatric evaluation, the child psychiatrist learned from her adoptive parents that Trina had been born prematurely to a teenage mother and placed in multiple foster homes until she was adopted. Trina was a small girl who appeared younger than her stated age, although her demeanor was bossy and pedantic. Trina's biologic family psychiatric history was unknown, she had at least one stigmata of fetal alcohol syndrome, but her IQ was in the average range. On mental status examination in the hospital, Trina reported that things were fine, that she was not depressed, and that she did not get along with kids her age but that she had a few friends. Trina admitted that she had a bad temper and that she did not remember what she did after she was in a rage. Trina's affect was odd, and she seemed to enjoy having the psychiatrist as her audience. Trina denied suicidal ideation and denied having been a danger to herself or her adoptive parents. Trina became irritable when questioned about the reasons for her current admission. The psychiatric inpatient team recommended a more structured school program, such as a partial hospital or day program. The diagnosis of bipolar disorder remained in question, as she did not meet the narrow phenotype for this disorder. A discharge diagnosis of Disruptive Mood Dysregulation Disorder was made.

CASE 2—ADOLESCENT PRESENTATION

Anna is a 16-year-old junior in high school who has been in psychiatric treatment since the age of 9 years when she was diagnosed and treated for ADHD, which she continued for the next 5 years. Anna had many friends and always got along well with her parents and her younger sister. At the age of 14 years, Anna experienced a sudden severe and debilitating depressive episode leading to an inability to get up in the morning. She stopped going to school, felt slowed down, and stayed in bed all day. Anna believed that her parents were trying to poison her and heard voices telling her that she should die, both of which she kept to herself. Anna's parents were surprised by the change in her behavior since, prior to that, Anna had been a good student and an active and popular teen. Initially, Anna's parents believed that she was just going through an adolescent phase that would pass soon. Anna's ADHD had been under good control and was responsive to Concerta 36 mg for the past 5 years. Anna's Concerta had been discontinued last year because she was a good student without it, and she was having some difficulty with insomnia. Anna's depressive episode, which emerged abruptly, did not pass, and in fact it got worse over the course of a few weeks. Anna experienced suicidal thoughts, and one night she made a suicide attempt by taking a "bunch" of acetaminophen, a few Concerta capsules, and a mix of cold medications she found in the bathroom. Anna came out of the bathroom and, after about 15 minutes, began vomiting. Anna's parents were shocked when she revealed that she had taken a mixture of pills because she was trying to kill herself. Anna's parents called 911 and were relieved to find out that she was medically stabilized in the emergency department and would be admitted to the university hospital adolescent psychiatric inpatient unit. Anna was monitored carefully for persisting or recurrent suicidal ideation, however, after her admission, she reported that she no longer wished to die. For the first week in the hospital, Anna was prescribed aripiprazole 2 mg by mouth per day while a trial of sertraline was initiated. Aripiprazole was discontinued after 2 weeks when sertraline was titrated up to 200 mg/day. Anna seemed to be improving each week after the initiation of sertraline, and she no longer reported delusions or hallucinations. Anna was able to get up and comply with the hospital activities and do some schoolwork, although she was not back to her previous level of energy or euthymic mood. Anna was continuing to improve, however, and she was discharged after 4 weeks and was able to return to school and continue with outpatient treatment. It took Anna about 9 more months to fully recover from her depressive episode. Anna remained on sertraline and saw her psychiatrist and therapist regularly. A few weeks after Anna turned 16 years old, she became increasingly irritable, argumentative, and began to wear heavy makeup and challenged her parents' rules about everything, which was not typical for her. Anna reported that she could not sleep at all, and she was talking faster and more than she usually did. Anna's parents noticed that she was up most of the night on social media and was interacting with both friends and strangers. Anna started to spend a lot of time with a different group of friends and seemed to erratically drop friends and make new ones. Anna began to break rules in school and at home and was extremely belligerent when it was brought to her attention. One night, Anna had secretly arranged online to meet an older man at a neighborhood shopping mall who turned out to be selling drugs and wanted Anna to help him. Anna was alternating between laughing hysterically and yelling at him which led to an angry altercation. The police were called, and Anna continued to laugh and yell incoherently and tried to run into the busy street, so the police placed Anna on a 72-hour hold for danger to self and took her to the nearest emergency department. Anna was placed in restraints when she tried to run out of the hospital and was admitted to the adolescent psychiatric inpatient unit with a diagnosis of mania. Anna's parents were notified. Upon admission, Anna was administered risperidone 0.5 mg to start, which she was willing to take by mouth. Anna displayed a partial response to risperidone 2.5 mg per day. Lithium augmentation was added to Anna's risperidone, starting with 300 mg by mouth twice daily. Anna remained in the hospital for 6 weeks until she was stable enough to be discharged and return to school and usual engagement with family and friends. A diagnosis of bipolar I disorder was made. Anna continued on risperidone and lithium after discharge while she adjusted to home and school.

COURSE AND PROGNOSIS

There are several pathways regarding the course and prognosis of children and adolescents diagnosed with early-onset bipolar disorder or disruptive mood dysregulation disorder. Those who present with severe mood dysregulation prepubertally, without discrete mood cycles, are more likely to develop anxiety and depressive disorders as they mature. Youths who present in adolescence with a recognizable manic episode are most likely to continue to meet the criteria for bipolar I disorder in adulthood. In both cases, long-term impairment is considerable.

A literature review of the long-term course of early-onset bipolar disorder by Cirone and colleagues (2021) found that there was a high degree of diagnostic stability, particularly among adolescents who were diagnosed with a bipolar disorder, within the bipolar spectrum over a period of 10 years. Those diagnosed with bipolar not otherwise specified (NOS) had a tendency to convert to bipolar disorder 1 over time. Significant comorbidity with ADHD, anxiety, and substance abuse was found across many studies, as well as significant impairment in psychosocial and school functioning, despite cognitive function within the average ranges. The persistence of mood symptoms, even at subsyndromic levels, was associated with functional impairment. The data reviewed in this study documented a high rate of suicidal behavior in youth with bipolar disorder. A higher rate of recovery was associated with strongly positive family relationships, which also was associated with lower rates of suicide. This review documented the high rate of suicidal behavior in youth with bipolar disorder. 14.7% of children and adolescents with a diagnosis of early-onset bipolar disorder had reported a suicide attempt over 3.5 years. Cirone and colleagues reported that studies reviewed indicated that 18% to 20% of youth diagnosed with early-onset bipolar disorder reported a suicide attempt over a 5-year period of observation. These reports are consistent with the high rates of suicide attempts made by adults with bipolar illness. In the studies of youth with early-onset bipolar disorder, the suicide attempt rate was reported to be higher among female patients. Suicide attempts in this population were also associated with the presence of depressive symptoms and their severity. A longitudinal study of 263 child and adolescent inpatients and outpatients with bipolar disorder followed for an average of 2 years found that approximately 70% recovered from their index episode within that period. Half of these patients had at least one recurrence of a mood disorder during this time, more frequently a depressive episode than a mania. There were no differences in the rates of recovery for children and adolescents whose diagnosis was bipolar I disorder, bipolar II disorder, or bipolar disorder NOS. However, those whose diagnosis was bipolar disorder NOS had a significantly longer duration of illness before recovery, with less frequent recurrences once they recovered. About 19% of patients changed polarity once per year or less, 61% shifted five or more times per year, about half cycled more than 10 times per year, and about one-third cycled more than 20 times per year. Predictors of more rapid cycling included lower socioeconomic status (SES), presence of lifetime psychosis, and bipolar disorder NOS diagnosis. Over the follow-up period, about 20% of subjects with bipolar II disorder converted to bipolar I disorder, and 25% of the bipolar disorder NOS subjects developed bipolar I disorder or bipolar II disorder during the follow-up period.

Like the natural history of bipolar disorders in adults, children have a wide range of symptom severity in manic and depressed episodes. The more frequent diagnostic conversions from bipolar II disorder to bipolar I disorder among children and adolescents, compared with adults, highlight the lack of stability of the bipolar II disorder diagnosis in youth. This is also the case concerning conversion from bipolar disorder NOS to other bipolar disorders. When bipolar disorder occurs in young children, recovery rates are lower. There is a higher likelihood of mixed states and rapid cycling, and higher rates of polarity changes compared with those who develop bipolar disorders in late adolescence or early adulthood. It is important to note the impact of strongly positive family relationships on the course and prognosis of early-onset bipolar disorder, which are strongly associated with fewer relapses and decreased suicide attempts.

TREATMENT

Treatment of early-onset bipolar disorder incorporates multimodal interventions including pharmacotherapy, psychoeducation, psychosocial interventions with the family, and school interventions to optimize a child's school adjustment and achievement.

Pharmacotherapy

Second-generation antipsychotic (SGA) agents and mood-stabilizing agents, mainly lithium, are the most well-studied agents providing efficacy in the treatment of manic/mixed or depressive episodes in early-onset bipolar disorders. Hobbs and colleagues (2022) reviewed effective pharmacologic agents in the treatment of early-onset bipolar disorder and created an updated algorithm for treatment. Currently, lithium and five SGAs are Food and Drug Administration (FDA) approved in the treatment of early-onset manic and mixed mood episodes. These include risperidone in 2007, aripiprazole and olanzapine in 2008, quetiapine in 2009, and asenapine in 2015. Lurasidone and olanzapine-fluoxetine are FDA approved for the treatment of early onset bipolar disorder, depressed mood.

Table 12-3 shows the SGAs approved by the FDA for either mania and mixed mood states or depressive mood states.

FDA approval of SGAs was based on randomized clinical trials (RCTs) demonstrating efficacy in the treatment of early-onset bipolar disorder. Eight RCTs have shown the efficacy of SGA agents in the treatment of bipolar disorder in youth between the ages of 10 and 17 years. These studies compared an atypical antipsychotic to placebo, or compared an atypical antipsychotic to a mood stabilizer, or added an antipsychotic to a mood-stabilizing agent. The atypical antipsychotics included olanzapine, quetiapine, risperidone, aripiprazole, and ziprasidone. All five of the atypical antipsychotic studies demonstrated significant efficacy in the treatment of early-onset bipolar manic or mixed states. A recent trial comparing quetiapine and valproate found that both were efficacious, but the quetiapine was superior in the speed of its effect. In another trial comparing risperidone and sodium valproate treatment for bipolar disorder in youth, risperidone had more rapid improvement and a higher final reduction in manic symptoms compared to sodium valproate.

Mood-stabilizing agents other than lithium, such as divalproex, carbamazepine, topiramate, and lamotrigine, have not shown sufficiently high efficacy in the treatment

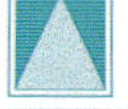

Table 12-3.
FDA-Approved Medications for Early-Onset Bipolar Disorder

Medication	Class	Age Range	Mood Episode
Lithium	Mood stabilizer	7–17 yr	Manic, or mixed episode
Risperidone (Risperdal)	Second-generation antipsychotic	10–17 yr	Manic or mixed episode
Olanzapine (Zyprexa)	Second-generation antipsychotic	10–17 yr	Manic or mixed episode
Aripiprazole (Abilify)	Second-generation antipsychotic	10–17 yr	Manic or mixed episode
Quetiapine (Seroquel)	Second-generation antipsychotic	10–17 yr	Manic or mixed episode
Asenapine (Saphris)	Second-generation antipsychotic	10–17 yr	Manic or mixed episode
Lurasidone (Latuda)	Second-generation antipsychotic	10–17 yr	Depressive episode
Olanzapine-fluoxetine (OFC) (Zyprexa-Prozac)	Second-generation antipsychotic–SSRI antidepressant	10–17 yr	Depressive episode

of early-onset bipolar illness to be considered for FDA approval. In trials using lithium and sodium valproate for the treatment of early-onset bipolar disorder, responses were mixed, with lithium results being less robust compared with atypical antipsychotics. Controlled trials have provided some evidence suggesting that lithium is efficacious in the management of aggression behavior disorders. The Collaborative Lithium Trials (CoLT) established a set of protocols in 2008 to establish the safety and potential efficacy of lithium in youth, and to develop studies to provide evidence-based dosing of lithium for youth. A group of researchers studied the first-dose pharmacokinetics of lithium carbonate in youth and found that clearance and volume correlate with total body weight in youth, and particularly with fat-free mass. The difference in body size was consistent with the pharmacokinetics of lithium metabolism in children and adults. Lithium is currently FDA approved for manic or mixed episodes of early-onset bipolar disorder in children and adolescents of 7 years of age and older. The Treatment of Early-Age Mania (TEAM) study, evaluating lithium, risperidone, and divalproex sodium (divalproex), reported that response rates for children who were switched from either lithium or divalproex sodium to risperidone due to partial or no response, showed a higher response rate than they did to the others. The TEAM study concluded, in 2015, that risperidone appears to be more useful than lithium or divalproex in children with early-onset bipolar disorder, manic/mixed episodes who were partial responders to the other medications. This study provided data which contributed to the FDA approval for risperidone in the treatment of early-onset bipolar disorder manic/mixed episode.

Lurasidone and olanzapine-fluoxetine combination (OFC) are currently FDA approved for depressed episodes of early-onset bipolar disorder in children 10 to 17 years.

Hobbs and colleagues (2022) offer algorithms for the treatment of both manic/mixed and depressive episodes in youth with early-onset bipolar disorder. These algorithms are updated from the 2005 American Academy of Child and Adolescent Psychiatry algorithm for the treatment of early-onset bipolar disorder. A portion of their algorithms in the treatment of manic/mixed episodes in youth without psychosis recommends the following:

- Monotherapy with an FDA-approved SGA (risperidone, aripiprazole, quetiapine, asenapine, or olanzapine).
- If there is no response, switch to another FDA-approved SGA.
- If there is no response to a second FDA-approved SGA and no psychosis present, discontinue the medication, and a trial of lithium is recommended.
- If there is a partial response to the SGA, can augment it with lithium.
- If there is not an increased response with lithium augmentation, possible augmentation with lamotrigine (with a slow titration to minimize the risk of Stevens–Johnson syndrome).

Hobbs and colleagues (2022) offer an updated algorithm for the pharmacologic treatment of depressive episodes in youth with early-onset bipolar disorder. A portion of their algorithm recommends the following:

- Lurasidone is chosen as a first-line treatment for depressive episodes in youth with early-onset bipolar disorder, depressed episode. Lurasidone is chosen over OFC since lurasidone has been reported to have fewer metabolic side effects.
- If lurasidone results in a partial response, it can be augmented with lithium.
- If there is no further improvement with lithium, it can be discontinued and lurasidone can be augmented with lamotrigine.
- If some depressive symptoms still remain with the combination of lurasidone and lamotrigine, a Selective Serotonin Reuptake Inhibitor (SSRI) such as escitalopram or fluoxetine can be added. It is important to monitor carefully for possible manic/mixed switch with the addition of an SSRI.
- If there was no response to lurasidone, OFC can be initiated.
- If partial response is achieved with OFC, it can be augmented with lamotrigine.
- If depression remains without improvement, an SSRI can be initiated with a non–FDA-approved mood stabilizing agent, such as lithium or another SGA.

Current evidence suggests a faster response and a more robust effect with atypical antipsychotics compared to mood-stabilizing agents in the treatment of early-onset bipolar disorder. However, after a youth with early-onset bipolar disorder has been stabilized and recovered from a given mood episode with an SGA agent, to minimize long-term metabolic adverse effects of SGAs, it is recommended to consider tapering it off and initiating lithium as a long-term maintenance treatment.

Psychosocial Treatment

Psychosocial treatment for youth and their families is an important addition to pharmacologic management of early-onset bipolar disorders. Miklowitz and colleagues (2021) provided a review and meta-analysis of psychosocial adjunctive therapies for youth experiencing early-onset bipolar disorder mood episodes and those at risk for the development of bipolar disorder or future recurrences. Effective psychosocial interventions for the prevention of episodes or recurrences were found to be in the form of family or group psychoeducation with guided skills training and tasks to enhance coping skills, monitoring, and managing prodromal symptoms. Effective psychosocial interventions for recovery from moderate or severe depressive or manic symptoms, cognitive restructuring, regulating daily rhythms, and communication training appeared to lead to stabilization.

Family-focused therapy (FFT) is the most well-studied psychosocial intervention for the prevention of recurrence or management of prodromal symptoms. This treatment consists of several sessions of psychoeducation, then sessions focusing on current stressors and a mood management plan, and then several sessions of communication enhancement training and problem-solving skills training. The use of this type of intervention for youths diagnosed with bipolar disorder or at risk for bipolar disorder (by family history or subthreshold symptoms) is of value. Adjunctive family-focused psychoeducational treatment modified for children and adolescents reduces the relapse rate. Children and adolescents treated with mood-stabilizing agents in addition to psychosocial intervention showed improvement in depressive symptoms, manic symptoms, and behavioral disturbance over 1 year.

A year-long trial of a modified Family Focused Treatment–High Risk in youth with bipolar disorder showed significant improvement in mood disturbance, especially depressive mood and hypomania, and improved psychosocial functioning. Family-focused treatment for high-risk youth is a promising intervention that deserves further investigation as a longitudinal follow-up to determine the course of youth at risk to develop bipolar disorder.

EPIDEMIOLOGY

The prevalence rates of bipolar disorder among youth vary significantly depending on the age group studied, and on whether the diagnostic criteria are applied narrowly, restricting it to discrete mood episodes, or more broadly, to include nonepisodic mood dysregulation, explosive behavior, and chronic irritability. Evidence from epidemiologic studies indicates that the risk for onset of bipolar disorder is highest in late adolescence and early adulthood. In younger children, bipolar disorder is rare, with no cases of bipolar I disorder identified in children between the ages of 9 and 13 years by the Great Smokey Mountain Study. However, severe mood dysregulation, explosive tantrums, and irritability, often a prominent feature in prepubertal children who received a diagnosis of bipolar disorder, was found in 3.3% of an epidemiologic sample. Disruptive mood dysregulation disorder was adopted as an alternative diagnosis to bipolar disorder in young children who were previously diagnosed by some as displaying a prepubertal form of bipolar disorder characterized by chronic irritability, severe mood dysregulation, and explosive episodes. In adolescents, bipolar disorder is more frequent, found to range from 0.06% to 0.1% of the general population of 16-year-olds in studies using a narrow definition of bipolar I disorder. The prevalence of subthreshold symptoms of bipolar illness was 5.7% in one study to at least 10% in another. Follow-up studies into adulthood revealed that the subthreshold manic symptoms predicted high levels of impairment with progression to depression and anxiety disorders, not bipolar I or II disorders.

Community use of the diagnosis of bipolar disorder in youth had increased markedly in the early to mid-2000s in both outpatient and inpatient psychiatric settings. One survey suggested there was a 40-fold increase in the diagnosis of early-onset bipolar disorder at outpatient clinics from the 1990s to the 2000s. Longitudinal prospective studies of children diagnosed with the broader nonepisodic form of bipolar disorder have not supported the validity of the diagnosis as leading to bipolar disorder in adolescence or adulthood. In recent times, with the inclusion of disruptive mood dysregulation disorder in DSM-5 and DSM-5-TR, the epidemiologic landscape is changing for identifying early-onset bipolar disorder in prepubertal children.

ETIOLOGY

Genetic Factors

Higher rates of bipolar disorder occur in first-degree relatives of the narrow phenotype of early-onset bipolar disorder compared to adult-onset of bipolar disorder. The high rates of comorbid ADHD among youth with early-onset bipolar disorder, diagnosed before the age of 18 years, have led to questions regarding the cotransmission of bipolar disorder and ADHD in families. Children diagnosed using the broader phenotype of bipolar disorder, that is, severe mood dysregulation, chronic irritability, and explosive outbursts, without discrete episodes of mania, do not have higher rates of bipolar disorder in family members. This suggests that the narrow and broad phenotypes of bipolar disorder are likely to be distinct disorders. Nearly 25% of adolescent offspring of parents diagnosed with bipolar I disorder experience a mood disorder by 17 years old. Most of the risk in the offspring of parents with mood disorders is for unipolar major depressive disorder. Disruptive behavior disorders were increased, in a longitudinal study, in the offspring of families with a member diagnosed with bipolar disorder compared to controls. The combination of ADHD and bipolar disorder comorbidity is not found as frequently in relatives of children with ADHD alone but is increased in offspring of parents with both disorders.

Bipolar disorder is believed to have a significant heritable component, however, its mode of inheritance remains unknown. Several research groups have concluded that early-onset bipolar disorder is a more severe form of the illness, characterized by more mixed episodes, greater psychiatric comorbidity, more lifetime psychotic symptoms, poorer response to prophylactic lithium treatment, and a greater heritability. The European collaborative study of early-onset bipolar disorder (France, Germany, Ireland, Scotland, Switzerland, England, and Slovenia) carried out a genome-wide linkage analysis of both the narrow and the broad phenotype of early-onset bipolar disorder. This group concluded that a genetic factor located in the 2q14 region is either specifically involved in the etiology of early-onset bipolar disorder, or that a gene in this region exerts influence as a modifier of other genes in the development of bipolar disorder in this age group. Other linkage regions that were found by this collaborative did not pertain only to the early-onset group of bipolar disorder, suggesting that there may be some genetic factors common to early-onset and adult-onset bipolar disorder. This conclusion is consistent with the increased incidence of adult-onset bipolar disorder among siblings of early-onset disease. Further genome-wide studies are needed to elucidate the genetic etiology of early-onset bipolar disorder.

Neurobiologic Factors

Converging data suggest that early-onset bipolar disorder is associated with both structural and functional brain alterations in prefrontal cortical and subcortical regions associated with the processing and regulation of emotional stimuli. MRI studies suggest that altered development of white matter and a decreased amygdalar volume are found more frequently in this population than in the general population.

Functional MRI (fMRI) studies are essential in that they can identify altered brain function in vulnerable populations such as youth with early-onset bipolar disorder at baseline. They can also elucidate functional changes toward normalization in brain functioning after various treatments, and potentially identify pretreatment neural predictors of good response to various treatments. An fMRI study of pediatric bipolar patients documented pretreatment brain activity and posttreatment effects of a trial of risperidone versus sodium valproate. This double-blind study included 24 unmedicated manic patients with a mean age of 13 years, randomized to either risperidone or sodium valproate treatment, and 14 healthy controls examined over 6 weeks. Before treatment, the patient group showed increased amygdala activity compared to healthy controls, which was poorly controlled by the higher ventrolateral prefrontal cortex (VLPFC) and the dorsolateral prefrontal cortex (DLPFC), which exert influence on the amygdala to control emotional regulation and processing. Increased amygdala activity at baseline predicted poorer treatment response to both risperidone and sodium valproate in the patient group. Patients were given an affective color-matching word task involving matching positive words (i.e., happiness, achievement, success), negative words (i.e., disappointment, depression, or rejection), or neutral words, with one of two colored circles displayed on a screen while administering the fMRI. Higher pretreatment right amygdala activity during a word task with positive and negative words in the risperidone group and higher pretreatment left amygdala activity with a positive word task in the sodium valproate group predicted a poor response on the Young Mania Rating Scale. Increased amygdala activity in early-onset bipolar patients might be a potential biomarker predicting resistance and poor treatment response to both risperidone and sodium valproate.

Neuropsychologic Studies

Impairments in verbal memory, processing speed, executive function, working memory, and attention are common in early-onset bipolar disorder. Data suggest that on tasks of working memory, processing speed, and attention, youth with comorbid bipolar disorder and ADHD demonstrate more pronounced impairments compared with those without ADHD. Other studies found that children with bipolar disorder make a higher number of emotion recognition errors compared with controls. The children more frequently identified faces as "angry" when presented with adult faces; however, these errors did not occur when they looked at children's faces. Impaired perception of facial expression also occurs in studies of adults with bipolar disorder.

Further Readings

Amerio A, Ossola P, Scagnelli F, et al. Safety and efficacy of lithium in children and adolescents: a systematic review in bipolar illness. *Eur Psychiatry*. 2018;54:85–97.

Arman S, Haghshenas M. Metabolic effects of adding Topiramate on Aripiprazole in bipolar patients aged between 6–18 years, a randomized, double-blind, placebo-controlled trial. *J Res Med Sci*. 2022;27:23.

Barton J, Mio M, Timmins V, Mitchell RHB, Goldstein BI. Prevalence and correlates of childhood-onset bipolar disorder among adolescents. *Early Interv Psychiatry*. 2023;17(4):385–393.

Besag FMC, Vasey MJ, Sharma AN, Lam ICH. Efficacy and safety of lamotrigine in the treatment of bipolar disorder across the lifespan: a systematic review. *Ther Adv Psychopharmacol*. 2021;11:20451253211045870.

Carlson GA. Pediatric bipolar disorder: a recurrent or chronic debate? *Bipolar Disord*. 2022;24(3):229–231.

Carlson GA, Pataki C. Affective disorders with psychosis in youth: an update. *Child Adolesc Psychiatr Clin N Am*. 2020;29(1):91–102.

Chiang KS, Miklowitz DJ. Psychotherapy in bipolar depression: effective yet underused. *Psychiatr Ann*. 2023;53(2):58–62.

Cirone C, Secci I, Favole I, et al. What do we know about the long-term course of early onset bipolar disorder? a review of the current evidence. *Brain Sci*. 2021;11(3):341.

DelBello MP, Kadakia A, Heller V, et al. Systematic review and network meta-analysis: efficacy and safety of second-generation antipsychotics in youths with bipolar depression. *J Am Acad Child Adolesc Psychiatry*. 2022;61(2):243–254.

Duffy A, Carlson G, Dubicka B, Hillegers MHJ. Pre-pubertal bipolar disorder: origins and current status of the controversy. *Int J Bipolar Disord*. 2020;8(1):18.

Findling RL, McNamara NK, Pavuluri M, et al. Lithium for the maintenance treatment of bipolar I disorder: a double-blind, placebo-controlled discontinuation study. *J Am Acad Child Adolesc Psychiatry*. 2019;58(2):287–296.e4.

Goldstein TR, Merranko J, Hafeman D, et al. A risk calculator to predict suicide attempts among individuals with early-onset bipolar disorder. *Bipolar Disord*. 2022;24(7):749–757.

Hobbs E, Reed R, Lorberg B, Robb AS, Dorfman J. Psychopharmacological treatment algorithms of manic/mixed and depressed episodes in pediatric bipolar disorder. *J Child Adolesc Psychopharmacol*. 2022;32(10):507–521.

Janiri D, Moccia L, Montanari S, et al. Use of lithium in pediatric bipolar disorders and externalizing childhood-related disorders: a systematic review of randomized controlled trials. *Curr Neuropharmacol*. 2023;21(6):1329–1342.

Leibenluft E, Kircanski K. Chronic irritability in youth: a reprise on challenges and opportunities toward meeting unmet clinical needs. *Child Adolesc Psychiatr Clin N Am*. 2021;30(3):667–683.

Marazziti D, Mucci F, Falaschi V, Dell'Osso L. Asenapine for the treatment of bipolar disorder. *Expert Opin Pharmacother*. 2019;20(11):1321–1330.
Mathieu F, Dizier M-H, Etain B, et al. European collaborative study of early-onset bipolar disorder: evidence for heterogeneity on 2q14 according to age at onset. *Am J Med Genet B Neuropsychiatr Genet*. 2010;153B(8):1425–1433.
Miklowitz DJ, Efthimiou O, Furukawa TA, et al. Adjunctive psychotherapy for bipolar disorder: a systematic review and component network meta-analysis. *JAMA Psychiatry*. 2021;78(2):141–150.
Miklowitz DJ, Schneck CD, Walshaw PD, et al. Effects of family-focused therapy vs enhanced usual care for symptomatic youths at high risk for bipolar disorder: a randomized clinical trial. *JAMA Psychiatry*. 2020;77(5):455–463.
Miklowitz DJ, Weintraub MJ, Walshaw PD, et al. Early family intervention for youth at risk for bipolar disorder: psychosocial and neural mediators of outcome. *Curr Neuropharmacol*. 2023;21(6):1379–1392.
Parry P, Allison S, Bastiampillai T. 'Pediatric bipolar disorder' rates are still lower than claimed: a re-examination of eight epidemiological surveys used by an updated meta-analysis. *Int J Bipolar Disord*. 2021;9(1):21.
Pataki C, Carlson GA. The comorbidity of ADHD and bipolar disorder: any less confusion? *Curr Psychiatry Rep*. 2013;15(7):372.
Patel RS, Veluri N, Patel J, Patel R, Machado T, Diler R. Second-generation antipsychotics in management of acute pediatric bipolar depression: a systematic review and meta-analysis. *J Child Adolesc Psychopharmacol*. 2021;31(8):521–530.
Post RM, Altshuler LL, Kupka R, et al. Double jeopardy in the United States: Early onset bipolar disorder and treatment delay. *Psychiatry Res*. 2020;292:113274.
Singh MK, Post RM, Miklowitz DJ, et al. A commentary on youth onset bipolar disorder. *Bipolar Disord*. 2021;23(8):834–837.
Stringaris A, Baroni A, Haimm C, et al. Pediatric bipolar disorder versus severe mood dysregulation: risk for manic episodes on follow-up. *J Am Acad Child Adolesc Psychiatry*. 2010;49(4):397–405.
Valizadeh P, Cattarinussi G, Sambataro F, Brambilla P, Delvecchio G. Neuroimaging alterations associated with medication use in early-onset bipolar disorder: an updated review. *J Affect Disord*. 2023;339: 984–997.
Van Meter A, Moreira ALR, Youngstrom E. Updated meta-analysis of epidemiologic studies of pediatric bipolar disorder. *J Clin Psychiatry*. 2019;80(3):18r12180.
Walkup JT, Wagner KD, Miller L, et al. Treatment of early-age mania: outcomes for partial and nonresponders to initial treatment. *J Am Acad Child Adolesc Psychiatry*. 2015;54(12):1008–1019.
Yee CS, Hawken ER, Baldessarini RJ, Vázquez GH. Maintenance pharmacological treatment of juvenile bipolar disorder: review and meta-analyses. *Int J Neuropsychopharmacol*. 2019;22(8):531–540.

13

Disruptive Mood Dysregulation Disorder

Disruptive mood dysregulation disorder (DMDD), according to the DSM-5-TR, describes recurrent severe, developmentally inappropriate temper outbursts which occur at least three times per week, along with a persistently irritable or angry mood between temper outbursts (Table 13-1). The disorder is not diagnosed in children less than 6 years of age, and symptoms must be present for at least a year, with the onset of symptoms by the age of 10 years. Prior to its first inclusion in the DSM-5 in 2013, clinicians often diagnosed children displaying persistence of DMDD symptoms with bipolar disorder or a combination of oppositional defiant disorder (ODD), attention deficit hyperactivity disorder (ADHD), and intermittent explosive disorder. Longitudinal data suggest that these children do not typically develop classic bipolar disorder in late adolescence or early adulthood. Instead, studies suggest that youth with chronic irritability and severe mood dysregulation are at higher risk for future unipolar depressive disorders and anxiety disorders. Some experts believe that hyperarousal is typically a part of this disorder, but DSM-5-TR does not include it in the diagnostic criteria. Currently, according to DSM-5-TR, neither bipolar disorder, ODD, nor intermittent explosive disorder may be diagnosed along with DMDD.

DIAGNOSIS AND CLINICAL FEATURES

The DSM-5-TR diagnostic criteria for DMDD require outbursts that appear to be grossly out of proportion to the situation. Children with these temper outbursts present with verbal rages or physical aggression toward people and/or property and are inappropriate for the child's

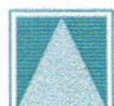

Table 13-1.
Disruptive Mood Dysregulation Disorder

	DSM-5-TR	ICD-10	ICD-11
Diagnostic name	Disruptive Mood Dysregulation Disorder	Other Persistent Mood (Affective) Disorders	Oppositional Defiant Disorder with Chronic Irritability-Anger, Unspecified
Duration	Outbursts occurring ≥3 times per week for a duration of ≥12 mo, during which there was no period greater than 3 mo during which all symptom criteria were not met		
Symptoms	Recurrent verbal or physical outbursts out of proportion to the triggering event Not consistent with expected response per developmental level Mood between outbursts is irritable or mad most of the time		
Required number of symptoms	All of the above		
Exclusions	<6 yr—diagnosis before age 6 >10 yr—symptoms beginning after age 10 Other medical condition Substance or medication, including withdrawal Other mental illness Cannot co-occur with: • Oppositional defiant disorder • Intermittent explosive disorder • Bipolar disorder		

developmental level. Temper outbursts occur, on average, three or more times per week, with variations in mood between outbursts, but with a persistence of negative mood. Symptoms must emerge before age of 10 years, be present for at least 12 months, and occur within at least two settings (i.e., home and school). This diagnosis is not made in children younger than 6 years or older than 18 years without childhood onset. In between temper outbursts, the child's mood is pervasively irritable and angry; this is observable by others, such as parents, teachers, or peers. A definitive diagnosis of bipolar disorder would take precedence over this one, and DMDD is not diagnosed if these symptoms occur only during a major depressive episode.

Gina, an 11-year-old girl was brought to the emergency department by the local psychiatric mobile response team (PMRT) after they were called by her school. The school was unable to contain her aggressive tantrum in which she was screaming and banging her head while kicking, biting, and throwing things at her teacher. Her rages and inappropriate tantrums were happening more frequently since she entered middle school as a sixth grader this year. Gina was being restrained in the patient room, pounding her hands on the gurney, crying, and yelling "Get me out of here!" when her mother arrived. Gina's mother had bruises on both legs from Gina's kicks, and she appeared distressed. Gina's mother walked away from her daughter who was safely restrained in the emergency department and burst into tears. "I don't know how to deal with her anymore." She told the doctor that, for the past three years, Gina had been having severe recurrent tantrums four to five times per week which were getting more frightening because she was growing fast. "She tantrums like a 4-year-old, and even when she is not having a tantrum, she is perpetually angry and irritable." She reported that Gina had lost all her friends due to her short fuse and frequent verbal and physical outbursts. She was almost always irritable, even on her birthday. Gina's mother kept hoping that, with a little more maturity, Gina would outgrow these tantrums and irritability. Gina's mother now worried that something might be physically wrong with her, but physical examination and routine blood tests revealed no abnormalities. Gina's tantrums had lessened somewhat during the 2-month summer vacation last year, despite the persistence of pervasive negative mood; however, as soon as school resumed, she was back to consistent marked irritability. After an interview with Gina, the doctor determined that she was not acutely suicidal and did not have a plan or intent to harm anyone. However, she required urgent intervention to help her and her family manage the outbursts. Gina calmed down in the emergency room after 2 hours and was discharged to home with urgent referrals to a child and adolescent psychiatrist. This psychiatrist evaluated her, diagnosed DMDD and a comorbid anxiety disorder related to school anxiety, and began a trial of fluoxetine to treat the anxiety and mood dysregulation. Gina also started cognitive-behavioral therapy (CBT) with a clinical psychologist who met with her both individually and with her parents. Gina resisted psychotherapy; however, after several sessions, she began to accept the help and liked her therapist. Gina's parents felt more hopeful than they had in a long time, and they learned that Gina's problems were not "all their fault." After titrating her fluoxetine to 20 mg per day, it became clear that her anxiety and irritability had diminished noticeably. Gina still had problems with peers, and she still had one or two tantrums per week; however, the tantrums were less prolonged and less intense. Gina seemed genuinely happy when a classmate invited her to a birthday party, and she was able to interact successfully with her peers during the party without any conflicts. Gina continues to benefit from CBT, and she remains on fluoxetine 20 mg a day. Gina is still a somewhat moody girl; however, she is doing well in school, has rekindled several friendships, and can participate in family gatherings without a major tantrum.

DIFFERENTIAL DIAGNOSIS

Bipolar Disorder

DMDD is not episodic, yet it has some overlapping symptoms with bipolar disorder. It had been theorized by some clinicians and researchers that the chronic and persistent symptoms of mood disturbance and irritability could be an early developmental presentation of bipolar disorder. Disruptive mood dysregulation, however, does not meet formal diagnostic criteria for mania in bipolar disorder, because irritability in DMDD is chronic and nonepisodic. It has been shown that children with DMDD typically do not develop bipolar disorder in the future, so it is distinguished from even early-onset bipolar disorder.

Oppositional Defiant Disorder

DMDD has some overlapping symptoms with ODD in that they both include irritability, temper outbursts, and anger. ODD includes symptoms of annoyance and defiance, which DMDD does not have. DMDD requires that irritable outbursts be present in at least two settings, whereas ODD requires that they be present in only one setting.

COMORBIDITY

DMDD often co-occurs with symptoms of other psychiatric disorders, although ODD may not be diagnosed concurrently. The most common comorbidities are ADHD (94%), ODD symptoms (84%), anxiety disorders (47%), and major depressive disorder (20%). The relationship of severe mood dysregulation and DMDD to bipolar disorder has been a topic of clinical investigation. DMDD is not episodic and may coexist with ADHD. Current evidence does not support its continuity with an emerging bipolar disorder.

EPIDEMIOLOGY

Most of the epidemiologic data applied to DMDD come from children and adolescents with severe mood dysregulation, which includes hyperarousal symptoms. When

DMDD was included in DSM-5 as a psychiatric disorder, the hyperarousal symptoms were omitted. Because DMDD differs from severe mood dysregulation disorder only in the absence of hyperarousal symptoms, the epidemiologic data from the severe mood dysregulation disorder studies is a useful proxy for DMDD. Severe mood dysregulation has a lifetime prevalence of 3% in children aged 9 to 19 years. Within that percentage, males (78%) are more prevalent than females (22%). The mean age of onset is 5 to 11 years of age.

COURSE AND PROGNOSIS

DMDD is a chronic disorder in children and adolescents. Longitudinal studies thus far have shown that patients with DMDD in childhood have a high risk of progressing to major depressive disorder, dysthymic disorder, and anxiety disorders over time in adulthood.

TREATMENT

The current treatment of disruptive mood dysregulation focuses on symptomatic interventions for anxiety and mood disorders. DMDD also commonly co-occurs with ADHD, so when that is the case, the ADHD can be treated. When DMDD and ADHD are comorbid, selective serotonin reuptake inhibitors (SSRIs) and stimulants would likely be the pharmacologic agents of first choice. There are scant treatment studies of DMDD in the literature. One controlled trial of youths with symptoms of severe mood dysregulation and ADHD symptoms who did not respond to stimulants demonstrated a response to sodium valproate combined with behavioral psychotherapy, as compared to placebo and behavioral psychotherapy. There are treatment studies underway of youth who exhibit symptoms of severe mood dysregulation utilizing an SSRI plus a stimulant compared to a stimulant and placebo.

Psychosocial interventions such as cognitive-behavioral therapy DMDD, and psychosocial interventions targeting children diagnosed with bipolar disorder may be beneficial.

Further Readings

Bhatara VS, Bernstein B, Fazili S. Complementary and integrative treatments of aggressiveness/emotion dysregulation: associated with disruptive disorders and disruptive mood dysregulation disorder. *Child Adolesc Psychiatr Clin N Am*. 2023;32(2):297–315.

Blader JC, Schooler NR, Jensen PS, Pliszka SR, Kafantaris V. Adjunctive divalproex versus placebo for children with ADHD and aggression refractory to stimulant monotherapy. *Am J Psychiatry*. 2009;166(12):1392–1401.

Brænden A, Zeiner P, Coldevin M, Stubberud J, Melinder A. Underlying mechanisms of disruptive mood dysregulation disorder in children: a systematic review by means of research domain criteria. *JCPP Adv*. 2022;2(1):e12060.

Brotman MA, Schmajuk M, Rich BA, et al. Prevalence, clinical correlates, and longitudinal course of severe mood dysregulation in children. *Biol Psychiatry*. 2006;60(9):991–997.

Bruno A, Celebre L, Torre G, et al. Focus on disruptive mood dysregulation disorder: a review of the literature. *Psychiatry Res*. 2019;279:323–330.

Copeland WE, Angold A, Costello J, Egger H. Prevalence, comorbidity, and correlates of DSM-5 proposed disruptive mood dysregulation disorder. *Am J Psychiatry*. 2013;170(2):173–179.

Fristad MA, Verducci JS. Walters K, Young ME. Impact of multifamily psychoeducational psychotherapy in treating children aged 8 to 12 years with mood disorder. *Arch Gen Psychiatry*. 2009;66(9):1013–1021

Gupta M, Gupta N. Disruptive mood dysregulation disorder: does variance in treatment responses also add to the conundrum? The widening gap in the evidence is a signal needing attention. *CNS Spectr*. 2022;27(6):659–661.

Havens JF, Marr MC, Hirsch E. Editorial: from bipolar disorder to disruptive mood dysregulation disorder: challenges to diagnostic and treatment specificity in traumatized youths. *J Am Acad Child Adolesc Psychiatry*. 2022;61(3):364–365.

Hawes MT, Carlson GA, Finsaas MC, Olino TM, Seely JR, Klein DN. Dimensions of irritability in adolescents: longitudinal associations with psychopathology in adulthood. *Psychol Med*. 2020;50(16):2759–2767.

Hendrickson B, Girma M, Miller L. Review of the clinical approach to the treatment of disruptive mood dysregulation disorder. *Int Rev Psychiatry*. 2020;32(3):202–211.

Kircanski K, Craske MG, Averbeck BB, Pine DS, Leibenluft E, Brotman MA. Exposure therapy for pediatric irritability: theory and potential mechanisms. *Behav Res Ther*. 2019;118:141–149.

Laporte PP, Matijasevich A, Munhoz TN, et al. Disruptive mood dysregulation disorder: symptomatic and syndromic thresholds and diagnostic operationalization. *J Am Acad Child Adolesc Psychiatry*. 2021;60(2):286–295.

Leibenluft E, Kircanski K. Chronic irritability in youth: a reprise on challenges and opportunities toward meeting unmet clinical needs. *Child Adolesc Psychiatr Clin N Am*. 2021;30(3):667–683.

Leibenluft E. Severe mood dysregulation, irritability, and the diagnostic boundaries of bipolar disorder in youths. *Am J Psychiatry*. 2011; 168(2):129–142.

Margulies DM, Weintraub S, Basile J, Grover PJ, Carlson GA. Will disruptive mood dysregulation disorder reduce false diagnosis of bipolar disorder in children? *Bipolar Disord*. 2012;14(5):488–496.

Stringaris A, Barona A, Haimm C, et al. Pediatric bipolar disorder versus severe mood dysregulation: risk for manic episodes on follow-up. *J Am Acad Child Adolesc Psychiatry*. 2010;49(4):397–405.

West AE, Pavuluri MN. Psychosocial treatments for childhood and adolescent bipolar disorder. *Child Adolesc Psychiatr Clin N Am*. 2009; 18(2):471–482.

Yearwood EL, Meadows-Oliver M. Mood dysregulation disorders. In: Yearwood EL, Pearson GS, Newland JA, eds. *Child and Adolescent Behavioral Health: A Resource for Advance Practice Psychiatric and Primary Care Practitioners in Nursing*. John Wiley & Sons Inc.; 2012:165.

Zonneyvlle-Bender MJS, Matthys W, van de Wiel NM, Lochman JE. Preventive effects of treatment of disruptive behavior disorder in middle childhood on substance use and delinquent behavior. *J Am Acad Child Adolesc Psychiatry*. 2007;46(1):33–39.

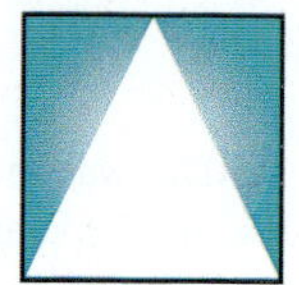

14 Disruptive Behavior Disorders of Childhood: Disruptive, Impulse Control, and Conduct Disorders

Disruptive behaviors, characterized by persistent patterns of oppositional and aggressive behaviors, are among the most frequent reasons for child and adolescent psychiatric evaluations. Displays of impulsive, oppositional, defiant, and aggressive behaviors are developmentally normative in young children of preschool age. Most youths who continue to display oppositional and defiant behavior patterns in middle childhood will find other forms of expression as they mature and no longer demonstrate these behaviors in adolescence or adulthood. The origin of stable patterns of oppositional, defiant, and conduct disordered behavior is widely accepted as a convergence of multiple contributing factors, including biologic, temperamental, learned, and psychological conditions. Risk factors for the development of aggressive behavior in youth include childhood maltreatment such as physical or sexual abuse, neglect, emotional abuse, and overly harsh and punitive parenting.

OPPOSITIONAL DEFIANT DISORDER

Oppositional defiant disorder (ODD) describes enduring patterns of negativistic, disobedient, and hostile behavior toward authority figures, as well as an inability to take responsibility for mistakes, leading to placing blame on others. Children with ODD frequently argue with adults and become easily annoyed by others. Children with ODD may have difficulty in the classroom and with peer relationships, but generally do not resort to physical aggression or significantly destructive behavior.

In contrast, children with conduct disorder engage in repeated acts of aggression, either covertly or overtly, that may cause physical harm to themselves and others and violate the rights of others.

In ODD, a child's temper outbursts, active refusal to comply with rules, and annoying behaviors exceed expectations for these behaviors for children of the same age. The disorder is an enduring pattern of negativistic, hostile, and defiant behaviors in the absence of significant violations of the rights of others.

Diagnosis and Clinical Features

Children with ODD often argue with adults, lose their temper, and are angry, resentful, and easily annoyed by others at a level and frequency that is outside of the expected range for their age and developmental level. Frequently, youth with ODD actively defy adults' requests or rules and deliberately annoy other persons. They tend to blame others for their own mistakes and misbehavior, more often than is appropriate for their developmental age. Manifestations of the disorder are almost invariably present in the home, but they may not be present at school or with other adults or peers. In some cases, the child has symptoms outside the home from the start; in others, it starts at home and later moves beyond that. Typically, symptoms of the disorder are most evident in interactions with adults or peers whom the child knows well. Thus, a child with ODD may not show signs of the disorder when examined clinically. Although children with ODD may be aware that others disapprove of their behavior, they may still justify it as a response to unfair or unreasonable circumstances. This disorder appears to cause more distress to those around the child than to the child. Table 14-1 compares the diagnostic criteria for ODD according to DSM-5-TR, ICD-10, and ICD-11.

The DSM-5-TR has divided ODD into three symptom clusters: angry/irritable mood, argumentative/defiant

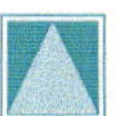

Table 14-1.
Comparative Diagnostic Criteria for Oppositional Defiant Disorder in DSM-5-TR, ICD-10 and ICD-11

	DSM-5-TR	ICD-10	ICD-11
Diagnostic name	Oppositional Defiant Disorder	Oppositional Defiant Disorder	Oppositional Defiant Disorder
Duration	≥6 mo If <5 yr, occurs most days If ≥5 yr, occurs ≥1 time/wk		Extended period
Symptoms	Loses temper Sensitive/easily annoyed Angry/resentful Argues with authorities Disobeys authorities or rules Annoys others on purpose Blames others Spiteful or vindictive ≥2×/past 6 mo	Conduct disorder, usually in younger children, with: • Disobedience • Defiance • Disruptive behavior • No delinquency or severe aggression or dissocial behaviors	Noncompliant, defiant, and disobedient behaviors inappropriate for age with: Difficulty getting along with others • Provocative, spiteful, or vindictive • Extremely irritable or angry
Required number of symptoms	≥4		
Psychosocial consequences	Distress or psychosocial impairment		Distress or psychosocial impairment
Exclusions	Substance or medication-induced, including withdrawal Other mental disorder		Relationship problems (i.e., response to overly harsh parents or teachers)
Symptoms specifiers			With or without chronic irritability-anger With limited prosocial emotions With typical prosocial emotions
Severity specifiers	**Mild:** occurs in 1 setting **Moderate:** occurs in ≥2 settings **Severe:** occurs in ≥3 settings		

behavior, and vindictiveness. A child may meet diagnostic criteria for ODD with a 6-month pattern of at least four symptoms from any of the three symptom clusters above. Note that, for spiteful or vindictive behaviors, the child must demonstrate these behaviors at least twice over a 6 month period. For children under 5 years, the pattern of behaviors should occur on most days for at least 6 months. For children 5 years or older, the pattern of behaviors should occur at least once per week for 6 months. Angry/irritable children with ODD often lose their tempers, are easily annoyed, and feel irritable much of the time. Argumentative/defiant children display a pattern of arguing with authority figures and adults such as parents, teachers, and relatives. Children with ODD may actively refuse to comply with requests, deliberately break the rules, and purposely annoy others. These children often do not take responsibility for their actions and often blame others for their misbehavior. Children with the vindictive type of ODD are spiteful and have shown vindictive or spiteful actions at least twice in 6 months to meet the diagnostic criteria.

Persistent ODD or irritability usually interferes with interpersonal relationships and school performance. Peers often reject these children, and they may become isolated and lonely. Despite adequate intelligence, they may do poorly or fail in school due to their lack of cooperation, reduced participation, and inability to accept help. Secondary to these difficulties are low self-esteem, poor frustration tolerance, depressed mood, and temper outbursts. Adolescents who are ostracized may turn to alcohol and illegal substances as a modality to fit in with peers. Chronically irritable children often develop mood disorders in adolescence or adulthood.

Pathology and Laboratory Examination

No specific laboratory tests or pathologic findings help diagnose ODD. Because some children with ODD become physically aggressive and violate the rights of others as they age, they may share some characteristics with people with high levels of aggression, such as low central nervous system (CNS) serotonin.

Differential Diagnosis

Oppositional behaviors are both healthy and adaptive within an expected range at specific developmental stages. We should distinguish periods of normative negativism from ODD. Developmentally appropriate oppositional behavior is neither considerably more frequent nor more intense than that seen in other children of the same mental age. According to the DSM-5-TR, ODD is not diagnosed in the presence of disruptive mood dysregulation disorder. (See Chapter 13 for a further discussion of disruptive mood dysregulation disorder.)

Oppositional defiant behavior occurring temporarily in reaction to a stressor should be diagnosed as an adjustment disorder. When features of ODD appear during conduct disorder, schizophrenia, or a mood disorder, we should not diagnose ODD. Oppositional and negativistic behaviors can also be present in attention-deficit/hyperactivity disorder (ADHD), cognitive disorders, and mental retardation. Whether ODD is diagnosed along with ADHD depends on the severity, pervasiveness, and duration of such behavior. Some young children who receive a diagnosis of ODD go on in several years to meet the criteria for conduct disorder. Some investigators believe that the two disorders may be developmental variants of each other, with conduct disorder being the natural progression of oppositional defiant behavior when a child matures. Most children with ODD, however, do not later meet the criteria for conduct disorder, and up to one-fourth of children with ODD may not meet the diagnosis several years later.

The predominance of aggression in children with ODD increases the risk that it may progress to conduct disorder. Children with ADHD and ODD are also at higher risk to develop conduct disorder before the age of 12 years. Some children who develop conduct disorder have a history of ODD. Subtypes of ODD may exist. Children who show some symptoms of conduct disorder (e.g., fighting, bullying) along with ODD are at higher risk to progress to meeting criteria for conduct disorder in childhood. When both ODD and conduct disorder are present, according to DSM-5-TR, they may be diagnosed concurrently.

Jenna, aged 7 years, was brought to the clinic for evaluation of irritability, negativity, and defiant behavior by her mother. She complained that Jenna had frequent, prolonged tantrums, triggered by not "getting her way," and often blaming these tantrums on her mother for being "unfair." Jenna had been having troubles in school as well, and her teacher had reported to the family that she seemed to have a habit of provoking other students as well as the teacher by making noises, pushing the chair of the student in front of her seat, and tapping her desk in class. Jenna often argued with her teacher loudly. Recently, at home, Jenna was kicking her foot against her mother's chair, and she asked her to stop. She looked at her directly and continued to kick her chair until her mother became angry and sent her to her room. Jenna refused to stay in her room, stating that she wasn't doing anything and that her mother was just picking on her. Jenna's mother reported that she has given up on asking her to help with chores because it inevitably results in an argument. Jenna appeared sullen and irritable during the interview. She insisted that her behaviors are all her mother's fault, and she is always nagging her unfairly. During the interview with her mother, Jenna interrupted her many times to argue and disagree. Despite Jenna's behavioral problems, she has been able to succeed academically and scored in the high average range on standardized tests. Jenna's mother reports that, as far back as in kindergarten, she was rejected by peers because she was always getting angry, had difficulty sharing her things, and was bossy. Jenna's mother reports that ever since her sister was born when Jenna was 3 years old, she has been angry and negative toward her for no apparent reason. Jenna's parents separated and divorced when she was 4. Jenna has had no contact with her father since then. Her mother was depressed for a year after the divorce and sought treatment, which helped. Jenna's mother has always felt guilty that Jenna's father is not in her life, and Jenna blames her mother for her father's absence. Jenna and her mother were referred for Parent–Child Interaction Therapy (PCIT).

COURSE AND PROGNOSIS

The course of ODD depends on the severity of the symptoms and the ability of the child to develop more adaptive responses to authority. The stability of ODD varies over time, with approximately 25% of children with the disorder no longer meeting diagnostic criteria. Persistence of oppositional defiant symptoms poses an increased risk of additional disorders, such as mood disorders, conduct disorder, and substance use disorders. Positive outcomes are more likely for intact families who can modify their expression of demands and give less attention to the child's argumentative behaviors.

An association exists between ODD and ADHD, as well as with mood disorders. In children who have a long history of aggression and ODD, there is a higher risk of the development of conduct disorder and later substance use disorders. Parental psychopathology, such as antisocial personality disorder and substance abuse, appears to be more common in families with children who have ODD than in the general population, which creates additional risks for chaotic and troubled home environments. The prognosis for ODD in a child depends somewhat on family functioning and the development of comorbid psychopathology.

TREATMENT

The primary treatment of ODD is family intervention using both direct training of the parents in child management skills and careful assessment of family interactions. The goals of this intervention are to reinforce more prosocial behaviors and to diminish undesired behaviors at the same time. Cognitive-behavioral therapists emphasize teaching parents how to alter their behavior to discourage the child's oppositional behavior by diminishing attention to it, and Parent–Child Interaction Therapy (PICT) focuses on selectively reinforcing and praising appropriate behavior and ignoring or not reinforcing undesired behavior.

Children with oppositional defiant behavior may also benefit from individual psychotherapy in which they role-play and "practice" more adaptive responses. In the therapeutic relationship, the child can learn new strategies to develop a sense of mastery and success in social situations with peers and families. In the safety of a more "neutral" relationship, children may discover that they are capable of less provocative behavior. Often, therapists must help restore the child's self-esteem before they can make more positive responses to external control. Parent–child conflict strongly predicts conduct problems; patterns of harsh physical and verbal punishment particularly evoke the emergence of aggression in children. Replacing harsh, punitive parenting and increasing positive parent–child interactions may positively influence the course of oppositional and defiant behaviors.

EPIDEMIOLOGY

Oppositional and negativistic behavior, in moderation, is developmentally normal in early childhood. The reported prevalence of ODD ranges from 1% to 11%, depending on the age and gender of the sample, with an average prevalence of about 3.3%. ODD is reported to occur at increased rates in boys before puberty, and an equal sex ratio is reported after puberty. The prevalence of oppositional defiant behavior in males and females diminishes in youth older than 12 years of age.

Epidemiologic studies of negativistic traits in nonclinical populations found some oppositional and defiant behavior in 16% to 22% of school-age children. Although oppositional defiant symptoms can begin as early as 3 years of age, it typically is noted by 8 years of age and usually not later than early adolescence.

ETIOLOGY

The most dramatic example of typical oppositional behavior peaks between 18 and 24 months, the "terrible twos," when toddlers are dramatically expressing their growing autonomy. Impairment begins when this developmental phase persists abnormally, authority figures overreact, or oppositional behavior recurs considerably more frequently than in most children of the same chronologic and developmental age. Among the criteria included in ODD, anger and irritability appears to be the one most predictive of later psychiatric disorders, and some elements may be attributed to temperament.

Children exhibit a range of temperamental predispositions to strong will, stable preferences, or high assertiveness. Parents who model more extreme ways of expressing and enforcing their own will may contribute to the development of chronic struggles with their children, which the children then reenact with other authority figures. What begins for an infant as an effort to establish self-determination may become transformed into an exaggerated behavioral pattern. In late childhood, environmental trauma, illness, or intellectual disability can trigger oppositionality as a defense against helplessness, anxiety, and low self-esteem. Typical oppositional behaviors occur in adolescence as an expression of the need to separate from the parents and to establish an autonomous identity.

Intermittent Explosive Disorder

Intermittent explosive disorder (IED) is characterized by recurrent verbal or physical outbursts, which typically begin in childhood or adolescence. Children and adolescents with IED have discrete episodes of outbursts which appear to be an overreaction to an observed provocation. The episodes appear within minutes or hours of a small provocation and tend to remit spontaneously. After an explosive episode, some youth show genuine regret or guilt. Significant impulsive or aggressive behaviors are generally absent between events. Clinicians should not diagnose IED if the behaviors can be accounted for by another disorder. To make a diagnosis of IED, a child or adolescent exhibits recurrent outbursts such as temper tantrums, which may include verbal or physical aggression toward others. During an outburst, a child or adolescent with IED may also cause harm to an animal or property. Typically, these outbursts occur several times in a week and appear to be spontaneous and impulsive. Table 14-2 compares the diagnostic criteria for IED according to DSM-5-TR, ICD-10, and ICD-11.

Diagnosis

As with most child and adolescent psychiatric disorders, the symptoms of IED cause significant distress or impairment in psychosocial and academic functioning and are not better accounted for by another psychiatric disorder. In order to meet criteria for this disorder, a child or adolescent must be older than 6 years (or of comparable developmental level).

The diagnosis of IED is made based on a history of recurrent episodes of loss of control associated with aggressive outbursts. One discrete episode does not justify the diagnosis. A child or adolescent may experience anxiety, guilt, or sadness following an outburst, but this is not a constant finding.

Physical Findings and Laboratory Examination

Blood chemistry (liver and thyroid function tests, fasting blood glucose, electrolytes), urinalysis (including drug toxicology) may help rule out other causes of aggression or impulsive behavior. These laboratory tests are not typically abnormal in children and adolescents with IED.

Differential Diagnosis

IED is diagnosed in the absence of other disorders associated with the occasional loss of control of aggressive

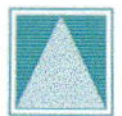

Table 14-2.
Intermittent Explosive Disorder

	DSM-5-TR	ICD-10	ICD-11
Diagnostic name	Intermittent Explosive Disorder	Other Habit and Impulse Disorders	Intermittent Explosive Disorder
Duration	See below		≤3 mo or 1 yr if outbursts are severe
Symptoms	Age ≥6 Recurrent spontaneous outbursts that are an overreaction to an event, with: • Verbal/physical aggression 2×/wk for ≥3 mo • 3 episodes resulting in harm/destruction over 1 yr period	Pattern of repeated maladaptive behaviors, not better explained by another disorder, associated with prodromal tension and release at time of act	Age ≥6 Brief impulsive/reactive episodes of verbal/physical aggression Out of proportion to the circumstance and developmental age
Required number of symptoms	All of the above		
Psychosocial consequences	Distress or psychosocial impairment		Distress or psychosocial impairment
Exclusions	Other medical condition Substance or medication-induced, including withdrawal Other mental disorder		Other medical condition Substance or medication-induced, including withdrawal Other mental disorder
Course specifiers	***Persistent:*** >12 mo		
Severity specifiers	***Severe*** if all symptom criteria met at relatively high level		

impulses have been ruled out as the primary cause. These other disorders include disruptive mood dysregulation disorder, ADHD, and bipolar spectrum disorders.

The episodic and discrete nature of IED differentiates it from conduct disorder and which are more pervasive patterns of behavior in which aggression is a consistent feature, and not just associated with discrete outbursts.

COMORBIDITY

Approximately 80% of individuals with IED meet the criteria for another psychiatric disorder. These include externalizing disorders, intellectual disabilities, autism spectrum disorders, anxiety disorders, and bipolar disorders.

COURSE AND PROGNOSIS

IED may begin at any stage of life but usually appears during childhood or adolescence. The onset can be sudden or insidious, and the course can be waxing and waning or chronic. IED is more common in males than females.

TREATMENT

There are currently no evidence-based treatment recommendations for IED in children and adolescents. Given the high rate of comorbidity, especially of ADHD, and other disruptive behavior disorders, pharmacotherapy of comorbid ADHD may be successful and lead to a decrease in aggressive behaviors.

A randomized clinical trial by McCloskey and colleagues (2022) comparing cognitive-behavioral therapy (CBT) to supportive therapy in adults, 44 participants with IED (22 men and 22 women) aged 20 to 55 years were administered 12 50-minute individual sessions of either a multicomponent cognitive-behavioral intervention for IED (n = 19) or the same number of sessions of supportive psychotherapy (n = 25). Participants in both treatments tended to improve over time, however, CBT was superior to supportive psychotherapy in decreasing aggressive behavior especially toward others. These findings support the use of a multicomponent cognitive-behavioral intervention in treating aggression in IED.

A goal of psychosocial treatment is to have the patient recognize and verbalize the thoughts or feelings that precede the explosive outbursts instead of acting them out. CBT and contingency management may be most helpful intervention.

Stimulant medication and other pharmacologic treatments for ADHD are indicated when ADHD is comorbid with IED.

Selective serotonin reuptake inhibitors (SSRIs) are may be useful in reducing impulsivity and aggression, especially when there is mood dysregulation.

Second-generation antipsychotics have been utilized in children and adolescents with recurrent severe aggressive behaviors with some positive response. However, given the metabolic side effects of these medications, when there are comorbid disorders that respond to other treatments, antipsychotics should not be used as a first line treatment.

Alex, a 13-year-old boy, was referred for psychiatric evaluation by his parents after repeated phone calls from his middle school with complaints that he was becoming enraged with his teachers and peers with little or no provocation. Alex's parents knew that Alex had always had a "short fuse" and often slammed doors or stormed out of the room if they made a minor request, but they were not worried because within a few minutes of an outburst, Alex was usually pleasant and in a good mood. Alex had always been a good student and had many friends in school. Alex always ate lunch with peers and spent recess playing basketball. In spite of his social nature, Alex's outbursts were becoming more frequent and unmanageable in school. Alex's outbursts in school appeared to be abrupt and based on minor requests from peers such as "stop kicking my chair." In that incident, Alex stood up and suddenly pulled his classmate's chair so hard that the student fell out of his chair, and Alex screamed at him, "You deserved that!" Alex's peers were beginning to avoid him due to his recurrent outbursts. A recent incident with his teacher occurred after she voiced a direction to the class that "... it's time to turn in your classwork." Alex suddenly got up out of his seat and ripped up his classwork, cursed at the teacher, and stormed out of the classroom. Alex's school was very distressed by his behavior and suspended him for several days after the incident with his teacher. Alex's school arranged a conference with Alex's parents and informed them that Alex would need to be evaluated in order to return to school because he had become a threat to the other students and to his teacher. Upon evaluation with a child and adolescent psychiatrist, he was diagnosed with intermittent explosive disorder. He did not meet criteria for any other psychiatric disorder. Alex was referred, along with his parents, to a cognitive-behavioral therapist who worked individually with Alex and also with Alex and his parents. Alex began to learn that there are more effective ways to deal with his frustration and was able to return to school with better coping strategies.

CONDUCT DISORDER

Aggressive patterns of behavior are among the most frequent reasons psychiatrists evaluate children and adolescents. Displays of impulsive and aggressive behaviors is developmentally normative in very young children; however, youths who continue to display excessive patterns of aggression and violations of fundamental rights of peers and family members when they reach school age and older are significantly impaired. Longitudinal studies have demonstrated that, for some youth, early patterns of aggressive disruptive behavior may become a lifelong pervasive repertoire culminating in antisocial personality disorder as an adult. The etiology of enduring patterns of aggressive behavior is widely accepted as a convergence of multiple contributing factors, including biologic, temperamental, learned, and psychological conditions. Risk factors for the development of aggressive behavior in youth include childhood maltreatment such as physical or sexual abuse, neglect, emotional abuse, and overly harsh and punitive parenting.

Youth with conduct disorder often demonstrate behaviors in the following four categories: physical aggression or threats of harm to people, destruction of their property or that of others, theft or acts of deceit, and frequent violation of age-appropriate rules. Conduct disorder is associated with many other psychiatric disorders, including ADHD, depression, and learning disorders. It is also associated with certain psychosocial factors, including childhood maltreatment, harsh or punitive parenting, family discord, lack of appropriate parental supervision, lack of social competence, and low socioeconomic level. The DSM-5-TR criteria require three persistent specific behaviors of 15 conduct disorder symptoms listed, over the past 12 months, with at least one of them present in the past 6 months. Conduct disorder symptoms include bullying, threatening, or intimidating others, and staying out at night despite parental prohibition. DSM-5-TR also specifies that when truancy from school is a symptom, it begins before 13 years of age. The disorder may be diagnosed in a person older than 18 years only if the person does not meet the criteria for antisocial personality disorder.

DSM-5-TR includes specifiers denoting the severity of the disorder, including "mild" in which there are few conduct problems above those needed to make the diagnosis and behaviors cause only minor harm to others. In "moderate" cases, symptoms exceed the minimum; however, there is less confrontation that may cause harm to individuals than in "severe" cases. According to DSM-5-TR, the "severe" level shows many conduct problems over the minimal diagnostic criteria or conduct problems that cause considerable harm to others. The work of Frick and colleagues (2021; 2019) has shown that children with high levels of callous–unemotional (CU) traits characterize a subgroup of youth with conduct disorders who show a unique causal processes underlying their problem behavior and are at a particularly high risk for serious impairment relative to others with these disorders. As a result, these traits have been integrated into major diagnostic classification systems for conduct disorders. DSM-5-TR identifies this enduring trait with pattern with the following specifier: "With limited prosocial emotions." To qualify for this specifier, multiple sources must confirm that the child or adolescent shows a persistent interpersonal and emotional pattern that can be characterized by at least two of the following: (1) lack of remorse or guilt, (2) callous lack of empathy, (3) unconcerned about performance, (4) shallow or deficient affect. Individuals with conduct disorder who qualify for this specifier are more likely to have a childhood-onset type and meet the criteria for a "severe" disorder. Children with conduct disorders engage in severe, repeated acts of aggression that can cause physical harm to themselves and others and frequently violate the rights of others. Children with conduct disorder usually have behaviors characterized by aggression to persons or animals, destruction of property, deceitfulness or theft, and multiple violations of rules, such as truancy from school. These behavioral patterns cause distinct difficulties in school life as well as in peer relationships. Conduct disorder has three subtypes based on the age of onset of the disorder. Childhood-onset subtype, in which at least one symptom has emerged repeatedly before age of 10 years; adolescent-onset type, in which no characteristic persistent symptoms occur until after age of 10 years; and unspecified-onset, in which age of onset is unknown. Although some young children show persistent patterns of behavior consistent with violating the rights of others or destroying property, the diagnosis of conduct disorder in children appears to increase with age. Epidemiologic surveys indicate that geographic locations representing a broad range of different cultures are not associated with significant variability in prevalence rates of either ODD or conduct disorder. A longitudinal study of population density and antisocial behaviors in youth found no relationship in children 4 to 13 years of age between conduct problems and density of the living area. However, higher rates of conduct problems were self-reported by youths 10 to 17 years who lived in higher-density communities.

DIAGNOSIS AND CLINICAL FEATURES

Conduct disorder does not develop overnight. Instead, many symptoms evolve until a consistent pattern develops that involves violating the rights of others. Very young children are unlikely to meet the criteria for the disorder because they are not developmentally able to exhibit the symptoms typical of older children with conduct disorder. A 3-year-old does not break into someone's home, steal with confrontation, force someone into sexual activity, or deliberately use a weapon that can cause serious harm. School-age children, however, can become bullies, initiate physical fights, destroy property, or set fires. Table 14-3 compares the diagnostic criteria for conduct disorder according to DSM-5-TR, ICD-10, and ICD-11.

The average age of onset of conduct disorder is younger in boys than in girls. Boys most commonly meet the diagnostic criteria by 10 to 12 years of age, whereas girls meet them closer to 14 to 16 years of age.

Children who meet the criteria for conduct disorder express their overt aggressive behavior in various forms. Aggressive antisocial behavior can take the form of bullying, physical aggression, and cruel behavior toward peers. Children may be hostile, verbally abusive, impudent, defiant, and negativistic toward adults. Persistent lying, frequent truancy, and vandalism are common. In severe cases, destructiveness, stealing, and physical violence often occur. Some adolescents make little effort to conceal their antisocial behavior. Sexual behavior and regular use of tobacco, liquor, or illicit psychoactive substances begin unusually early for such children and adolescents. Suicidal thoughts, gestures, and acts are frequent in children and adolescents with conduct disorder who are in conflict with peers, family members, or the law and are unable to problem-solve their difficulties.

Some children with aggressive behavioral patterns have impaired social attachments, as evidenced by their difficulties with peer relationships. Some may befriend a much older or younger person or have superficial relationships with other antisocial youngsters. Many children with conduct problems have poor self-esteem, although they may project an image of toughness. They may lack the skills to communicate in socially acceptable ways and appear to have little regard for the feelings, wishes, and welfare of others. Children and adolescents with conduct disorders often feel guilt or remorse for some of their behaviors but frequently blame others to avoid punishment.

Many children and adolescents with conduct disorder suffer from the deprivation of having few of their dependency needs met and may have had either overly harsh parenting or a lack of appropriate supervision. The deficient socialization of many children and adolescents with conduct disorder can be expressed in physical violation of others and, for some, in sexual violation of others. Severe punishments for behavior in children with conduct disorder almost invariably increase their maladaptive expression of rage and frustration rather than ameliorating the problem.

In evaluation interviews, children with aggressive conduct disorders are typically uncooperative, hostile, and provocative. Some have a superficial charm and compliance until they discuss their problem behaviors. Then, they often deny any problems. If the interviewer persists, the child may attempt to justify misbehavior or become suspicious and angry about the source of the examiner's information and perhaps bolt from the room. Most often, the child becomes angry with the examiner and expresses resentment of the examination with open belligerence or sullen withdrawal. Their hostility is not limited to adult authority figures, but they also direct it to their peers and younger children. They often bully those who are smaller and weaker. By boasting, lying, and expressing little interest in a listener's responses, such children reveal their lack of trust in adults to understand their position.

Evaluation of the family situation often reveals severe marital disharmony, which initially may center on disagreements about the management of the child. Because of a tendency toward family instability, parent surrogates are often in the picture. Children with conduct disorder are more likely to be unplanned or unwanted babies. The parents of children with conduct disorder, especially the father, have higher rates of antisocial personality disorder or alcohol use disorder. Aggressive children and their families show a stereotyped pattern of impulsive and unpredictable verbal and physical hostility. A child's aggressive behavior rarely seems directed toward any definable goal and offers little pleasure, success, or even sustained advantages with peers or authority figures.

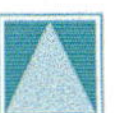

Table 14-3.
Conduct Disorder

	DSM-5-TR	ICD-10	ICD-11
Diagnostic name	Conduct Disorder	Conduct Disorder	Conduct-Dissocial Disorder
Duration	≥1 symptom for ≥6 mo Other symptoms ≥1 yr	6 mo or longer	≥12 mo, persistent and recurrent behavior
Symptoms	Bullying others Initiating physical fights Use of a weapon causing serious harm Physical cruelty toward others Physical cruelty toward animals Stealing while physically confronting a victim Forcing sexual activity on another Deliberately setting a fire Deliberately destroying someone's property Breaking into another's property Lying to obtain goods or favors or to avoid obligations Stealing items of high value without necessarily confronting victim Staying out at night against parental restrictions ≤ age 13 ≥2 episodes of running away (or 1× if prolonged) Frequent truancy ≤age 13	Repeated and pervasive pattern of antisocial behavior, aggression and defiance that are significantly deviant for age-appropriate expectations. Actions may involve cruelty, bullying, destructiveness, lying, running away/truancy, and anger.	Violating rights of others/laws/norms, including: • Aggression toward people/animals • Destruction of property • Deceit/theft • Serious rule violations
Required number of symptoms	3		
Psychosocial consequences			Distress or psychosocial impairment
Symptoms specifiers	• **With limited prosocial emotions:** demonstrating at least two of the following over 12 mo and in multiple contexts: • *Lack of remorse or guilt* • *Callous—lack of empathy* • *Unconcerned about performance* • *Shallow or deficient affect*	**Conduct disorder confined to the family** context (within nuclear family) **Unsocialized conduct disorder** (predominant aggression, often toward other children) **Socialized conduct disorder** (despite aggression, there is good integration into their peer group)	With limited prosocial emotions With typical prosocial emotions
Course specifiers	**Childhood-onset type** (symptoms present prior to age 10) **Adolescent-onset type** (no symptoms prior to age 10)		Childhood onset Adolescent onset
Severity specifiers	**Mild:** few symptoms in excess of number needed to make diagnosis, with relatively minor resultant harm to others **Moderate**: intermediate symptoms and consequences **Severe:** many issues in excess of minimum needed for diagnosis, with resultant harm to others being considerable		

In other cases, conduct disorder includes repeated truancy, vandalism, and physical severe aggression or assault against others by a gang, such as mugging, gang fighting, and beating. Some adolescents who become part of a gang have the skills for age-appropriate social interactions; others are recruited because they are socially isolated and willing to oblige gang leadership in return for becoming part of the group. Gang members may feel true concern for the welfare of their friends or their respective gang members; however, it may become dangerous for them to blame other gang members or inform on them. In some cases, gang members have a history of adequate conformity during early childhood that ended when the youth became a member of the delinquent peer group, usually in preadolescence or during early adolescence. Other members of gangs have prior history of neglect or abuse, and may evidence childhood histories of marginal or poor school performance, significant behavior problems, anxiety, and depressive symptoms. Patterns of paternal discipline are rarely ideal and can vary from harshness and excessive strictness to inconsistency or relative absence of supervision and control.

Pathology and Laboratory Examination

No specific laboratory test or neurologic pathology helps make the diagnosis of conduct disorder. Some evidence indicates that amounts of certain neurotransmitters, such as serotonin in the CNS, are low in some people with a history of violent or aggressive behavior toward others or themselves. Whether this association is related to the cause or is the effect of violence or is unrelated to the violence is not clear.

DIFFERENTIAL DIAGNOSIS

Disturbances of conduct, including impulsivity and aggression, may occur in many childhood psychiatric disorders, ranging from ADHD, to ODD, to disruptive mood dysregulation disorder, to major depression, to bipolar disorder, specific learning disorders, and psychotic disorders. Therefore, clinicians must obtain a comprehensive history of the chronology of the symptoms to determine whether the conduct disturbance is a transient or an enduring pattern. Isolated acts of aggressive behavior do not justify a diagnosis of conduct disorder; an entrenched pattern must be present. The relationship of conduct disorder to ODD is still under debate. Typically, we think of ODD as a mild precursor of conduct disorder, without the violation of rights, likely to be diagnosed in younger children who may be at risk for conduct disorder. Children who progress from ODD to conduct disorder over time maintain their oppositional characteristics, and some evidence indicates that the two disorders are independent. Currently, in the DSM-5-TR, ODD and conduct disorder are considered distinct, but they can coexist. Many children with ODD do not develop conduct disorder, and conduct disorder emerging in adolescence is not necessarily preceded by ODD. The main distinguishing clinical feature between these two disorders is that in conduct disorder, the youths violate the fundamental rights of others, whereas, in ODD, hostility and negativism fall short of seriously violating the rights of others.

Mood disorders are often present in children who exhibit irritability and aggressive behavior. We should rule out both major depressive disorder and bipolar disorder, but the full syndrome of conduct disorder can occur during the onset of a mood disorder. Substantial comorbidity exists between conduct disorder and depressive disorders. A recent report concludes that the high correlation between the two disorders arises from shared risk factors for both disorders rather than a causal relation. Thus, a series of factors, including family conflict, adverse life events, an early history of conduct disturbance, level of parental involvement, and affiliation with delinquent peers, contribute to the development of affective disorders and conduct disorder. This comorbidity is not the case with ODD, which we cannot diagnose if it occurs exclusively during a mood disorder.

ADHD and learning disorders are commonly associated with conduct disorder. Usually, the symptoms of these disorders predate the diagnosis of conduct disorder. Substance use disorders are also more common in adolescents with conduct disorder than in the general population. Evidence indicates an association between fighting behaviors as a child and substance use as an adolescent. Once there is a pattern of drug use, this pattern may interfere with the development of positive mediators, such as social skills and problem-solving, which could enhance the remission of the conduct disorder. Thus, once substance abuse develops, it may promote the continuation of the conduct disorder. Obsessive-compulsive disorder (OCD) also frequently seems to coexist with disruptive behavior disorders. All the disorders described here should be noted when they co-occur. Children with ADHD often exhibit impulsive and aggressive behaviors that may not meet the full criteria for conduct disorder.

Troy, age 13 years, was referred for psychiatric evaluation after being picked up by police in the middle of the night while attempting to break into a convenience store. Troy became combative and violent when the police found him, so they placed him on an involuntary hold and brought him to the nearest hospital emergency room. Troy explained that he would rather live on the street than at home because he likes being with his friends. Troy reported that he hates being at home because his father hits him and his mother constantly yells at him. Troy's mother was contacted by the emergency room and reported that Troy has left and stayed out overnight multiple times in the past year, but that he usually returns the next morning. Troy's mother complains Troy is always in trouble. Troy has a long history of fighting with peers, destroying property at home and repeated shoplifting, which started when he was 8 years old. Troy's mother reports that she doesn't understand why he seems unconcerned when he has hurt a peer badly in a fight, and he does not seem to show any empathy at home even when he has harmed his siblings. The police have been involved on many occasions, including for violent fights between family members, truancy, staying out all night, stealing from a neighborhood store, and smoking marijuana. Troy has a quick temper, and his mother knows he was involved in several serious fights over the past year in the neighborhood. Troy is particularly cruel to his younger brother with autism spectrum disorder, continually taunting and teasing him without any regard to his feelings.

Troy's mother stated that he continually lies, sometimes for no apparent reason. When he was 6 years of age, he was fascinated with fire and set several small fires at home, fortunately with no serious injury or damage. Troy's mother was tearful when she disclosed that Troy seems to be turning out just like his father who is an alcoholic and has spent time incarcerated for burglary, assault, and battery. Troy's mother discloses that his father exhibits the same callous and unemotional reaction to others' pain. Troy's mother reports that she has never understood that trait in her husband or her son. When Troy was interviewed in the emergency department by a child and adolescent psychiatrist, Troy initially refused to answer questions and turned away scowling, but gradually began to talk. Troy presented a tough image with an indifferent attitude toward the interviewer. Troy endorsed physical abuse by his father and disclosed that that he ran away from home to get away from his father. On further questioning, Troy disclosed that his father started beating him with a belt when he was as young as 6 years of age. When questioned about fights with peers, Troy justified his behaviors as just having fun. Troy reported that others provoked the fights. Troy denied using weapons in fights, although he bragged about breaking the nose of another youth.

Troy's school records indicated that he required an Individualized Educational Plan (IEP) starting when he was in the second grade and was evaluated for the hyperactive and impulsive symptoms of attention-deficit/hyperactivity disorder (ADHD) when he was in first grade. Troy was diagnosed by a child and adolescent psychiatrist with ADHD and prescribed methylphenidate. Troy's family was against medication for children and, after a brief trial, discontinued treatment. Troy has not received any treatment for ADHD since the first grade. Troy is currently in seventh grade special education classes, and he has a history of failing and repeating fifth grade. Troy is failing several classes, and he may have to repeat seventh grade. Troy admits to frequent truancy this year and reports that he has problems with completing schoolwork. His previous psychiatric evaluation indicated that the department of child and family services (Child Protective Services) evaluated the family for possible neglect when he was 9 years of age after he and his younger brother with autism were found wandering around on the street late one evening without supervision. Troy's family was referred for counseling and attended the required sessions but did not seem to improve their parenting. Both of Troy's parents have a history of drug and alcohol abuse. Troy's birth was unplanned, and his mother used drugs during pregnancy. Troy's parents had separated soon after his birth, when his mother returned to live with her parents briefly, but ultimately they got back together when Troy was about a year old and continue to live together with recurrent domestic violence.

COMORBIDITY

ADHD and conduct disorder often coexist, with ADHD often predating the development of conduct disorder, and not infrequently substance abuse. CNS injury, dysfunction, or damage predisposes a child to impulsivity and behavioral disturbances, which sometimes evolve into conduct disorder.

COURSE AND PROGNOSIS

Poor prognostic signs for conduct disorder include young age at onset, high number of severe symptoms, and CU lack of empathy. Although children with CU traits represent only a subset of childhood-onset conduct disorder, when these traits are present, they are indicators that increasing empathy is a necessary part of a treatment program for these children. Youth with more severe conduct disorder seem to be most vulnerable to comorbid disorders later in life, such as mood disorders and substance use disorders. A longitudinal study found that, while assaultive behavior in childhood predicts a higher risk of incarceration later in life, the diagnosis of conduct disorder itself does not correlate with imprisonment. Mild symptoms, an absence of coexisting psychiatric disorders, and average to high-average intellectual functioning are good prognostic signs.

TREATMENT

Psychosocial Interventions

PCIT, developed by Hembree-Kigin and McNeil (1995), is considered a first-line psychosocial intervention for young children with frequent temper tantrums, oppositional and defiant behavior, and verbal or physical aggression.

For children with conduct disorders who show significant levels of CU responses and a lack of expected empathy for their developmental level, psychosocial interventions must focus on enhancing empathy.

Kimonis et al. (2019) developed a modified PCIT treatment, called PCIT-CU, with a focus on increasing empathy in this subgroup of children. The modifications included:

- Coaching parents to engage in warm and emotionally responsive parenting.
- Shifting parental emphasis from punishment to rewarding desired behaviors.
- Enhancing attention to critical facial cues (i.e., micro expressions) that signal distress in others to improve emotional recognition in the child.

- Improving emotional understanding by linking emotional expressions in others to the situation in which they occur and identifying situations that trigger anger and frustration in the child.
- Teaching and positively reinforcing prosocial and empathic behavior in the child, with parental modeling, role-play, and social stories.
- Increasing frustration tolerance in the child through modeling, role-play, and reinforcing use of learned cognitive-behavioral strategies to decrease the incidence of aggressive behavior.

Kimonis and colleagues reported on an open trial of their PCIT-CU intervention in 23 children (aged 3 to 6 years) with conduct disorders and elevated CU traits who were referred to a university mental health clinic. The authors reported that 74% of the subjects completed the program and noted high levels of parent-reported satisfaction with the program. Further, the intervention produced decreases in child conduct problems and CU traits and increases in empathy. Kimonis and colleagues reported a high rate of maintaining gains in a 3-month follow-up.

A variety of parent management training (PMT) and problem-solving skills training (PSST) approaches have been used to help children with conduct disturbances.

PSST, developed in 1987 by Kazdin, is a 12-week sequential program that helps children develop problem-solving solutions when faced with conflictual situations. Assignments called "supersolvers" provide vignette situations in which children can practice these techniques. Therapists can add a companion program, PMT, to the intervention, but PSST can be useful even without the parent component. Another CBT-based intervention, the Incredible Years (IY), targeting young children from 3 to 8 years, is administered over 22 weeks and delivers sessions to the child and has a parent training component and teacher training. Another CBT-based intervention is the Anger Coping Program, an 18-session intervention for school-age children in grades 4 to 6 focused on a child's increased development of emotion recognition and regulation and managing anger. Anger coping strategies include distraction, self-talk, perspective taking, goal setting, and problem-solving.

Overall, treatment programs have been more successful in decreasing overt symptoms of conduct, such as aggression, than the covert symptoms, such as lying or stealing. Treatment strategies for young children that focus on increasing social behavior and social competence reduce aggressive behavior. In one study, 548 third graders were administered a school-based intervention instead of a regular health curriculum in several public schools in North Carolina, called *Making Choices: Social Problem-Solving Skills for Children* (MC), along with supplemental teacher and parent components. Compared with third graders receiving the routine health curriculum, children exposed to the MC program were rated lower on the posttest social and overt aggression, and higher on social competence. Also, they scored higher on information-processing skills. These findings support the notion that school-based prevention programs have the potential to strengthen social and emotional skills and diminish aggressive behavior among normal populations of school-age children. School settings can also use behavioral techniques to promote socially acceptable behavior toward peers and to discourage covert antisocial incidents.

Early sustained preventive interventions (e.g., at a kindergarten age) can significantly alter the course and prognosis of aggressive behavior. A screening program used with kindergarteners predicted lifetime disruptive behavior disorder by age 18 years, with the highest risk group demonstrating an 82% chance of a disruptive behavior diagnosis without intervention. One prevention program, *The Fast Track Preventive Intervention,* randomized 891 kindergarteners to either a 10-year prevention program or a control condition. The 10-year intervention included parent behavior management, child social cognitive skills, reading, home visiting, mentoring, and classroom curricula. The children in the Fast Track Intervention were less likely to develop conduct disorder during those 10 years and for 2 years thereafter.

Psychopharmacological Interventions

The efficacy of psychopharmacological interventions includes several placebo-controlled studies of risperidone for aggression in youth as well as conduct disorders. According to a review by Khan and colleagues (2019), based on at least seven randomized clinical trials, there is some evidence of limited efficacy with risperidone in reducing conduct problems and aggression in children and adolescents (5 to 18 years) when prescribed short term (6 to 12 weeks). Risperidone was found superior to placebo in reducing aggressive behavior in a large 6-month placebo-substitution study. Risperidone was approved by the Food and Drug Administration (FDA) for the treatment of irritability in children 5 years to 17 years with autism spectrum disorder in 2006. In this population, risperidone is used to manage aggression and mood swings. Aripiprazole was also approved by the FDA in 2009 for the treatment of irritability in children 6 years to 17 years old. One randomized, double-blind, placebo-controlled trial with quetiapine also showed some efficacy for aggressive behavior. Early studies of antipsychotics, most notably haloperidol, reported decreased aggressive and assaultive behaviors in children with a variety of psychiatric disorders. Atypical antipsychotics risperidone, olanzapine, quetiapine, ziprasidone, and aripiprazole have generally replaced the older antipsychotics in clinical practice due to their comparable efficacy and improved side effect profiles. Side effects of second-generation antipsychotics include sedation, increased prolactin levels (with risperidone use), and extrapyramidal symptoms, including akathisia. In general, however, the atypical antipsychotics appear to be well tolerated.

According to the review by Khan and colleagues (2019), other classes of pharmacologic agents, including mood stabilizers, anticonvulsants, stimulant agents, and selective norepinephrine reuptake inhibitors, have been reported to show a low level of evidence as a sole treatment for aggression or conduct disorder. A study of sodium valproate in youth with conduct disorder showed that those who responded most robustly exhibited aggression characterized by agitation, dysphoria, and distress. A double-blind, placebo-controlled study of carbamazepine did not show the superiority of carbamazepine over placebo in decreasing aggression. A pilot study found that clonidine may decrease aggression. The SSRIs, including fluoxetine, sertraline, paroxetine, and citalopram, are used clinically to target symptoms of impulsivity, irritability, and mood lability, which frequently accompany conduct disorder. Conduct disorder often coexists with ADHD, learning disorders, anxiety disorders, and mood disorders, all of which have some evidence-based interventions.

EPIDEMIOLOGY

The worldwide prevalence of conduct disorder has been estimated to range from 2% to 2.5%, with a prevalence of 3% to 4% in boys and 1% to 2% in girls. Although these estimates suggest that conduct disorder is not highly prevalent, retrospective studies of lifetime prevalence and prospective studies of cumulative prevalence have suggested that up to 10% of children and adolescents meet criteria for conduct disorder during their youth.

In the United States, lifetime prevalence of conduct disorder has been reported to range from 6% to 16% for males, and from 2% to 9% for females. The ratio of conduct disorder in males compared to females ranges from 4:1 to as much as 12:1. In school-age children, the point prevalence of conduct disorder has been reported to be approximately 1% to 2%. The prevalence of conduct disorder and antisocial behavior is associated with psychosocial factors including socioeconomic status, genetic contributions, as well as psychiatric disorders in parents.

ETIOLOGY

A meta-analysis of longitudinal studies indicates that the critical risk factors that predict conduct disorder include genetic contributions to impulsivity and CU traits, physical or sexual abuse or neglect, poor parental supervision, and harsh and punitive parental discipline. Low IQ and poor school achievement are also risk factors for the development of conduct disorder.

According to the comprehensive review by Fairchild and colleagues (2019), multivariate twin studies have identified at least two separate genetic factors that contribute to conduct disorder; one is related to rule breaking, and the other to overt aggression. Conduct disorder is not a unified construct in terms of its genetic expression. Heritability estimates for conduct problems are higher in males than in females, but the implicated genetic factors seem to be similar. The genetic contribution to conduct disorder appears to increase from childhood to adolescence; however, the genetic contribution is not stable over time, suggesting that a variety of different genes may contribute to conduct disorder, and they may become activated at different stages of development. Twin studies have demonstrated differential levels of genetic influence on the severity of certain symptoms within conduct disorder, with a higher heritability reported for aggressive behaviors than for nonaggressive behaviors. The heritability of CU traits has been estimated at 45% to 67%, which is higher than for the entire constellation of symptoms that constitute conduct disorder.

Parental Factors

Harsh, punitive parenting characterized by severe physical and verbal aggression is associated with the development of children's maladaptive aggressive behaviors. Chaotic home conditions are associated with conduct disorder and delinquency. Divorce itself is not necessarily a risk factor, but the persistence of hostility, resentment, and bitterness between divorced parents may be the more significant contributor to maladaptive behavior. Parental psychopathology, child abuse, and severe neglect increase the risk of conduct disorder. Antisocial behavior patterns, alcohol use disorder, and substance use disorder in the parents are associated with a higher risk of conduct disorder in their children. Parents who are so abusive or neglectful that their children are removed for their own safety may have parents that were scarred by their upbringing and are both victims and perpetrators of maltreatment.

Studies indicate that parents of children with conduct disorder have high rates of severe psychiatric disorders including psychotic disorders. Data show that children who exhibit a persistent pattern of aggressive behavior often experience physical and/or emotional abuse and harsh parenting.

Genetic Factors

A study of more than 6,000 male, female, and opposite-sex twins found that genetic and environmental factors accounted for proportionally the same amount of variance in males and females. Genetic or shared environmental factors exert different effects on males and females in childhood conduct disorder, but by adulthood, the gender-specific influences on antisocial behavior are no longer apparent. The sex-specific effects on antisocial behavior in youth along with the replicated finding of a potential role for the X-linked monoamine oxidase A gene in the etiology of antisocial behavior leads to the need for further genetic investigation of conduct disorder on the X chromosome and for analyses of these behaviors to be done separately by gender.

Sociocultural Factors

Youth living in population-dense areas have higher rates of aggression and delinquency. Unemployed parents, lack of a supportive social network, and lack of positive participation in community activities seem to predict conduct disorder. Associated findings that may influence the development of conduct disorder in urban areas are exposure to and prevalence of substance use. A survey of alcohol use and mental health in adolescents found that weekly alcohol use among adolescents is associated with increased delinquent and aggressive behavior. Significant interactions between frequent alcohol use and age indicated that those adolescents with weekly alcohol use at younger ages were most likely to exhibit aggressive behaviors and mood disorders. Although drug and alcohol use does not cause conduct disorder, it increases the risks associated with it. Drug intoxication itself can also aggravate the symptoms. Thus, all factors that increase the likelihood of regular substance use may promote and expand the disorder.

Violent Video Games and Violent Behavior

Longitudinal studies corroborate the contribution of media violence, including video gaming in middle-school children, with the expression of aggression in those adolescents. A review of the literature on the effect of violent video games on children and adolescents revealed that violent video game playing is related to aggressive affect, physiologic arousal, and aggressive behaviors. It stands to reason that the degree of exposure to violent games and the more restriction of activity would be related to a greater preoccupation with violent themes.

Psychological Factors

Poor emotion regulation among youth is associated with higher rates of aggression and conduct disorder. Emotion regulation is associated with social competence and can be observed even in children of preschool age—those children with greater degrees of emotion dysregulation exhibit higher levels of aggression. Poor modeling of impulse control and the chronic lack of having their own needs met leads to a less developed sense of empathy.

Neurobiologic Factors

Neuroimaging studies utilizing MRI have used voxel-based morphometry methods to compare structural brain differences between children with conduct disorder and healthy controls. Studies have reported that children with conduct disorder had decreased gray matter in limbic brain structures and the bilateral anterior insula and left amygdala compared to healthy controls. A study investigated structural brain differences in children comorbid for ODD or conduct disorder and ADHD compared to those with ADHD alone and healthy controls. Findings included decreased gray matter in ADHD and ADHD comorbid for ODD or conduct disorder compared to controls in regions including bilateral temporal and occipital cortices and the left amygdala.

Neuroimaging studies suggest that the most consistent structural abnormalities in conduct disorder are reduced cortical thickness in the ventromedial prefrontal cortex, orbitofrontal cortex, superior temporal cortex, fusiform gyrus, precentral gyrus, and precuneus. These regions are implicated in moral and affective decision-making, face processing, motor functions, and self-referential processing.

Neurotransmitter studies in children with conduct disorder suggest a low level of plasma dopamine β-hydroxylase, an enzyme that converts dopamine to norepinephrine, leading to a hypothesis of decreased noradrenergic functioning in conduct disorder. Other studies of conduct-disordered juvenile offenders have found high plasma serotonin levels in the blood. Evidence indicates that blood serotonin levels correlate inversely with levels of 5-hydroxyindoleacetic acid (5-HIAA) in the cerebrospinal fluid (CSF) and that low 5-HIAA levels in CSF correlate with aggression and violence.

Neurologic Factors

An electroencephalography (EEG) study investigating resting frontal brain electrical activity, emotional intelligence, aggression, and rule-breaking in 10-year-old children found that aggressive children had significantly higher relative right frontal brain activity at rest compared with nonaggressive children. Frontal resting brain electrical activity likely reflects the ability to regulate emotion. Boys tended to show lower emotional intelligence than girls and more significant aggressive behavior than girls. No relationship, however, was found between emotional intelligence and pattern of frontal EEG activation.

Child Abuse and Maltreatment

Evidence shows that children chronically exposed to violence, physical or sexual abuse, and neglect, particularly at a young age, are at high risk for demonstrating aggression. A study of female caregivers exposed to intimate partner violence revealed a strong association with offspring aggression and mood disturbance. Severely abused children and adolescents tend to be hypervigilant; in some cases, they misperceive benign situations as directly threatening and respond defensively with violence. Not all expressed aggressive behavior in adolescents is synonymous with conduct disorder; however, youth with a repetitive pattern of hypervigilance and violent responses are likely to violate the rights of others.

Further Readings

Bonham MD, Shanley DC, Waters AM, Elvin OM. Inhibitory control deficits in children with oppositional defiant disorder and conduct disorder compared to attention deficit/hyperactivity disorder: a systematic review and meta-analysis. *Res Child Adolesc Psychopathol.* 2021;49(1):39–62.

Boxer P, Huesmann LR, Bushman BJ, O'Brien M, Moceri D. The role of violent media preference in cumulative developmental risk for violence and general aggression. *J Youth Adolesc.* 2009;38(3):417–428.

Burke JD, Evans SC, Carlson GA. Debate: oppositional defiant disorder is a real disorder. *Child Adolesc Ment Health.* 2022;27(3):297–299.

Ciesinski NK, Zajac MK, McCloskey MS. Predictors of treatment outcome in cognitive behavioral therapy for intermittent explosive disorder: a preliminary analysis. *J Consult Clin Psychol.* 2024;92(1):54–60.

Coccaro EF. Psychiatric comorbidity in intermittent explosive disorder. *J Psychiatr Res.* 2019;118:38–43.

Colins OF, Fanti KA, Andershed H. The DSM-5 limited prosocial emotions specifier for conduct disorder: comorbid problems, prognosis, and antecedents. *J Am Acad Child Adolesc Psychiatry.* 202160(8):1020–1029.

Conduct Problems Prevention Research Group. The effects of the Fast Track Preventive Intervention on the development of conduct disorder across childhood. *Child Dev.* 2011;82(1):331–345.

Copeland W, Shanahan L, Costello EJ, Angold A. Cumulative prevalence of psychiatric disorders by young adulthood: a prospective cohort analysis from the Great Smoky Mountains Study. *J Am Acad Child Adolesc Psychiatry.* 2011;50(3):252–261.

Correll CU, Kratochvil CJ, March JS. Developments in pediatric psychopharmacology: focus on stimulants, antidepressants, and antipsychotics. *J Clin Psychiatry.* 2011;72(5):655–670.

Fairchild G, Hawes DJ, Frick PJ, et al. Conduct disorder. *Nat Rev Dis Primers.* 2019;5(1):43.

Frick PJ, Kemp EC. Conduct disorders and empathy development. *Annu Rev Clin Psychol.* 2021;17:391–416.

Hawes DJ, Gardner F, Dadds MR, et al. Oppositional defiant disorder. *Nat Rev Dis Primers.* 2023;9(1):31.

Hembree-Kigin TL, McNeil CB. *Parent–Child Interaction Therapy.* Springer; 1995.

Huebner T, Vloet TD, Marx I, et al. Morphometric brain abnormalities in boys with conduct disorder. *J Am Acad Child Adolesc Psychiatry.* 2008;47(5):540–547.

Kaur M, Floyd A, Balta AM. Oppositional defiant disorder: evidence-based review of behavioral treatment programs. *Ann Clin Psychiatry.* 2022;34(1):44–58.

Kazdin AE, Esveldt-Dawson K, French NH, Unis AS. Effects of parent management training and problem-solving skills training combined in the treatment of antisocial child behavior. *J Am Acad Child Adolesc Psychiatry.* 1987;26(3):416–424.

Khan S, Down J, Aouira N, et al. Current pharmacotherapy options for conduct disorders in adolescents and children. *Expert Opinion on Pharmacotherapy.* 2019;20(5):571–583.

Kimonis ER, Fleming G, Briggs N, et al. Parent–child interaction therapy adapted for preschoolers with callous–unemotional traits: an open trial pilot study. *J Clin Child Adolesc Psychol.* 2019;48(Suppl. 1): S347–S361.

Kohlhoff J, Cibralic S, Wallace N, et al. A randomized controlled trial comparing parent child interaction therapy–toddler, circle of security-parenting™ and waitlist controls in the treatment of disruptive behaviors for children aged 14–24 months: study protocol. *BMC Psychol.* 2020; 8(1):93.

LeBlanc JC, Binder CE, Armenteros JL, et al. Risperidone reduces aggression in boys with a disruptive behavior disorder and below average intelligence quotient: analysis of two placebo-controlled randomized trials. *Int Clin Psychopharmacol.* 2005;20(5):275–283.

Levantini V, Muratori P, Bertacchi I, et al. The "measure of empathy in early childhood": psychometric properties and associations with externalizing problems and callous unemotional traits. *Child Psychiatry Hum Dev.* 2024.

Masi G, Carucci S, Muratori P, Balia C, Sesso G, Milone A. Contemporary diagnosis and treatment of conduct disorder in youth. *Expert Rev Neurother.* 2023;23(12):1277–1296.

McCloskey MS, Chen EY, Olino TM, Coccaro EF. Cognitive-behavioral versus supportive psychotherapy for intermittent explosive disorder: a randomized controlled trial. *Behav Ther.* 2022;53(6):1133–1146.

Meier MH, Slutske WS, Heath AC, Martin NG. Sex differences in the genetic and environmental influences on childhood conduct disorder and adult antisocial behavior. *J Abnorm Psychol.* 2011;120(2):377–388.

Murray J, Farrington DP. Risk factors for conduct disorder and delinquency: key findings from longitudinal studies. *Can J Psychiatry.* 2010;55(10):633–642.

Padhy R, Saxena K, Remsing L, Heumer J, Plattner B, Steiner H. Symptomatic response to sodium divalproex in subtypes of conduct disorder. *Child Psychiatry Hum Dev.* 2011;42(5):584–593.

Paiva GCC, de Paula JJ, Costa DS, et al. Parent training for disruptive behavior symptoms in attention deficit hyperactivity disorder: a randomized clinical trial. *Front Psychol.* 2024;15:1293244.

Paul P, Bennett CN. Review of neuropsychological and electrophysiological correlates of callous-unemotional traits in children: implications for EEG neurofeedback intervention. *Clin EEG Neurosci.* 2021;52(5):321–329.

Pelletier J, Collett B, Gimpel G, Crowley S. Assessment of disruptive behaviors in preschoolers: psychometric properties of the disruptive behavior disorders rating scale and school situations questionnaire. *J Psychoeduc Assess.* 2006;24:3–18.

Reyes M, Buitelaar J, Toren P, Augustyns I, Eerdekens M. A randomized, double-blind, placebo-controlled study of risperidone maintenance treatment in children and adolescents with disruptive behavior disorders. *Am J Psychiatry.* 2006;163(3):402–410.

Salvatore JE, Dick DM. Genetic influences on conduct disorder. *Neurosci Biobehav Rev.* 2018;91:91–101.

Van Huylle CA, Waldman ID, D'Onofrio BM, Rodgers JL, Rthouz PJ, Lahey BB. Developmental structure of genetic influences on antisocial behavior across childhood and adolescence. *J Abnorm Psychol.* 2009;118(4):711–721.

Webster-Stratton C, Reid JM. The Incredible Years parents, teachers and children training series. In: Weisz JR, Kadin AE, eds. *Evidence-Based Psychotherapies for Children and Adolescents.* 2nd ed. Guildford; 2010:194–210.

Zahrt DM, Melzer-Lange MD. Aggressive behavior in children and adolescents. *Pediatr Rev.* 2011;32(8):325–332.

Zuddas A, Zanni R, Usala T. Second generation antipsychotics (SGAs) for non-psychotic disorders in children and adolescents: a review of the randomized controlled studies. *Eur Neuropsychopharmacol.* 2011;21(8):600–620.

15

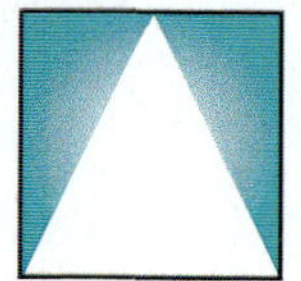

Anxiety Disorders: Separation Anxiety Disorder, Generalized Anxiety Disorder, Social Anxiety Disorder, Selective Mutism

Anxiety disorders are among the most common disorders in youth, affecting 10% to 20% of children and adolescents at some point in their development. Although observable expressions of anxiety mark developmental milestones in infants, children, and adolescents, anxiety disorders in youth can be impairing academically, personally, and socially with family and friends. Anxiety disorders in childhood and adolescence are associated with a higher risk of additional anxiety disorders, depressive disorders, and panic attacks. Fear is an expected response to a real or perceived threat; however, anxiety is the anticipation of future danger. The main characteristic of all the anxiety disorders is a recurrent emotional and physiologic arousal in response to excessive perceptions of perceived threat or danger. Anxiety disorders commonly found in youth include separation anxiety disorder, generalized anxiety disorder, social anxiety disorder, and selective mutism. We classify them by how the anxiety is experienced, the situations that trigger it, and the course that it tends to follow.

Separation anxiety disorder, generalized anxiety disorder, and social anxiety disorder in children are often considered together in the evaluation process and differential diagnosis, and in developing treatment strategies, because they are highly comorbid and have overlapping symptoms. A child with separation anxiety disorder, generalized anxiety disorder, or social anxiety disorder has a 60% chance of having at least one of the other two disorders as well. Of children with one of the above anxiety disorders, 30% have all three of them. Children and adolescents may also have additional comorbid anxiety disorders such as specific phobia or panic disorder. Separation anxiety disorder, generalized anxiety disorder, and social anxiety disorder are distinguished from each other by the types of situations that elicit excessive anxiety and avoidance behaviors. Table 15-1 highlights the overlapping symptoms and differences between separation anxiety disorder, generalized anxiety disorder, and social anxiety disorder.

SEPARATION ANXIETY DISORDER

Separation anxiety is a universal human developmental phenomenon emerging in infants at about 8 months to 1 year, marking a child's awareness of separation from his or her mother or primary caregiver. Normative separation anxiety peaks between 8 and 18 months and will diminish by about 2½ years of age, enabling young children to develop a sense of comfort away from their parents in preschool. Separation anxiety or stranger anxiety most likely evolved as a human response that has survival value. The expression of transient separation anxiety is also typical in young children entering school for the first time. Approximately 15% of young children display intense and persistent fear, shyness, and social withdrawal when faced with unfamiliar settings and people. Young children with this pattern of significant behavioral inhibition are at higher risk for the development of separation anxiety disorder, generalized anxiety disorder, and social anxiety disorder. Behaviorally inhibited children, as a group, exhibit characteristic physiologic traits, including higher than average resting heart rates, higher morning cortisol levels than

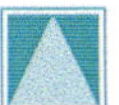

Table 15-1.
Features of DSM-5-TR Childhood Anxiety Disorders

Criteria	Separation Anxiety Disorder (SAD)	Social Anxiety Disorder (Soc AD)	Generalized Anxiety Disorder (GAD)
Duration needed for diagnosis	At least 4 wk	Typically, at least 6 mo	More days than not for 6 mo
Circumstances in which symptoms emerge	Extreme distress when separated from attachment figures	Marked fear in new social situations with peers and adults	Excessive worry about school and other performance, causing at least one symptom (restlessness, fatigue, poor concentration, irritability, muscle tension, or sleep disturbance
Symptoms that typically occur with friends	Worries that attachment figures are not safe	Feelings of discomfort and fear eating in front of them, talking to them	Worries that peers do not like them and seeks reassurance
Symptoms that often occur in school	May refuse to go to school, worries about harm to family while in school	Worries about feeling embarrassed while answering questions out loud, may speak quietly	Worries about failing exams, natural disasters, or contracting an infectious illness from being exposed to a sick peer
Sleep	Refusal or reluctance to sleep away from home or away from attachment figures	May have difficulty falling asleep	May have difficulty falling asleep due to worries about natural disasters or performance concerns the following day in school
Physiologic symptoms	Headaches, stomachaches, tearfulness, palpitations when separation is anticipated	May exhibit stiff posture, blushing, avoidance of conversation, soft voice in social situations	Shortness of breath, palpitations, hyperventilation when required to perform an activity in front of others
Differential diagnosis	Soc AD, GAD, depressive disorder	SAD, GAD, depressive disorder	Soc AD, SAD, depressive disorder

average, and low heart rate variability. Separation anxiety disorder is developmentally inappropriate and excessive anxiety related to separation from the primary attachment figure. According to the DSM-5-TR, separation anxiety disorder is a level of fear or anxiety regarding separation from their parents or primary caregiver which is beyond developmental expectations.

Furthermore, there may be a pervasive worry that harm will come to a parent upon separation, which leads to extreme distress and sometimes nightmares. The DSM-5-TR requires the presence of at least three symptoms related to excessive worry about separation from a significant attachment figure for at least 4 weeks. The worries often take the form of refusal to go to school, fears and distress on separation, repeated complaints of physical symptoms such as headaches and stomachaches when anticipating separation, and nightmares related to separation issues. Table 15-2 highlights the symptoms of separation anxiety disorder according to DSM-5-TR, ICD-10, and ICD-11.

GENERALIZED ANXIETY DISORDER

Children with generalized anxiety disorder have significant distress in activities of daily life, often focused on the child's fears of incompetence in many areas, including school performance and in social settings. Children with generalized anxiety disorder, according to DSM-5-TR, experience at least one of the following symptoms: restlessness, being easily fatigued, "mind going blank," irritability, muscle tension, or sleep disturbance. Children with generalized anxiety disorder tend to feel fearful in multiple settings and expect more negative outcomes when faced with academic or social challenges, compared with peers. Children and adolescents with generalized anxiety disorder may experience symptoms of autonomic hyperarousal such as tachycardia, shortness of breath, or dizziness, and are more likely than nonanxious youth to experience sweating, nausea, or diarrhea when they become anxious. Children and adolescents with generalized anxiety disorder tend to be overly concerned about potential natural disasters such as earthquakes or floods, and these worries can interfere with their daily activities. Finally, children and adolescents with generalized anxiety disorder are continuously worried about the quality of their performance in academics, sports, and other activities, and often seek excessive reassurance about their performance. Table 15-3 highlights the symptoms of generalized anxiety disorder according to DSM-5-TR, ICD-10, and ICD-11.

SOCIAL ANXIETY DISORDER

Children who experience intense distress in social situations, especially in new situations that can occur at school and outside of school, are impaired by their fear

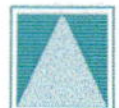

Table 15-2.
Separation Anxiety Disorder

	DSM-5-TR	ICD-10	ICD-11
Diagnostic name	Separation Anxiety Disorder	Separation Anxiety Disorder of Childhood	Separation Anxiety Disorder
Duration	Symptoms persist over ≥4 wk in children or ≥6 mo in adults		≥Several months
Symptoms	Recurrent distress on separation or anticipated separation from the attachment figure Worry of losing attachment figure or of their being harmed Worry about unexpected events that will result in forced separation from the attachment figure Hesitance to leave home or be away from the attachment figure Fear of being alone in a setting without an attachment figure Difficulty sleeping without being near attachment figure Nightmares related to fear of separation Physical symptoms occurring during separation or anticipation of separation	Fear of separation causes anxiety Anxiety arises during early childhood Severity is out of proportion and of longer duration than would be expected by normal developmental/ age standards	Marked/excessive fear/anxiety about separation from an attachment figure Symptoms vary by developmental level but may include: • Persistent thoughts of being separated due to some harm/ unexpected event • Reluctance/refusal to go to school or work • Excess distress related to a separation from an attachment figure • Recurrent nightmares about separation • Physical symptoms associated with separation (gastrointestinal, headaches)
Required number of symptoms	≥3 of the symptoms above meeting the required duration		
Psychosocial consequences	Distress or psychosocial impairment	Impaired functioning	Distress or psychosocial impairment
Exclusions	Another mental disorder		Another mental disorder
Comments		Note: Classified under (Emotional disorders with onset specific to childhood)	

of scrutiny or humiliation and have the diagnosis of social anxiety disorder. These symptoms must be present in peer settings, not only in interactions with adults. Their distress may be expressed in the form of crying, tantrums, avoidance, or freezing. Children who experience severe social anxiety leading to becoming "mute" in distressing social situations are diagnosed with a related but independent disorder, selective mutism, according to DSM-5-TR, which will be described separately. According to DSM-5-TR, social anxiety disorder is characterized by consistent anxiety and distress in one or more social situations recurrently. Situations in which a child with social anxiety disorder feels exposed to possible scrutiny by others can provoke fear or anxiety, and the child will often try to avoid these feared social situations. A child or adolescent with social anxiety disorder may exhibit the symptoms only related to performance, which targets a specific type of performing, such as fear of public speaking. The performance-only type typically manifests in school or academic settings in which one must make public presentations, such as in front of classmates in school. Children and adolescents with the performance-only form of social anxiety disorder do not experience significant distress in social situations that don't involve performing.

Social anxiety disorder has significant implications for future accomplishments, since it is associated with higher levels of distress in school, work, and in leisure activities. Despite the significant impairment caused by social anxiety disorder, up to half of the individuals with the disorder do not receive treatment. Table 15-4 highlights the symptoms of social anxiety disorder in the DSM-5-TR, ICD-10, and ICD-11.

DIAGNOSIS AND CLINICAL FEATURES

Separation anxiety disorder, generalized anxiety disorder, and social anxiety disorder are highly related in children and adolescents because, in many youth,

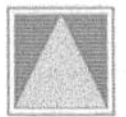

Table 15-3.
Generalized Anxiety Disorder

	DSM-5/DSM-5-TR	ICD-10	ICD-11
Diagnostic name	Generalized Anxiety Disorder	Generalized Anxiety Disorder	Generalized Anxiety Disorder
Duration	≥6 mo, more days than not		Persists for several months, more days than not
Symptoms	Excessive anxiety or worry about a wide range of situations Difficulty controlling or managing worry Symptoms of anxiety/worry, including: • Restlessness • Fatigue • Poor concentration • Irritability • Muscle tension • Sleep disturbance	Persistent and generalized anxiety Anxiety not associated with a particular object, event, or situation Predominant symptoms may include worry, shaking, muscle tension, sweating, lightheadedness, palpitations, and GI symptoms	Free-floating anxiety or excessive worry about negative events Anxiety is accompanied by symptoms such as: • Motor restlessness, muscle tension • Autonomic overactivity • Feeling nervous, restless, or on edge • Difficulty concentrating • Irritability • Insomnia
Required number of symptoms	Both excessive worry and difficulty controlling worry must be present, in addition to ≥3 of the associated symptoms of anxiety/worry		
Psychosocial consequences	Distress or psychosocial impairment		Distress or psychosocial impairment
Exclusions	Other medical condition Substance or medication, including withdrawal Other mental illness		Other medical condition Substance or medication, including withdrawal Other mental illness

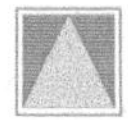

Table 15-4.
Social Anxiety Disorder

	DSM-5-TR	ICD-10	ICD-11
Diagnostic name	Social Anxiety Disorder (Social Phobia)	Social Phobias	Social Anxiety Disorder
Duration	Persistent and lasting typically ≥6 mo		Persistent and lasting ≥several months
Symptoms	Anxiety related to social situations, given the fear of being judged or scrutinized by others Fear of allowing anxiety to show and be noticed by others, be perceived negatively, or will lead to embarrassment or rejection Avoidance of feared social situations Anxiety and fear are out of proportion to the social context	Fear of being judged or scrutinized by other people Fear of judgment or embarrassment leads to avoidance of social situations It can be associated with low self-esteem Panic attacks may develop	Anxiety occurs in ≥1 social interaction or while performing Fear or concern of being negatively evaluated by others The feared situation is avoided or endured with intense anxiety
Required number of symptoms	All of the above		
Psychosocial consequences	Marked distress and/or impairment		Marked distress and/or impairment
Exclusions	Other medical condition Substance or medication, including withdrawal Other mental illness		Other mental illness
Symptoms specifiers	**Performance only** (anxiety related specifically to publicly performing or speaking)		

overlapping symptoms and comorbid disorders occur. Generalized anxiety disorder is the most common anxiety disorder among youth, more common in adolescents than in younger children. In approximately one-third of these cases, a child or adolescent with generalized anxiety disorder will also exhibit separation anxiety disorder and social anxiety disorder.

Diagnostic criteria for separation anxiety disorder, according to the DSM-5-TR, include three symptoms such as persistent and excessive worry about losing major attachment figures; about possible harm befalling attachment figures upon separation; about future separation from a significant attachment figure; persistent reluctance or refusal to go to school or elsewhere because of fear of separation; persistent and excessive fear or reluctance to be alone or without major attachment figures at home or without significant adults in other settings; persistent reluctance or refusal to go to sleep without being near a major attachment figure or to sleep away from home; repeated nightmares involving the theme of separation; repeated complaints of physical symptoms, including headaches and stomachaches, when separation from significant attachment figures is anticipated; and recurrent excessive distress when separation from home or significant attachment figures is anticipated or involved. Symptoms must be present for 4 weeks in children or adolescents. Table 15-2 lists the comparative diagnostic criteria for separation anxiety disorder in DSM-5-TR, ICD-10, and ICD-11.

The following case history demonstrates separation anxiety disorder along with autonomic arousal symptoms.

Janet was a 7-year-old girl who was referred due to refusing to go to school. Janet refused to sleep in her room alone at night, which her mother accommodated, and she exhibited violent tantrums each morning in order to avoid going to school. Janet expressed recurrent fears that her mother would get into a car accident and die when they weren't together. She also worried that there would be a fire in their home while she was in school, and her mother would die. Janet's developmental history revealed that she was anxious and irritable as an infant and toddler. She cried for hours when her parents occasionally hired a babysitter at night, and she had long crying jags in school when she was sent to preschool. Janet's mother had a history of generalized anxiety disorder, and her father had recurrent major depression. When her parents separated when Janet was 6 years of age, she became more concerned and territorial over her mother. Janet always kept track of her mother's whereabouts and insisted that she stay at home because she would not be safe if she went out.

Nighttime was a particularly difficult time at home. When Janet's mother tried to get her to remain in her room, Janet would whine and cry and insist that her mother lie in bed with her until she falls asleep. Janet reported frequent nightmares that her mother died and that monsters prevented her from rescuing her mother, taking her away from her family forever.

During the daytime, Janet would shadow her mother around the house. Janet would agree to play a game with her sister in the house only if her mother was nearby. When Janet's mother went upstairs, she would interrupt the game and follow her upstairs. Janet refused to sleep at a friend's house. Frequently, as the evening progressed at home, Janet described a queasy sensation in her stomach mixed with feelings of sadness.

On school days, Janet often complained of stomachaches and tried to stay home. Janet appeared distressed and panicky and would become aggressive toward her mother when she attempted to drop her off at school. Once at school, she seemed calmer and less distressed, but frequently was seen in the nurse's office, complaining of nausea and seeking to be sent home. (Adapted from Gail A Bernstein, M.D. and Anne E. Layne, Ph.D.)

The essential feature of separation anxiety disorder is extreme anxiety precipitated by separation from the primary caregiver, home, or familiar surroundings. In contrast, in generalized anxiety disorder, fears are focused on adverse outcomes from natural disasters or various events, including academics, peer relationships, and family activities. In generalized anxiety disorder, a child or adolescent experiences at least one recurrent physiologic symptom, such as restlessness, poor concentration, irritability, or muscle tension. In social anxiety disorder, the child's fears peak during social situations involving exposure to unfamiliar people or situations. Children and adolescents with social anxiety disorder have extreme concerns about being embarrassed, humiliated, or negatively judged. In each of the preceding anxiety disorders, the child's experience can approach a feeling of terror or panic. The distress experienced by youth with anxiety disorders is higher than that normally expected for the child's developmental level and is not otherwise explainable. Morbid fears, preoccupations, and ruminations characterize anxiety disorders. Children with anxiety disorders overestimate the probability of danger and the likelihood of a negative outcome. Many children with anxiety disorders are preoccupied with their health and worry that their families or friends will become ill. Fears of getting lost, being kidnapped, and losing the ability to be in contact with their families are predominant among children with separation anxiety disorder.

Adolescents with anxiety disorders may not directly express their worries; however, their behavioral patterns often reflect either separation anxiety or other anxiety if they exhibit discomfort about leaving home, engage excessively in solitary activities because of fears about how they will perform in front of peers, or experience distress when away from their families. Separation anxiety disorder in children is often manifested at the thought of travel or in the course of travel away from home. Children may refuse to go to camp, a new school, or even a friend's house. Frequently, a continuum exists between mild anticipatory anxiety before separation to pervasive anxiety after the separation has occurred. Premonitory signs include irritability, difficulty eating, whining, staying in a room alone, clinging to parents, and following a parent everywhere. Often, when a family moves, a child displays separation anxiety by intense clinging to the mother figure. Children with anxiety disorders may retreat from social or group activities and express feelings of loneliness because of their self-imposed isolation.

Sleep difficulties are common in children and adolescents with anxiety disorders. In youth with severe separation anxiety, a child or adolescent may require having someone remain with him or her until he or she falls asleep. An anxious child may awaken and go to a parent's bed or even sleep at the parent's door to diminish anxiety. Nightmares and morbid fears may be expressions of anxiety.

Associated features of anxiety disorders include fear of the dark and imaginary vague images. Children may have the feeling that eyes are staring at them and monsters are reaching out for them in their bedrooms. Children with separation anxiety disorder, generalized anxiety disorder, and social anxiety disorder often complain of somatic symptoms and may be more sensitive to changes in their bodies compared to youth without anxiety disorders. Children with separation anxiety disorder, generalized anxiety disorder, or social anxiety disorder are often more emotionally sensitive than peers and more easily brought to tears. Frequent somatic complaints accompanying anxiety disorders include gastrointestinal symptoms, nausea, vomiting, and stomachaches; unexplained pain in various parts of the body; sore throats; and flu-like symptoms. Older children and adolescents with anxiety disorders typically complain of somatic experiences such as cardiovascular and respiratory symptoms—palpitations, dizziness, faintness, and feelings of strangulation. Physiologic signs of anxiety are a part of the diagnostic criteria for generalized anxiety disorder, but they are more often also experienced by children with separation anxiety and social anxiety disorder than the general population. The following case history demonstrates a young adolescent with generalized anxiety disorder.

Jose was a 14-year-old boy referred by his pediatrician to see a child and adolescent psychiatrist for an evaluation due to missing many days at school because of chronic functional gastrointestinal complaints. Gastrointestinal workup had not revealed any medical diagnoses. On interview, Jose appeared withdrawn and tentative but cooperative with questions. Jose endorsed multiple worries that included concerns about his health, his parents' safety, his school performance, and fears that his peers don't really like him. Jose's most significant worries were related to illnesses and safety, including worries about getting into a car accident or being hit by lightning. Jose's mother reported that Jose had become very reluctant to see friends, whether inside or outside, because he feared he would contract COVID-19 even when his peers were well. Jose would become distraught if he heard news reports about catastrophic events locally and around the world (e.g., kidnapping, crime, terrorism). Jose's family and teachers described Jose as overly perfectionistic about his schoolwork and often concerning himself with family finances, his parents' job security, and worries that his parents might become ill. Symptoms that Jose reported daily primarily involved abdominal pain, feeling dizzy and nauseated, and insomnia. Jose perseverated on his worries, repetitively verbalizing his worries even after receiving reassurance. Jose disclosed that he worried for hours each day and could not "turn off" his distressing worries.

Jose's medical history was unremarkable, except for frequent complaints of gastrointestinal pain and discomfort since kindergarten. Jose had been a shy young child, although all of his developmental milestones were achieved as expected. Jose was described as very compliant and had no history of behavior problems. Jose was very concerned about his academic performance from an early age despite the fact that he was an excellent student and received As in most subjects with an occasional B. Jose was shy in new social situations and slow to warm up, but he was well liked by peers. Jose's family history included maternal recurrent depression as well as a history of generalized anxiety disorder, social anxiety, and separation anxiety disorder as a child. Jose had two younger brothers who were high achievers and did not display significant anxiety symptoms. (Adapted from Gail A Bernstein, M.D. and Anne E. Layne, Ph.D.)

The next case history demonstrates a school-aged child with comorbid anxiety and depressive disorders.

Kelly was a 10-year-old fifth grader who lived with her biologic parents and two sisters, ages 8 and 5 years. Kelly was a highly articulate child who has always been a good student, although she never volunteered answers in school unless her teachers call on her. Kelly got along well with her sisters when at home, but she has always declined invitations to go to friends' homes for a sleepover and has turned down opportunities to go to parties. Over the past year, as her peers are getting together more on the weekends, she has become more self-conscious and isolative. Kelly reports that she gets too nervous and blushes when she is with friends outside of the classroom at school and she cannot think of anything to say to them. Kelly reports that she is embarrassed to go shopping or to the movies, even when her friends' parents accompany them, because she fears they might run into other neighborhood peers along the way and she will feel "stupid" because they will see how shy she is and make fun of her. Recently, Kelly's former best friend asked her why she stopped eating lunch with her and her new friends in school. Kelly disclosed that she avoided eating lunch with her because she always invited other friends to join them, and Kelly was too uncomfortable around new people. Kelly explained that she felt humiliated when they would talk about their weekend plans, and even when they invited her to join, she would just look the other way and ignore the conversation. Kelly had become isolated, even in school, and admitted to her mother that she was lonely. Kelly was brought for an evaluation after her 8-year-old sister reported to her mother that Kelly spent all of her time alone in school. Kelly's sister reported that, whenever she and Kelly saw each other at school, she looked sad and stressed out, and wasn't talking to her friends. Kelly was down, always in poor spirits, and had stopped interacting with her sisters very often. On some occasions, Kelly's younger sister invited Kelly to parties or friends' homes, but Kelly usually declined and often became tearful. Kelly was evaluated by a child psychiatrist who made the diagnoses of social anxiety disorder, generalized anxiety disorder, and major depression and recommended a combination of cognitive-behavioral therapy (CBT) for anxiety and depression and a trial of fluoxetine. Kelly and her family decided to try the medication while they looked for a therapist. Kelly was started on 10 mg of fluoxetine, and over the next month was titrated up to a dose of 20 mg. By the third week of the medication, Kelly was noticeably less resistant to going out with her sisters to places and seemed less stressed when they met other peers. Kelly's younger sister noticed that she did not seem as sad and started to sit with peers at lunch in the school cafeteria. Kelly reported that she did not feel as self-conscious as she used to in class and was willing to try to go to a friend's house. She still resisted going to a birthday party of a peer that she did not know very well. Kelly continued on the medication and began weekly CBT, and within 2 months, she was significantly less anxious in social situations. Kelly still occasionally complained of a stomachache but didn't let that stop her from activities. Kelly's family was impressed when she requested a birthday party for her 11th birthday and decided to invite 10 friends.

Pathology and Laboratory Examination

No specific laboratory measures help in the diagnosis of separation anxiety disorder, generalized anxiety disorder, or social anxiety disorder.

DIFFERENTIAL DIAGNOSIS

The presence of separation anxiety is a developmentally expected feature in a developing infant and does not represent an impairing condition. Thus, clinical judgment must be used in distinguishing developmentally normal anxiety from separation anxiety disorder in each age group. In school-aged children, a child experiencing more than typical distress is apparent when refusing school regularly. For children who resist school, it is essential to distinguish whether fear of separation, worry about performance, academic difficulties, or specific fears of humiliation in front of peers or the teacher are driving the resistance.

When depressive disorders occur in children, we should evaluate for possible comorbidities, such as anxiety disorders, as well. Comorbid diagnoses of an anxiety disorder and depressive disorder are made when a patient meets both criteria, as the two diagnoses often coexist. Panic disorder with agoraphobia is uncommon before 18 years of age; the fear is of being incapacitated by a panic attack rather than of separation from parental figures. School refusal is a frequent symptom in separation anxiety disorder but is not pathognomonic of it. Children with diagnoses such as specific phobias, social anxiety disorder, or fear of failure in school because of a learning disorder may also lead to school refusal. When school refusal occurs in an adolescent, the severity of the dysfunction is generally higher than when it emerges in a young child. Table 15-1 presents similar and distinguishing characteristics of childhood separation anxiety disorder, generalized anxiety disorder, and social anxiety disorder.

COURSE AND PROGNOSIS

The course and the prognosis of separation anxiety disorder, generalized anxiety disorder, and social anxiety disorder are varied and are related to the age of onset, the duration of the symptoms, and comorbid anxiety and depressive disorders. Children who maintain attendance in school, after-school activities, and peer relationships generally have a better prognosis than children or adolescents who refuse to attend school and withdraw from social activities. The multisite randomized clinical trial Child/Adolescent Anxiety Multimodal Study (CAMS), which was initiated in 2002 and continued enrolling subjects for the next 6 years, was the largest multi-site double-blind study providing evidence of effective acute treatment for children and adolescents with one or more anxiety disorders. CAMS subjects were randomized into four groups consisting of active sertraline medication alone, CBT alone, both together, and placebo. The double-blind aspect was limited to the active medication versus the placebo group. The study period was 12 weeks of double-blind, placebo-controlled study followed by a 6-month follow-up period. The investigators found that predictors of future remission included younger age of initiation of treatment, lower severity of anxiety, absence of a comorbid depressive or anxiety disorder, and the absence of social anxiety disorder as the primary anxiety disorder. Early age of onset and older age at diagnosis in this study predicted slower recovery. Studies have revealed an increased risk of and significant overlap between separation anxiety disorder and future depressive disorders. In cases with multiple comorbidities, the prognosis is more guarded. Longitudinal data indicate that some children with severe school refusal continue to resist attending school into adolescence and remain impaired for many years.

TREATMENT

The treatment of child and adolescent separation anxiety disorder, generalized anxiety disorder, and social anxiety disorder are often considered together, given the frequent overlapping symptomatology and co-occurrence of these disorders. The multimodal comprehensive treatment approach, which paved the way for the evidence-based treatment of children and adolescents with anxiety disorders, usually includes psychotherapy, most often CBT, family education, family psychosocial intervention, and pharmacologic interventions, such as selective serotonin reuptake inhibitors (SSRIs). Details of the CAMS are as follows: a double-blind, placebo-controlled, multi-site study that included 488 children and adolescents with separation anxiety disorder, generalized anxiety disorder, or social anxiety disorder. The investigators treated them with either CBT alone, SSRI medication (sertraline) alone, both CBT and sertraline, or placebo. After an acute treatment phase of 12 weeks, those in the combined CBT plus sertraline group had an 80.7% response rate of much or very much improved on the clinical global improvement (CGI) rating. Response rates for the CBT-only and sertraline-only groups were 59.7% and 54.9%, respectively. The placebo response was 23.7%. Over time, during an open follow-up, the combination of CBT plus sertraline continued to provide the most efficacies. All three treatments—CBT, sertraline, and their combination—were superior to placebo and thus effective treatments in childhood anxiety, but combined treatment was most likely to help children and adolescents with anxiety disorders. A trial of CBT is often administered before medication when a child can function sufficiently at school, home, and in treatment. For children with more severe impairment, a combination of treatments is recommended. CBT is a first-line evidence-based treatment for childhood anxiety disorders. A meta-analysis reviewed 16 randomized controlled trials of CBT for childhood anxiety disorders and found CBT to be consistently superior to a wait-list control group or a psychological placebo group. Exposure-based CBT has received the most empiric support among psychotherapeutic interventions for anxiety disorders in youth and is superior to wait-list control groups in reducing impairment and symptoms of anxiety.

Several psychosocial interventions have been designed specifically for anxiety disorders in young children. In a randomized clinical trial of CBT for 4- to 7-year-old children, the children received a manualized intervention called "Being Brave: A Program for Coping with Anxiety for Young Children and their Parents." The intervention used a combination of parent-only sessions and child-and-parent sessions. Response rate, measured as much or very much improved on the CGI Scale for Anxiety, was 69% among completers versus 32% of the wait-list controls. The treated children showed significantly better CGI improvement for social anxiety disorder, separation anxiety disorder, and specific phobia, but not generalized anxiety disorder. This treatment, a developmentally modified parent–child CBT, shows promise in young children.

Coaching Approach Behavior and Leading by Modeling (the CALM program) is an intervention aimed at treating anxiety disorders in children younger than 7 years of age who are too young for traditional CBT. The CALM program draws on previous work with children aged 2 to 7 years through interventions that target a child's undesired behavior by modifying parents' behavior, called Parent–Child Interaction Therapy (PCIT). The CALM program is a 12-session manual-based intervention that provides live, individualized coaching via a bug-in-the-ear receiver worn by the parent during sessions. It incorporates exposure tasks and promotes "brave" behavior with parent coaching. A pilot study using the CALM program with nine patients with a mean age of 5.4 years found that all treatment completers (seven patients and families) were global responders, and all but one showed functional improvement. Adapting the PCIT model for anxiety disorders in young children appears to be a promising approach to treating anxiety in early childhood.

A meta-analysis of randomized controlled trials (RCTs) of antidepressant agents for childhood anxiety provides evidence that multiple SSRIs, including fluoxetine, sertraline, and fluvoxamine, are efficacious in the treatment of childhood anxiety. Based on this evidence, SSRIs became the first choice of medication in the treatment of anxiety disorders in children and adolescents. When serotonin-norepinephrine reuptake inhibitor (SNRI) medications came onto the market, they provided an additional option in the treatment of youth anxiety disorders.

The Federal Drug Administration (FDA) has recently approved escitalopram as well as duloxetine, an SNRI medication, for the treatment of generalized anxiety in children 7 years and older. Escitalopram is also FDA approved for the treatment of major depressive disorder in children 12 years and older. Fluoxetine is FDA approved for the treatment of major depressive disorder in children 8 years and older.

A multisite investigation by the NIMH Research Units in Pediatric Psychopharmacology (RUPP) confirmed the safety and efficacy of fluvoxamine in the treatment of childhood separation anxiety disorder, generalized anxiety disorder, and social anxiety disorder as early as 2000. This double-blind, placebo-controlled study of 128 children and adolescents revealed that 76% of children in the group treated with fluvoxamine showed significant improvement compared with 29% of those in the placebo group. Response to medication was noticeable after only 2 weeks of treatment. Fluvoxamine dosages ranged from 50 to 250 mg/day in children and up to 300 mg/day in adolescents. Children and adolescents with less comorbid depressive symptoms had the best response. Youths who responded continued fluvoxamine for 6 months, and almost all of them continued to be responders at the 6-month mark.

Several other randomized clinical trials have also supported the efficacy of SSRIs in the treatment of child and adolescent anxiety disorders. A randomized, controlled trial found fluoxetine, at a dose of 20 mg/day, to be safe and effective for children with these disorders, with minor side effects including gastrointestinal distress, headache, and drowsiness. Also, a randomized clinical trial for the treatment of generalized anxiety disorder in children lends support for the efficacy of sertraline.

The FDA has placed a "black box" warning on antidepressants, including all of the SSRI agents, used in the treatment of any childhood disorder, because of concerns about increased suicidality; however, no individual childhood anxiety study has found a statistically significant increase in suicidal thoughts or behaviors.

Currently, tricyclic antidepressant drugs are not recommended in the treatment of anxiety and depressive disorders in youth due to their potentially serious cardiac adverse effects. Other agents, including buspirone and β-adrenergic receptor antagonists such as propranolol, have been used clinically in children with anxiety disorders, but currently, no data support their efficacy. Diphenhydramine may be used in the short term for insomnia in children with anxiety disorders. Open trials and one double-blind, placebo-controlled study suggested that alprazolam, a benzodiazepine, may help to control anxiety symptoms in separation anxiety disorder. Clonazepam has been studied in open trials and may be useful in controlling symptoms of panic and other anxiety symptoms. Benzodiazepines are not generally recommended in long-term treatment of anxiety disorders in children and adolescents.

SSRIs, SNRIs, and CBT, alone and in combination, have demonstrated efficacy in the treatment of anxiety disorders in many youth, but approximately 20% to 35% of children and adolescents with anxiety disorders do not appear to benefit. Childhood anxiety disorders tend to wax and wane over time, and persistent school refusal associated with separation anxiety disorder is a serious and impairing condition. A comprehensive treatment plan involves the child, the parents, and the child's peers and school. Family participation in treatment is critical in the management of severe separation anxiety disorder, especially in children who refuse to attend school, so that firm encouragement of school attendance is maintained while providing appropriate support. When initiation of a return to a full school day is overwhelming, the treatment team and school may optimally help arrange a program so the child can progressively increase the time spent at school. Graded exposure to the feared situation is an essential component of behavioral interventions useful for separation anxiety. When school refusal in a child or adolescent is treatment resistant, a child or adolescent may require hospitalization to begin exposure to a modified school program while away from home.

Evidence-based treatments for anxiety disorders in youth support CBT and treatment with an SSRI or SNRI medication. In young children, CBT is preferred as the initial form of treatment. When symptoms remain after a trial of CBT, SSRIs are usually added. When symptoms are severe, a combination of CBT and SSRI medication is usually recommended.

EPIDEMIOLOGY

The prevalence of anxiety disorders reported has varied depending on the age group of the children surveyed, and the diagnostic instruments used. The lifetime prevalence of any anxiety disorder in children and adolescents ranges from 10% to 27%. In adolescents, the lifetime prevalence of anxiety disorders is up to about 33%. Anxiety disorders are not uncommon in preschoolers as well. An epidemiologic survey using the Preschool Age Psychiatric Assessment (PAPA) found that 9.5% of preschoolers met criteria for any anxiety disorder, with 6.5% exhibiting generalized anxiety disorder, 2.4% meeting criteria for separation anxiety disorder, and 2.2% meeting criteria for social anxiety disorder. Separation anxiety disorder is estimated to be about 4% in children and young adolescents. Separation anxiety disorder is more common in young children than in adolescents and occurs equally in boys and girls. The onset may occur during preschool years but is most common in children 7 to 8 years of age. The rate of generalized anxiety disorder in school-aged children is estimated to be approximately 3%, the rate of social anxiety disorder is 1%, and the rate of simple phobias is 2.4%. In adolescents, lifetime prevalence for panic disorder is 0.6%; the prevalence of generalized anxiety disorder is 3.7%. Anxiety disorders appear to emerge most often in children 5 to 7 years old and 13 to 18 years old.

ETIOLOGY

Biopsychosocial Factors

Multiple investigations have found evidence for the influences of parental psychopathology and parenting styles on the emergence of anxiety disorders in childhood. Longitudinal studies have found that parental overprotection correlates with an increased risk of the development of anxiety disorders in children, and insecure parent–child attachment is associated with higher-than-expected rates of anxiety disorders in childhood. It is also well known that maternal depression and anxiety have led to an increased risk of anxiety and depression in children. Psychosocial factors, in conjunction with a child's temperament, influence the degree of separation anxiety evoked in situations of brief separation and exposure to unfamiliar environments. The temperamental trait of shyness and withdrawal in unfamiliar situations is associated with a higher risk of developing separation anxiety disorder, generalized anxiety disorder, social anxiety disorder, or all three during childhood and adolescence.

External life stresses often coincide with the development of the disorder. The death of a relative, a child's illness, a change in a child's environment, or a move to a new neighborhood or school is frequent in the histories of children with separation anxiety disorder. In a vulnerable child, these changes probably intensify anxiety.

Neurophysiologic correlations exist with behavioral inhibition (extreme shyness); children with this constellation have a higher resting heart rate and an acceleration of heart rate with tasks requiring cognitive concentration. Additional physiologic correlates of behavioral inhibition include elevated salivary cortisol levels, elevated urinary catecholamine levels, and more significant papillary dilation during cognitive tasks.

Neuroimaging studies of adolescents with anxiety show increased activation of the amygdala compared to nonanxious adolescents when presented with anxiety-provoking stimuli. Furthermore, anxious adolescents maintain the hyperactivation of the amygdala over time, rather than showing an attenuation of the effect as in nonanxious adolescents. Structural studies of the amygdala in adolescents with anxiety have led to conflicting results, with some studies finding increased amygdala volumes, whereas other studies are finding decreased amygdala volumes.

Social Learning Factors

Fear, in response to a variety of unfamiliar or unexpected situations, may be unwittingly communicated from parents to children by direct modeling. If a parent is fearful, the child will probably have a phobic adaptation to new situations, especially to a school environment. There is much data to suggest that overprotective parenting promotes increased interpersonal sensitivity in healthy children and increases the risk of social anxiety disorder in children with behavioral inhibition or other anxiety disorders such as separation anxiety disorder. Some parents appear to teach their children to be anxious by overprotecting them from expected dangers or by exaggerating the dangers. For example, a parent who cringes in a room during a lightning storm teaches a child to do the same. A parent who is afraid of mice or insects conveys fright to a child.

Conversely, a parent who becomes angry with a child when the child expresses fear of a given situation, for example, when exposed to animals, may promote a phobic concern in the child by exposing the child to the intensity of the anger expressed by the parent. When parents have anxiety disorders, this magnifies the social learning factors in the development of anxiety reactions. These factors may be pertinent in the development of separation anxiety disorder as well as in generalized anxiety disorder and social anxiety disorder. A recent study found no association between psychosocial hardships, such as ongoing family conflict, and behavioral inhibition among young children. It appears that temperamental predisposition to anxiety disorders emerges as a highly heritable constellation of traits and due to psychosocial stressors.

Genetic Factors

Genetic studies suggest that genes account for at least one-third of the variance in the development of anxiety disorders. Heritability for anxiety disorders in children and adolescents ranges from 36% to 65%, with the highest estimates found in younger children with anxiety disorders. Two heritable characteristics—behavioral inhibition (the tendency toward fear and withdrawal in new situations) and physiologic hyperarousal—have both been found to impart significant risk factors for the future development of an anxiety disorder. However, although the temperamental constellation of behavioral inhibition, excessive shyness, the tendency to withdraw from unfamiliar situations, and the eventual emergence of anxiety disorders have a genetic contribution, one-third to two-thirds of young children with behavioral inhibition do not appear to go on to develop anxiety disorders.

Family studies have shown that the offspring of adults with anxiety disorders are at an increased risk of having an anxiety disorder themselves. Separation anxiety disorder and depression in children overlap, and the presence of an anxiety disorder increases the risk of a future episode of a depressive disorder. The current consensus on the genetics of anxiety disorders suggests that what is inherited is a general predisposition toward anxiety, causing heightened levels of arousal, emotional reactivity, and increased negative affect, all of which increase the risk of developing separation anxiety disorder, generalized anxiety disorder, and social anxiety disorder.

SELECTIVE MUTISM

Selective mutism, believed to be related to social anxiety disorder, is included as an independent disorder in the DSM-5-TR. Selective mutism is characterized in a child by persistent muteness, that is lack of speaking, in one or more specific social situations, most typically, the school setting. A child with selective mutism may remain wholly silent or near silent, in some cases only whispering in a school setting. Although selective mutism often begins before age 5 years, it may not be apparent until the child is expected to be reading or speaking aloud in school. The current conceptualization of selective mutism focuses on a convergence of underlying social anxiety, along with an increased risk of expressive speech and language problems leading to a lack of speaking in specific social situations. Typically, children with selective mutism are either completely silent during stressful situations, or verbalize almost inaudibly single-syllable words. Despite an increased risk for delayed speech and language acquisition, children with this disorder are fully capable of speaking competently when not in a socially anxiety-producing situation. Some children with the selective mutism will communicate with eye contact or nonverbal gestures but not verbally when at school. Otherwise, children with selective mutism speak fluently at

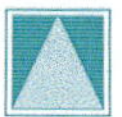

Table 15-5.
Selective Mutism

	DSM-5-TR	ICD-10	ICD-11
Diagnostic name	Selective Mutism	Elective Mutism	Selective Mutism
Duration	≥1 mo (not exclusively during the first month of school)		≥1 mo (not exclusively during the first month of school)
Symptoms	Persistent lack of speech in particular social situations despite being able to speak in other situations	Presence of selectively speaking related to specific emotions, resulting in a child that has previously demonstrated the ability to speak not speaking in particular social situations It may be associated with other symptoms of anxiety, social withdrawal, and sensitivity	Selectivity in speaking with language competence in some situations but not others
Psychosocial consequences	Psychosocial impairment		Psychosocial impairment
Exclusions	Another mental disorder Communication disorder Lack of proficiency with the spoken language in a given situation	Pervasive developmental disorders Developmental disorders of speech and language Transient mutism as part of separation anxiety in young children	Another mental disorder
Comments		Note: Classified as a disorder of social functioning with onset specific to childhood and adolescence	

home and in many familiar settings. Selective mutism is believed to be related to social anxiety disorder because of its expression primarily in selective social situations.

DIAGNOSIS AND CLINICAL FEATURES

The diagnosis of selective mutism is not difficult to make after it is known that a child has adequate language skills in some environments but not in others. The mutism may have developed gradually or suddenly after a disturbing experience. The age of onset can range from 4 to 8 years. Mute periods are most manifested in school or outside the home; in rare cases, a child is mute at home but not in school. Children who exhibit selective mutism may also have symptoms of separation anxiety disorder, school refusal, and delayed language acquisition. Because social anxiety symptoms are typically present in children with selective mutism, behavioral disturbances, such as temper tantrums and oppositional behaviors, may also occur in the home. Compared to children with generalized anxiety disorder or separation anxiety disorder, children with selective mutism tend to have less social competence and more social anxiety. Table 15-5 compares the criteria for selective mutism according to DSM-5-TR.

Lily is a 5-year-old Korean American kindergarten student who lives with her biologic mother, father, and siblings. Lily and her parents speak Korean almost all the time at home, but she and her sisters speak in English to each other most of the time. Although Lily learned and spoke English fluently by the time she was 3 years old, Lily's parents reported that, ever since Lily entered preschool at the age of 3 years, she has not spoken at all at school despite speaking well at home. At home, Lily is animated and quite talkative with her immediate family and a few young cousins. Lily speaks softly to adult relatives outside of her immediate family, and her communication is often limited to one-word responses to their questions. Lily's parents report that she also exhibits excessive fear and anxiety in social situations, and she often "freezes" in situations when the attention is on her. At the time of her evaluation, Lily had not received prior treatment. Lily met all of her developmental milestones on time and appeared to have above-average intelligence. Lily enjoys dancing, singing, and imaginative play with her sisters.

During the initial evaluation, Lily made intermittent eye contact with the clinician and responded to questions with nods but not verbal responses. Lily's parents reported that this behavior is typical of her when in a new situation and that she communicates nonverbally and makes intermittent eye contact until she "gets to know someone." Lily has been described as slow to warm up. Lily's parents provided a videotape of her playing at home with her sisters. Lily was animated and speaking spontaneously and fluently without apparent impairment. Lily received a diagnosis of selective mutism and was noted to have some symptoms of social anxiety disorder. CBT to address her selective mutism was recommended.

When treatment began, Lily did not communicate verbally, but she did communicate non verbally by nodding her head to indicate yes or no. Lily's therapist gradually developed a rapport with Lily, coloring together and doing simple puzzles at first. The therapist used animal puppets to help Lily to "warm up" without speaking directly to the therapist. After three sessions, Lily was willing began to answer some of the therapist's questions in a whisper. Lily received stickers for completing each speaking assignment given to her by her therapist, first in a whisper and then in a very soft voice, and, after filling up the sticker charts, she received a small reward such as a coloring book.

After being able to speak to her therapist in a low speaking voice, Lily's therapist, with the help of Lily's parents and an agreement with her teacher, began to give Lily some simple assignments involving communicating with her teacher and classmates. These tasks were implemented gradually and included waving to the teacher, playing an audiotape of her saying "hello" to the teacher, and then whispering "hello" to the teacher. Once Lily was able to say "hello" to the teacher in a regular voice, she was asked to say the same to one of her classmates that she liked. After 14 sessions, Lily began to speak in complete sentences during class when called on. Although Lily did not volunteer to answer, she was able to respond verbally when called on. Lily then went on to practice speaking some words to her classmates. Lily's most impressive therapeutic achievement during her therapy was to stand in front of her whole class and say good morning to the class.

During the last few sessions of therapy, Lily's mother continued to take an increasingly active role in providing speaking assignments to Lily and following up on them with praise. When Lily entered the first grade, after a couple of weeks of nodding and speaking very softly, Lily was able to transition to a full speaking voice in school. After completion of therapy, Lily's mother continued to monitor Lily's speaking behaviors and to promote speaking in new situations by encouraging and rewarding the desired speaking behaviors. Lily's parents were very pleased when Lily began to ask to have playdates with several of her peers in school. (Adapted from Lindsey Bergman, Ph.D. and John Piacentini, Ph.D.)

Pathology and Laboratory Examination

No specific laboratory measures are useful in the diagnosis or treatment of selective mutism.

DIFFERENTIAL DIAGNOSIS

Differential diagnosis of children who are silent or speak only in whispers in specific social situations focuses on evaluating the child for specific communication disorder, autism spectrum disorder, and social anxiety disorder. Social anxiety disorder may be comorbid with selective mutism. Once confirming that a child is fully capable of speaking when comfortable, such as at home, but not in stressful situations, such as in school, an anxiety disorder is strongly considered. Shy and slow to warm up children may exhibit a transient reticence to speak in new, anxiety-provoking situations; however, this typically resolves on its own in several weeks. Shy, inhibited children often have histories of not speaking in the presence of strangers and of clinging to their mothers in new situations. Most children who appear to be mute on entering school improve spontaneously and may be described as having transient adaptation shyness. It is important to distinguish between selective mutism and intellectual disabilities, autism spectrum disorder, and expressive language disorder. In those disorders, a child may have an inability, rather than a refusal, to speak. In rare cases of mutism secondary to conversion disorder, the mutism is pervasive; these rare cases typically do not occur in very young children. Children introduced into an environment in which their first language is not spoken, even if they are proficient in the new language, may take some time to adjust to speaking the second language.

COURSE AND PROGNOSIS

Children with selective mutism are often excessively shy during the preschool years, but the onset of the full disorder is usually not evident until age 5 or 6 years. Many very young children with early symptoms of selective mutism in a transitional period when entering preschool have a spontaneous improvement over several months and never fulfill the criteria for the disorder. A typical pattern for a child with selective mutism is to speak almost exclusively at home with the nuclear family but not elsewhere, especially not at school. Consequently, a child with selective mutism may have academic difficulties or even failure due to a lack of participation. Children with selective mutism are typically shy, anxious, and at increased risk for a depressive disorder. Many children with early-onset selective mutism remit with or without treatment. Recent data suggest that fluoxetine may influence the course of selective mutism, and treatment enhances recovery. Children in whom the disorder persists often have difficulty forming social relationships. Teasing and scapegoating by peers may cause them to refuse to go to school. Some children with any form of severe social anxiety are rigid, compulsive, negativistic, and prone to temper tantrums and oppositional and aggressive behavior at home. Other children with the disorder tolerate the feared situation by communicating with gestures, such as nodding, shaking the head, and saying "Uh-huh" or "No." In one follow-up study, about one-half of children with selective mutism improved within 5 to 10 years. Children who do not improve by the age of 10 years appear to have a long-term course and a worse prognosis. As many as one-third of children with selective mutism, with or without treatment, may develop other psychiatric disorders, particularly other anxiety disorders and depression.

TREATMENT

The first line of treatment for a very young child who presents with selective mutism is a course of CBT. For more severe cases in which a child is not responsive to an adequate trial of CBT, optimal treatment is often a multimodal approach using psychoeducation for the family, CBT, and SSRIs as needed. Preschool children may also benefit from a therapeutic nursery. For school-aged children as well, individual CBT is the first-line treatment. Family education and cooperation are beneficial. Although randomized clinical trials are limited in the treatment of selective mutism in children, given its overlapping symptoms with social anxiety disorder, the recommended treatment protocols are similar. Evidence indicates that children with social anxiety disorder respond to various SSRIs, and, currently, CBT treatments have also demonstrated efficacy in children with anxiety disorders.

A recent report of 21 children with selective mutism treated in an open trial with fluoxetine suggested that this medication may be useful for childhood selective mutism. Reports have confirmed the efficacy of fluoxetine in the treatment of adult social anxiety disorder and at least one double-blind, placebo-controlled study using fluoxetine with children with mutism. A large National Institute of Mental Health–funded study of anxiety disorders in children and adolescents, called RUPP, has shown distinct superiority of fluvoxamine over placebo in the treatment of a variety of childhood anxiety disorders. Children with selective mutism may benefit similarly to those with social anxiety disorder, given the current belief that it is a subgroup of social anxiety disorder. SSRI medications that have been shown in randomized, placebo-controlled trials to have benefit in the treatment of children with social anxiety disorder include fluoxetine (20 to 60 mg/day), fluvoxamine (50 to 300 mg/day), sertraline (25 to 200 mg/day), and paroxetine (10 to 50 mg/day).

EPIDEMIOLOGY

The prevalence of selective mutism varies with age, with younger children at increased risk for the disorder. According to the DSM-5-TR, the point prevalence of selective mutism using clinic or school samples ranges between 0.03% and 1%, depending on whether a clinical or community sample is studied. A sizeable epidemiologic survey in the United Kingdom reported a prevalence rate of selective mutism to be 0.69% in children 4 to 5 years of age. Another survey in the United Kingdom identified 0.06% of 7-year-olds as having selective mutism. Young children are more vulnerable to the disorder than older ones. Selective mutism appears to be more common in girls than in boys. Clinical reports suggest that many young children spontaneously "outgrow" this disorder as they age; the longitudinal course of the disorder remains to be studied.

ETIOLOGY

Genetic Contribution

Selective mutism may have many of the same etiologic factors leading to the emergence of social anxiety disorder. In contrast to other childhood anxiety disorders, however, children with selective mutism are at higher risk for delayed onset of speech or speech abnormalities that may be contributory. However, in addition to the speech and language factor, one survey found that 90% of children with selective mutism met diagnostic criteria for social anxiety disorder. These children showed high levels of social anxiety without notable psychopathology in other areas, according to parent and teacher ratings. Thus, selective mutism may not represent a distinct disorder but may be a subtype of social anxiety disorder. Maternal anxiety, depression, and heightened dependence needs occur in families of children with selective mutism, similar to families with children who exhibit other anxiety disorders.

Parental Interactions

Parental anxiety disorders leading to observable anxiety in parenting may unwittingly reinforce anxious responses to new situations, including selective mutism in children. Children with selective mutism usually speak freely at home and only exhibit symptoms when under social pressure either in school or other social situations. Some children seem predisposed to selective mutism after early emotional or physical trauma; thus, some clinicians refer to the phenomenon as *traumatic mutism* rather than selective mutism.

Speech and Language Factors

Selective mutism is conceptualized as an anxiety-based refusal to speak; however, a higher-than-expected proportion of children with the disorder have a history of speech delay. An intriguing finding suggests that children with selective mutism are at higher risk for a disturbance in auditory processing, which may interfere with the efficient processing of incoming sounds. For the most part, however, speech and language problems in children with selective mutism are subtle and cannot account for the diagnosis.

FURTHER READINGS

Bai S, Rolon-Arroyo B, Walkup JT, et al. Anxiety symptom trajectories from treatment to 5- to 12-year follow-up across childhood and adolescence. *J Child Psychol Psychiatry*. 2023;64(9):1336–1345.

Bandelow B, Allgulander C, Baldwin DS, et al. World Federation of Societies of Biological Psychiatry (WFSBP) guidelines for treatment of anxiety, obsessive-compulsive and posttraumatic stress disorders—version 3. Part I: anxiety disorders. *World J Biol Psychiatry*. 2023;24(2):79–117.

Baumel WT, Strawn JR. Neurobiology of treatment in pediatric anxiety disorders. *Child Adolesc Psychiatr Clin N Am*. 2023;32(3):589–600.

Bilek E, Tomlinson RC, Whiteman AS, et al. Exposure-focused CBT outperforms relaxation-based control in an RCT of treatment for child and adolescent anxiety. *J Clin Child Adolesc Psychol*. 2022;51(4):410–418.

Carbone D, Schmidt LA, Cunningham CC, et al. Behavioral and socioemotional functioning in children with selective mutism: a comparison with anxious and typically developing children across multiple informants. *J Abnorm Child Psychol*. 2010;38(8):1057–1067.

Castagna PJ, Farahdel E, Potenza MN, Crowley MJ. The current state-of-the-art in pharmacotherapy for pediatric generalized anxiety disorder. *Expert Opin Pharmacother*. 2023;24(7):835–847.

Comer JS, Puliafico AC, Aschenbrand SG, et al. A pilot feasibility evaluation of the CALM Program for anxiety disorders in early childhood. *J Anxiety Disord*. 2012;26(1):40–49.

Compton SN, Walkup JT, Albano AM, et al. Child/Adolescent Anxiety Multimodal Study (CAMS): rationale, design, and methods. *Child Adolesc Psychiatry Ment Health*. 2010;4:1.

Cornacchio D, Furr JM, Sanchez AL, et al. Intensive group behavioral treatment (IGBT) for children with selective mutism: a preliminary randomized clinical trial. *J Consult Clin Psychol*. 2019;87(8):720–733.

Davis TE III, May A, Whiting SE. Evidence-based treatment of anxiety and phobia in children and adolescents: current status and effects on the emotional response. *Clin Psychol Rev*. 2011;31(4):592–602.

Fagan HA, Baldwin DS. Pharmacological treatment of generalised anxiety disorder: current practice and future directions. *Expert Rev Neurother*. 2023;23(6):535–548.

Ginsburg GS, Kendall PC, Sakolsky D, et al. Remission after acute treatment in children and adolescents with anxiety disorders: findings from the CAMS. *J Consult Clin Psychol*. 2011;79(6):806–813.

Hirshfeld-Becker DR, Masek B, Henin A, et al. Cognitive behavioral therapy for 4- to 7-year-old children with anxiety disorders: a randomized clinical trial. *J Consult Clin Psychol*. 2010;78(4):498–510.

Koskela M, Ståhlberg T, Yunus WMAWM, Sourander A. Long-term outcomes of selective mutism: a systematic literature review. *BMC Psychiatry*. 2023;23(1):779.

Naveed S, Amray AN, Jahan N, Moti-Wala FB, Majeed MH. Psychopharmacology in pediatric mixed anxiety disorder: an evidence-based review. *Innov Clin Neurosci*. 2019;16(9-10):36–43.

Nicotra CM, Strawn JR. Advances in pharmacotherapy for pediatric anxiety disorders. *Child Adolesc Psychiatr Clin N Am*. 2023;32(3): 573–587.

Oerbeck B, Overgaard KR, Stein MB, Pripp AH, Kristensen H. Treatment of selective mutism: a 5-year follow-up study. *Eur Child Adolesc Psychiatry*. 2018;27(8):997–1009.

Otani K, Suzuki A, Matsumoto Y, Kamata M. Parental overprotection increases interpersonal sensitivity in healthy subjects. *Compr Psychiatry*. 2009;50(1):54–57.

Rapee RM, Creswell C, Kendall PC, Pine DS, Waters AM. Anxiety disorders in children and adolescents: a summary and overview of the literature. *Behav Res Ther*. 2023;168:104376.

Rodrigues Pereira C, Ensink JBM, Güldner MG, Lindauer RJL, De Jonge MV, Utens EMWJ. Diagnosing selective mutism: a critical review of measures for clinical practice and research. *Eur Child Adolesc Psychiatry*. 2023;32(10):1821–1839.

Rynn M, Puliafico A, Heleniak C, Rikhi P, Ghalib K, Vidair H. Advances in pharmacotherapy for pediatric anxiety disorders. *Depress Anxiety*. 2011;28(1):76–87.

Schneider S, Blatter-Meunier J, Herren C, Adornetto C, In-Albon T, Lavallee K. Disorder-specific cognitive-behavioral therapy for separation anxiety disorder in young children: a randomized waiting-list–controlled group. *Psychother Psychosom*. 2011;80(4):206–215.

Schwenck C, Gensthaler A, Vogel F, Pfeffermann A, Laerum S, Stahl J. Characteristics of person, place, and activity that trigger failure to speak in children with selective mutism. *Eur Child Adolesc Psychiatry*. 2022;31(9):1419–1429.

Seligman LD, Hovey JD, Ibarra M, Hurtado G, Marin CE, Silverman WK. Latino and non-latino parental treatment preferences for child and adolescent anxiety disorders. *Child Psychiatry Hum Dev*. 2020;51(4):617–624.

Strawn JR, Mills JA, Poweleit EA, Ramsey LB, Croarkin PE. Adverse effects of antidepressant medications and their management in children and adolescents. *Pharmacotherapy*. 2023;43(7):675–690.

Strawn JR, Moldauer L, Hahn RD, et al. A multicenter double-blind, placebo-controlled trial of escitalopram in children and adolescents with generalized anxiety disorder. *J Child Adolesc Psychopharmacol*. 2023;33(3):91–100.

Vogel F, Gensthaler A, Stahl J, Schwenck C. Fears and fear-related cognitions in children with selective mutism. *Eur Child Adores Psychiatry*. 2019;28(9):1169–1181.

Walkup JT, Albano AM, Piacentini J. Cognitive behavioral therapy, sertraline, or a combination in childhood anxiety. *N Engl J Med*. 2008; 359(26):2753–2766.

Walter HJ, Bukstein OG, Abright AR, et al. Clinical practice guideline for the assessment and treatment of children and adolescents with anxiety disorders. *J Am Acad Child Adolesc Psychiatry*. 2020;59(10): 1107–1124.

Warner EN, Ammerman RT, Glauser TA, Pestian JP, Agasthya G, Strawn JR. Developmental epidemiology of pediatric anxiety disorders. *Child Adolesc Psychiatr Clin N Am*. 2023;32(3):511–530.

16

Obsessive-Compulsive Disorder, Trichotillomania, and Body Dysmorphic Disorder

OBSESSIVE-COMPULSIVE DISORDER IN CHILDHOOD AND ADOLESCENCE

Obsessive-compulsive disorder (OCD) is common in both youth and adults, with prevalence rates ranging between 1% and 3%. Data suggest that up to 25% of cases of OCD have their onset by 14 years of age. The overall clinical presentation of OCD in youth is like that in adults; however, compared to adults, children and adolescents with OCD more often do not consider their obsessional thoughts or repetitive behaviors to be unreasonable. In milder cases of OCD, a trial of cognitive-behavioral therapy (CBT) is the initial intervention. OCD in youth is often treated successfully with selective serotonin reuptake inhibitors (SSRIs) or CBT alone or in combination. The results of the first large-scale, randomized, placebo-controlled study, called the Pediatric OCD Treatment Study (POTS), demonstrated that the highest rates of remission in pediatric OCD are with a combination of both serotonergic agents and CBT treatment. A meta-analysis in 2022 by Tao and colleagues comparing pharmacologic interventions, psychological interventions, and combined treatment for OCD in youth confirmed the same result.

Children and adolescents with obsessions or compulsions are typically brought for psychiatric evaluation and treatment due to the excessive time that they devote to their intrusive thoughts and repetitive rituals. Some children view their compulsive rituals as reasonable responses to their extreme fears and anxieties. Nevertheless, they are aware of their discomfort and inability to carry out usual daily activities promptly due to the compulsions, such as getting ready to leave their homes to go to school each morning.

The obsessions reported most in children and adolescents include extreme fears of contamination—exposure to dirt, germs, or disease—followed by worries related to harm befalling themselves, family members, or fear of harming others due to losing control over aggressive impulses. Also commonly reported are obsessional needs for symmetry or exactness, hoarding, and excessive religious or moral concerns. Typical compulsive rituals among children and adolescents involve cleaning, checking, counting, repeating behaviors, or arranging items. Associated features in children and adolescents with OCD include avoidance, indecision, doubt, and slowness to complete tasks. In most cases of OCD among youth, obsessions and compulsions are present. According to the DSM-5-TR, diagnosis of OCD is identical to that of adults, with two specifiers that are especially pertinent for youth. One is to indicate if the child has fair, poor, or absent insight, which is relevant to young children who may not recognize that their obsessions and compulsions may not be based on "fact." An additional specifier relevant to youth is whether the individual has a current or past history of a tic disorder, which is more common in males who also meet criteria for Tourette disorder.

Table 16-1 outlines comparative diagnostic criteria for OCD in DSM-5-TR, ICD-10, and ICD-11.

Many children and adolescents who develop OCD have an insidious onset and may hide their symptoms as long as possible so that their rituals will not be challenged or disrupted. A minority of children, particularly males with early onset, may have a rapid unfolding of multiple symptoms within a few months. OCD is often comorbid with anxiety disorders, Attention-Deficit/Hyperactivity Disorder (ADHD), and tic disorders, especially Tourette disorder children with comorbid OCD and tic disorders are more likely to exhibit counting, arranging, or ordering compulsions and less likely to manifest excessive washing and cleaning compulsions. The high comorbidity of OCD, Tourette disorder, and ADHD has led investigators to postulate a shared genetic vulnerability to all three of these disorders. It is crucial to search for comorbidity in children and adolescents with OCD so that the treatments can be optimal.

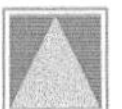

Table 16-1.
Comparative Diagnostic Criteria for Obsessive-Compulsive Disorder

	DSM-5-TR	ICD-10	ICD-11
Diagnostic name	Obsessive-Compulsive Disorder	Obsessive-Compulsive Disorder	Obsessive-Compulsive Disorder
Duration	Persistent		Persistent
Symptoms	Obsessions (Intrusive thoughts that accompany behaviors and that individuals may attempt to ignore or counteract through action) Compulsions (repetitive actions, commonly driven by an obsessive thought, performed to relieve anxiety or fear)	Recurrent obsessional thoughts and/or compulsive acts Obsessions: ideas, images, or impulses occurring recurrently Compulsions: repeated, stereotyped behaviors meant to neutralize a thought/anxiety or prevent a perceived adverse event Attempts at resisting thoughts and behaviors are frequently unsuccessful and cause worsening anxiety	Obsessions: repetitive/persistent thoughts/images/impulses, experienced as intrusive and unwanted, associated with anxiety Compulsions: repetitive behaviors/rituals in response to obsessions
Required number of symptoms	Obsessive thoughts, compulsions, or both	Presence of obsessions, compulsions, or both	
Psychosocial consequences	Symptoms and behaviors consume ≥1 hr per day or cause distress or psychosocial impairment		Symptoms and behaviors consume ≥1 hr per day or cause distress or psychosocial impairment
Exclusions	Other medical condition Substance or medication, including withdrawal Other mental illness	Obsessive-compulsive personality disorder	Other medical condition Substance or medication, including withdrawal
Symptoms specifiers	Tic related: current or prior tic disorder With good or fair insight With poor insight With absent insight and/or delusional beliefs	Predominantly obsessional thoughts or ruminations Predominantly compulsive acts (obsessional rituals) Mixed obsessional thoughts and acts	Fair to good insight Poor to absent insight

Jesse, an 11-year-old boy in the sixth grade, was brought for evaluation by his parents, who expressed concerns over his repeated questions and anxiety regarding developing COVID-19. Jesse was a high-functioning boy who abruptly began to exhibit extremely disruptive behaviors related to his fears of "catching" COVID-19 and his resulting refusal to go to school or be near other people. His school refusal began approximately 2 to 3 months before the evaluation. Jesse's behaviors included relentless concerns about contracting illness, washing rituals, repeated expressions of uncertainty over his behavior, seeking reassurance, repeating rituals, and avoidance.

Jesse repeatedly expressed his fear and belief that he had just been exposed to COVID-19 through exposure to multiple strangers who he believed were infected. For example, while riding in the car, if Jesse saw a stranger from the window who appeared to him to be "ill," he experienced a surge of extreme anxiety and obsessively agonized about whether the stranger had COVID-19 and had exposed him to it. Despite his parents' reassurances about his safety and lack of exposure to illness, Jesse insisted on vigorously washing for approximately 1 hour each time he returned home after being out. Jesse also expressed doubts about his own behavior. He often asked his parents, "Did I do something to infect myself with COVID-19?" Reassurance was only slightly calming. While Jesse had previously been an excellent student, he began to lose the ability to focus on schoolwork. While reading passages from assigned materials, Jesse frequently experienced severe anxiety, worrying about whether he was getting sick, which was followed by wondering if he had missed a word or misunderstood the sentence, so he then proceeded to reread the material. Completing a page of written material began to take Jesse 30 to 60 minutes. Over several weeks, he was less and less able to complete assignments, following which he became very distressed over his deteriorating grades.

During Jesse's evaluation, his family history suggested that, prior to the COVID-19 pandemic, Jesse's older sister had experienced a period in which she, too, had similar but milder anxieties, with less interference in functioning, and she had never received any treatment for those symptoms.

At the intake interview, Jesse presented as a preoccupied, worried, and sad boy who was cooperative with questioning; however, he wore several masks. He did not volunteer much information, and he allowed his parents to recount the extent of his symptoms. Jesse believed that his relentless concerns were reasonable and that he required repeated reassurance from his parents in order to continue his daily activities. Jesse met full diagnostic criteria for OCD. Symptoms of depression were present but not sufficient for major depressive disorder.

Jesse began CBT with a psychologist; however, Jesse was so fearful of deviating from his rituals that he was unable to participate fully in his treatment, and he became despondent about his future. Jesse refused to go to school due to his increasing distress associated with getting sick from his classmates and his shame about his diminishing academic performance. Given his limited progress during the first 2 months of CBT, he was evaluated by a psychiatrist who added fluoxetine, titrated to 40 mg/day. Over 3 weeks, there was some improvement, and Jesse was more amenable to cooperating with his CBT treatment. CBT and SSRI treatment continued over the next 3 months regularly. Over time, Jesse finally began to show some flexibility in his adamant belief that he was perpetually exposed and infected with COVID-19, and he was able to decrease the amount of time he spent with washing rituals. Once he had found some relief from his symptoms, Jesse was able to focus more on his schoolwork, peers, and his family life. Follow-up over the next year was positive; Jesse maintained his gains from treatment with only minimal interference from residual OCD symptoms. Jesse's academic achievement improved, he was able to engage in activities with friends, and he spent almost no time preoccupied with obsessional thoughts of having contracted the virus, and/or washing rituals.

Pathology and Laboratory Examination

No specific laboratory measures are useful in the diagnosis of OCD.

Even when the onset of obsessions or compulsions appears to be associated with a recent infection with group A beta-hemolytic stretptococcus (GABHS), the antigens and antibodies to the bacteria do not indicate a causal relationship between GABHS and OCD.

Differential Diagnosis

Developmentally appropriate rituals in the play and behavior of young children should not be confused with OCD in that age group. Preschoolers often engage in ritualistic play and request a predictable routine such as bathing, reading stories, or selecting the same stuffed animal at bedtime to promote a sense of security and comfort. These routines allay developmentally normal fears and lead to reasonable completion of daily activities. On the other hand, extreme fears drive the obsessions or compulsions, and this significantly interferes with daily function because of the excessive time that they consume and the extreme distress that ensues when they are interrupted. The rituals of preschoolers generally become less rigid by the time they enter grade school, and school-age children do not typically experience a surge of anxiety when they encounter small changes in their routine.

Children and adolescents with generalized anxiety disorder, separation anxiety disorder, and social anxiety disorder experience intense worries that they repeatedly express; however, these are mundane compared to obsessions, which are often so extreme that they appear bizarre. A child with generalized anxiety disorder typically worries repeatedly about performance on academic examinations, whereas a child with OCD may experience repeated intrusive thoughts that he may harm someone he loves. The compulsions of OCD are not present in other anxiety disorders; however, children with autism spectrum disorders often display repetitive behaviors that may resemble OCD. In contrast with the rituals of OCD, children with autism spectrum disorder are not responding to anxiety but are more often exhibiting stereotyped behaviors that are self-stimulating or self-comforting.

Children and adolescents with tic disorders such as Tourette disorder may display complex repetitive, compulsive behaviors like the compulsions seen in OCD. Children and adolescents with tic disorders are at higher risk for the development of concurrent OCD.

Severe OCD symptoms may be difficult to distinguish from delusional symptoms, especially when the obsessions and compulsions are bizarre. In most adults, and often in youth with OCD, despite an inability to control their obsessions or resist completing compulsions, insight into their lack of reasonableness is preserved. That is, an individual's conviction in their beliefs often does not reach delusional intensity. When insight is present and underlying anxiety can be described, even in the face of significant dysfunction due to bizarre obsessions and compulsions, the diagnosis of OCD is suspect.

Course and Prognosis

OCD with onset in childhood and adolescence is most often a chronic, waxing and waning disorder with variability in severity and outcome. Follow-up studies suggest that up to 40% to 50% of children and adolescents recover from OCD with minimal residual symptoms. A study of childhood OCD treatment with sertraline resulted in close to 50% of participants experiencing complete remission and partial remission in another 25% with a follow-up time of 1 year. Predictors of the best outcome were in those children and adolescents without comorbid disorders, including tic disorders and ADHD. A study of 142 children and adolescents with OCD followed over 9 years at the Maudsley Hospital in England found 41% to have a persistence of OCD, with 40% exhibiting an additional psychiatric diagnosis at follow-up. The main predictor for persistent OCD was the duration of illness at the time of the initial assessment. Approximately half of the follow-up group was still receiving treatment, and half believed that they needed continued treatment.

Neuropsychological functioning may also play a role in outcome and prognosis. A study of 63 youth with OCD who completed the Rey–Osterrieth Complex Figure (ROCF), along with specific subtests of the Wechsler Intelligence Scale for Children, Third Edition (WISC-III), found that 5-minute recall accuracy from the ROCF was positively correlated with response to treatment, particularly CBT. These findings imply that poorer performance on the ROCF and poor response to therapy may be in part due to executive functioning difficulties and that treatment may need to be modified to account for these obstacles.

Overall, the prognosis is hopeful for most children and adolescents with mild to moderate OCD. In up to 10% of cases, severe OCD may represent a prodrome of a psychotic disorder in children and adolescents. In youth with subthreshold OCD symptoms, there is a high risk of developing full OCD disorder within 2 years. Childhood OCD is responsive to available treatments, resulting in improvement, if not complete remission, at least for a period of time in most cases.

Treatment

CBT and SSRIs are both beneficial treatments for OCD in youth, with the combination being most efficacious. CBT geared toward children of varying ages is based on the principle of developmentally appropriate exposure to the feared stimuli coupled with response prevention, leading to diminishing anxiety over time on exposure to feared situations. CBT manuals can ensure that the therapist can make developmentally appropriate interventions and that the child and parents receive comprehensive education.

Treatment guidelines for children and adolescents with mild to moderate OCD recommend a trial of CBT before initiating medication. However, the POTS, a multisite National Institute of Health (NIH)-funded investigation of sertraline and CBT, each alone and in combination, for the treatment of childhood-onset OCD, revealed that the combination was superior to either treatment alone. Each treatment alone also provided encouraging levels of response. The mean daily dose of sertraline was 133 mg/day in the group administered the combination treatment, and 170 mg/day for the sertraline alone group. Improvement with the pharmacologic intervention of childhood OCD usually occurs within 8 to 12 weeks of treatment. Most children and adolescents who experienced remission with acute treatment using SSRIs were still responsive over a year. Among youth with OCD who obtain a partial response to a therapeutic trial of SSRI treatment, augmentation with a short-term OCD-specific CBT leads to a significantly greater response. Evidence shows that higher treatment expectations by patients and families link to better treatment response, greater compliance with home-based CBT assignments, less drop out of treatment, and reduced impairment. The finding that the combination of CBT and SSRI medications in the treatment of OCD in youth is most effective was confirmed in a meta-analysis of treatment studies of youth OCD in 2022.

In addition to individual CBT, both family and group CBT interventions are efficacious in the treatment of childhood OCD. Family CBT (FCBT) intervention in the treatment of OCD in youth increases the response rates. A controlled comparison of FCBT and psychoeducation and relaxation (PRT) in 71 families of children with OCD showed that clinical remission rates in the FCBT group were significantly higher than those in the PRT group. The FCBT treatment reduced parent involvement and accommodation in their affected child's symptoms, which led to decreased symptomatology.

A randomized controlled study investigating webcamera–delivered FCBT (W-CBT) compared to a waitlist condition assigned 31 families to one of the above conditions. Assessments were conducted immediately before and after treatment and at a 3-month follow-up for the W-CBT group. The W-CBT group was superior to the waitlist control group on all primary outcome measures, with large effect sizes. Eighty-one percent of the W-CBT group responded, compared to 13% of the waitlist group. The children maintained the gains at the 3-month follow-up assessment. The authors conclude that W-CBT may be efficacious in the treatment of OCD in youth and may be a promising tool for future dissemination.

Exposure and response prevention (ERP) was studied in a group format in youth with OCD in a community-based program. Group-based ERP was effective in reducing OCD symptom severity and depressive symptoms, but not anxiety symptoms, in a naturalistic treatment setting for children with OCD and comorbid anxiety or depressive features.

Multiple randomized clinical trials establish the efficacy of SSRIs for OCD in youth. A meta-analysis of 13 studies of SSRIs, including sertraline, fluvoxamine, fluoxetine, and paroxetine, has provided evidence of the efficacy of SSRIs with a moderate effect size. A randomized controlled clinical trial of citalopram versus fluoxetine in youth with OCD found that citalopram was as safe and effective as fluoxetine for the treatment of OCD in children and adolescents. There have been no apparent differences in the rate of response for the individual SSRIs.

Currently, three SSRIs: sertraline (at least 6 years), fluoxetine (at least 7 years), and fluvoxamine (at least 8 years), as well as clomipramine (at least 10 years), have received FDA approval for the treatment of OCD in youth. The black-box warning for antidepressants used in children for any disorder, including OCD, is applicable so that close monitoring for suicidal ideation or behavior is mandated when using these agents in children.

Typical side effects that emerge with the use of SSRIs include insomnia, nausea, agitation, tremor, and fatigue. Dosage ranges for the various SSRIs found to have efficacy in randomized clinical trials are the following: fluoxetine (20 to 60 mg), sertraline (50 to 200 mg), fluvoxamine (up to 200 mg), and paroxetine (up to 50 mg).

Clomipramine was the first antidepressant studied in the treatment of OCD in childhood and the only tricyclic antidepressant that has FDA approval for the treatment of anxiety disorders in childhood. Clomipramine was efficacious in doses up to 200 mg, or 3 mg/kg, whichever is less. Nevertheless, clomipramine is not recommended as a first-line treatment due to its higher potential risks compared to other SSRIs, including the cardiovascular risk of hypotension and arrhythmia and seizure risk.

Pediatric patients with OCD who respond only partially to medications tend to have at least moderate to severe OCD symptoms, high ratings of global impairment, and significant comorbidity even after their partial response to an adequate trial of medication. Augmentation strategies with medications to enhance serotonergic effects, such as with atypical antipsychotics (e.g., risperidone), have demonstrated increased response when SSRIs yield a partial response. Aripiprazole augmentation in 39 adolescents with OCD who did not respond to two trials of monotherapy with SSRIs led to 59% of patients being rated as improved or very much improved. Patients who responded to aripiprazole were less impaired at baseline in functional impairment but not in the clinical severity of their OCD. Aripiprazole's final mean dose was 12.2 mg/day. This agent may be useful for pediatric OCD and warrants further controlled trials.

Epidemiology

OCD is common among children and adolescents, with a point prevalence of about 0.5% and a lifetime prevalence of 1% to 3%. The rate of OCD among youth rises exponentially with increasing age, with rates of 0.3% in children between the ages of 5 and 7 years, rising to rates between 0.6% and 1% among teens. Rates of OCD among adolescents are higher than those for schizophrenia or bipolar disorder. Among young children with OCD, there appears to be a slight male predominance, which diminishes with age.

Etiology

Genetic Factors. Genetic factors contribute significantly to the development of OCD in early-onset illness. The rate of OCD among first-degree relatives of children and adolescents who develop OCD is 10 times greater than for the general population. Twin studies have shown that the concordance rates for OCD are higher for monozygotic twins (0.57) than for dizygotic twins (0.22); however, nongenetic factors play a role that may be equal to or greater than genetic contributions in some cases. OCD is a heterogeneous disorder that has been recognized for decades to run in families. Also, the presence of subclinical symptom constellations in family members appears to breed true. Genetic linkage studies have revealed evidence of susceptibility loci on chromosomes 1q, 3q, 6q, 7p, 9p, 10p, and 15q. The OCD collaborative genetics study found that the *Sapap3* gene was associated with grooming disorders and may be a promising candidate gene for OCD. There is evidence that the glutamate receptor–modulating genes may also be associated with and play a role in the emergence of OCD. Family studies have suggested a relationship between OCD and tic disorders such as Tourette disorder. OCD and tic disorders likely share susceptibility factors, which may include both genetic and nongenetic factors.

Neuroimmunology. Immunologic contributions to the emergence of OCD are hypothesized to be related to an inflammatory process in the basal ganglia associated with an immune response to a systemic infection that may trigger OCD and tics. A prototype of this hypothesis has been the controversial association of OCD symptoms in a small subgroup of children and adolescents following documented exposure to or infection with GABHS. Under this hypothesis, cases of infection-triggered OCD have been termed Pediatric Autoimmune Neuropsychiatric Disorders Associated with Streptococcus (PANDAS), and parallel an autoimmune process leading to a movement disorder much like Sydenham chorea following rheumatic fever. The presentation of OCD in children and adolescents in association with acute exposure to GABHS represents a minority of OCD cases in youth, without evidence that it is causative, and remains controversial.

Neurochemistry. The evidence that SSRIs diminish symptoms of OCD, along with findings of altered sensitivity to the acute administration of 5-hydroxytryptamine (5-HT) agonists in individuals with OCD, supports the probability of serotonin's role in OCD. Also, the dopamine system is likely influential in OCD, especially in light of the frequent comorbidity of OCD with tic disorders in childhood. Clinical observations have indicated that obsessions and compulsions worsen with stimulants, as with patients who have comorbid ADHD. Dopamine antagonists, administered along with SSRIs, may augment the effectiveness of SSRIs in the treatment of OCD. Evidence suggests that multiple neurotransmitter systems may play a role in OCD.

Neuroimaging. Both CT and MRI of untreated children and adults with OCD have revealed smaller volumes of basal ganglia segments compared to healthy controls. A meta-analysis of voxel-based morphometry (VBM) to assess gray matter density compared 343 OCD patients with 318 healthy controls and found that gray matter density in OCD patients was smaller in parietofrontal cortical regions (including the supramarginal gyrus, the dorsolateral prefrontal cortex, and the orbitofrontal cortex), but larger in the basal ganglia (the putamen) and anterior prefrontal cortex, compared to healthy controls. Increased gray matter volume in the basal ganglia of

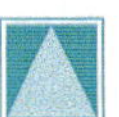

Table 16-2.
Comparative Diagnostic Criteria for Trichotillomania (Hair-Pulling Disorder)

	DSM-5-TR	ICD-10	ICD-11
Diagnostic name	Trichotillomania (Hair-Pulling Disorder)	Trichotillomania	Body-Focused Repetitive Behavior Disorders
Symptoms	Recurrent hairpulling causing hair loss Repeated attempts to change/end behaviors	Presence of noticeable hair loss due to recurrent hairpulling Hair-pulling behavior preceded by increased anxiety that is relieved by hairpulling	Recurrent and habitual actions directed at the integument (e.g., hairpulling, skin-picking, lip-biting) Typically accompanied by unsuccessful attempts to decrease or stop the behaviors
Required number of symptoms	All of the above		
Psychosocial consequences	Distress or psychosocial impairment		Distress or psychosocial impairment
Exclusions	Other medical condition Substance or medication, including withdrawal	Pre-existing inflammation of the skin Response to delusion or hallucination Stereotyped movement disorder	Cultural behaviors (i.e., self-flagellation as part of religious ceremonies)

patients with OCD has been reported in other studies as well. These structural abnormalities in the prefrontal-basal ganglia are likely to be integrally involved in the pathophysiology of OCD. It is not clear whether the increases in gray matter in individuals with OCD occur before or after the symptoms emerge. In children, there is evidence of increased thalamic volume. Adult studies have provided evidence of hypermetabolism of frontal cortical-striatal-thalamo-cortical (CSTC) networks in untreated individuals with OCD. Of interest, imaging studies of before and after treatment have revealed that both medication and behavioral interventions lead to a reduction of orbitofrontal and caudate metabolic rates in children and adults with OCD.

TRICHOTILLOMANIA

Trichotillomania (hair-pulling disorder) is a body-focused repetitive behavior disorder characterized by repetitive hairpulling, leading to variable hair loss that may be visible to others. It resembles both obsessive-compulsive and impulse control disorders: increased tension before the hairpulling leads to the behavior and then subsequent relief or satisfaction. Trichotillomania is characterized by pulling out one's hair. The pulling is not for cosmetic reasons, but instead, individuals often describe an irresistible urge to pull out their hair. This hairpulling results in noticeable hair loss and is associated with repeated attempts to decrease or stop hairpulling. Patients with hair-pulling disorder may experience an increasing sense of tension before engaging in the behavior and achieve a sense of release or gratification from pulling out their hair. All areas of the body may be affected, most commonly the scalp. Other areas involved are eyebrows, eyelashes, and beard; trunk, armpits, and pubic areas are less commonly involved.

There are (at least) two types of hairpulling. *Focused pulling* is the use of an intentional act to control unpleasant personal experiences, such as an urge, bodily sensation (e.g., itching or burning), or thought. In contrast, *automatic pulling* occurs outside the person's awareness and, most often, during sedentary activities. Most patients have a combination of these types.

Trichophagy, or mouthing of the hair, may follow the hair plucking. Youth with trichotillomania may also engage in other body-focused repetitive behavior disorders which may cause self-injury, such as nail-biting, scratching, gnawing, or excoriation of their skin.

Table 16-2 shows comparative diagnostic criteria for trichotillomania.

Comorbidity

Comorbid conditions include other body-focused repetitive behavior disorders, with excoriation (skin-picking) disorder the most common. OCD is also more prevalent in hair-pulling disorder than in the general population. More than half of treatment-seeking individuals with hair-pulling disorder have a comorbid psychiatric disorder, with mood and anxiety disorders the most common after skin-picking.

Epidemiology

Studies of select populations, such as college students, indicate that the point prevalence of trichotillomania is around 0.5% to 2%. Age of onset is typically at menarche, and female:male ratio is about 4:1 in adults. Pediatric samples include an equal distribution between males and females.

Course and Prognosis

There are relatively little data on the long-term course of trichotillomania. In the absence of intervention, its course is likely often chronic. However, some data indicate that in some cases, spontaneous remission does occur.

Treatment

Early data indicated that trichotillomania, like OCD, responds more robustly to clomipramine than to desipramine. Unfortunately, subsequent trials of SSRIs and venlafaxine in trichotillomania have not consistently demonstrated efficacy. A trial of N-acetyl cysteine (NAC), up to 3,600 mg/day, a nutraceutical that acts on the glutamatergic system, has shown some promise. NAC has been found to improve skin-picking in youth.

A double-blind placebo-controlled study in adults with trichotillomania or excoriation disorder, by Grant and colleagues (2023), found that memantine, an N-Methyl-D-Aspartate (NMDA) receptor antagonist, showed some promise of improvement in both disorders.

Habit reversal training (HRT) is a set of cognitive-behavioral techniques that have been shown somewhat efficacious in the treatment of childhood trichotillomania. Components of HRT include awareness training, competing for response training, and social support. Controlled trials of augmentation of habit reversal therapy/self control (HRT/SC) with acceptance and commitment therapy, dialectical behavior therapy, or cognitive therapy have also suggested efficacy in trichotillomania.

Etiology

From a cognitive-affective neuroscience perspective, neuropsychological investigations of trichotillomania have suggested deficits in working memory and visual–spatial learning. Structural and functional brain imaging studies have suggested some involvement of cortico-striato-thalamo-cortical (CSTC) circuits relevant to habit learning, although data is sparse. There is also evidence of the involvement of brain regions associated with reward processing and affect regulation. Family and twin studies provide evidence for genetic susceptibility, as well as a relationship to OCD and other body-focused repetitive behaviors.

BODY DYSMORPHIC DISORDER

Youth with body dysmorphic disorder (BDD) have persistent preoccupations about one or more perceived defects or flaws in one's appearance. The defects or flaws appear slight or are not observable to others. Their concerns about their appearance result in a range of mental acts or behaviors, including comparing themselves with others, checking in the mirror, or camouflaging their perceived flaws.

BDD frequently begins in childhood, with most patients having some symptoms by the age of 18 years. Rautio and colleagues (2022) reported on the clinical findings in 136 adolescents with BDD. Their report included 136 girls, 32 boys, and 4 transgender individuals (age range 10 to 19 years). Most of the adolescents displayed moderately severe symptoms, with more than half showing poor or absent insight about their beliefs. Comorbid psychiatric disorders were found in 71.5% of the study population. Eleven percent of the study group had histories of suicidal thoughts or behaviors. Girls reported significantly more severe BDD symptoms, more depression, suicidal thoughts, and histories of self-harm compared to boys.

The most common concerns involve the face and head, particularly specific parts (e.g., the skin, nose shape and size, or hair), although symptoms may focus on any area of the body. More than a quarter of patients are concerned with the symmetry of their appearance. Table 16-3 shows comparative diagnostic criteria for BDD.

Commonly associated symptoms include ideas of reference, frequent mirror checking or avoidance of reflective surfaces, and attempts to hide the presumed deformity. The ideas of reference are typically focused on others noticing the alleged flaw. The effects on a person's life can be significant, and it is essential to assess avoidance due to BDD symptoms, which can range from minor social avoidance to being housebound.

Comorbidity

BDD is frequently associated with comorbid depression, with a lifetime rate of 75%, as well as with suicidality, with 80% having experienced suicidal ideation. About one-third of BDD patients have a lifetime history of OCD, and around 30% of BDD patients experience panic attacks triggered by appearance concerns. BDD is also associated with high levels of rejection sensitivity and low self-esteem. Many patients with BDD use substances to self-medicate symptoms of social anxiety or emotional pain.

Epidemiology

Point prevalence estimates of BDD in the United States have ranged from 1.7% to 2.4%, indicating that this is one of the more common obsessional disorders.

The mean age of onset of BDD is typically in adolescence. As in the case of OCD, community studies indicate a higher prevalence of females with BDD, while clinical reports indicate a roughly even male:female ratio.

Course and Prognosis

The course of BDD is generally chronic, and in the absence of intervention, symptoms may persist for decades. Earlier age of onset and more severe symptoms at intake may predict a worse course.

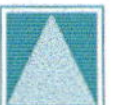

Table 16-3.
Comparative Diagnostic Criteria for Body Dysmorphic Disorder

	DSM-5-TR	ICD-10	ICD-11
Diagnostic name	Body Dysmorphic Disorder	Body Dysmorphic Disorder	Body Dysmorphic Disorder
Symptoms	Preoccupation with physical appearance and subjective flaws Presence of repetitive behaviors at some point during the disorder • Checking • Grooming • Skin-picking • Recurrent thoughts/perseveration on comparing physical appearance to that of others	Excessive preoccupation with image or appearance	Persistent preoccupation with ≥1 perceived defects or flaws in appearance Excessive self-consciousness about the perceived defect(s) Accompanied by any of the following: • Repetitive/excessive behaviors (repeatedly examining) • Excessive attempts to hide or alter the defect • Avoiding social or other situations
Required number of symptoms	Both of the above causing significant impairment and/or distress and excluding other causes of symptoms		
Psychosocial consequences	Distress or psychosocial impairment	Distress or psychosocial impairment	
Exclusions	An eating disorder (if the primary focus is body fat or weight)		Other medical illness Substance
Symptoms specifiers	With muscle dysmorphia: preoccupation with perceived low muscle mass or small body build With good or fair insight With poor insight With absent insight and/or delusional beliefs		Fair to good insight Poor to absent insight

Treatment

SSRIs have been shown to have some efficacy in the treatment of BDD. There is some evidence that, as in the case of OCD, doses higher than those ordinarily used in the treatment of depression may be needed to treat BDD, as are longer durations of treatment. There is little controlled data on using dopamine receptor blockers as augmenting agents; what exists is not encouraging. However, clinicians have reported anecdotal evidence for using aripiprazole as an augmenting agent.

Further Readings

Cervin M. Obsessive-compulsive disorder: diagnosis, clinical features, nosology, and epidemiology. *Psychiatr Clin North Am*. 2023;46(1):1–16.

Grant JE, Chamberlain SR, Redden SA, Leppink EW, Odlaug BL, Kim SW. N-Acetylcysteine in the treatment of excoriation disorder: a randomized clinical trial. *JAMA Psychiatry*. 2016;73(5):490–496.

Grant JE, Chesivoir E, Valle S, Ehsan D, Chamberlain SR. Double-blind placebo-controlled study of memantine in trichotillomania and skin-picking disorder. *Am J Psychiatry*. 2023;180(5):348–356.

Henein A, Pascual-Sanchez A, Corciova S, Hodes M. Obsessive-compulsive disorder in treatment seeking children & adolescents during the COVID-19 pandemic. *Eur Child Adolesc Psychiatry*. 2024;33(2):629–632.

Henkel ED, Jaquez SD, Diaz LZ. Pediatric trichotillomania: review of management. *Pediatr Dermatol*. 2019;36(6):803–807.

Hoffman J, Williams T, Rothbart R, et al. Pharmacotherapy for trichotillomania. *Cochrane Database Syst Rev*. 2021;9(9):CD007662.

Lee DK, Lipner SR. The potential of *N*-acetylcysteine for treatment of trichotillomania, excoriation disorder, onychophagia, and onychotillomania: an updated literature review. *Int J Environ Res Public Health*. 2022;19(11):6370.

Mataix-Cols D. Editorial: body dysmorphic disorder in children and adolescents: time to act. *J Am Acad Child Adolesc Psychiatry*. 2024:S0890-8567(24)00252-1.

Parli GM, Gales MA, Gales BJ. N-acetylcysteine for obsessive-compulsive and related disorders in children and adolescents: a review. *Ann Pharmacother*. 2023;57(7):847–854.

Pazuniak M, Pekrul SR. Obsessive-compulsive disorder in autism spectrum disorder across the lifespan. *Child Adolesc Psychiatr Clin N Am*. 2020;29(2):419–432.

Pediatric OCD Treatment Study (POTS) Team. Cognitive-behavior therapy, sertraline, and their combination for children and adolescents with obsessive-compulsive disorder: the Pediatric OCD Treatment Study (POTS) randomized controlled trial. *JAMA*. 2004;292(16):1969–1976.

Rajabi S, Kamran L, Joukar KamalAbadi M. Epidemiology of body dysmorphic disorder among adolescents: a study of their cognitive functions. *Brain Behav*. 2022;12(4):e01710.

Rautio D, Jassi A, Krebs G, et al. Clinical characteristics of 172 children and adolescents with body dysmorphic disorder. *Eur Child Adolesc Psychiatry*. 2022;31(1):133–144.

Ricketts EJ, Peris TS, Grant JE, et al. Clinical characteristics of youth with trichotillomania (hair-pulling disorder) and excoriation (skin-picking) disorder. *Child Psychiatry Hum Dev*. 2024;55(4):975–986.

Schachar RJ, Dupuis A, Anagnostou E, et al. Obsessive-compulsive disorder in children and youth: neurocognitive function in clinic and community samples. *J Child Psychol Psychiatry*. 2022;63(8):881–889.

Schuyler M, Geller DA. Childhood obsessive-compulsive disorder. *Psychiatr Clin North Am*. 2023;46(1):89–106.

Tao Y, Li H, Li L, et al. Comparing the efficacy of pharmacological and psychological treatment, alone and in combination, in children and adolescents with obsessive-compulsive disorder: a network meta-analysis. *J Psychiatr Res*. 2022;148:95–102.

Uhre CF, Ritter M, Jepsen JRM, et al. Atypical neurocognitive functioning in children and adolescents with obsessive-compulsive disorder (OCD). *Eur Child Adolesc Psychiatry*. 2024;33(7):2291–2300.

17 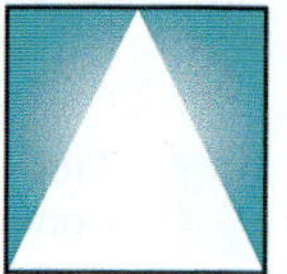

Early-Onset Schizophrenia

Early-onset schizophrenia is diagnosed in youth before the age of 18 years using the same DSM-5-TR criteria used for adults. Childhood-onset schizophrenia is defined as a schizophrenia diagnosis being made before the age of 13 years. Schizophrenia typically presents in middle to late adolescence with prevalence estimates in the United States of approximately 0.7%. Childhood onset is much rarer; reports have estimated prevalence to range from about 0.025% to less than 0.04%. Early-onset schizophrenia is characterized by a more chronic course, with severe social and cognitive consequences and increased negative symptoms compared to adult-onset schizophrenia. Childhood-onset schizophrenia is believed to represent a subgroup of early-onset schizophrenia with a higher heritable etiology, and higher than average rates of premorbid developmental abnormalities that appear to be markers of abnormal brain development. Early-onset schizophrenia is associated with severe clinical course, poor psychosocial functioning, and increased evidence of brain abnormalities. Children with childhood-onset schizophrenia have more significant deficits in measures of IQ, memory, and tests of perceptuomotor skills compared with individuals with adolescent-onset schizophrenia. Increased impairment in childhood-onset schizophrenia on cognitive measures such as working memory and perceptuomotor skills may be premorbid markers of illness rather than sequelae of the disorder. Although cognitive impairments are more considerable in younger patients with schizophrenia, the clinical symptom presentation of schizophrenia remains remarkably similar across the ages, and the diagnosis of childhood-onset schizophrenia is continuous with that in adolescents and adults, with one exception: in childhood-onset schizophrenia, a failure to achieve expected social and academic functioning may replace a deterioration in functioning.

It is important to note that about 17% of children and about 8% of adolescents in the general population report psychotic-like symptoms such as possible hallucinations and/or odd beliefs, according to a review by Sunshine and McClellan (2012); however, the majority do not have schizophrenia or another psychotic disorder and will not develop one.

DIAGNOSIS AND CLINICAL FEATURES

All the symptoms included in adult-onset schizophrenia may be present in children and adolescents with the disorder. Youth with early-onset schizophrenia are more likely to have a premorbid history of social rejection, poor peer relationships, clingy withdrawn behavior, and academic trouble than those with adult-onset schizophrenia. Some children with schizophrenia evaluated in middle childhood have early histories of delayed motor milestones and language acquisition which overlap with symptoms of autism spectrum disorder (ASD).

The onset of schizophrenia in childhood is frequently insidious, starting with inappropriate affect or unusual behavior; it may take months or years for a child to meet all the diagnostic criteria for schizophrenia.

Auditory hallucinations commonly occur in children with schizophrenia. The voices may reflect an ongoing critical commentary or command hallucinations that may instruct children to harm or kill themselves or others. Hallucinatory voices may sound human or animal, or "bizarre," for example, identified as "a computer in my head," "Martians," or the voice of someone familiar, such as a relative. The childhood-onset schizophrenia project at the National Institute of Mental Health (NIMH) found high rates across all hallucination modalities. However, there were unexpectedly high rates of tactile, olfactory, and visual hallucinations among this study group of patients with childhood-onset schizophrenia. Visual hallucinations were associated with lower IQ and earlier age at onset of disease. Visual hallucinations are often frightening; affected children may "see" images of the devil, skeletons, scary faces, or space creatures. Transient phobic visual hallucinations, such as images of ghosts, monsters, or other frightening images, may occur in severely anxious and traumatized children, especially at night, who do not develop major psychotic disorders. Visual, tactile, and olfactory hallucinations may be a marker of more severe psychosis.

Delusions occur in up to half of children and adolescents with schizophrenia, in various forms, including persecutory, grandiose, and religious. Delusions increase in frequency with increased age. Blunted or inappropriate affect emerges almost universally in children with schizophrenia. Children and adolescents with schizophrenia may giggle inappropriately or cry without being able to explain why. Formal thought disorders, including loosening of associations and thought blocking, are common features among youth with schizophrenia. Illogical thinking and poverty of thought are also often present. Unlike adults with schizophrenia, children with schizophrenia do not tend to display poverty of speech content, but they speak less than other children of the same intelligence and are ambiguous in the way they refer to persons, objects, and events. The communication deficits observable in children with schizophrenia include unpredictably changing the topic of conversation without introducing the new topic to the listener (loose associations). Youth with schizophrenia also exhibit illogical thinking and speaking and tend to underuse self-initiated repair strategies to aid in their communication. When the meaning of speech is unclear or vague, typical youth will attempt to clarify their communication with repetitions, revision, and more detail. Youth with schizophrenia, however, often fail to clarify unclear verbal communication by revising the wording, fillers, or starting over. These deficits are examples of negative symptoms in early-onset schizophrenia.

Core phenomena for schizophrenia seem to be universal across the age span; however, a child or adolescent's developmental level significantly influences the presentation of the symptoms. Delusions of young children are less complex, therefore, than those of older children; for example, age-appropriate content, such as animal imagery and monsters, is likely to be a source of delusional fear in young children. According to the DSM-5-TR, a child with schizophrenia may experience deterioration of function, along with the emergence of psychotic symptoms, or the child may never achieve the expected level of functioning. Youth may meet criteria for schizoaffective disorder, using the same criteria as those used for adults. In schizoaffective disorder, symptoms meet criteria for a major depressive episode or manic episode at the same time that the symptoms meeting criteria for schizophrenia are present. Tables 17-1 and 17-2 show comparative diagnostic criteria for schizophrenia and schizoaffective disorder respectively.

Table 17-1.
Comparative Diagnostic Criteria for Schizophrenia

	DSM-5-TR	ICD-10	ICD-11
Diagnostic name	Schizophrenia	Schizophrenia	Schizophrenia
Duration	Symptoms present continuously for ≥6 mo		≥1 mo
Symptoms	Presence of: • Delusions • Hallucinations • Disorganized speech • Disorganized behavior and/or catatonia • Negative symptoms (such as flattened affect, lack of motivation)	Distortions in thinking and/or perception, in addition to negative changes in affect, frequently involving affective blunting. Symptoms may or may not be associated with cognitive dysfunction over time. Common symptoms include: • Thought echo • Thought insertion or withdrawal • Thought broadcasting • Delusional perception • Delusions or control, influence, or passivity • Hallucinatory voices • Disordered/disorganized thinking • Negative symptoms	Disturbance in multiple mental modalities, including: • Thinking (delusions, disorganized thought) • Perception (hallucinations) • Self-experience (of being externally controlled) • Cognition (attention, verbal memory, social cognition) • Volition (motivation) • Affect (blunted) • Behavior (bizarre, inappropriate, or purposeless) • Catatonia may be present
Required number of symptoms	≥2 of the above symptoms, among which ≥1 symptom must be delusions, hallucinations, or disorganized speech		
Psychosocial consequences	Level of functioned decreased in ≥1 more major areas of function (e.g., work, interpersonal, self-care)		

(continued)

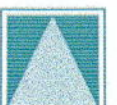

Table 17-1.
Comparative Diagnostic Criteria for Schizophrenia (Continued)

	DSM-5-TR	ICD-10	ICD-11
Exclusions	Another medical condition Substance/medication, including withdrawal Other mental illness (i.e., bipolar disorder, schizoaffective disorder if mood episode history is present)	Organic neurologic disease Schizoaffective disorder Epilepsy Psychoactive substances	Another medical condition Substance/medication, including withdrawal
Symptoms specifiers	**With catatonia** defined as the presence of ≥3 of the following: • Reduced psychomotor activity/stupor • Catalepsy (posture induced passively is held against gravity) • Waxy flexibility (resistance to passive motion) • Mutism • Negativism • Posturing • Odd mannerisms • Stereotypic behaviors • Agitation • Grimacing • Echolalia (copying another's speech) • Echopraxia (copying another's movements)	**Paranoid schizophrenia** **Hebephrenic schizophrenia has** prominent negative changes in affect, with inappropriate mood, social isolation, unpredictable behavior. **Catatonic schizophrenia has** prominent psychomotor changes associated with catatonia, such as posturing, odd mannerisms/affect, and stupor vs. agitation. **Undifferentiated schizophrenia** **Residual schizophrenia** Chronic illness with evidence of cognitive changes as a result of long-standing disease **Simple schizophrenia** Slow progressive development of changes in behavior and functioning, with affective blunting developing often without clear preceding psychotic symptoms **Other schizophrenia** **Schizophrenia unspecified**	Positive symptoms Negative symptoms Depressive mood symptoms Manic mood symptoms Psychomotor symptoms Cognitive symptoms
Course specifiers	**First episode, currently in acute episode** **First episode, currently in partial remission** (with partial remission defined as improvement in symptoms such that diagnostic criteria may no longer be fully met) **First episode, currently in full remission** (with full remission defined as lack of any symptoms) **Multiple episodes, currently in acute episode** (at minimum has history of two episodes, separated by remission) **Multiple episodes, currently in partial remission** **Multiple episodes, currently in full remission** **Continuous** **Unspecified**		First/multiple episode(s), currently symptomatic First/multiple episode(s), in partial remission First/multiple episode(s), in full remission First/multiple episode(s), unspecified

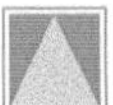

Table 17-2.
Comparative Diagnostic Criteria for Schizoaffective Disorder

	DSM-5-TR	ICD-10	ICD-11
Diagnostic name	Schizoaffective Disorder	Schizoaffective Disorders	Schizoaffective Disorder
Duration	Mood episode symptoms must be present for more days than not during the total duration of the illness, though there must also be a period of ≥2 wk during which delusions or hallucinations are present in the absence of mood episodes.		≥1 mo
Symptoms	Presence of symptoms meeting criteria for a major depressive episode or manic episode while also exhibiting symptom criteria for schizophrenia	Episode presentation of symptoms of affective disturbance and schizophrenic symptoms that do not meet criteria for either schizophrenia or depressive/manic episodes	Diagnostic requirements of schizophrenia and a manic, mixed, or moderate or severe depressive episode are met within the same episode of illness, either simultaneously or within a few days of each other
Exclusions	Another medical condition Other mental illness A substance or medication, including withdrawal		Another medical condition Other mental illness A substance or medication, including withdrawal
Symptoms specifiers	**Bipolar type:** manic episode present **Depressive type:** depressive episode present **With catatonia,** defined as the presence of ≥3 of the following: • Reduced psychomotor activity/stupor • Catalepsy (posture induced passively is held against gravity) • Waxy flexibility (resistance to passive motion) • Mutism • Negativism • Posturing • Odd mannerisms • Stereotypic behaviors • Agitation • Grimacing • Echolalia (copying another's speech) • Echopraxia (copying another's movements)	**Schizoaffective disorder, manic type** **Schizoaffective disorder, depressive type** **Schizoaffective disorder, mixed type** **Schizoaffective disorder, unspecified** **Other schizoaffective disorder**	Positive symptoms Negative symptoms Depressive mood symptoms Manic mood symptoms Psychomotor symptoms Cognitive symptoms
Course specifiers	**First episode, currently in acute episode** **First episode, currently in partial remission** (with partial remission defined as improvement in symptoms such that diagnostic criteria may no longer be fully met) **First episode, currently in full remission** (with full remission defined as lack of any symptoms) **Multiple episodes, currently in acute episode** (history of ≥2 episodes, separated by remission) **Multiple episodes, currently in partial remission** **Multiple episodes, currently in full remission** **Continuous** **Unspecified**		

Peter was evaluated psychiatrically and hospitalized when he was a 13-year-old seventh grader. Peter had a longstanding history of mood dysregulation, and poor social skills which led to being bullied, academic problems, and recurrent temper outbursts. A few months after the school year started, Peter began withdrawing from family meals and isolating himself in his room. Over the next 6 months, his symptoms became worse, with increased suspiciousness of family members and classmates, fearfulness, and beliefs that he was communicating with Satan. Peter appeared to be responding to auditory hallucinations that he believed were coming from avatars in his computer games and commanded him to harm his parents. Peter had been refusing to eat dinner at home, reporting to his mother that the food had a strange smell that he believed meant it was poisoned. At night, Peter would see frightening figures in his room. Peter's parents noted Peter's bizarre behaviors, such as mumbling to himself and perseverating about devils and demons when talking to his family. On one occasion he assaulted his younger brother, saying he was evil and needed to be destroyed. During this episode, he scratched himself with a kitchen knife to "please Satan." Peter's parents called 911 and Peter was placed on an involuntary hold by police for danger to self and others and brought to the hospital emergency room where he was admitted to the psychiatric unit.

Peter was the product of full-term pregnancy and normal delivery. His speech and motor developmental milestones were delayed by about 6 months. However, his pediatrician reassured his parents that this was within the limits of healthy development. As a younger child, Peter tended to be quiet and socially awkward and had trouble keeping up with his classmates. Peter's intellectual function was evaluated and found to be in the average range; however, academic achievement testing revealed that Peter was functioning below grade level. Peter had been a lonely and isolated child, with significant difficulty making friends.

During his hospitalization, Peter's psychiatrist prescribed Aripiprazole and increased the dose to 30 mg/day over the next 10 days. Peter's auditory hallucinations were moderately improved after 3 weeks of treatment. Peter continued to be suspicious and mistrustful of his physicians and family. While hospitalized, Peter attended biweekly group therapy sessions and individual therapy sessions three times per week. Peter's family remained perplexed as to what had caused severe deterioration and blamed themselves for allowing him so much time with online computer games. The inpatient treatment team met with his parents for weekly sessions during his hospitalization. It reassured them that they had not caused his illness and that their continued support would increase his chances of improvement and of remaining well. After being discharged from the hospital 30 days later, Peter was placed in a special education program within a nonpublic school, where he was assigned a school counselor who met with him regularly. Peter's family found a private therapist with expertise in cognitive behavioral therapy and working with teens with psychotic symptoms to help Peter with his fears and suspicions. At the time of discharge from the hospital, Peter's symptoms were much improved; however, he still experienced auditory hallucinations at night. Over the next 2 years, Peter had several relapses of frank psychosis, especially when he used marijuana daily, and each time he was hospitalized he was able to be stabilized. Several other second-generation antipsychotics were tried, including olanzapine, and risperidone to determine if they were more effective. Although Peter improved with each antipsychotic, none led to long-lasting stability. When he was 15 years old, Peter's parents decided to place him in a local residential treatment center to maintain his stability. While in the treatment center, Peter continued to receive individual therapy and family therapy, and his family remained very supportive. Even with these interventions, Peter's mental status recurrently deteriorated, leading to disorganized thinking, paranoid delusions, and inappropriate affect. When Peter became frankly psychotic, he had periods of pacing and muttering to himself, with little to no social interaction with others unless initiated by adults. After observing Peter's mood, behavior, and thought processes for approximately 6 months, in the residential treatment facility, Peter's psychiatrist decided to initiate a trial of clozapine, when Peter was 15½ years old. Peter achieved significant improvement with clozapine therapy which was much more effective than his previous antipsychotic medications. Despite considerable improvement, Peter remained mildly symptomatic. (Adapted from Jon M. McClellan, M.D.)

Pathology and Laboratory Examinations

No specific laboratory tests are diagnostically specific for childhood-onset schizophrenia.

DIFFERENTIAL DIAGNOSIS

Making a diagnosis of childhood-onset schizophrenia is challenging. Very young children who report hallucinations, apparent thought disorders, language delays, and an inability to differentiate reality from fantasy may be manifesting phenomena better accounted for by nonpsychotic disorders such as posttraumatic stress disorder (PTSD) or ASD.

The differential diagnosis of early-onset schizophrenia includes ASD, bipolar disorders, depressive disorders with psychotic features, PTSD, and substance-induced disorder. Children with childhood-onset schizophrenia have frequent comorbidities, including attention-deficit hyperactivity disorder (ADHD), oppositional defiant disorder, and major depression.

Childhood Psychotic Phenomena without a Psychotic Disorder

Auditory and visual hallucinations can appear as self-limited events in nonpsychotic young children who are experiencing extreme stress or anxiety related to unstable home lives, abuse, or neglect, or in children experiencing a significant loss.

Major Depression with Psychotic Features

Psychotic phenomena are common among children with major depressive disorder, in which both hallucinations and, less commonly, delusions may occur. The congruence of mood with psychotic features is most pronounced in depressed children, although children with schizophrenia may also seem sad. The hallucinations and delusions of schizophrenia are more likely to have a bizarre quality than those of children with depressive disorders.

Bipolar Disorder

In children and adolescents with bipolar I disorder, it often is challenging to distinguish a first episode of mania with psychotic features from schizophrenia if the child has no history of previous depressions. Grandiose delusions and hallucinations are typical of manic episodes, but clinicians often must follow the natural history of the disorder to confirm the presence of a mood disorder. ASDs share some features with schizophrenia, most notably difficulty with social relationships, an early history of delayed language acquisition, and ongoing communication deficits.

Autism Spectrum Disorder

Blunted affect, social isolation, eccentric thoughts, ideas of reference, and bizarre behavior occur in both early-onset schizophrenia and ASD; however, in schizophrenia, overt psychotic symptoms, such as hallucinations, delusions, or incoherence emerge at some point. Hallucinations alone, however, are not evidence of schizophrenia; patients must show either a deterioration of function or an inability to meet an expected developmental level to warrant the diagnosis of schizophrenia.

However, hallucinations, delusions, and formal thought disorder are core features of schizophrenia and not the usual features of ASD. ASD is usually diagnosed by 3 years of age, whereas schizophrenia with childhood-onset usually manifests after 5 years of age.

TRAUMA/POSTTRAUMATIC STRESS DISORDER

Children and adolescents with PTSD often report flashbacks or experiences of reliving traumatic experiences which have some features in common with psychotic-like phenomena. Children with PTSD don't typically display disorganized thoughts, persistent bizarre auditory hallucinations, or blunted affect. A history of trauma does not preclude schizophrenia; in fact the risk of developing schizophrenia is elevated in youth who have experienced childhood adverse events.

SUBSTANCE-INDUCED DISORDERS AND GENERAL MEDICAL DISORDERS

Among adolescents, use of alcohol and other substances sometimes can result in a deterioration of function, psychotic symptoms, and paranoid delusions. Amphetamines, lysergic acid diethylamide (LSD), and phencyclidine (PCP) may lead to a psychotic state. Sudden, flagrant onset of paranoid psychosis may suggest substance-induced psychotic disorder. Medical conditions that can induce psychotic features include thyroid disease, systemic lupus erythematosus, and temporal lobe disease.

COURSE AND PROGNOSIS

The course and outcome of early-onset schizophrenia is dependent on numerous variables, including the child's premorbid level of functioning, the age of onset, IQ, response to psychosocial and pharmacologic interventions, degree of remission after the first psychotic episode, and degree of family support. Early age at onset and comorbid developmental delays, learning disorders, lower IQ, premorbid behavioral disorders, and chronicity or long length of a first psychotic episode are likely to compromise prognosis. Psychosocial and family stressors are known to influence the relapse rate in adults with schizophrenia, and high expression of negative emotion (EE) likely affects children with childhood-onset schizophrenia, as well. Consistent family emotional support with low levels of expressed emotion, particularly negative, predicts fewer relapses in youth with schizophrenia.

An important factor in the outcome is the accuracy and stability of the diagnosis of schizophrenia. One study reported that one-third of children who received an initial diagnosis of schizophrenia later had a manic episode and the diagnosis was changed to bipolar disorder in adolescence. Children and adolescents with bipolar I disorder may have a better long-term prognosis than those with schizophrenia. The NIMH-funded Treatment of Early-Onset Schizophrenia study reported the outcome of neurocognitive functioning in 8- to 19-year-old youth with schizophrenia or schizoaffective disorders who participated in a randomized, double-blind clinical trial comparing molindone, olanzapine, and risperidone. The three medication groups yielded no group differences in neurocognitive functioning over a year; however, when data from the three groups were combined, a significant modest improvement was observed in several domains of neurocognitive functioning. The authors concluded that antipsychotic intervention in youth with early-onset schizophrenia spectrum disorders led to modest improvement in neurocognitive function.

TREATMENT

The treatment of childhood-onset schizophrenia requires a multimodal approach, including psychoeducation for families, pharmacologic interventions, psychotherapeutic interventions, social skills interventions, and appropriate educational placement.

Antipsychotic medication treatments are a central component of treatment for early-onset schizophrenia. Randomized controlled trials support the efficacy of the

SGAs for early-onset schizophrenia, with seven currently approved by the FDA for the treatment of early-onset schizophrenia in adolescents 13 years and older.

Randomized clinical trials (RCTs) have demonstrated benefits of several different psychosocial interventions for youth presenting with prodromal psychotic symptoms, with improvements found in cognitive and social behaviors. These interventions include CBT, group skills training, cognitive remediation therapy (CRT), multifamily psychoeducation, and supportive counseling on the prevention of psychosis. In youth with prodromal states, the specific psychosocial interventions have been shown to be more effective than standard treatments in delaying the onset of a full psychotic disorder over a 2-year follow-up period. Psychosocial interventions in adults with schizophrenia and their families have been found to mediate psychosis and to decrease the relapse rate and severity of illness over time. Family education and ongoing therapeutic family interventions are critical in maintaining the maximum level of support for the patient. Monitoring the most appropriate educational setting for a child with childhood-onset schizophrenia is essential, especially given the frequent social skills deficits, attention deficits, and academic difficulties that often accompany childhood-onset schizophrenia.

Pharmacotherapy

SGAs, or serotonin-dopamine antagonists, are the current mainstay pharmacologic treatments for children and adolescents with schizophrenia. Currently, seven SGAs are FDA approved for adolescents 13 years and older with schizophrenia: lurasidone, aripiprazole, risperidone, olanzapine, quetiapine, paliperidone, and brexpiprazole. These approvals were based largely on data from RCTs showing superiority of these SGAs over placebo in early-onset schizophrenia. Table 17-3 details the SGAs with FDA approval in the treatment of early-onset schizophrenia.

RCTs did not show superiority of ziprasidone or asenapine over placebo in trials conducted by Findling and colleagues in 2013. Worldwide the most frequently prescribed SGAs in the treatment of early-onset schizophrenia are aripiprazole, quetiapine, and risperidone. Clozapine, a serotonin receptor antagonist with some dopamine (D_2) antagonism, has been used successfully in treatment-resistant schizophrenia in adults for improving both negative and positive symptoms. It remains an off-label choice of last resort in youth based on its potentially serious side effects. Evidence from multisite RCTs supports efficacy of risperidone, olanzapine, aripiprazole, and clozapine in the treatment of early-onset schizophrenia. Two RCTs using risperidone in adolescents with schizophrenia found risperidone at doses up to 3 mg/day to be superior to placebo. A multisite randomized 6-week controlled trial of olanzapine in adolescents with schizophrenia found that it was more efficacious than a placebo. An RCT of aripiprazole at two fixed doses found that it was superior to placebo in the treatment of positive symptoms of adolescent schizophrenia; however, more than 40% of subjects in the active medication group did not achieve remission. Finally, clozapine is more effective than haloperidol in improving both positive and negative symptoms in treatment-resistant schizophrenia in youth. A randomized study compared clozapine to high doses of olanzapine and found that response rates were about twice as high for clozapine as olanzapine (66% vs. 33%) when the investigators defined response as 30% or better reduction in symptoms on the Brief Psychiatric Rating Scale and improvement on the Clinical Global Impression Scale. The Treatment of Early-Onset Schizophrenia Spectrum Disorders Study (TEOSS) described by Findling and colleagues (2010) compared the efficacy of risperidone and olanzapine with those of molindone, a mid-potency first-generation antipsychotic. In this study, lacking a placebo group, each of these agents provided a similar therapeutic effect; however, fewer than half of the patients responded optimally.

A double-blind, randomized 8-week controlled trial compared the efficacy and safety of olanzapine to clozapine in childhood-onset schizophrenia. Children with childhood-onset schizophrenia who were resistant to at least two previous treatments with antipsychotics were randomized to treatment for 8 weeks with either olanzapine or clozapine followed by a 2-year open-label follow-up. Using the Clinical Global Impression of Severity of Symptoms Scale and Schedule for the Assessment of Negative/Positive Symptoms, clozapine was associated with a reduction in all outcome measures. In contrast,

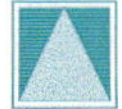

Table 17-3.
FDA-Approved Medications for Early-Onset Schizophrenia

Medication	Class	Age range	Disorder
Risperidone (Risperdal)	Second-generation antipsychotic	13–17 yr	Schizophrenia
Olanzapine (Zyprexa)	Second-generation antipsychotic	13–17 yr	Schizophrenia
Aripiprazole (Abilify)	Second-generation antipsychotic	13–17 yr	Schizophrenia
Quetiapine (Seroquel)	Second-generation antipsychotic	13–17 yr	Schizophrenia
Paliperidone (Invega)	Second-generation antipsychotic	12–17 yr	Schizophrenia
Lurasidone (Latuda)	Second-generation antipsychotic	13–17 yr	Schizophrenia
Brexpiprazole (Rexulti)	Second-generation antipsychotic	13–17 yr	Schizophrenia

olanzapine showed improvement on certain measures but not on all. The only statistically significant measure in which clozapine was superior to olanzapine was in alleviating negative symptoms compared with baseline. Clozapine was associated with more adverse events, such as lipid abnormalities and a seizure in one patient.

Several studies have provided evidence that risperidone, a benzisoxazole derivative, is as effective as the older high-potency first-generation antipsychotics, such as haloperidol, and causes less frequent severe side effects in the treatment of schizophrenia in older adolescents and adults. Published case reports and limited more extensive controlled studies have supported the efficacy of risperidone in the treatment of psychosis in children and adolescents. Risperidone can cause weight gain and dystonic reactions and other extrapyramidal adverse effects in children and adolescents. Olanzapine is generally well tolerated for extrapyramidal adverse effects compared with first-generation antipsychotics and risperidone, but it is associated with moderate sedation and significant weight gain.

In the IMPACT trial, described by Correl and colleagues (2020), in which youth with severe mental disorders received treatment with several different SGAs, subjects who were overweight or obese were either switched to another SGA with less metabolic side effects, or metformin was added to their regimen, or they were provided with healthy lifestyle education. The groups who were switched to another antipsychotic with lower metabolic risk and those provided with metformin as an add-on showed reduction in their body mass index (BMI); however, those provided with healthy lifestyle education did not decrease their BMI.

SGAs in youth are associated with a number of potential adverse effects, including weight gain, sedation, metabolic problems, and extrapyramidal side effects. Safety monitoring for youth being treated with antipsychotic medications should include a comprehensive metabolic panel including fasting glucose, lipid profile, body mass index, hemoglobin A1C, liver function tests, complete blood count, blood pressure, and weight at the onset of treatment. These laboratory tests should be repeated every 6 months to 1 year while the youth remains on antipsychotic medication.

Psychosocial Interventions

Psychosocial interventions aimed at family education and patient and family support are critical components of the treatment plan for childhood-onset schizophrenia. Psychosocial interventions that have been shown to be helpful in young adults can be applied to children and adolescents with schizophrenia, including cognitive-behavioral approaches, family therapy, psychoeducation, and social skills training. These interventions have been shown to have positive results in mediating distress from hallucinations and delusions in schizophrenia and diminishing the number of relapses in young adults with onset of schizophrenia.

An RCT by Morrison and colleagues in the United Kingdom (2020) is underway, comparing the efficacy of antipsychotic medication monotherapy, a psychological intervention (CBT + family intervention), and a combination of the two therapies for youth 14 to 18 years of age with a first episode of psychosis. The main aim of the study was to establish the feasibility of RCT in adolescents with first-episode psychosis. Findings of the current trial suggest that all three arms of the study (antipsychotic monotherapy, CBT + family intervention, and the combination of these interventions) appear to be safe and provided benefit for both negative and positive symptoms. There was no indication during the trial that the psychological interventions in the absence of antipsychotic treatment caused harm.

The first known randomized controlled pilot study utilizing CBT in adolescents with early-onset psychosis was conducted by Muller and colleagues (2020) in Germany. This study enrolled 25 adolescents with early-onset schizophrenia who were randomized to either 9 months (20 sessions) of CBT + treatment as usual (TAU) or TAU alone. TAU typically consisted of antipsychotic medication treatment and supportive therapeutic interventions. The primary goal of this study was to assess the efficacy of modified CBT for the reduction of positive symptoms, along with TAU, compared to TAU alone. Secondary goals of the study included assessing levels of negative symptoms, symptom remission, depression, psychosocial functioning, and quality of life. This pilot study also aimed to assess the tolerability, feasibility, and safety of CBT combined with TAU compared to TAU alone. The results indicated improvement in positive psychotic symptoms in both groups without differences reaching statistical significance; however, a trend for advantage in the CBT + TAU group was found in the reduction of delusions compared to the TAU alone group. Follow-up assessments were conducted at 9 months and again at 24 months. The secondary goals of the study were assessment of negative symptoms, psychosocial functioning, and quality of life after treatment. At each assessment, both groups showed improvements in positive and negative symptoms, as well as in depression, psychosocial functioning, and quality-of-life measures, which were still present at 24-month follow-up. Both treatment conditions were well accepted and tolerated by the subjects. The authors concluded that, while antipsychotic medication and supportive interventions accounted for much of the improvements in both groups, the persistence of clinically meaningful effects, especially regarding improvements in negative symptoms, psychosocial functioning, and quality of life, suggests an additional benefit of CBT + TAU.

CRT consists of 40 hours of sessions in which patients with schizophrenia are coached in order to improve verbal memory, problem-solving skills, and processing speed, according to Data and colleagues (2020). There have not been RCTs to support its efficacy; however, there is a suggestion that it may be useful as an adjunctive early intervention.

Psychotherapists who work with children and adolescents with early-onset schizophrenia must take into account a youth's developmental level in order to support the child's developmentally appropriate reality testing and understand the youth's developmentally appropriate sense of self. Long-term supportive family interventions and cognitive-behavioral and remediation interventions, combined with pharmacotherapy, are likely to be the most effective approach to early-onset schizophrenia.

EPIDEMIOLOGY

Early-onset schizophrenia affects approximately 0.7% of the population, and childhood-onset schizophrenia affects less than 0.04% of the population. Thus, early-onset schizophrenia is about five times more common in adolescents compared to prepubertal children. Early-onset and especially childhood-onset schizophrenia resemble the more severe forms of adult schizophrenia, although higher rates of comorbidity are found in youth with schizophrenia. Comorbid disorders include ADHD, depressive disorders, anxiety disorders, speech and language disorders, and motor disturbances.

Boys have a slight preponderance among children diagnosed with schizophrenia, with an estimated ratio of about 1.67 boys to 1 girl. Boys are generally identified and diagnosed with schizophrenia at a younger age than girls. Schizophrenia is rarely diagnosed in children younger than 5 years of age. The prevalence of schizophrenia among the parents of children with schizophrenia is about 8%, which is about twice the prevalence in the parents of patients with adult-onset schizophrenia.

ETIOLOGY

Early-onset schizophrenia is a highly heritable neurodevelopmental disorder in which interactions between genes and the environment result in abnormal early brain development. Early-onset schizophrenia is characterized by a complex genetic architecture with both inherited and de novo genetic mutations distributed in almost all chromosomes, according to Fernandez and colleagues (2019). The consequences of the aberrant brain development in schizophrenia may not be fully evident until adolescence or early adulthood; however, data support the hypothesis that white matter abnormalities and disturbances in myelination in childhood lead to abnormal connectivity between brain regions. The aberrant connectivity in various regions of the brain is likely a significant contributing factor in the psychotic symptoms and cognitive deficits in childhood-onset schizophrenia.

Genetic Factors

In recent years, according to a review by Besterman (2023), rare genetic variants that are highly penetrant, as well as more commonly found genetic variants with much lower penetrance, may contribute to an increased risk of the emergence of schizophrenia. Estimates of heritability for childhood-onset schizophrenia have been as high as 80% and may be attributable to more than 200 distinct possible genomic loci that may be involved. Large genomic deletions and duplications, such as copy number variations (CNVs), represent well-documented neurodevelopmental disorder risk factors, and de novo single-nucleotide variations (SNVs) in genes involved in brain development are also believed to be contributing factors in the etiology of early-onset schizophrenia according to a review by Fernandez and colleagues. Specific CNVs associated with schizophrenia include 22q11.2 deletion, 3q29 deletion, 1q21.1 deletion, and 16p11.2 duplication. Early-onset schizophrenia is associated with other neurodevelopmental disorders such as ASD and ADHD. According to the review by Fernandez and colleagues, 66 copy number variations (CNVs) in 16 autosomal chromosomes and in 2 sex chromosomes, and 36 different SNVs were reported in 12 autosomal chromosomes and 1 sex chromosome. Mutations were distributed in various chromosomes illustrating the genetic heterogeneity of early-onset schizophrenia. It is highly notable that more than 90% of CNVs reported to be involved in early-onset schizophrenia have also been reported to be involved in ASD, suggesting that there may be genetic overlap between these disorders. Although genomic research has increased significantly in recent years, its utility in determining the most effective clinical treatments is still limited but broadening with increasing research. It is well known that youth with early-onset schizophrenia have higher rates of schizophrenia among their relatives than patients with adult-onset schizophrenia.

Endophenotype Markers for Childhood-Onset Schizophrenia. Currently, no reliable method can identify persons at the highest risk for schizophrenia in a given family. Neurodevelopmental abnormalities and higher-than-expected rates of neurologic soft signs and impairments in sustaining attention and in strategies for information processing appear among children at high risk. Increased rates of disturbed communication styles exist in family members of individuals with schizophrenia. Reports have documented higher-than-expected neuropsychological deficits in attention, working memory, and premorbid IQ among children who later develop schizophrenia and its spectrum disorders.

Magnetic Resonance Imaging Studies

The NIMH prospective study of more than 100 patients with childhood-onset schizophrenia and their typically developing siblings has demonstrated progressive loss of gray matter, delayed and disrupted white matter growth, and a decline in cerebellar volume in those with childhood-onset schizophrenia. Siblings of affected children also showed some of these brain disruptions, however, the gray matter abnormalities were normalized over time in the siblings, indicating a protective mechanism not present in children with schizophrenia. The hippocampal volume loss across the age span appears to be static among children with childhood-onset schizophrenia. The magnetic resonance imaging (MRI) component of the study, which followed children with schizophrenia and their healthy siblings for two decades, documented that in childhood-onset schizophrenia, progressive brain gray matter loss occurs continuously over time. This gray matter shrinkage occurs with ventricular increases, with a pattern of loss originating in the parietal region and proceeding frontally to dorsolateral prefrontal and temporal cortices, including superior temporal gyri. Studies of childhood-onset schizophrenia at the NIMH provided evidence that early loss of parietal gray matter followed by frontal and parietal gray matter loss is more pronounced in childhood-onset schizophrenia than in schizophrenia with later onset. Other research utilized diffusion tensor images from children with childhood-onset schizophrenia versus controls and found increased diffusivities in the posterior corona radiata in children with childhood-onset schizophrenia, which implicated abnormal connectivity with the parietal lobes. These results contrasted with findings among subjects with later onset of schizophrenia in whom there were more abnormalities in the frontal lobes. A retrospective clinical review by Levman and colleagues (2023) found abnormal morphology in the brains of youth with early-onset schizophrenia compared to healthy controls. Abnormalities included increased regionally distributed surface curvature measurements in the early-onset schizophrenia cohort relative to neurotypical controls. This includes an abnormally increased surface curvature in the right pars orbitalis, left subcentral gyrus, right pars triangularis, right posterior cingulate, right orbital gyrus, right frontal pole, left inferior occipital gyrus, right lateral orbitofrontal gyrus, and the left medial occipito-temporal and lingual sulci, and right insular sulci.

ATTENUATED PSYCHOSIS SYNDROME (A CONDITION FOR FURTHER STUDY)

Attenuated psychosis syndrome (APS) was a new diagnostic category proposed as a condition for further study first in 2013 in DSM-5. It represents a set of symptoms which are prodromal and may progress to a full diagnosis of schizophrenia in the future. It continues to be a condition for further study in the DSM-5-TR. APS consists of at least one of the following: attenuated delusions, attenuated hallucinations, or attenuated disorganized speech. Symptoms in this syndrome must be present at least once per week over the past month, have worsened over the past year, and are impairing enough to warrant clinical attention. It is a syndrome characterized by subthreshold psychotic symptoms, less severe than those found in psychotic disorders, but which are often present in prodromal psychotic states.

Debate and controversy among clinicians and researchers have surrounded the inclusion of APS in the DSM-5 and the DSM-5-TR. Some believe that the identification and treatment of a prodromal syndrome of a psychotic disorder might delay the onset and course of the full psychotic illness. However, others believe that identification of a prodromal syndrome, which may rarely, if ever, progress to a full psychotic illness, would lead to unnecessary exposure to antipsychotic agents with unpredictable and possibly harmful effects. There is agreement, however, that patients with subthreshold prodromal psychotic symptoms are often impaired and need psychological and psychiatric intervention.

A meta-analysis reported that the rate of onset of psychotic disorders in those patients with prodromal psychotic symptoms was 18% at 6 months, 22% at 1 year, 29% at 2 years, and 36% at 3 years. In a follow-up study, of those with prodromal symptoms who went on to develop a threshold psychotic illness, 73% met the criteria for schizophrenia.

In children and adolescents, psychotic symptoms are not necessarily a hallmark of a threshold psychotic disorder compared to adults. For example, in 50% of children with major depressive episodes, psychotic symptoms were present. Also, epidemiologic studies have found that globally, auditory hallucinations occur in 9% to 21% of children and 8.4% of adolescents. Thus, in youth, the association between subthreshold psychotic symptoms and the emergence of future psychotic illness may not be a reliable predictor. Nevertheless, identification and follow up of youth with APS may provide an increased understanding of the longitudinal significance of these symptoms.

Diagnosis

APS, according to DSM-5-TR, is based on the presence of at least one of the following: delusions, hallucinations, or disorganized speech, which causes functional impairment. Although the symptoms may not have progressed to full psychotic severity, they must have been present at least once per week for 1 month and must have emerged or worsened in the past year. The symptoms must cause impairment and warrant clinical attention.

Attenuated delusions are described as suspicious, persecutory, or grandiose, resulting in a lack of trust in others, and a sense of danger. Attenuated delusions, in contrast to delusions of threshold illness, may lead to loosely organized beliefs about hostile intentions of others or danger; however, the delusions are not as fixed as they become in full-blown psychotic illness. Attenuated hallucinations include altered sensory perceptions such as the perception of murmurs, rumblings, or shadows that are disturbing, but which youth may doubt and challenge. Disorganized communication or speech may present as vague or confusing explanations or circumstantial or tangential communication. When severe but still in the attenuated range, thought blocking or loose associations may emerge; however, in contrast to psychotic illness, redirection is possible, and one can usually achieve a logical conversation. Although impairment is present in APS, the individual retains awareness and insight into the mental changes that are occurring.

Treatment

According to a review of ultra–high-risk patients who display prodromal symptoms of psychosis by Nelson and McGorry in 2020, approximately 30% went on to develop a psychotic illness over a period of several years, which is more than 1,000 times as likely as a first episode of a psychotic illness in the general population. Among the 70% of patients with ultra–high-risk who did not go on to develop a psychotic illness, about half of them developed a mood disorder, and about one-third developed an anxiety disorder.

Treatment recommendations that have emerged by consensus include the following approaches:

1. Individual CBT with or without family participation.
2. Focus on the presenting problems, including mood and anxiety symptoms or disorders.
3. Academic, educational, and social skill interventions to maintain function in these areas.
4. If psychological interventions are ineffective or only partially beneficial, or there are safety concerns, the addition of an SGA is recommended, starting with a low dose.
5. If symptoms remain, close monitoring is recommended for a period of several years.

Etiology

Genetic Factors. Family studies have demonstrated that genetic factors influence vulnerability for schizophrenia spectrum disorders and other psychotic disorders. To the extent that APS and schizophrenia are related, genetic contributions are likely to be significant. Adoption and twin studies have confirmed that monozygotic twins have about a 50% concordance rate for schizophrenia compared to dizygotic twins, who have a concordance rate of about 10%. Also, adopted children of parents with schizophrenia do not have higher rates of schizophrenia; but biologic children of schizophrenic parents do. However, genetic factors do not account fully for the emergence of schizophrenia spectrum disorders since there is only a 50% concordance of exhibiting these disorders among monozygotic twins. Environmental factors also play an essential role.

Environmental Factors. Early environmental factors that increase the risk of developing schizophrenia include fetal malnutrition, hypoxia at birth, and possibly prenatal infections. Other environmental factors include trauma, stress, social adversity, and isolation. Finally, gene–environment interactions may influence an individual's sensitivity to adverse environmental events.

Further Readings

Adnan M, Motiwala F, Trivedi C, Sultana T, Mansuri Z, Jain S. Clozapine for management of childhood and adolescent-onset schizophrenia: a systematic review and meta-analysis. *J Child Adolesc Psychopharmacol.* 2022;32(1):2–11.

American Academy of Child and Adolescent Psychiatry (AACAP) Committee on Quality Isuues (CQI). Practice parameter for the assessment and treatment of children and adolescents with schizophrenia. *J Am Acad Child Adolesc Psychiatry.* 2013;52(9):976–990.

Arango C, Ng-Mak D, Finn E, Byrne A, Loebel A. Lurasidone compared to other atypical antipsychotic monotherapies for adolescent schizophrenia: a systematic literature review and network meta-analysis. *Eur Child Adolesc Psychiatry.* 2020;29(9):1195–1205.

Barnes TR, Drake R, Paton C, et al. Evidence-based guidelines for the pharmacological treatment of schizophrenia: updated recommendations from the British Association for Psychopharmacology. *J Psychopharmacol.* 2020;34(1):3–78.

Besterman AD. A genetics-guided approach to the clinical management of schizophrenia. *Schizophr Res.* 2024;267:462–469.

Catalan A, Salazar de Pablo G, Vaquerizo Serrano J, et al. Annual research review: prevention of psychosis in adolescents—systematic review and meta-analysis of advances in detection, prognosis and intervention. *J Child Psychol Psychiatry.* 2021;62(5):657–673.

Correll CU, Findling RL, Tocco M, Pikalov A, Deng L, Goldman R. Safety and effectiveness of lurasidone in adolescents with schizophrenia: results of a 2-year, open-label extension study. *CNS Spectr.* 2022;27(1):118–128.

Correll CU, Fusar-Poli P, Leucht S, et al. Treatment approaches for first episode and early-phase schizophrenia in adolescents and young adults: a Delphi Consensus Report from Europe. *Neuropsychiatr Dis Treat.* 2022;18:201–219.

Correll CU, Sikich L, Reeves G, et al. Metformin add-on vs. antipsychotic switch vs. continued antipsychotic treatment plus healthy lifestyle education in overweight or obese youth with severe mental illness: results from the IMPACT trial. *World Psychiatry.* 2020;19(1):69–80.

Driver DI, Thomas S, Gogtay N, Rapoport JL. Childhood-onset schizophrenia and early-onset schizophrenia spectrum disorders: an update. *Child Adolesc Psychiatr Clin N Am.* 2020;29(1):71–90.

Fernandez A, Drozd MM, Thümmler S, et al. Childhood-onset schizophrenia: a systematic overview of its genetic heterogeneity from classical studies to the genomic era. *Front Genet.* 2019;10:1137.

Findling RL, Johnson JL, McCLellan J, et al. Double-blind maintenance safety and effectiveness findings from the Treatment of Early-Onset Schizophrenia Spectrum Disorders (TEOSS) study. *J Am Acad Child Adolesc Psychiatry.* 2010;49(6):583–594

Goldman R, Loebel A, Cucchiaro J, Deng L, Findling RL. Efficacy and safety of lurasidone in adolescents with schizophrenia: a 6-week, randomized placebo-controlled study. *J Child Adolesc Psychopharmacol.* 2017;27(6):516–525.

Gupta N, Gupta M, Esang M. Lost in translation: challenges in the diagnosis and treatment of early-onset schizophrenia. *Cureus.* 2023; 15(5):e39488.

Harvey PD, Isner EC. Cognition, social cognition, and functional capacity in early-onset schizophrenia. *Child Adolesc Psychiatr Clin N Am.* 2020;29(1):171–182.

Iasevoli F, Razzino E, Altavilla B, et al. Relationships between early age at onset of psychotic symptoms and treatment resistant schizophrenia. *Early Interv Psychiatry.* 2022;16(4):352–362.

Keepers GA, Fochtmann LJ, Anzia JM, et al; (Systematic Review). The American Psychiatric Association practice guideline for the treatment of patients with schizophrenia. *Focus (Am Psychiatr Publ).* 2020;18(4):493–497.

Kelleher I, Murtagh A, Molloy C, et al. Identification and characterization of prodromal risk syndromes in young adolescents in the community: a population-based clinical interview study. *Schizophr Bull.* 2012;38(2):239–246.

Levman J, Kabaria P, Nangaku M, Takahashi E. Morphological abnormalities in early-onset schizophrenia revealed by structural magnetic resonance imaging. *Biology (Basel).* 2023;12(3):353.

Loewy RL, Corey S, Amirfathi F, et al. Childhood trauma and clinical high risk for psychosis. *Schizophr Res*. 2019;205:10–14.

Lopez-Morinigo JD, Leucht S, Arango C. Pharmacological treatment of early-onset schizophrenia: a critical review, evidence-based clinical guidance and unmet needs. *Pharmacopsychiatry*. 2022;55(5):233–245.

Morrison AP, Pyle M, Maughan D, et al; MAPS group. Antipsychotic medication versus psychological intervention versus a combination of both in adolescents with first-episode psychosis (MAPS): a multicentre, three-arm, randomised controlled pilot and feasibility study. *Lancet Psychiatry*. 2020;7(9):788–800.

Müller H, Kommescher M, Güttgemanns J, et al. Cognitive behavioral therapy in adolescents with early-onset psychosis: a randomized controlled pilot study. *Eur Child Adolesc Psychiatry*. 2020;29(7):1011–1022.

Nelson B, McGorry P. The prodrome of psychotic disorders: identification, prediction, and preventive treatment. *Child Adolesc Psychiatr Clin N Am*. 2020;29(1):57–69.

Patel PK, Leathem LD, Currin DL, Karlsgodt KH. Adolescent neurodevelopment and vulnerability to psychosis. *Biol Psychiatry*. 2021;89(2):184–193.

Pontillo M, Averna R, Tata MC, Chieppa F, Pucciarini ML, Vicari S. Neurodevelopmental trajectories and clinical profiles in a sample of children and adolescents with early- and very-early-onset schizophrenia. *Front Psychiatry*. 2021;12:662093.

Shaw P, Sporn A, Gogtay N, et al. Childhood onset schizophrenia: a double-blind clozapine-olanzapine comparison. *Arch Gen Psychiatry*. 2006;63(7):721–730.

Stanton KJ, Denietolis B, Goodwin BJ, Dvir Y. Childhood trauma and psychosis: an updated review. *Child Adolesc Psychiatr Clin N Am*. 2020;29(1):115–129.

Sunshine A, McClellan J. Practitioner review: psychosis in children and adolescents. *J Child Psychol Psychiatry*. 2023;64(7):980–988.

Taylor JH, Appel S, Eli M, et al. Time to clinical response in the treatment of early onset schizophrenia spectrum disorders study. *J Child Adolesc Psychopharmacol*. 2021;31(1):46–52.

Yee CS, Bahji A, Lolich M, Vázquez GH, Baldessarini RJ. Comparative efficacy and tolerability of antipsychotics for juvenile psychotic disorders: a systematic review and network meta-analysis. *J Clin Psychopharmacol*. 2022;42(2):198–208.

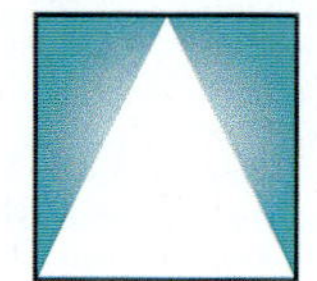

18 Tic Disorders: Tourette Disorder and Chronic Motor or Vocal Tic Disorder

TOURETTE DISORDER

Tics are neuropsychiatric events characterized by brief, rapid motor movements or vocalizations in response to irresistible premonitory urges. Although frequently rapid, tics may include more complex patterns of movements and longer vocalizations. Converging evidence from many lines of research suggests that the production of tics involves dysfunction in the basal ganglia region of the brain, particularly of dopaminergic transmission in the cortico-striatothalamic circuits. Because tic disorders are significantly more common in children than in adults, the postulated alterations in dopamine circuitry in many affected children appear to improve over time. Tics may be transient or chronic, with a waxing and waning course. Tics typically emerge at age 5 to 6 years of age and tend to reach their highest severity between 10 and 12 years. About one-half to two-thirds of children with tic disorders will be much improved or in remission by adolescence or early adulthood. We distinguish tic disorders by the type of tics, their frequency, and the pattern in which they emerge over time. Motor tics most commonly affect the muscles of the face and neck, such as eye-blinking, head-jerking, mouth-grimacing, or headshaking. Typical vocal tics include throat-clearing, grunting, snorting, and coughing. Tics are repetitive muscle contractions resulting in movements or vocalizations that are involuntary. However, patients can sometimes voluntarily suppress them. Children and adolescents may exhibit tic behaviors that occur after a stimulus or in response to a premonitory internal urge.

The most widely studied and most severe tic disorder is Gilles de la Tourette syndrome, also known as Tourette disorder. Georges Gilles de la Tourette (1857–1904) first described a patient with a syndrome, which became known as Tourette disorder in 1885, while he was studying with Jean-Martin Charcot in France. De la Tourette noted a syndrome in several patients that included multiple motor tics, coprolalia, and echolalia. Tics often consist of motions we might use in volitional movements. One-half to two-thirds of children with Tourette disorder exhibit a reduction in or complete remission of tic symptoms during adolescence. There are many common comorbid psychiatric disorders and behavioral problems likely to emerge along with Tourette disorder. For example, the relationship between Tourette disorder, attention-deficit/hyperactivity disorder (ADHD), and obsessive-compulsive disorder (OCD) is not clear. Epidemiologic surveys indicate that more than half of children with Tourette disorder also meet criteria for ADHD. There appears to be a bidirectional relationship between Tourette disorder and OCD, with 20% to 40% of Tourette disorder patients meeting full criteria for OCD. First-degree relatives of patients with OCD have higher rates of tic disorders compared to the general population.

There are a few small reports suggesting that the obsessive-compulsive symptoms most likely to occur in Tourette disorder are characteristically related to ordering and symmetry, counting, and repetitive touching. In contrast, OCD symptoms in the absence of tic disorders usually stem from fears of contamination and fear of harming self or others. Motor and vocal tics can be simple or complex. *Simple motor tics* are those composed of repetitive, rapid contractions of functionally similar muscle groups—for example, eye-blinking, neck-jerking, shoulder-shrugging, and facial-grimacing. Common *simple vocal tics* include coughing, throat-clearing, grunting, sniffing, snorting, and barking. *Complex motor tics* appear to be more purposeful and ritualistic than simple tics. Common *complex motor tics* include grooming behaviors, the smelling of objects, jumping, touching behaviors, echopraxia (imitation of observed behavior), and copropraxia (display of obscene gestures). *Complex vocal tics* include repeating words or phrases out of context, coprolalia (use of obscene words or phrases), palilalia (a person repeating their own words), and echolalia (repetition of the last-heard words of others).

Although older children and adolescents with tic disorders may be able to suppress their tics for minutes or hours, young children are often not cognizant of their tics or experience their urges to perform their tics as irresistible. Sleep, relaxation, or absorption in activity can all attenuate tics. Tics often disappear during sleep.

Diagnosis and Clinical Features

A diagnosis of Tourette disorder depends on a history of multiple motor tics that generally emerge over months or years and the emergence of at least one vocal tic at some point. According to the DSM-5, tics may wax and wane in frequency but must have persisted for more than a year since the first tic emerged to meet the diagnosis. The average age of onset of tics is between 4 and 6 years of age, although in some cases, tics may occur as early as 2 years of age. The peak age for the severity of tics is between 10 and 12 years of age. For a diagnosis of Tourette disorder, the onset must occur before the age of 18 years. Table 18-1 compares the diagnostic approaches to Tourette disorder.

In Tourette disorder, typically, the initial tics are in the face and neck. Over time, the tics tend to occur in a downward progression. The most commonly described tics are those affecting the face and head, the arms and hands, the body and lower extremities, and the respiratory and alimentary systems. In these areas, the tics take the form of grimacing; forehead puckering; eyebrow-raising; eyelid-blinking; winking; nose-wrinkling; nostril-trembling; mouth-twitching; displaying the teeth; biting the lips and other parts; tongue-extruding; protracting the lower jaw; nodding, jerking, or shaking the head; twisting the neck; looking sideways; head-rolling; hand-jerking; arm-jerking; plucking fingers; writhing fingers; fist-clenching; shoulder-shrugging; foot, knee, or toe shaking; walking peculiarly; body writhing; jumping; hiccupping; sighing; yawning; snuffing; blowing through the nostrils; whistling; belching; sucking or smacking sounds; and clearing the throat. Several assessment instruments are currently available that are useful in making diagnoses of tic disorders, including comprehensive self-report assessment tools, such as the *Tic Symptom Self Report* and the *Yale Global Tic Severity Scale,* administered by a clinician (Table 18-2).

In some studies, more than 25% of children with Tourette disorder received stimulants for a diagnosis of ADHD before receiving a diagnosis of Tourette disorder. The most frequent initial symptom is an eye-blink tic, followed by a head tic or a facial grimace. Most complex motor and vocal symptoms emerge several years after the initial symptoms. Coprolalia, a very unusual symptom involving shouting or speaking socially unacceptable or obscene words, occurs in less than 10% of patients and rarely in the absence of comorbid psychiatric disturbance. Mental coprolalia—in which a patient experiences a sudden, intrusive, socially unacceptable thought or obscene word—occurs more often than coprolalia. In severe cases, physical self-injury has occurred due to tic behaviors.

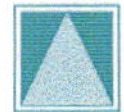

Table 18-1.
Comparative Diagnostic Criteria for Tourette Disorder

	DSM-5-TR	ICD-10	ICD-11
Diagnostic name	Tourette's disorder	Combined vocal and multiple motor tic disorder (de la Tourette)	Tourette syndrome
Duration	Despite waxing or waning, symptoms have been present for ≥1 year since the initial onset		≥1 year. Onset in developmental period.
Symptoms	Presence of both motor and vocal tics over the course of illness, with onset <age 18	Tic disorder involving multiple motor ticks and ≥1 more vocal tics; symptoms present in childhood or adolescence and tend to persist into adulthood	The presence of both motor tic(s) and phonic tic(s) that may or may not manifest concurrently or continuously during the symptomatic course. Motor and phonic tics are defined as sudden, rapid, nonrhythmic, and recurrent movements or vocalizations, respectively.
Exclusions	Other medical condition Substance or medication induced, including withdrawal		Another medical condition (e.g., Huntington disease) Substance or medication on (e.g., amphetamine), including withdrawal effects (e.g., from benzodiazepines)
Comments	If symptoms of ONLY motor OR vocal tics, the diagnosis would be "Persistent (Chronic) Motor or Vocal Tic Disorder"		

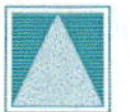

Table 18-2.
Clinical Assessment Tools in Tic Disorders

Domain	Type	Reliability and Validity	Sensitive to Change
Tics			
Tic Symptom Self-Report	Parent/self	Good	Yes
Yale Global Tic Severity Scale	Clinician	Excellent	Yes
Attention-Deficit/Hyperactivity Disorder			
Swanson, Nolan, and Pelham-IV	Parent/teacher	Excellent	Yes
Abbreviated Conners' Questionnaire	Parent/teacher	Excellent	Yes
Obsessive-Compulsive Disorder			
Yale–Brown Obsessive Compulsive Scale and Children's Yale–Brown Obsessive Compulsive Scale	Clinician	Excellent	Yes
National Institute of Mental Health Global Obsessive Compulsive Rating Scale	Clinician	Excellent	Yes
General			
Child Behavior Checklist	Parent/teacher	Excellent	No

Ezra, age 10 years, came to the Tic Disorder Clinic for an evaluation of motor tics in the head and neck, occasional coughing and grunting, and a new symptom of throat-clearing many times per day. Ezra had a history of attention-deficit/hyperactivity disorder (ADHD), which included significant hyperactivity and impulsive and oppositional behavior. He is a fifth-grade student in a regular class at the local public school. Ezra was barely passing several subjects in school, blurted things out in class, often argued with adults, and had few friends. His tics were moderate.

At age 5, due to his activity level and poor concentration, Ezra's pediatrician made a diagnosis of ADHD and recommended a trial of Concerta (methylphenidate extended-release tablets) at 36 mg/day, which he began in the first grade. Within a week of starting medication, Ezra's overly active and impulsive behavior showed a dramatic improvement; however, he remained argumentative and oppositional. In the spring of his first-grade year, however, Ezra began showing motor and phonic tics consisting of head-jerking, facial movements, coughing, and grunting. He discontinued the Concerta to see if this made a difference and, although the tics transiently decreased, they came back in full force within a month.

During his evaluation at the Tic Disorder Clinic, Ezra was a healthy child who was the product of an uncomplicated pregnancy, labor, and delivery, and whose developmental milestones were appropriate. Intellectual testing completed by the school psychologist revealed a full-scale IQ of 105. Ezra's mother noted that he has had longstanding trouble falling asleep but sleeps through the night. Ezra had always been described as argumentative and easily frustrated with frequent outbursts of temper; however, when he was not having a tantrum, his mood was generally upbeat.

Ezra had frequent vocal tics, including grunting, coughing, and noticeable throat clearing. Ezra denied depressed mood or suicidal ideation, although he reported distress about everyday issues such as being teased by peers, not having enough friends, and his poor school performance. Ezra denied recurring worries about contamination or harm coming to him or family members, or fears of acting on unwanted impulses. Other than mild touching habits involving the need to touch objects with each hand three times or in combinations of three, Ezra denied repetitive rituals. Several motor tics occurred during the evaluation session, including blinking, head-jerking, and shoulder tics. Ezra was restless and easily distracted throughout the session and often needed assistance with entertaining himself when not directly involved in the conversation.

Given the history of enduring motor and phonic tics, confirmed by direct observation, the diagnoses of Tourette disorder and ADHD were confirmed.

Ezra and his family met with the child and adolescent psychiatrist to learn about the waxing and waning nature of tic symptoms and the natural history of Tourette disorder. Ezra began seeing a behavioral psychologist specializing in habit reversal training. In this treatment, Ezra learned to engage in a behavior physically incompatible with his tic (a competing response) each time he experienced the urge to perform this tic. The competing response for Ezra's shoulder tic, which consisted of raising his shoulders as far as he could, was to gently press his shoulders down and extend his neck each time he felt the urge to engage in this tic. With repeated practice of his competing response, his urge to engage in this tic greatly diminished to the point where he was able to manage the urge without performing the tic. Ezra responded well to his behavioral therapy, and over 8 weeks, he had learned how to become aware of the urges that occurred before his tics and to replace his usual tics with less-distressing and less-disruptive behaviors. (Adapted from L. Scahill M.S.N., Ph.D. and JF Leckman, M.D.)

Pathology and Laboratory Examination

No specific laboratory diagnostic test exists for Tourette disorder, but many patients with Tourette disorder have nonspecific abnormal electroencephalogram (EEG) findings. Computed tomography (CT) and magnetic resonance imaging (MRI) scans have revealed no specific structural lesions, although about 10% of all patients with Tourette's disorder show some nonspecific abnormality on CT scans.

Differential Diagnosis

We should differentiate tics from other movements and movement disorders (e.g., dystonic, choreiform, athetoid, myoclonic, and hemiballismic movements) and the neurologic diseases that they may characterize (e.g., Huntington disease, parkinsonism, Sydenham chorea, and Wilson disease), as listed in Table 18-3. We should also distinguish tremors, mannerisms, and stereotypic movement disorder (e.g., head-banging or body-rocking) from tic disorders. Stereotypic movement disorders, including movements such as rocking, hand-gazing, and other self-stimulatory behaviors, seem to be voluntary and often produce a sense of comfort, in contrast to tic disorders. Although tics in children and adolescents may or may not feel controllable, they rarely produce a sense of well-being. Compulsions are sometimes difficult to distinguish from complex tics and may be on the same continuum biologically. Tic disorders may also occur comorbidly with mood disturbances. In a recent survey, the greater the severity of tics, the higher the probability of both aggressive and depressive symptoms in children. When a child experiences an exacerbation of tic symptoms, behavior and mood also seem to deteriorate.

Course and Prognosis

Tourette disorder is a childhood-onset neuropsychiatric disorder characterized by both motor and vocal tics, which usually emerge in early childhood, with a natural history leading to reduction or complete resolution of tics symptoms in many cases by adolescence or early adulthood. During childhood, individual tic symptoms may decrease, persist, or increase, and new symptoms may replace old ones. Impairment may be associated with the motor and vocal tic symptoms of Tourette disorder; however, in some cases, interference in function is exacerbated by comorbid ADHD and OCD, both of which frequently coexist with the disorder. Although many children with Tourette disorder will experience a decline in the frequency and severity of tic symptoms during adolescence, at present no clinical measures exist

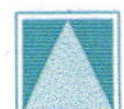

Table 18-3.
Differential Diagnosis of Tic Disorders

Disease or Syndrome	Age at Onset	Associated Features	Course	Predominant Type of Movement
Hallervorden–Spatz	Childhood–adolescence	May be associated with optic atrophy, club feet, retinitis pigmentosa, dysarthria, dementia, ataxia, emotional lability, spasticity, autosomal recessive inheritance	Progressive to death in 5–20 yr	Choreic, athetoid, myoclonic
Dystonia musculorum deformans	Childhood–adolescence	Autosomal recessive inheritance commonly, primarily among Ashkenazi Jews; a more benign autosomal dominant form also occurs	Variable course, often progressive but with rare remissions	Dystonia
Sydenham chorea	Childhood, usually 5–15 yr	More common in females, usually associated with rheumatic fever (carditis elevated ASO titers)	Usually self-limited	Choreiform
Huntington disease	Usually 30–50 yr but childhood forms are known	Autosomal dominant inheritance, dementia, caudate atrophy on CT scan	Progressive to death in 10–15 yr after onset	Choreiform
Wilson disease (hepatolenticular degeneration)	Usually 10–25 yr	Kayser–Fleischer rings, liver dysfunction, inborn error of copper metabolism; autosomal recessive inheritance	Progressive to death without chelating therapy	Wing-beating tremor, dystonia
Hyperreflexias (including latah, myriachit, Jumping Frenchman of Maine)	Generally, in childhood (dominant inheritance)	Familial; may have generalized rigidity and autosomal inheritance	Nonprogressive	Excessive startle response; may have echolalia, coprolalia, and forced obedience

(*continued*)

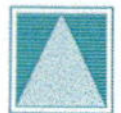

Table 18-3.
Differential Diagnosis of Tic Disorders (Continued)

Disease or Syndrome	Age at Onset	Associated Features	Course	Predominant Type of Movement
Myoclonic disorders	Any age	Numerous causes, some familial, usually no vocalizations	Variable, depending on cause	Myoclonus
Myoclonic dystonia	5–47 yr	Nonfamilial, no vocalizations	Nonprogressive	Torsion dystonia with myoclonic jerks
Paroxysmal myoclonic dystonia with vocalization	Childhood	Attention, hyperactive, and learning disorders; movements interfere with ongoing activity	Nonprogressive	Bursts of regular, repetitive clonic (less tonic) movements and vocalizations
Tardive Tourette syndrome	Variable (after antipsychotic medication use)	Reported to be precipitated by discontinuation or reduction of medication	May terminate after increase or decrease of dosage	Orofacial dyskinesias, choreoathetosis, tics, vocalization
Neuroacanthocytosis	Third or fourth decade	Acanthocytosis, muscle wasting, parkinsonism, autosomal recessive inheritance	Variable	Orofacial dyskinesia and limb chorea, tics, vocalization
Encephalitis lethargica	Variable	Shouting fits, bizarre behavior, psychosis, Parkinson disease	Variable	Simple and complex motor and vocal tics, coprolalia, echolalia, echopraxia, palilalia
Gasoline inhalation	Variable	Abnormal EEG; symmetrical theta and theta bursts frontocentrally	Variable	Simple motor and vocal tics
Postangiographic complications	Variable	Emotional lability, amnestic syndrome	Variable	Simple motor and complex vocal tics, palilalia
Postinfectious	Variable	EEG: occasional asymmetrical theta bursts before movements, elevated ASO titers	Variable	Simple motor and vocal tics, echopraxia
Posttraumatic	Variable	Asymmetrical tic distribution	Variable	Complex motor tics
Carbon monoxide poisoning	Variable	Inappropriate sexual behavior	Variable	Simple and complex motor and vocal tics, coprolalia, echolalia, palilalia
XYY genetic disorder	Infancy	Aggressive behavior	Static	Simple motor and vocal tics
XXY and 9_p mosaicism	Infancy	Multiple physical anomalies, mental retardation	Static	Simple motor and vocal tics
Duchenne muscular dystrophy (X-linked recessive)	Childhood	Mild intellectual disability	Progressive	Motor and vocal tics
Fragile X syndrome	Childhood	Intellectual disability, facial dysmorphism, seizures, autistic features	Static	Simple motor and vocal tics, coprolalia
Developmental and perinatal disorders	Infancy, childhood	Seizures, EEG and CT abnormalities, psychosis, aggressivity, hyperactivity, Ganser syndrome, compulsivity, torticollis	Variable	Motor and vocal tics, echolalia

ASLO, antistreptolysin O; CT, computed tomography; EEG, electroencephalogram.

to predict which children may have persistent symptoms into adulthood. Children with mild forms of Tourette disorder often have satisfactory peer relationships, function well in school, and develop adequate self-esteem, and may not require treatment.

Treatment

Psychoeducation is a useful intervention in order for families to gain an understanding of the variability of tics, the natural history of the disorder, and ways to support stress reduction. Families need to be well-informed advocates for their children since it is easy to misinterpret tics as a child's purposeful misbehavior, rather than a response to an irresistible urge. The subjective distress of the child and the functional disruptions caused by the disorder argue for active treatment. In mild cases, children with tic disorders who are functioning well socially and academically may not seek, nor require treatment. In more severe cases, peers may ostracize children with tic disorders, and the tics can disrupt academic work. We should consider a variety of interventions, including psychosocial, pharmacologic, and school-based. A scale to measure tic severity, the *Premonitory Urge for Tics Scale* (PUTS), is internally consistent and correlates with overall tic severity in youths over 10 years of age.

The European clinical guidelines for Tourette disorder and other tic disorders recommends that both behavioral and pharmacologic interventions be considered in more severe cases, with behavioral interventions typically the first line of treatment. Tics require treatment when they cause social and emotional problems, depression, or isolation. Children who are prone to severe persistent complex motor tics or loud vocal tics may be the objects of bullying and social rejection. Tic reduction in school may help preserve healthy social relationships and diminish depressive and anxiety symptoms. Tics may also lead to impairment in academic achievement. School difficulties in children with Tourette disorder are not uncommon, and reduction in tics may support increased academic success. Tics may also lead to physical discomfort, based on the repetitive musculoskeletal exertion, especially concerning head and neck tics. In some children with Tourette disorder, tics can worsen headaches and migraines. Behavioral and pharmacologic interventions can both target tic reductions, which can lead to improved quality of life.

Evidence-Based Behavioral and Psychosocial Treatment. The Canadian guidelines for the evidence-based treatment of tic disorders: behavioral therapy, deep brain stimulation and transcranial magnetic stimulation, and a large multi-site RCT of "Comprehensive Behavioral Intervention for Tics" (CBIT) both found converging evidence supporting *habit-reversal training* and *exposure and response prevention* as efficacious treatments for tic reduction. In an RCT of CBIT, 61 children received habit reversal training as their main component of treatment, and they also received relaxation treatment and a functional intervention to identify situations that worsened or sustained tics and strategies to decrease exposure to these situations. The control group of 65 children received supportive psychotherapy and psychoeducation. After 10 weeks of treatment, the intervention group had a significantly reduced Yale Global Tic Severity Scale Total Tic Score compared with the control group.

HABIT REVERSAL. The primary components of habit reversal are awareness training, in which the child uses self-monitoring to enhance awareness of tic behaviors and the premonitory urges or sensations, indicating that a tic is about to occur. In competing-response training, the patient learns to voluntarily perform a behavior that is physically incompatible with the tic, contingent on the onset of the premonitory urge or the tic itself, blocking expression of the tic. The competing-response strategy relies on the self-reported observations of patients that tics occur in response to irresistible premonitory urges in order to diminish the urge. Performing the tic satisfies or reduces the premonitory urges, thus reinforcing the tics, and over time they become repeated entrenched behaviors. Competing-response training is different from voluntary tic suppression in that the patient initiates a voluntary behavior to manage the premonitory urge and thus disrupts the reinforcement of the tic, rather than merely trying to suppress the tic. Successful competing-response training significantly reduces the premonitory urge and can decrease or eliminate the urge. For motor tics, the patient may choose a less noticeable behavior, whereas for vocal tics, slow rhythmic breathing is the most common voluntary competing response. Patients can perform competing responses without disrupting usual activities.

EXPOSURE AND RESPONSE PREVENTION. The rationale for this treatment relies on the notion that tics occur as a conditioned response to unpleasant premonitory urges, and since the tics reduce the urge, they become associated with the premonitory urge. Each time the tic reduces the urge, this strengthens the association. Rather than using competing responses, as in habit-reversal training, exposure and response prevention asks the patient to suppress tics for increasingly prolonged periods in order to break the association between the urges and the tics. Theoretically, if a patient learns to resist performing the tic in response to the urge for long enough periods, the urge may become more tolerable, or attenuate, and the need to perform the tic may diminish.

Many other behavioral interventions, such as relaxation training, self-monitoring, bio (neuro) feedback, and cognitive-behavioral treatment (CBT), are not useful for reducing tics on their own. However, it may help to include some of these strategies in comprehensive treatment programs for children with tic disorders who are receiving habit-reversal training. Habit reversal has been the most extensively researched behavioral treatment for tic disorders; it is highly effective and is currently the first-line behavioral treatment for tic disorders.

Evidence-Based Pharmacotherapy. Several reviews of pharmacologic treatments for tics suggest that the following classes of pharmacologic agents have an evidence base for treating tics: typical and atypical antipsychotics; noradrenergic agents; and alternative treatments such as tetrabenazine, topiramate, and tetrahydrocannabinol (THC).

ATYPICAL AND TYPICAL ANTIPSYCHOTIC AGENTS. Risperidone, with its high affinity for dopamine D_2 and serotonin 5-HT_2 receptors, is the most well-studied atypical antipsychotic in the treatment of tics. There is considerable evidence for its efficacy. Multiple randomized, controlled studies in children and adolescents have shown favorable results compared to placebo as well as in head-to-head studies with the typical antipsychotics haloperidol and pimozide. Risperidone was associated with fewer adverse events compared to typical antipsychotics; however, it can cause weight gain, metabolic side effects, and hyperprolactinemia. In a randomized, double-blind, parallel-group study of Tourette disorder comparing risperidone to pimozide, risperidone showed superiority in reducing comorbid obsessive-compulsive symptoms as well as reducing tics. In other randomized clinical trials, risperidone reduced tics in children, adolescents, and adults with mean daily doses of 2.5 mg with a range of 1 to 6 mg.

Haloperidol and pimozide are the two most well-investigated and FDA-approved antipsychotic agents in the treatment of Tourette disorder. However, atypical antipsychotics such as risperidone are often first-line agents due to their safer side-effect profiles. Both haloperidol and pimozide are efficacious in multiple randomized clinical trials in the treatment of Tourette disorder. Both haloperidol and pimozide present significant risks for extrapyramidal side effects; in a long-term naturalistic follow up study, haloperidol produces more significant acute dyskinesia and dystonia compared to pimozide.

Risperidone and pimozide had equal efficacy in one study of children, adolescents, and adults with Tourette disorder.

Aripiprazole has become a pharmacologic agent of interest in the treatment of tic disorders due to its mode of action; in addition to its D_2 receptor antagonistic actions, aripiprazole is also a partial D_2 and 5-HT_{1A} receptor agonist and a 5-HT_{2A} antagonist. A multisite double-blind controlled study of aripiprazole in children with Tourette disorder in China found a reduction in tic behaviors in about 60% of the aripiprazole group compared to about 64% reduction in a group treated with tiapride, a benzamide with selective D_2 receptor antagonism. There was no significant difference between the two groups. Although sedation and sleep disturbance are common side effects with aripiprazole, weight gain is less pronounced than with risperidone.

Olanzapine and ziprasidone are also efficacious in the treatment of tic disorders in at least one RCT. Sedation and weight gain were prominent side effects with olanzapine, and potential QT prolongation was an issue with ziprasidone. Quetiapine is a potentially useful agent in the treatment of tics, with its higher affinity for 5-HT_2 receptors than for D_2 receptors. However, randomized clinical trials are needed. Clozapine, contrary to many other atypical antipsychotics, is not useful in the treatment of tics.

NORADRENERGIC AGENTS. Noradrenergic agents, including clonidine and guanfacine, as well as atomoxetine, are frequently used in children as primary treatments or adjunctive treatments for comorbid ADHD and tics. Several studies have provided moderate evidence for the efficacy of clonidine, an α_2-adrenergic agent, in the treatment of tics in children, adolescents, and adults with tic disorders. The largest randomized trial with oral clonidine compared to placebo found a modest reduction in tics with clonidine. A multisite randomized, double-blind placebo-controlled trial using the clonidine patch in the treatment of tic disorders in children found a significant improvement in tic symptoms (about 69%) compared to about 47% of the children in the control group. The usual dose range for clonidine is from 0.05 mg orally three times daily to 0.1 mg four times daily, and for guanfacine, it is from 1 to 4 mg/day. When used in these dosage ranges, adverse effects of the α-adrenergic agents may include drowsiness, headache, irritability, and occasional hypotension.

Guanfacine has been used by clinicians, however it's efficacy regarding reducing tics is controversial. In one randomized clinical trial treating 34 children with ADHD and tics, guanfacine was superior to placebo in the reduction of tics. In another double-blind placebo-controlled trial of 24 children with Tourette disorder, guanfacine was not superior to placebo.

Atomoxetine, a selective norepinephrine reuptake inhibitor, was found to reduce both tics and ADHD symptoms in a multicenter industry trial of 148 children. Atomoxetine also reduced both tics and ADHD in a subgroup of patients in this study who had Tourette disorder. Additional studies are needed to confirm the safety and efficacy of atomoxetine in the treatment of children with Tourette disorder.

Given the frequent comorbidity of tic behaviors and obsessive-compulsive symptoms or disorders, the SSRIs have been used alone or in combination with antipsychotics in the treatment of Tourette disorder. They seem to be useful; however, there have not been controlled trials yet to determine the effect of SSRIs on tic reduction.

Data suggest that methylphenidate, in most cases, does not increase the rate or intensity of motor or vocal tics in most children with hyperactivity and tic disorders.

ALTERNATIVE AGENTS: TETRABENAZINE, TOPIRAMATE, AND TETRAHYDROCANNABINOL

Tetrabenazine. A vesicular monoamine transporter type 2 inhibitor, tetrabenazine depletes presynaptic dopamine and serotonin and blocks postsynaptic dopamine receptors. There are no randomized clinical trials of this agent in the treatment of Tourette disorder in children; however, clinical experience suggests that this agent may have benefit in tic reduction. In a follow-up of 2 years of treatment in 77 children and adolescents, one study reports tic reduction improvement in 80% of subjects. Side effects of this agent include sedation, parkinsonism, depression, insomnia, anxiety, and akathisia.

Topiramate. A GABAergic drug, used primarily as an anticonvulsant, topiramate, was effective for reducing tics in a small randomized clinical trial of children and adults with Tourette disorder. Side effects were minimal. Although this does not confirm its efficacy, GABA-modulating agents deserve further study in the treatment of tic disorders.

Tetrahydrocannabinol. A small, randomized trial suggested that THC may be safe and efficacious in the treatment of tics without neuropsychological impairment. In this trial, reported adverse effects included dizziness, fatigue, and dry mouth. Potential additional side effects include anxiety, depressive symptoms, tremor, and insomnia. This small trial does not confirm efficacy for this agent in the treatment of tics. Instead, it raises questions about the potential improvements in treatment-resistant tic disorders using this agent.

Epidemiology

The estimated prevalence of Tourette disorder ranges from 3 to 8 per 1,000 school-age children. Males are affected between two and four times more often than females. The unique features of Tourette disorder, in which tics wax and wane and may change in character, frequency, and severity over relatively short periods, have made ascertainment of its prevalence challenging. Furthermore, remission of tics is particularly age-dependent in that tics tend to emerge and increase from ages 5 to 10 years of age, and in many cases, decrease in frequency and severity after the age of 10 to 12 years. At age 13 years, however, using stringent criteria, the prevalence rate for Tourette disorder drops to 0.3%. The lifetime prevalence of Tourette disorder is estimated to be approximately 1%.

Etiology

Genetic Factors. Twin studies, adoption studies, and segregation analysis studies all support a genetic basis, albeit a complex one, for Tourette disorder. Twin studies indicate that concordance for the disorder in monozygotic twins is significantly higher than that in dizygotic twins. Tourette disorder and chronic motor or vocal tic disorder are likely to occur in the same families; this lends support to the view that the disorders are part of a genetically determined spectrum. The sons of mothers with Tourette disorder seem to be at the highest risk for the disorder. Evidence in some families suggests an autosomal dominant transmission for Tourette disorder. Tourette disorder appears to be inherited through an autosomal pattern in some families, intermediate between dominant and recessive. A study of 174 unrelated probands with Tourette disorder identified a higher than chance occurrence of a rare sequence variant in SLITRK1, believed to be a candidate gene on chromosome 13q31.

Up to half of all patients with Tourette disorder also have ADHD, and up to 40% of those with Tourette disorder also have OCD. These frequent comorbidities with Tourette disorder can lead to a plethora of overlapping symptoms. Family studies have provided compelling evidence for the association between tic disorders and OCD. First-degree relatives of persons with Tourette disorder are at high risk for the development of Tourette disorder, chronic motor or vocal tic disorder, and OCD.

Neuroimaging Studies. A functional (fMRI) study of brain activity 2 seconds before and after a tic found that paralimbic and sensory association areas were involved. Furthermore, evidence suggests that voluntary tic suppression involves deactivation of the putamen and globus pallidus, along with partial activation of regions of the prefrontal cortex and caudate nucleus. Compelling, but indirect, evidence of dopamine system involvement in tic disorders includes the observations that pharmacologic agents that antagonize dopamine (haloperidol, pimozide, and fluphenazine) suppress tics and those agents that increase central dopaminergic activity (methylphenidate, amphetamines, and cocaine) tend to exacerbate tics. The relation of tics to neurotransmitter systems is complex and not yet well understood; for example, in some cases, antipsychotic medications, such as haloperidol, are not effective in reducing tics, and the effect of stimulants on tic disorders reportedly varies. In some cases, Tourette disorder has emerged during treatment with antipsychotic medications.

More direct analyses of the neurochemistry of Tourette disorder have been possible utilizing brain proton magnetic resonance spectroscopy (MRS). Neuroimaging studies using cerebral blood flow in PET and SPECT suggest that alterations of activity may occur in various brain regions in patients with Tourette disorder compared to controls, including the frontal and orbital cortex, striatum, and putamen.

Immunologic Factors and Postinfection. An autoimmune process and, in particular, one that is secondary to group A β-hemolytic streptococcal infection, has been hypothesized as a potential mechanism for the development of tics and obsessive-compulsive symptoms in some cases. Data have been conflicting and controversial, and this mechanism appears to be unlikely as an etiology of Tourette disorder in most cases. One case-control study found little evidence of the development or exacerbation of tics, or obsessions or compulsions, in children with well-documented and treated group A β-hemolytic streptococcal infections.

PERSISTENT (CHRONIC) MOTOR OR VOCAL TIC DISORDER

Chronic motor or vocal tic disorder is defined as the presence of either motor tics or vocal tics, but not both. Tics may wax and wane but must have persisted for more than 1 year since the first tic onset to meet the diagnosis for persistent (chronic) motor or vocal tic disorder. According to DSM-5-TR, this disorder must have its onset before the age of 18 years. We would not diagnose chronic motor or vocal tic disorder if the patient already has Tourette disorder.

Diagnosis and Clinical Features

The onset of chronic motor or vocal tic disorder typically occurs in early childhood. Chronic vocal tics are considerably rarer than chronic motor tics. Chronic vocal tics, in the absence of motor tics, are typically less conspicuous than the vocal tics in Tourette disorder. The vocal tics are usually not loud or intense and are not mainly from the vocal cords; they consist of grunts or other noises caused by thoracic, abdominal, or diaphragmatic contractions. Table 18-4 shows comparative diagnostic criteria for persistent (chronic) tic disorder in the DSM-5-TR, ICD-10, and ICD-11.

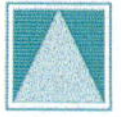

Table 18-4.
Comparative Diagnostic Criteria for Persistent (Chronic) Tic Disorder

	DSM-5-TR	ICD-10	ICD-11
Diagnostic name	Persistent (Chronic) Motor or Vocal Tic Disorder	Tic Disorder	• Chronic Motor Tic Disorder • Chronic Phonic Tic Disorder
Duration	Despite waxing or waning, symptoms have been present >1 yr since the initial onset		≥1 yr
Symptoms	Presence of either motor or vocal tics over the course of illness, but not both. Onset before the age of 18	Presence of a tic, defined as an involuntary, fast, repeated and nonrhythmic motor movement or vocal production that is sudden and seemingly purposeless. Such tics are experienced as urges that are strong, but that can be suppressed variably	Motor and vocal tics are defined as sudden, rapid, nonrhythmic, and recurrent movements or vocalizations, respectively
Exclusions	Other medical condition Substance or medication-induced, including withdrawal		
Course specifiers		Transient tic disorder (lasting <12 mo) Chronic motor or vocal tic disorder (lasting longer than a year)	
Severity specifiers			
Comments	If symptoms are less than 1 yr, the diagnosis would be **Provisional Tic Disorder** **Other Specified Tic Disorder** is reserved for cases in which symptoms do not meet full criteria, and the clinician chooses not to specify reasons for the disorder, or there is insufficient information	Chronic motor or vocal tic disorder (lasting longer than a year)	

Differential Diagnosis

We should differentiate chronic motor tics from a variety of other motor movements, including choreiform movements, myoclonus, restless legs syndrome, akathisia, and dystonias. Involuntary vocal utterances can occur in certain neurologic disorders, such as Huntington disease and Parkinson disease.

Course and Prognosis

Children whose tics emerge between the ages of 6 and 8 years seem to have the best outcomes. Symptoms often last for 4 to 6 years and remit in early adolescence. Children whose tics involve the limbs or trunk may have less prompt remission than those with only facial tics.

Treatment

The treatment of chronic motor or vocal tic disorder depends on several factors, including the severity and frequency of the tics; the patient's subjective distress; the effects of the tics on school or work, job performance, and socialization; and the presence of any other concomitant mental disorder. Psychotherapy may help minimize the secondary social difficulties caused by severe tics. Behavioral techniques, particularly habit reversal treatments, are effective in treating chronic motor or vocal tic disorder. When severe, atypical antipsychotics such as risperidone may reduce the tics. If not effective, typical antipsychotics such as pimozide or haloperidol may be helpful. Behavioral interventions are the first line of treatment.

Epidemiology

The rate of chronic motor or vocal tic disorder is 100 to 1,000 times greater than that of Tourette disorder in school-age children. School-age boys are at the highest risk. The estimated prevalence of chronic motor or vocal tic disorder is from 1% to 2%.

Etiology

Chronic motor or vocal tic disorder, as well as Tourette disorder, tend to aggregate in the same families. Twin studies have found a high concordance for either Tourette disorder or chronic motor tics in monozygotic twins. This finding supports the importance of hereditary factors in the transmission of tic disorders.

Further Readings

Andrén P, Jakubovski E, Murphy TL, et al. European clinical guidelines for Tourette syndrome and other tic disorders-version 2.0. Part II: psychological interventions. *Eur Child Adolesc Psychiatry*. 2022;31(3):403–423.

Andrén P, Wachtmeister V, Franzé J, et al. Effectiveness of behaviour therapy for children and adolescents with Tourette syndrome and chronic tic disorder in a naturalistic setting. *Child Psychiatry Hum Dev*. 2021;52(4):739–750.

Coffey B, Jankovic J, Claassen DO, et al. Efficacy and safety of fixed-dose deutetrabenazine in children and adolescents for tics associated with Tourette syndrome: a randomized clinical trial. *JAMA Netw Open*. 2021;4(10):e2129397.

Essoe JK, Grados MA, Singer HS, Myers NS, McGuire JF. Evidence-based treatment of Tourette's disorder and chronic tic disorders. *Expert Rev Neurother*. 2019;19(11):1103–1115.

Farhat LC, Behling E, Landeros-Weisenberger A, et al. Comparative efficacy, tolerability, and acceptability of pharmacological interventions for the treatment of children, adolescents, and young adults with Tourette's syndrome: a systematic review and network meta-analysis. *Lancet Child Adolesc Health*. 2023;7(2):112–126.

Garcia-Delgar B, Servera M, Coffey BJ, et al; EMTICS collaborative group. Tic disorders in children and adolescents: does the clinical presentation differ in males and females? A report by the EMTICS group. *Eur Child Adolesc Psychiatry*. 2022;31(10):1539–1548.

Giedinghagen A. The tic in TikTok and (where) all systems go: Mass social media induced illness and Munchausen's by internet as explanatory models for social media associated abnormal illness behavior. *Clin Child Psychol Psychiatry*. 2023;28(1):270–278.

Han VX, Kozlowska K, Kothur K, et al. Rapid onset functional tic-like behaviours in children and adolescents during COVID-19: Clinical features, assessment and biopsychosocial treatment approach. *J Paediatr Child Health*. 2022;58(7):1181–1187.

Jiang J, Chen M, Huang H, Chen Y. The aetiology of Tourette syndrome and chronic tic disorder in children and adolescents: a comprehensive systematic review of case-control studies. *Brain Sci*. 2022;12(9):1202.

Mataix-Cols D, Isomura K, Brander G, et al. Early-life and family risk factors for tic disorder persistence into adulthood. *Mov Disord*. 2023;38(8):1419–1427.

Müller-Vahl KR, Szejko N, Verdellen C, et al. European clinical guidelines for Tourette syndrome and other tic disorders: summary statement. *Eur Child Adolesc Psychiatry*. 2022;31(3):377–382.

Nissen JB, Carlsen AH, Thomsen PH. One-year outcome of manualised behavior therapy of chronic tic disorders in children and adolescents. *Child Adolesc Psychiatry Ment Health*. 2021;15(1):9.

Openneer TJC, Huyser C, Martino D, Schrag A; EMTICS Collaborative Group; Hoekstra PJ, Dietrich A. Clinical precursors of tics: an EMTICS study. *J Child Psychol Psychiatry*. 2022;63(3):305–314.

Pringsheim T, Ganos C, Nilles C, et al. European Society for the Study of Tourette Syndrome 2022 criteria for clinical diagnosis of functional tic-like behaviours: international consensus from experts in tic disorders. *Eur J Neurol*. 2023;30(4):902–910.

Ricketts EJ, Woods DW, Espil FM, et al. Childhood predictors of long-term tic severity and tic impairment in Tourette's disorder. *Behav Ther*. 2022;53(6):1250–1264.

Roessner V, Eichele H, Stern JS, et al. European clinical guidelines for Tourette syndrome and other tic disorders-version 2.0. Part III: pharmacological treatment. *Eur Child Adolesc Psychiatry*. 2022;31(3):425–441.

Tan CY, Chiu NC, Zeng YH, et al. Psychosocial stress in children with Tourette syndrome and chronic tic disorder. *Pediatr Neonatol*. 2024; 65(4):336–340.

Wattanarojjanakit P, Chuthapisith J, Khongkhatithum C. Anxiety and parenting style in children and adolescents with tic disorders. *Pediatr Neurol*. 2023;146:139–143.

Zinna S, Luxton R, Papachristou E, Dima D, Kyriakopoulos M. Comorbid chronic tic disorder and Tourette syndrome in children requiring inpatient mental health treatment. *Clin Child Psychol Psychiatry*. 2021;26(3):894–905.

19

Elimination Disorders

INTRODUCTION

Mastering control over bowel and bladder function is a complex developmental milestone that involves motor and sensory functions, coordinated through frontal lobe activities and regulated by neurons in the pons and midbrain area. It develops gradually in a toddler over several months. Infants generally void small volumes of urine approximately every hour, commonly stimulated by feeding, and may have incomplete bladder emptying. As the infant matures into a toddler, bladder capacity increases, and between 1 and 3 years of age, cortical inhibitory pathways develop that allow the child to have voluntary control over reflexes that control the bladder muscles. The ability to have muscular control over the bowel usually occurs before bladder control. The typical sequence is the development of nocturnal fecal continence, diurnal fecal continence, diurnal bladder control, and nocturnal bladder control. Toilet training is affected by many factors, including intellectual capacity, social maturity, cultural determinants, and the psychological interactions between the child and parents. It relies on maturing neurobiologic systems, so children with developmental delays may display delayed bowel and bladder continence. When children regularly exhibit incontinence, it troubles both the children and their families and may be misunderstood as voluntary misbehavior.

Encopresis (repeated passage of feces into inappropriate places) and enuresis (repeated urination into bed or clothes) are the two elimination disorders described in DSM-5-TR. ICD-10 contains the diagnoses of nonorganic encopresis and enuresis, categorized among the "other behavioral and emotional disorders with onset usually occurring in childhood and adolescence." ICD-11 uses the terms encopresis and enuresis and contains criteria similar to DSM-5-TR. We should not make these diagnoses until age of 4 years for encopresis and after age of 5 years for enuresis, the ages at which a typically developing child masters these skills. Healthy development encompasses a range of time in which a child can devote the attention, motivation, and physiologic skills to exhibit competency in elimination processes.

ENCOPRESIS

Clinical and Diagnostic Features

According to both DSM-5-TR and ICD-10 and 11, encopresis occurs when a child passes feces into inappropriate places regularly. Table 19-1 compares the diagnostic approaches for encopresis. Encopresis may be present in children who have bowel control and intentionally deposit feces in their clothes or other places for a variety of emotional reasons. Anecdotal reports have suggested that occasionally, encopresis is an expression of anger or rage toward a punitive or hostile parent. The inappropriate repetitive behavior elicits attention (albeit negative), and breaking this behavioral pattern is difficult. In other children, encopresis can occur during stress—for example, the birth of a new sibling—but in such cases, the behavior is usually transient.

Encopresis can also be present on an involuntary basis in the absence of physiologic abnormalities. In these cases, a child may not exhibit adequate control over the sphincter muscles, either because they are absorbed in another activity or unaware of the process. The feces may be of normal, near-normal, or liquid consistency. Some involuntary soiling occurs from the chronic retaining of stool, which may result in a liquid overflow. In rare cases, the involuntary overflow of stool results from psychological causes of diarrhea or anxiety disorder symptoms. DSM-5-TR includes specifiers to indicate whether or not the disorder consists of constipation and overflow incontinence.

Studies have indicated that children with encopresis who do not have gastrointestinal illnesses have high rates of abnormal anal sphincter contractions. This finding is particularly prevalent among children with encopresis with constipation and overflow incontinence who have difficulty relaxing their anal sphincter muscles when trying to defecate. Children with constipation who have problems with sphincter relaxation are not likely to respond well to laxatives in the treatment of their encopresis. Children with encopresis without abnormal sphincter tone will likely improve relatively quickly.

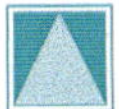

Table 19-1. Encopresis

	DSM-5-TR	ICD-10	ICD-11
Diagnostic name	Encopresis	Nonorganic Encopresis	Encopresis
Duration	≥1/mo for ≥3 consecutive months		≥1/mo for several months
Symptoms	Passing stool into clothes or onto the floor	A pattern of voluntarily or involuntarily passing feces in places that are inappropriate within the sociocultural context	Repeated and persistent passage of feces in inappropriate places Inappropriate for developmental age (4)
Exclusions	Age <4 Substance use Another medical condition other than ones causing constipation	Organic causes of encopresis	Other medical condition Substance or medication, including withdrawal
Severity specifiers	With constipation and overflow incontinence Without constipation and overflow incontinence		With constipation and overflow incontinence Without constipation and overflow incontinence

Jimmy is a 6-year-old boy with encopresis, nocturnal enuresis, insomnia, and nightmares. He was placed with his current foster family at age 3 years after being removed from his biologic family due to physical abuse and severe neglect. He had been exposed to methamphetamine and alcohol in utero. When he arrived at his foster home, Jimmy spoke only a few words, did not eat solid food, and wore diapers. He had little interest in learning toilet skills and was unconcerned about being in wet or soiled diapers. He would often smear and play with his feces at night when he couldn't sleep.

Over the past 3 years, Jimmy had learned to use the toilet but was inconsistent in using it without his caregivers' coaching. He had been diagnosed with autism spectrum disorder and was a client of the Regional Center. He was able to converse verbally, but echolalic phrases and poor prosody were evident in his language. Jimmy had learned to eat solid food, but was very picky and would mainly eat chicken nuggets. He resisted using the bathroom in his special education class and would often return home with soiled underwear, which he would routinely hide in his closet. Jimmy's pediatrician examined him and determined that he had chronic constipation. He started a treatment program of polyethylene glycol every morning with a behavioral component of sitting on the toilet for 10 minutes after every meal. After a week, Jimmy succeeded in having a bowel movement in the toilet. Jimmy was given a small reward for trying to have a bowel movement in the toilet each time he tried. In a few weeks, Jimmy began to initiate sitting on the toilet after meals, and his bowel function began to normalize.

Pathology and Laboratory Examination

There are no specific tests for encopresis, and testing is mainly to rule out medical illnesses, such as Hirschsprung disease. The physician should perform an abdominal examination to help determine whether fecal retention is responsible for encopresis with constipation and overflow incontinence, and an abdominal x-ray can help determine the degree of constipation present. Tests to assess whether sphincter tone is abnormal are generally not conducted in uncomplicated cases of encopresis.

Differential Diagnosis

In encopresis with constipation and overflow incontinence, constipation can begin as early as the child's first year and can peak between the second and fourth years. Soiling usually starts by age 4. There are frequent liquid stools and hard fecal masses in the colon and the rectum on abdominal palpation and rectal examination. Complications include impaction, megacolon, and anal fissures.

Aganglionic megacolon or Hirschsprung disease is a significant differential, in which a patient may have an empty rectum and no desire to defecate but may still have an overflow of feces. The disorder occurs in 1 in 5,000 children; signs appear shortly after birth. Faulty nutrition is rarely the cause of encopresis with constipation and overflow incontinence. Other conditions are rare as well, including structural disease of the anus, rectum, and colon, adverse drug effects, or nongastrointestinal medical (endocrine or neurologic) disorders.

Course and Prognosis

The outcome of encopresis depends on the etiology, the chronicity of the symptoms, and coexisting behavioral problems. Encopresis is sometimes self-limiting and rarely continues beyond middle adolescence. Encopresis in children who have associated physiologic factors, such as poor gastric motility and an inability to relax the anal sphincter muscles, is more challenging to treat than that in those with constipation but normal sphincter tone.

Encopresis is a particularly objectionable disorder to family members, who may assume that the behavior is due to "laziness," and family tensions are often high. Peers are intolerant of developmentally inappropriate behavior and typically taunt a child with encopresis. Many affected children have abysmally low self-esteem and feel constant social rejection. Psychologically, a child may appear blunted toward the symptoms or, less frequently, may be entrenched in a pattern of encopresis to express anger. The outcome of encopresis is influenced by a family's willingness and ability to participate in treatment without being overly punitive and by the child's ability and motivation to engage in treatment.

Treatment

A typical treatment plan for a child with encopresis includes daily oral administration of laxatives such as polyethylene glycol (PEG) at 1 g/kg per day and often a surgical disimpaction under general anesthesia before administering maintenance laxatives. Also, help is a cognitive-behavioral intervention to help the child begin regular attempts to have bowel movements in the toilet and to diminish anxiety related to bowel movements. Laxatives are not necessary for children who are not constipated and do have reasonable bowel control, but regular timed intervals on the toilet may be helpful with these children as well.

Often, there is considerable family discord and distress, and it is crucial to reduce family tensions about the symptoms and establish a nonpunitive atmosphere. Similarly, we should help to reduce the child's embarrassment at school. A treatment plan may include arranging for many changes of underwear with minimal embarrassment. The education of the family and correcting of misperceptions that a family may have must occur before treatment.

Research supports the use of interactive parent–child family guidance interventions based on psychological and behavioral interventions for children younger than age 9 years.

Supportive psychotherapy and relaxation techniques may help treat the anxieties and other sequelae of children with encopresis, such as low self-esteem and social isolation. Family interventions can be helpful for children who have bowel control but who continue to deposit their feces in inappropriate locations. An optimal outcome occurs when a child feels control over their bowel function.

Epidemiology

Encopresis affects about 3% of 4-year-olds and 1.6% of 10-year-old children. Incidence rates for encopretic behavior decrease drastically with increasing age. Between the ages of 10 and 12 years, it affects about 0.75% of typically developing children. Globally, the community prevalence of encopresis ranges from 0.8% to 7.8%. In Western cultures, bowel control is established in more than 95% of children by their fourth and 99% by their fifth birth. Encopresis is virtually absent in youth with normal intellectual function by the age of 16 years. Males are three to six times more likely to have encopresis than females. A significant relationship exists between encopresis and enuresis.

Etiology

Ninety percent of chronic childhood encopresis is likely functional. Children with this disorder typically withhold feces by contracting their gluteal muscles, holding their legs together, and tightening their external anal sphincter. In some cases, this is an entrenched behavioral response to previously painful bowel movements due to hard stool, leading to fear of defecation and withholding behaviors. Encopresis involves an often-complicated interplay between physiologic and psychological factors leading to an avoidance of defecation. However, when children chronically hold in bowel movements, the result is often fecal impaction and eventual overflow soiling. This pattern occurs in more than 75% of children with encopretic behavior. This standard set of circumstances in most children with encopresis supports a behavioral intervention focusing on ameliorating constipation while increasing appropriate toileting behavior. Inadequate training or the lack of proper toilet training may delay a child's attainment of continence.

Evidence indicates that some encopretic children have lifelong inefficient and ineffective sphincter control. Other children may soil involuntarily, either because of an inability to adequately control the sphincter or excessive fluid caused by a retentive overflow.

In about 5% to 10% of cases, medical conditions cause fecal incontinence, including abnormal innervation of the anorectal region, ultrashort-segment Hirschsprung disease, neuronal intestinal dysplasia, or spinal cord damage.

Encopresis may be more likely to occur among children with known sexual abuse and other psychiatric disorders. Encopresis, however, is not a specific indicator of sexual abuse.

It is evident that once a child has developed a pattern of withholding bowel movements and attempts to defecate have become painful, the child's fear and resistance to changing the pattern are high. Battles with parents who insist that their untreated child attempts to defecate may aggravate the condition and cause secondary behavioral difficulties. Untreated children with encopresis, however, frequently end up being socially ostracized and rejected. The social consequences of soiling can lead to the development of emotional problems. On the other hand, children with encopresis who clearly can control their bowel function adequately but chronically deposit feces of relatively normal consistency in abnormal places are likely to have pre-existing neurodevelopmental problems. Occasionally, a child has a specific fear of using the toilet, leading to a phobia.

In some cases, encopresis can be secondary, emerging after a period of healthy bowel habits in conjunction with a disruptive life event, such as the birth of a sibling or a move to a new home. When encopresis manifests after a long period of fecal continence, it may reflect a regressive developmental behavior based on a severe stressor, such as parental separation, loss of a best friend, or unexpected academic failure.

Megacolon. Most children with encopresis retain feces and become constipated, either voluntarily or secondary to painful defecation. In some cases, a subclinical pre-existing anorectal dysfunction exists that contributes to constipation. In either case, the resulting chronic rectal distention from large, hard fecal masses can cause loss of tone in the rectal wall and desensitization to pressure. Thus, children in this situation become even less aware of the need to defecate, and overflow encopresis occurs, usually with relatively small amounts of liquid or soft stool leaking out.

ENURESIS

Clinical and Diagnostic Features

Enuresis is the repeated voiding of urine into a child's clothes or bed; the voiding may be involuntary or intentional. The child must exhibit a developmental or chronologic age of at least 5 years. Children with enuresis are at higher risk for ADHD compared with the general population. They are also more likely to have comorbid encopresis. DSM-5-TR breaks down the disorder into three types: nocturnal, diurnal, and both (Table 19-2).

Pathology and Laboratory Examination

No single laboratory finding is pathognomonic of enuresis, but clinicians must rule out organic factors, such as urinary tract infections, which may predispose a child to enuresis. Structural obstructive abnormalities may be present in up to 3% of children with apparent enuresis. Usually, clinicians defer sophisticated radiographic studies in uncomplicated cases of enuresis with no signs of repeated infections or other medical problems.

Differential Diagnosis

Medical causes of bladder dysfunction must be investigated and ruled out. Urinary tract infections, obstructions, or anatomical conditions are often found in children who experience both nocturnal and diurnal enuresis combined with urinary frequency and urgency. We should consider various causes of genitourinary pathology. Depending on the signs and symptoms, these can include obstructive uropathy, spina bifida occulta, and cystitis—there are many other causes of polyuria and enuresis, such as diabetes mellitus and diabetes insipidus. Also, we should consider disturbances of consciousness and sleep, such as seizures, intoxication, sleepwalking disorder (during which a child urinates), and adverse effects from medications.

Course and Prognosis

Enuresis is often self-limited and may spontaneously remit. Most children who master control over their bladder gain self-esteem and improved social confidence.

Most children have primary enuresis and have not been dry for at least 6 months, whereas secondary enuresis has an onset after at least 6 months. Enuresis after at least 1 dry year usually begins between the ages of 5 and 8; if it occurs much later, especially during adulthood, we

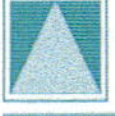

Table 19-2. Enuresis

	DSM-5-TR	ICD-10	ICD-11
Diagnostic name	Enuresis	Nonorganic Enuresis	Enuresis
Duration	Occurring ≥2/wk for a minimum of three consecutive months		Several times per week for several months
Symptoms	Urinating into bed or clothes either voluntary or unintentionally	Involuntary voiding of urine Abnormal for age	Repeated and persistent voiding of urine into bed or clothes Inappropriate for developmental age
Exclusions	Age <5 Substance use Other medical condition	Other medical condition	Other medical condition Substance or medication
Symptom specifiers	Nocturnal only Diurnal only Nocturnal and diurnal		

should investigate for other causes. Some evidence indicates that the late onset of enuresis in children is more frequently associated with a concomitant psychiatric difficulty than enuresis without at least 1 dry year. Relapses are common in those who remit, whether they have had treatment or not. The consequences of relapse include poor self-image, decreased self-esteem, social embarrassment and restriction, and intrafamilial conflict. The course is likely improved with the treatment of comorbid disorders such as ADHD.

Treatment

Spontaneous remission is common; however, interventions become necessary when enuresis causes functional impairment. The first step in any treatment plan is to review appropriate toilet training. If the parents have not attempted toilet training with the child, we should guide the parents and the patient in this undertaking. It is helpful to keep records, determine a baseline, and follow the child's progress; it may also be therapeutic. A star chart may benefit. Other practical techniques include restricting fluids before bed and using a night light to toilet-train the child. Alarm therapy has been a mainstay of treatment for enuresis. The alarm is a battery-operated device that can be attached to a child's underwear or a mat. The alarm is triggered as soon as voiding begins by emitting a loud noise that awakens the child. This method depends on the child's ability to wake up and respond to the alarm by getting up and voiding in the toilet. A child who can respond optimally is at least 6 or 7 years old.

Another simple intervention for children with enuresis and bowel dysfunction is to assess whether chronic constipation is contributing to urinary dysfunction and to consider increasing dietary fiber to diminish constipation.

Behavioral Therapy. Classical conditioning with the bell (or buzzer) and pad (alarm) apparatus is generally the most effective treatment for enuresis, with about half of treated patients remitting. Bladder training, which rewards delayed micturition, has also been used; however, it is decidedly inferior to the bell and pad.

Pharmacotherapy. We can consider medication when dietary and behavioral interventions are not sufficient and enuresis causes social, family, or functional impairment.

Desmopressin, an antidiuretic compound available as an intranasal spray, can reduce enuresis. The effectiveness varies widely in different studies. In most studies, enuresis recurs shortly after discontinuing the medication. Adverse effects of desmopressin include headache, nasal congestion, epistaxis, and stomachache. The most severe adverse effect reported was a hyponatremic seizure experienced by a child.

Antidepressants, particularly imipramine, were the first medications used for enuresis and are still sometimes used to take advantage of the anticholinergic side effects of the medication. However, there are considerable side effects, particularly cardiac effects. Reboxetine has fewer cardiac effects; however, it is unavailable in the United States.

Psychotherapy. Psychodynamic psychotherapy may help address coexisting psychiatric problems and the emotional and family difficulties that arise secondary to chronic enuresis. However, the behavioral therapy approaches described above are the treatments of choice.

Epidemiology

Enuresis's prevalence decreases with age: 5% to 10% in 5-year-olds, 1.5% to 5% in 9- to 10-year-olds, and about 1% in adolescents 15 years and older. Enuretic behavior is considered developmentally appropriate among young toddlers, precluding diagnoses of enuresis; however, enuretic behavior occurs in 82% of 2-year-olds, 49% of 3-year-olds, and 26% of 4-year-olds regularly.

Although most children with enuresis do not have a comorbid psychiatric disorder, children with enuresis are at higher risk for the development of another psychiatric disorder.

Nocturnal enuresis is about 50% more common in boys and accounts for about 80% of children with enuresis. Diurnal enuresis is also seen more often in boys, who frequently delay voiding until it is too late. A spontaneous resolution of nocturnal enuresis is about 15% per year.

Etiology

Enuresis involves complex neurobiologic systems, including contributions from cerebral and spinal cord centers, motor and sensory functions, and autonomic and voluntary nervous systems. Neurons regulate urination in the pons and midbrain regions. Bladder detrusor muscle contraction occurs on reaching bladder capacity, which can lead to enuresis in a sleeping child. Therefore, excessive volumes of urine produced at night may lead to enuresis at night in children without any physiologic abnormalities. Nighttime enuresis often occurs in the absence of a specific neurogenic cause. Daytime enuresis may develop based on behavioral habits developed over time.

Daytime enuresis may occur in the absence of neurologic abnormalities resulting from habitual, voluntary tightening of the external sphincter during urges to urinate. The pattern may become set in a young child who may start with a normal or overactive detrusor muscle in the bladder but with repeated attempts to prevent leaking or urination when there is an urge to void. Over time, the sensation of the urge to urinate diminishes, and the bladder does not empty regularly, leading to enuresis at night when the bladder is relaxed and can empty without resistance. This immature pattern of urinating can account for some cases of enuresis, especially when the pattern has been in place since early childhood. Most children are not enuretic by intention or even with awareness until after they are wet. Physiologic factors often play a role in the development of enuresis, and behavioral patterns are likely to maintain the maladaptive urination. Healthy bladder control, acquired gradually, is influenced by neuromuscular and cognitive development, socioemotional factors, toilet training, and genetic factors. Difficulties in one or more of these areas can delay urinary continence.

Genetic factors play a role in the expression of enuresis, given that the emergence of enuresis is significantly higher in first-degree relatives. A longitudinal study of child development found that children with enuresis were about twice as likely to have concomitant developmental delays as those who did not have enuresis. About 75% of children with enuresis have a first-degree relative who has or has had enuresis. A child's risk for enuresis is more than seven times higher if the father was enuretic. The concordance rate is higher in monozygotic twins than in dizygotic twins. There is a significant genetic component, and much can be accounted for by tolerance for enuresis in some families and other psychosocial factors.

Studies indicate that children with enuresis with a normal anatomical bladder capacity report an urge to void with less urine in the bladder than children without enuresis. Other studies report that nocturnal enuresis occurs when the bladder is full because of lower-than-expected levels of nighttime antidiuretic hormone. This low level of the hormone could lead to higher-than-usual urine output. Enuresis does not appear to be related to a specific stage of sleep or time of night; instead, bedwetting appears randomly. In most cases, the quality of sleep is average. Little evidence indicates that children with enuresis sleep more soundly than other children.

Psychosocial stressors appear to precipitate enuresis in a subgroup of children with the disorder. In young children, the disorder may relate to the birth of a sibling, hospitalization, the start of school, separation of a family due to divorce, or a move to a new environment.

Further Readings

Brazzeli M, Griffiths P, Cody JD, Tappin D. Behavioural and cognitive interventions with or without other treatments for the management of faecal incontinence in children. *Cochrane Database Syst Rev*. 2011;12:CD002240.

Brown ML, Pope AW, Brown EJ. Treatment of primary nocturnal enuresis in children: a review. *Child Care Health Dev*. 2010;37(2):153–160.

Friedman FM, Weiss JP. Desmopressin in the treatment of nocturia: clinical evidence and experience. *Ther Adv Urol*. 2013;5(6):310–317.

Har AF, Croffie JM. Encopresis. *Pediatr Rev*. 2010;31(9):368–374.

Harris J, Lipson A, Dos Santos J. Evaluation and management of enuresis in the general paediatric setting. *Paediatr Child Health*. 2023;28(6):362–376.

Mikkelsen EJ. Elimination disorders. In: Boland RJ, Verduin ML, eds. *Kaplan & Sadock's Comprehensive Textbook of Psychiatry*. 11th ed. Wolters Kluwer; 2025.

Mugie SM, Di Lorenzo C, Benninga MA. Constipation in childhood. *Nat Rev Gastroenterol Hepatol*. 2011;8(9):502–511.

Perrin N, Sayer L, While A. The efficacy of alarm therapy versus desmopressin therapy in the treatment of primary mono-symptomatic nocturnal enuresis: a systematic review. *Prim Health Care Res Dev*. 2015;16(1):21–31.

Rajindrajith S, Devanarayana NM, Benninga MA. Review article: faecal incontinence in children: epidemiology, pathophysiology, clinical evaluation and management. *Aliment Pharmacol Ther*. 2013;37(1):37–48.

Rowan-Legg A; Canadian Paediatric Society, Community Paediatrics Committee. Managing functional constipation in children. *Paediatr Child Health*. 2011;16(10):661–670.

Sinha R, Raut S. Management of nocturnal enuresis–myths and facts. *World J Nephrol*. 2016;5(4):328–338.

Yilmaz S, Bilgiç A, Hergüner S. Effect of OROS methylphenidate on encopresis in children with attention-deficit/hyperactivity disorder. *J Child Adolesc Psychopharmacol*. 2014;24(3):158–160.

20

Adolescent Substance Use Disorders

Substance use is a public health concern among American youth. The most common substances used by adolescents in the United States are tobacco, alcohol, and marijuana. There are many other substances that adolescents may abuse. These include cocaine, heroin, inhalants, phencyclidine (PCP), lysergic acid diethylamide (LSD), dextromethorphan, anabolic steroids, and various club drugs, including 3,4-methylenedioxymethamphetamine (MDMA or Ecstasy), flunitrazepam, gamma-hydroxybutyrate (GHB), and ketamine.

Approximately 20% of 8th graders in the United States have tried illicit drugs, and about 30% of 10th through 12th graders have used an illicit substance. Alcohol remains the most common substance used and abused by adolescents. Binge drinking occurs in about 6% of adolescents, and teens with alcohol use disorders are at higher risk of problems with other substances as well.

The Diagnostic and Statistical Manual of Mental Disorders, Fifth Edition (DSM-5-TR) combines abuse and dependence under the diagnosis of substance use disorder. It also contains diagnoses for intoxication, withdrawal, and substance-induced disorders. These apply to youths as well as adults. Some experts are concerned about the relevance of the criteria to adolescents, especially regarding tolerance and withdrawal. Some adolescents may develop tolerance to alcohol, for example, without any impairment. Withdrawal may have clinical significance. However, it does not correlate well with the level of severity.

Many risk and protective factors influence the age of onset and severity of substance use among adolescents. Psychosocial risk factors mediating the development of substance use disorders include parent modeling of substance use, family conflict, lack of parental supervision, peer relationships, and individual stressful life events. Protective factors that mitigate adolescent substance use include variables such as stable family life, strong parent–child bond, consistent parental supervision, investment in academic achievement, and a peer group that models prosocial family and school behaviors. Interventions that diminish risk factors are likely to mitigate substance use.

Approximately one in five adolescents has used marijuana or hashish. Approximately one-third of adolescents have used cigarettes by the age of 17 years. Studies of alcohol use among adolescents in the United States have shown that by 13 years of age, one-third of boys and almost one-fourth of girls have tried alcohol. By 18 years of age, 92% of males and 73% of females reported trying alcohol, and 4% reported using alcohol daily. Of high school seniors, 41% reported using marijuana; 2% reported using the drug daily.

Drinking among adolescents follows adult demographic drinking patterns: The highest proportion of alcohol use occurs among adolescents in the Northeast; Whites are more likely to drink than are other groups; among Whites, Roman Catholics are the least likely nondrinkers. The four most common causes of death in persons between the ages of 10 and 24 years are motor vehicle accidents (37%), homicide (14%), suicide (12%), and other injuries or accidents (12%). In pediatric trauma centers, more than one-third of adolescents need treatment for alcohol or drug use.

Studies considering alcohol and illicit drug use by adolescents as psychiatric disorders have demonstrated a higher prevalence of substance use, particularly alcoholism, among biologic children of alcoholics than among adopted youth. This finding is supported by family studies of genetic contributions, by adoption studies, and by observing children of substance users reared outside the biologic home.

Numerous risk factors influence the emergence of adolescent substance abuse. These include parental belief in the harmlessness of substances, lack of anger control in families of substance abusers, lack of closeness and involvement of parents with children's activities, maternal passivity, academic difficulties, comorbid psychiatric disorders such as conduct disorder and depression, parental and peer substance use, impulsivity, and early onset of cigarette smoking. The higher the number of risk factors, the more likely it is that an adolescent will be a substance user.

DIAGNOSIS AND CLINICAL FEATURES

Table 20-1 compares the text revision of the DSM-5-TR, and the 10th and 11th editions of the International Statistical Classification of Diseases and Related Health Problems (ICD-10, ICD-11) approaches to diagnosing substance use disorders.

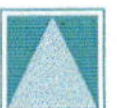

Table 20-1.
Substance Use Disorder

	DSM-5-TR	ICD-10	ICD-11
Diagnostic name	Substance Use Disorder (indicate specific substance) • Alcohol • Cannabis • Hallucinogens • Inhalants • Opioids • Sedatives, hypnotics, anxiolytics • Stimulants	Mental and Behavioral Disorders due to (indicate specific substance) Indicate if a dependence syndrome	Substance Dependence (indicate specific substance)
Duration	Symptoms occur within 12 mo		≥3 mo
Symptoms	Impaired control • Use of larger amounts/longer use than intended • Persistent desire or unsuccessful efforts to reduce the use • Significant time invested in obtaining, using, or recovering from a substance • Cravings to use • Social impairment • Use interfering in the fulfillment of responsibilities • Use despite social, personal, financial, health and other consequences of substance use • Reduction in other personal and interpersonal activities due to use • Risky use • Use in high risk or dangerous situations • Use despite recognition of potential physical or mental problems caused by substance use • Pharmacologic criteria • Tolerance • Withdrawal (does not apply to inhalants or hallucinogens)	Behavioral, cognitive, and physiologic manifestations of repeated substance use Frequently associated with cravings to use the drug and difficulties controlling use Pattern of persistent use despite recognition of adverse consequences of use Prioritization of substance use over other social, financial, and personal obligations Frequently accompanied by tolerance and withdrawal states	Recurrent (episodic or continuous) use of a substance with associated impairment. • Impaired control over the use • Preference of substance to other obligations and activities • Physiologic features, including tolerance or withdrawal
Required number of symptoms	≥2		≥2
Psychosocial consequences	Marked impairment and/or distress		
Exclusions		***Psychotic state*** ***Nonalcoholic Korsakov psychosis or syndrome***	An episode of harmful use A harmful pattern of use
Symptom specifiers	**In a controlled environment:** currently in an environment where access to substances is restricted **Substance-specific specifiers:** Tobacco Use Disorder On maintenance therapy Opioid Use Disorder On maintenance therapy Hallucinogen Use Disorder: Specify the hallucinogen Inhalant Use Disorder: Specify the inhalant	***Associated specifiers:*** **Psychotic disorder:** psychotic symptoms following a psychoactive substance, not due to acute intoxication alone or due to withdrawal alone. **Amnesic syndrome:** chronic impairment in memory due to the use	
Course specifiers	**In early remission:** no symptoms for 3–12 mo (except cravings) **In sustained remission:** no symptoms >1 yr (except cravings)		Current use Early full remission: 1–12 mo Sustained partial remission: mostly abstinent for ≥12 mo Sustained remission: fully abstinent for ≥12 mo

(continued)

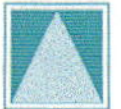

Table 20-1.
Substance Use Disorder (Continued)

	DSM-5-TR	ICD-10	ICD-11
Severity specifiers	**Mild**: 2–3 symptoms **Moderate**: 4–5 Symptoms **Severe**: ≥6 symptoms		
Comments		Note: ICD additionally defines "Harmful use" as a pattern of use causing harm to health, both physical and/or mental. This classification is independent of the presence of a dependence syndrome.	Alternative diagnoses include: Harmful use of a substance: ≥1 mo in which use of a substance causes physical or mental harm. A harmful pattern of use of a substance: regular or sporadic use of a substance that causes physical or mental harm

We should make a diagnosis of alcohol or drug use in adolescents through a careful interview, observations, laboratory findings, and history provided by reliable sources. Many nonspecific signs may point to alcohol or drug use, and clinicians must be careful to corroborate hunches before jumping to conclusions. Substance use exists on a continuum with experimentation (the mildest use), regular use without visible impairment, abuse, and, finally, dependence. Changes in academic performance, nonspecific physical ailments, changes in relationships with family members, changes in one's peer group, unexplained phone calls, or changes in personal hygiene may indicate substance use in an adolescent. Many of these also occur with depression, prodromal psychotic disorders, and adjustment issues, for example, to a new school.

Substance use is related to a variety of behaviors, including early sexual experimentation, risky driving, destruction of property, stealing, "heavy metal" or electronic dance music (EDM), and, occasionally, preoccupation with cults or Satanism. Although none of these behaviors necessarily predicts substance use, at the extreme, many of these behaviors reflect alienation from the mainstream of developmentally expected social behavior. Adolescents with inadequate social skills may use a substance as a modality to join a peer group. In some cases, adolescents begin their substance use at home with their parents, who also use substances to enhance their social interactions. Although no evidence indicates what determines a typical adolescent user of alcohol or drugs, many substance users seem to have underlying social skills deficits, academic difficulties, and less-than-optimal peer relationships.

Nicotine

Nicotine is one of the most addictive substances known; it involves cholinergic receptors and enhancing acetylcholine, serotonin, and β-endorphin release. Young teens who smoke cigarettes are also exposed to other drugs more frequently than nonsmoking peers.

Alcohol

Alcohol use in adolescents rarely results in the sequelae observed in adults with chronic use of alcohol, such as withdrawal seizures, Korsakoff syndrome, Wernicke aphasia, or cirrhosis of the liver. One report, however, has stated that adolescent alcohol exposure may result in diminished hippocampal brain volume. Because the hippocampus is involved with attention, it is conceivable that adolescent alcohol use could result in compromised cognitive function, especially concerning attention.

Marijuana

The short-term effects of the active ingredient in marijuana, tetrahydrocannabinol (THC), include impairment in memory and learning, distorted perception, diminished problem-solving ability, loss of coordination, increased heart rate, anxiety, and panic attacks. Abrupt cessation of heavy marijuana use by adolescents can result in a withdrawal syndrome characterized by insomnia, irritability, restlessness, drug craving, depressed mood, and nervousness, followed by anxiety, tremors, nausea, muscle twitches, increased sweating, myalgia, and general malaise. Typically, the withdrawal syndrome begins 24 hours after the last use, peaks at 2 to 4 days, and diminishes after 2 weeks. Marijuana use correlates with an increased risk of psychiatric disorders. Poor cognitive functioning has been associated with chronic marijuana use, although it is not clear whether marijuana impairs cognitive function. Deficits in verbal learning, memory, and attention occur in chronic marijuana users, and both acute and chronic marijuana use are associated with changes in cerebral blood flow to specific brain regions, which PET can detect. Functional imaging studies suggest that there is less activity in brain regions involved with attention and memory in chronic marijuana users. A 15-year follow-up of 50,465 Swedish males in the military reported that participants who had used marijuana by 18 years of age were 2.4 times more likely to develop schizophrenia. Risks associated with chronic marijuana use include higher rates of motor vehicle accidents, impaired respiratory function, increased risk of cardiovascular disease, and potential increased risk for psychotic symptoms and disorders.

Cocaine

Cocaine can be sniffed, snorted, injected, or smoked. *Crack* is the term given to cocaine that has been changed to a free base for smoking. Cocaine's effects include constriction of peripheral blood vessels, dilated pupils, hyperthermia, increased heart rate, and hypertension. High doses or prolonged use of cocaine can induce paranoid thinking. There is an immediate risk of death secondary to cardiac arrest or from seizures followed by respiratory arrest. In contrast to stimulants used to treat ADHD, such as methylphenidate, cocaine quickly crosses the blood–brain barrier and moves off the dopamine transporter within 20 minutes; methylphenidate remains bound to dopamine for long periods.

Heroin

Heroin, a derivative of morphine, is produced from poppy plant. Heroin usually appears as a white or brown powder that users can snort, but more commonly, they take it intravenously. Withdrawal symptoms include restlessness, muscle and bone pain, insomnia, diarrhea and vomiting, cold flashes with goosebumps, and kicking movements. Withdrawal occurs within a few hours after use; symptoms peak between 48 and 72 hours later and remit within about a week.

Club Drugs

Adolescents who frequent nightclubs, raves, bars, or music clubs also frequently use MDMA, GHB, flunitrazepam (Rohypnol), and ketamine. GHB, flunitrazepam (a benzodiazepine), and ketamine (an anesthetic) are primarily depressants and can be added to drinks without detection because they are often colorless, tasteless, and odorless. Congress passed The Drug-Induced Rape Prevention and Punishment Act after finding that these drugs were used in date rapes. MDMA is a derivative of methamphetamine, a synthetic with both stimulant and hallucinogenic properties. MDMA can inhibit serotonin and dopamine reuptake. MDMA can result in dry mouth, increased heart rate, fatigue, muscle spasms, and hyperthermia.

Lysergic Acid Diethylamide

LSD is odorless, colorless, and has a slightly bitter taste. Higher doses of LSD can produce visual hallucinations and delusions and, in some cases, panic. The sensations experienced after the ingestion of LSD usually diminish after 12 hours. Flashbacks can occur up to 1 year after use. LSD can produce tolerance; that is, after multiple uses, one needs more to feel the same degree of intoxication.

COMORBIDITY

Rates of alcohol and marijuana use are reportedly higher in relatives of youth with depression and anxiety disorders. On the other hand, mood disorders are common among those with alcoholism. Evidence indicates another strong link between early antisocial behavior, conduct disorder, and substance abuse. Substance abuse is a form of behavioral deviance that, unsurprisingly, is associated with other forms of social and behavioral deviance. Early intervention with children who show early signs of social deviance and antisocial behavior may conceivably impede the processes that contribute to later substance abuse.

It is essential to know about all comorbid disorders, which may show differential responses to treatment. Surveys of adolescents with alcoholism show rates of 50% or higher for additional psychiatric disorders, especially mood disorders. A recent survey of adolescents who used alcohol found that more than 80% met the criteria for another disorder. The disorders most frequently present were depressive disorders, disruptive behavior disorders, and drug use disorders. These rates of comorbidity are even higher than those for adults. The diagnosis of alcohol use disorder was likely to follow, rather than precede, other disorders; that a large proportion of adolescents with alcoholism have a previous childhood disorder may have both etiologic and treatment implications. In this survey, the onset of alcohol use disorders did not systematically precede other substance use disorders. In 50% of cases, alcohol use followed drug use. Alcohol use may be a gateway to drug use, but it is not in most cases. The presence of other psychiatric disorders was associated with an earlier onset of alcohol use disorder, but it did not seem to indicate a more protracted course of alcoholism.

TREATMENT

Interventions for substance use disorders in adolescents first require effective screening and identification of those teens in need of treatment. Once identifying a substance use disorder in a teen, we have a variety of treatment options.

Per the goals of the US Substance Abuse Mental Health Services Administration (SAMHSA), a school-based alcohol and drug Screening, Brief Intervention, and Referral to Treatment (SBIRT) has been initiated in a study with 629 adolescents aged 14 to 17 years in 13 participating high schools in New Mexico. Initially, school-based health centers provided substance use screenings for all students seen in the clinic for any reason. Once identified, substance-using adolescents were offered either brief intervention by clinic staff (85.1% of those identified), whereas 14.9% received brief treatment or referral to treatment. The brief intervention was based on motivational interviewing to help the student gain motivation for behavioral change, with a referral for more intensive treatment if needed.

Students who received the intervention, regardless of the severity of their substance use, reported decreases in self-reported drinking to intoxication at the 6-month follow-up.

The students reporting drug use self-reported using less at follow-up. Forty-two percent of the students reported alcohol use, and 37% reported intoxication. Eighty-five percent of study participants who reported drug use reported only marijuana use in the month before entering the study. The frequency of alcohol and marijuana as the most predominant substances in this age group is consistent with epidemiologic data. Overall, this school-based intervention had the advantage of being easily accessible to adolescents and provided a graded option for treatment according to the severity of substance use. This study suggests that school-based programs for identifying and providing brief interventions for high school students are viable and merit further study.

Treatment of substance use disorders in adolescents can directly prevent substance use behaviors, provide education for the patient and family, and address cognitive, emotional, and psychiatric factors that influence substance use in a variety of settings such as a residential milieu, group, and individual psychosocial session.

One validated instrument used as a guide for clinicians in the treatment of adolescent substance use designates levels of care appropriate for the symptoms. This instrument, called the *Child and Adolescent Levels of Care Utilization Services* (CALOCUS), outlines six levels of care:

0: Basic services (prevention)
1: Recovery maintenance (relapse prevention)
2: Outpatient (once per week visits)
3: Intensive outpatient (two or more visits per week)
4: Intensive integrated services (day treatment, partial hospitalization, wraparound services)
5: Nonsecure, 24-hour medically monitored service (group home, residential treatment facility)
6: Secure 24-hour medical management (inpatient psychiatric or highly programmed residential facility)

Treatment settings that serve adolescents with alcohol or drug use disorders include inpatient units, residential treatment facilities, halfway houses, group homes, partial hospital programs, and outpatient settings. Components of adolescent alcohol or drug use treatment include individual psychotherapy, drug-specific counseling, self-help groups (Alcoholics Anonymous [AA], Narcotics Anonymous [NA], Alateen, Al-Anon), substance abuse education and relapse prevention programs, and random urine drug testing. Family therapy and psychopharmacologic intervention are also helpful to add.

Before deciding on the most appropriate treatment setting for a particular adolescent, a screening process must take place in which structured and unstructured interviews help to determine the types of substances they are using as well as the quantities and frequencies. Determining coexisting psychiatric disorders is also critical. Rating scales can document the severity of abuse in the pretreatment and posttreatment periods. The *Teen Addiction Severity Index* (T-ASI), the *Adolescent Drug and Alcohol Diagnostic Assessment* (ADAD), and the *Adolescent Problem Severity Index* (APSI) are several severity-oriented rating scales. The T-ASI includes the dimensions of family function, school or employment status, psychiatric status, peer social relationships, and legal status.

After obtaining most of the information about substance use and the patient's overall psychiatric status, we must choose a treatment strategy and an appropriate setting must be determined. Two very different approaches to the treatment of substance use disorders are the Minnesota model and the multidisciplinary professional model. The Minnesota model relies on the premise of AA; it is an intensive 12-step program with a counselor who functions as the primary therapist. The program uses self-help participation and group processes. Inherent in this treatment strategy is the need for adolescents to admit that substance use is problematic and that help is necessary. Furthermore, they must be willing to work toward altering their lifestyle to eradicate substance use.

The multidisciplinary professional model consists of a team of mental health professionals, usually led by a physician. Following a case-management model, each team member has specific treatment areas for which they are responsible. Interventions may include CBT, family therapy, and pharmacologic intervention. This approach usually is suited for adolescents with comorbid psychiatric diagnoses.

Cognitive-behavioral approaches to psychotherapy for adolescents with substance use generally require that adolescents be motivated to participate in treatment and refrain from further substance use. The therapy focuses on relapse prevention and maintaining abstinence.

Psychopharmacologic interventions for adolescent alcohol and drug users are still in their early stages. The presence of mood disorders indicates the need for antidepressants, and generally, SSRIs are the first line of treatment. Occasionally, we might choose to substitute the illicit drug with another drug that is more amenable to the treatment situation, for example, using methadone instead of heroin. Adolescents are required to have documented attempts at detoxification and consent from an adult before they can enter such a treatment program.

Miles, a 17-year-old 12th grader, was admitted to an inpatient dual diagnosis (psychiatric and substance abuse treatment) program for the second time following a relapse, depression, and threats of suicide. Miles reported a long-standing history of ADHD, but he had been a good student and had not had any difficulties until middle school. Miles reported an onset of substance use at age 13 years, a rapid progression in substance involvement since age 14 years, and current use of marijuana daily, drinking alcohol up to five times each week, and experimentation with a variety of substances, such as LSD, Ecstasy, and heroin. After being discharged from the dual diagnosis inpatient program, Miles attended weekly teen group sessions focusing on his substance use problems. Family sessions led to the realization that Miles's mother had been depressed for some time, which contributed to the highly conflictual daily interactions between Miles, his sister, and his father. Miles's mother entered into her treatment and started family therapy. The family was interacting more peacefully for the next 2 months. Miles was improving regarding his substance use; however, his depressive symptoms increased following 8 weeks of abstinence. His psychiatrist started him on fluoxetine. After titrating the medication to 30 mg, Perter remained on it for 6 months, at which time he showed improvement in mood and treatment compliance. Miles continued to attend teen AA meetings and outpatient therapy. The family conflict soon recurred, however, and Miles became noncompliant with outpatient treatment, medication, and meetings. He resumed old relationships with substance-using peers and relapsed into daily marijuana use and occasional alcohol use. (Courtesy of Oscar G. Bukstein, M.D.)

Efficacious treatments for cigarette smoking cessation include nicotine-containing gum, patches, nasal sprays, or inhalers. Bupropion aids in diminishing cravings for nicotine and is beneficial in the treatment of smoking cessation.

Because comorbidity influences treatment outcomes, it is essential to pay attention to other disorders, such as mood disorders, anxiety disorders, conduct disorder, or ADHD, during the treatment of substance use disorders.

EPIDEMIOLOGY

Alcohol

The Centers for Disease Control and Prevention Youth Risk Behavior Survey found that 72.5% of high school students had tried at least one alcoholic drink. The SAMHSA 2022 National Survey on Drug Use and Health reported that among adolescents aged 12 to 20, about 15% used alcohol in the past month, and about 3% had binged alcohol in the past month. Findings from the Monitoring the Future Survey suggest that about 39% of adolescents have used alcohol before the eighth grade.

Marijuana

For the last two decades, marijuana has been one of the most widely used drugs by young people in developed countries, and recently, it has become highly used globally. Marijuana is the most commonly used illicit drug among high school students in the United States. The SAMHSA 2022 National Survey on Drug Use and Health reported that among adolescents aged 12 to 17, 11.5% had used marijuana in the past year. About 8% of 8th-grade students, 20% of 10th-grade students, and 30% of 12th-grade students reported using cannabis in the past year.

Marijuana is a "gateway drug" because the strongest predictor of future cocaine use is frequent marijuana use during adolescence. Prevalence rates for marijuana are highest among Native American males and females; these rates are nearly as high in White males and females and Mexican American males. The lowest annual rates occur in Latin American females, African American females, and Asian American males and females.

Cocaine

The annual cocaine use reported by high school seniors decreased by more than 30% between 1990 and 2000. Currently, about 0.5% of 8th-grade students, 1% of 10th-grade students, and 2% of 12th-grade students are estimated to have used cocaine. Crack cocaine use, however, is increasing in prevalence and is most common among those between the ages of 18 and 25.

Crystal Methamphetamine

Crystal methamphetamine, or "ice," was at a relatively low level of use in adolescence about one decade ago at 0.5% and has steadily increased to a recent rate of 1.5% among 12th graders.

Opioids

A survey of 7,374 high school seniors found that 12.9% reported nonmedical use of opioids. Of users, more than 37% reported intranasal administration of prescription opioids. From 2021 to 2022, there was a slight increase in the nonmedical use of prescription narcotics, with 1.7% of 12th-grade students reporting use in the past year.

Lysergic Acid Diethylamide (LSD)

About 3% of 8th-grade students, 6% of 10th-grade students, and 9% of 12th-grade students used LSD. Of 12th-grade students, 0.1% report daily use. The current LSD rates are lower than the rates of LSD use during the past two decades.

3,4-Methylenedioxymethamphetamine (MDMA)

MDMA has increased in popularity over the last decade. In the United States, 5% of 10th graders and 8% of 12th graders use the drug. This popularity is true even though its perceived danger has dramatically increased among adolescents. There have been accidental adolescent deaths due to MDMA.

Gamma-Hydroxybutyrate (GHB)

GHB, a club drug, has been found in surveys to have an annual prevalence rate of 1.1% for 8th graders, 1.0% for 10th graders, and a 1.6% rate of use for 12th graders.

Ketamine

Ketamine, another club drug, was found recently to have a rate of 1.3% annual prevalence for 8th graders, 2.1% for 10th graders, and 2.5% rate for 12th graders.

Flunitrazepam (Rohypnol)

Flunitrazepam (Rohypnol), a third club drug, has been found to have an annual prevalence rate of about 1% for all high school grades combined.

Anabolic Steroids

Despite reported knowledge of the risks of anabolic steroids among high school students, surveys over the last 5 years found rates of anabolic steroid use to be 1.6% among 8th graders and 2.1% among 10th graders. Up to 45% of 10th and 12th graders reported knowledge of the risks of anabolic steroids; however, over the last decade, it appears that high school seniors reported less disapproval of their use.

Inhalants

The use of inhalants in the form of glue, aerosols, and gasoline is relatively more common among younger than older adolescents. Among 8th-, 10th-, and 12th-grade students, 17.6%, 15.7%, and 17.6%, respectively, report using inhalants; 0.2% of 8th-grade students, 0.1% of 10th-grade students, and 0.2% of 12th-grade students report daily use of inhalants.

Multiple Substance Use

Among adolescents enrolled in substance abuse treatment programs, 96% are polydrug users; 97% of adolescents who abuse drugs also use alcohol.

ETIOLOGY

Genetic Factors

The concordance for alcoholism is reportedly higher among monozygotic than dizygotic twins. Studies of children of alcoholics reared away from their biologic homes have shown that these children have about a 25% chance of becoming alcoholics.

Psychosocial Factors

Among adolescents, substance use, particularly marijuana use, is strongly influenced by peers, and especially for those adolescents who report using marijuana for relaxation, the drug helps them to escape from stress and ease social interactions. There are data to suggest, however, that marijuana use is also associated with both social anxiety disorder and depressive symptoms. Among young adolescents who start using alcohol, tobacco, and marijuana at an early age, data suggest that they often come from families with low parental supervision. The risk of early initiation of substances is most significant for children below 11 years of age. Increased parental supervision during middle childhood years may diminish drug and alcohol sampling and ultimately diminish the risk of using marijuana, cocaine, or inhalants in the future.

Further Readings

Buckner JD, Heimberg RG, Schneier FR, Liu SM, Wang S, Blanco C. The relationship between cannabis use disorder and social anxiety disorder in the National Epidemiologic Study of Alcohol and Related Conditions (NESARC). *Drug Alcohol Depend.* 2012;124(1–2):128–134.

Centers for Disease Control and Prevention (CDC). Youth risk behavior survey: data summary and trends report, 2011–2021. www.cdc.gov/yrbs/dstr/pdf/YRBS_Data-Summary-Trends_Report2023_508.pdf

Fiorentini A, Volunteri LS, Dragogna F, et al. Substance-induced psychoses: a critical review of the literature. *Curr Drug Abuse Rev.* 2011; 4(4):228–240.

Fraser S, Hides L, Philips L, Proctor D, Lubman DI. Differentiating first episode substance induced primary psychotic disorders with concurrent substance use in young people. *Schizophr Res.* 2012;136(1–3): 110–115.

Giedd JN, Stockman M, Weddle C, et al. Anatomic magnetic resonance imaging of the developing child and adolescent brain. In: Reyna VF, Chapman SB, Dougherty MR, Copnfrey J, eds. *The Adolescent Brain: Learning, Reasoning, and Decision Making.* American Psychological Association; 2012.

Kaminer Y, Winters KC. Proposed DSM-5 substance use disorders for adolescents: if you build it, will they come? *Am J Addict.* 2012;21(3): 280–281.

Lenk KM, Erickson DJ, Winters KC, Nelson TF, Toomey TL. Screening services for alcohol misuse and abuse at four-year colleges in the U.S. *J Subst Abuse Treat.* 2012;43(3):352–358.

Lenoue S, Riggs PD. Adolescent substance use disorders. In: Boland RJ, Verduin ML, eds. *Kaplan & Sadock's Comprehensive Textbook of Psychiatry.* Eleventh edition. Wolters Kluwer; 2025.

McCabe SE, West BT, Teter CJ, Boyd CJ. Medical and nonmedical use of prescription opioids among high school seniors in the United States. *Arch Pediatr Adolesc Med.* 2012;166(9):797–802.

Mitchell SG, Gryczynski J, Gonzales A, et al. Screening, brief intervention, and referral to treatment (SBIRT) for substance use in a school-based program: services and outcomes. *Am J Addict.* 2012;21: S5–S13.

National Institute on Drug Abuse. Most reported substance use among adolescents held steady in 2022. 2022. https://nida.nih.gov/news-events/news-releases/2022/12/most-reported-substance-use-among-adolescents-held-steady-in-2022

Substance Abuse and Mental Health Services Administration. Highlights for the 2022 National Survey on Drug Use and Health. www.samhsa.gov/data/sites/default/files/reports/rpt42731/2022-nsduh-main-highlights.pdf

Winters KC. Advances in the science of adolescent drug involvement: implications for assessment and diagnosis—experience from the United States. *Curr Opin Psychiatry.* 2013;26(4):318–324.

Winters KC, Martim CS, Chung T. Substance use disorders in DSM-V when applied to adolescents. *Addiction.* 2011;106(5):882–884; discussion 895–897.

Yuma-Guerrero PJ, Lawson KA, Velasquez MM, von Sternberg K, Maxson T, Garcia N. Screening, brief intervention, and referral for alcohol use in adolescents: a systematic review. *Pediatrics.* 2012; 130(1):115–122.

21

Psychiatric Treatment for Children and Adolescents

Research on pediatric psychiatric treatments, both somatic and psychotherapeutic, is a rapidly growing area as many treatments, previously only studied in adults, are shown to be effective in children. Historically, there was a reluctance to investigate treatments, particularly psychopharmacological treatments, in children, given the concern of possible harm. It is reasonable to have such apprehensions as we are still learning about the effect of many treatments on the developing brain. However, this must balance against the harm done when inadequately treating psychiatric disorders in children. We now know that many disorders have a better prognosis when treated early. Fortunately, growing data suggests that many treatments appear safe and effective for children and adolescents. Still, much more research needs to be done, particularly on the long-term effects of treatment.

This section briefly reviews selected evidence-based psychiatric treatments in the pediatric population. An exhaustive review is beyond the scope of this book, and the reader is referred to the chapters on the various psychiatric disorders in children and adolescents for more information on effective treatments for each disorder.

SOMATIC TREATMENTS FOR CHILDREN AND ADOLESCENTS

Psychopharmacology

The use of psychiatric medications in children and adolescents has become increasingly common over the past few decades, reflecting a growing recognition of mental health disorders in pediatric populations and increased randomized clinical trials in this population. This recognition is supported by the increasing evidence showing that many classes of medication that are effective for adults are also helpful for children and adolescents. This evidence includes randomized placebo-controlled trials and multi-site, as well as National Institute of Mental Health (NIMH)–funded research comparing types of treatment with treatment combinations of pharmacologic interventions and psychosocial therapies.

However, psychiatric medications present unique challenges in this population. The prescriber must consider the stage of developmental, long-term safety concerns, and ethical issues surrounding informed consent and decision-making capacity. Similarly, the clinician must consider pharmacokinetics and pharmacodynamics in children. Children have greater hepatic capacity, more glomerular filtration, and less fatty tissue than adults. Thus, stimulants, antipsychotics, and tricyclic drugs are eliminated more rapidly by children than by adults; lithium may also be eliminated more rapidly, and children may be less able to store drugs in their fat. Because of children's quick elimination, the half-lives of many medications may be shorter in children than in adults. Because of these factors, the clinician may need to adjust a dose based on the patient's weight, especially in younger and smaller patients.

Little evidence indicates clinicians can predict a child's treatment response from the plasma level. Lithium is an exception, given its narrow therapeutic index.

This section reviews some significant medication groups relevant to child and adolescent psychiatry. Although we note the traditional drug classifications, we also include the approach from the Neuroscience-based Nomenclature (NbN), which is a system for classifying psychotropic medications based on their pharmacology and mode of action.

Medications for Attention-Deficit/Hyperactivity Disorder (ADHD). Stimulant pharmacologic agents remain the primary treatment of ADHD in children, adolescents, and adults. Stimulant options include amphetamine-based medications, including mixed amphetamine salts (e.g., Adderall), lisdexamfetamine, and methylphenidate-based medications.

Multiple studies support the efficacy of stimulant medications for ADHD. Stimulants reduce hyperactivity, inattentiveness, and impulsivity in about 75% of children with ADHD. The effects are not paradoxical because children without ADHD respond similarly.

The US Food and Drug Administration (FDA) has approved various stimulant medications for different age groups, and stimulant medications are available in multiple formulations, including immediate-release, extended-release, and transdermal paths. The most frequently researched and used stimulant is methylphenidate. Current practice is leaning toward more use of once-a-day, long-acting preparations of stimulants. The extended-release preparations, such as Concerta (extended-release methylphenidate) and Adderall XR, have the advantage of covering symptoms throughout the school day without the necessity of taking another dose and delivering medication more continuously. The methylphenidate transdermal patch (Daytrana) has the advantage of delivering medication until the patch is removed and for children who cannot swallow pills.

Common side effects of stimulants include decreased appetite, sleep disturbances, and potential impact on growth. Long-term safety and efficacy data are generally reassuring, although more studies are needed.

In addition to the stimulants, which are considered first-line medications for ADHD in children and adolescents, several nonstimulant medications are effective for ADHD. They are primarily used for children who have not responded well to stimulants or have experienced significant side effects using them. These medications likely help through their impact on blocking the action of norepinephrine.

Atomoxetine (Strattera) is a norepinephrine reuptake inhibitor. It is well absorbed after ingestion and reaches its maximal plasma concentration after about 1 to 2 hours. Common side effects of atomoxetine include abdominal discomfort, decreased appetite, dizziness, and irritability. Rarely, the medication may cause minor blood pressure and heart rate increases. Atomoxetine is metabolized by the cytochrome P450 (CYP) 2D6 hepatic enzyme system, and a fraction of patients are poor metabolizers, which may increase the plasma half-life by about fivefold. When combined with other medications that inhibit CYP 2D6, such as fluoxetine and paroxetine, diminished metabolism of atomoxetine can occur, and the dose may need to be decreased.

Clonidine and guanfacine are alpha-2 adrenergic agonists designed as antihypertensives but also have efficacy for ADHD through their effect on norepinephrine. These medications have shown moderate efficacy in reducing ADHD symptoms, especially hyperactivity and impulsivity. They are also beneficial for managing ADHD-related sleep difficulties and tics. The effectiveness of these drugs is generally considered lower than that of stimulants but higher than placebo. Common side effects include sedation, fatigue, dizziness, and dry mouth. Less frequently, they may cause changes in blood pressure and heart rate. While both medications work similarly, guanfacine is often preferred due to its longer half-life, allowing for once-daily dosing and potentially fewer side effects related to sedation and blood pressure changes.

The medications that are FDA-approved for ADHD are summarized in Table 21-1.

Medications for Psychotic Disorders. Although still commonly categorized as typical or atypical, these terms are becoming obsolete. The most widely used medications for schizophrenia in the United States are atypical agents, and not all these agents have similar receptor actions. A preferable approach may be that of the NbN, which includes the following categories: Dopamine–serotonin antagonists, Dopamine–serotonin–norepinephrine antagonist, dopamine partial agonists, and dopamine antagonists. Generally, the "typical" or first-generation antipsychotics are dopamine antagonists, although several are dopamine–serotonin antagonists. These latter medications, including thioridazine and thiothixene, differ from olanzapine in the ratio of receptor antagonism—the typical antipsychotics in this category are more potent dopamine antagonists than olanzapine. The remaining "atypical" or second-generation antipsychotics tend to have combined effects on multiple receptors, usually serotonin in addition to dopamine and, in some cases, norepinephrine as well.

Antipsychotics can treat various conditions in children and adolescents, including schizophrenia, bipolar disorder, and irritability associated with autism spectrum disorders (ASDs). Aggressive, explosive, and assaultive behaviors related to disruptive behavior disorders, psychotic disorders, and posttraumatic stress disorders (PTSDs) have been treated with antipsychotic agents with varying reports of success.

Among the second-generation antipsychotics, risperidone, aripiprazole, and olanzapine have FDA approval for various indications in children and adolescents. They are used for schizophrenia, bipolar disorder, and irritability in autism. The major side effects concerns are metabolic side effects, including weight gain and diabetes.

The first-generation antipsychotics are less commonly used in pediatric populations, given their side effects profiles. Among them, haloperidol may be the most frequently used, generally for severe behavioral problems or tic disorders. These agents are pure dopamine antagonists and commonly cause Parkinsonian symptoms. The most common Parkinsonian side effects are bradykinesia and tremors. More concerning is akathisia, and if this sense of inner restlessness cannot be treated through dose reduction or adjunctive medication (data is mixed, however, on the efficacy of adjuncts), it often requires a change in drug. Tardive dyskinesia is a concerning longer-term effect, and frequent examinations for signs of abnormal involuntary symptoms are needed to help prevent these from becoming permanent side effects. Most alarming is the neuroleptic malignant syndrome, which includes symptoms of a high fever, autonomic instability, and muscular rigidity and is a medical emergency necessitating immediate hospitalization for monitoring and treatment.

The antipsychotic medications FDA-approved for schizophrenia or psychosis are summarized in Table 21-2. As some other antipsychotic medications are approved for bipolar disorder instead, these are included among the mood stabilizers.

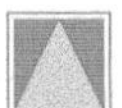

Table 21-1. Medications FDA-Approved for ADHD in Children and Adolescents

Medication	Brand Names	Current Terminology	Mode of Action	Age (yr)	Dosing (mg)[a] Initial Daily Dose	Target Daily Dose
		Dopamine Enhancers				
Amphetamine	Adzenys, Dynavel, Evekeo	Stimulant	Reuptake inhibitors (DAT, NET) and releaser (DA, NA)	3–18	2.5–5.0	2.5–40
Dextroamphetamine/ amphetamine salts	Adderall	Stimulant	Reuptake inhibitors (DAT, NET) and releaser (DA, NA)	3–18	2.5–5.0	2.5–40
Dextroamphetamine/ amphetamine salts extended release (ER/XR)	Adderall XR, Mydayis	Stimulant	Reuptake inhibitors (DAT, NET) and releaser (DA, NA)	6–18	5–20	5–40
Lisdexamfetamine	Vyvanse	Stimulant	Prodrug of dextroamphetamine Reuptake inhibitors (DAT, NET) and releaser (DA, NA)	6–18	30	30–70
Methylphenidate	Ritalin, Methylin, Quillivant	Stimulant	Reuptake inhibitors (DAT, NET)	6–18	2.5–5.0 bid	5–60
Methylphenidate extended release (ER)	Concerta, Quillivant ER	Stimulant	Reuptake inhibitors (DAT, NET)	6–18	18	18–72
Dexmethylphenidate	Focalin	Stimulant	Reuptake inhibitors (DAT, NET)	6–18	2.5 bid	5–20
Dexmethylphenidate extended release (ER/XR)	Focalin XR	Stimulant	Reuptake inhibitors (DAT, NET)	6–18	5	5–30
		Norepinephrine Receptor Inhibitor				
Atomoxetine	Straterra[c]	Selective norepinephrine reuptake inhibitor (SNRI)	Reuptake Inhibitor (NET)	6–18	<70k kg: 0.5 mg/kg >70 kg: 40 mg	<70 kg: Up to 1.4 mg/kg >70 kg: 40–80 mg
		Norepinephrine Blocker				
Clonidine[b]	Catapres,[c] Durnacol,[c] Other brands[c]	Norepinephrine blocker	Receptor agonist (alpha-2)	6–18	27–40.5 kg: 0.05 mg 40.5–45 kg: 0.05 mg >45 kg: 0.1 mg	27–40 kg: 0.05–0.2 mg 40.5–45 kg: 0.05–0.3 mg >45 kg: 0.1–0.4 mg
Clonidine extended release (ER)	Kapvay[c]	Norepinephrine blocker	Receptor agonist (alpha-2)	6–18	0.1	0.1–0.4
Guanfacine[b]	Tenex[c]	Norepinephrine blocker	Receptor agonist (alpha-2)	6–18	27–40.5 kg: 0.5 mg 40.5–45 kg: 0.5 mg >45 kg: 1 mg	27–40.5 kg: 0.5–2 mg 40.5–45 kg: 0.5–3 mg >45 kg: 1–4 mg
Guanfacine extended release (ER)	Intuniv	Norepinephrine blocker	Receptor agonist (alpha-2)	6–18	25–33.9 kg: 1 mg 34–41.4 kg: 1 mg 41.5–49.4 kg: 1 mg 49.4–58.4 kg: 1 mg	25–33.9 kg: 1–3 mg 34–41.4 kg: 1–4 mg 41.5–49.4 kg: 1–5 mg 49.4–58.4 kg: 1–6 mg

[a]For informational purposes only. Please consult the package insert of a product for specific dosage guidelines. The doses given refer to monotherapy. Combination treatment may require dose adjustments.

[b]The extended-release formulations of clonidine and guanfacine are FDA-approved for ADHD in children 6–18. The short-acting formulations are frequently used off-label.

[c]These brand formulations have been discontinued. Generic formulations are available.

bid, twice-daily dosage; DA, dopamine; DAT, dopamine transporter; NE, noradrenaline; NET, norepinephrine transporter.

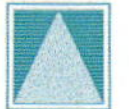

Table 21-2.
Medications FDA-Approved for Psychotic Disorders in Children and Adolescents

Medication	Brand Names	Current Terminology	Mode of Action	Age (yr)	Dosing (mg)[a] Initial Daily Dose	Target Daily Dose
Dopamine-Serotonin Antagonists						
Olanzapine	Zyprexa	Atypical (second generation) antipsychotic	Receptor antagonists (D2, 5HT2)	13–17	2.5–5	10 (2.5–5 mg increments)
Thioridazine	Mellaril	Typical (first generation) antipsychotic	Receptor antagonists (D2, 5HT2)	2–12	0.5–3 mg/kg/ day divided q8hr	Not to exceed 3 mg/kg/day
				>12	50–100	200–800
Thiothixene	Navane	Typical (first generation) antipsychotic	Receptor antagonists (D2, 5HT2)	>12	2–5	15–30. Not to exceed 60
Dopamine–Serotonin–Norepinephrine Antagonists						
Risperidone	Risperdal	Atypical (second generation) antipsychotic	Receptor antagonist (D2, 5-HT2, NE alpha-2)	≥13	0.5	3 (0.5–1 mg increments)
Paliperidone	Invega	Atypical (second generation) antipsychotic	Receptor antagonist (D2, 5-HT2, NE alpha-2)	≥12	3	<51 kg: 3 mg/day increments, not to exceed 6 ≥51: as above, not to exceed 12
Dopamine Partial Agonists						
Aripiprazole	Abilify	Atypical (second generation) antipsychotic	Receptor antagonist (D2, 5-HT2, NE alpha-2)	13–17	2	10–30 Increase to 5 after 2 days, 10 after 2 more, increase by 5 per day.
Dopamine Antagonists						
Haloperidol	Haldol	Typical (first generation) antipsychotic	Receptor antagonists (D2)	3–12	0.25–0.5 divided q8–12hr	0.05–0.15 mg/kg/day
				>12	0.5–2	Not to exceed 30
Perphenazine	Trilafon	Typical (first generation) antipsychotic	Receptor antagonists (D2)	>12	8–16 q6–12hr	Not to exceed 64 mg/day
Prochlorperazine	Compazine	Typical (first generation) antipsychotic	Receptor antagonists (D2)	2–6	2.5	Not to exceed 10 on the first day, not to exceed 20
				6–12	2.5	Not to exceed 10 on the first day, not to exceed 25
Trifluoperazine	Stelazine	Typical (first generation) antipsychotic	Receptor antagonists (D2)	6–12	1	Not to exceed 15
				>12	2–5	

[a]For informational purposes only. Please consult the package insert of a product for specific dosage guidelines.

Medications for Depression. Many of the antidepressants used in adults have evidence for their efficacy in children and adolescents, and several are FDA-approved for the treatment of major depressive disorder. This includes both serotonin blockers (selective serotonin reuptake inhibitors or SSRIs and related medications) and norepinephrine blockers (tricyclic antidepressants or TCAs); however, TCAs are not commonly used in this population given their more significant side effect profile, including anticholinergic effects and the risk of cardiotoxicity.

SSRIs currently are the drugs of choice in the pharmacologic treatment of depressive disorders in children and adolescents.

A substantial evidence base exists for the efficacy of SSRIs in the treatment of separation anxiety, generalized anxiety disorder (GAD), and social phobia in children and adolescents. Although frequently used, apart from duloxetine, the use of these agents is off-label.

One concern regarding using antidepressants in children is the black box warning for most antidepressants.

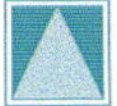

Table 21-3.
Medications FDA-Approved for Major Depressive Disorder in Children and Adolescents

Medication	Brand Names	Current Terminology	Mode of Action	Age (yr)	Dosing (mg)[a] Initial Daily Dose	Dosing (mg)[a] Target Daily Dose (Assuming Gradual Increases)
			Serotonin Enhancers			
Fluoxetine	Prozac, Sarafem	SSRI	Reuptake inhibitor (SERT)	>8	10–20 (start 10 in lower weight children, may increase after 1 wk)	10–20. Not to exceed 20.
Escitalopram	Lexapro	SSRI	Reuptake inhibitor (SERT)	≥12	10	10–20. Not to exceed 20.
			Norepinephrine Enhancers			
Desipramine	Norpramin	Tricyclic antidepressant	Reuptake inhibitor (NET)	≥12	25–50	100, Not to exceed 150.
Protriptyline	Vivactil	Tricyclic antidepressant	Reuptake inhibitor (NET)	≥12	15–20	15–20
			Serotonin–Norepinephrine Enhancers			
Amitriptyline	Elavil, Levate	Tricyclic antidepressant	Serotonin–norepinephrine enhancers	Adolescents	25–50	100
			Serotonin–Dopamine Blockers			
Trimipramine	Surmontil, Trimip, Tripramine	Tricyclic antidepressant	Reuptake inhibitor (NET)	≥12	50	100

[a]For informational purposes only. Please consult the package insert of a product for specific dosage guidelines.

The FDA required this warning in 2004 after a comprehensive review of clinical trial data suggesting an increased risk of suicidal thoughts and behaviors in young people taking antidepressants. The data reviewed by the FDA in 2004 did not suggest that there was an increase in completed suicide in this population. In 2007, the FDA expanded this wording to include young adults up to 24. Critics of this warning point out that the increase is slight and the risk of suicide in untreated depression is much greater; however, given the data of a modest but measurable risk, clinicians should be vigilant for signs of worsening depression, unusual changes in behavior, or the emergence of suicidal ideation in children, adolescents, and young adults taking antidepressants.

Apart from this concern, most side effects of SSRIs are tolerable. Some anecdotal reports indicate occasional SSRI-induced apathy in children and adolescents. Although rare, there is a risk of serotonin syndrome, which can range from mild symptoms (shivering, diarrhea) to severe (muscle rigidity, fever, and seizures). Patients exhibiting even minor symptoms require emergent evaluation. In milder cases, stopping the medication and giving supportive care is usually adequate for quickly alleviating the symptoms. In more severe cases, medications to address specific symptoms, such as benzodiazepines for agitation, muscle stiffness, and seizure-like symptoms, or cyproheptadine, which may block serotonin production and lessen the symptoms, may be helpful.

The antidepressants that are FDA-approved for the treatment of depression in children and adolescents are summarized in Table 21-3.

Medications for Obsessive-Compulsive Disorder (OCD). Several SSRIs and one TCA are also FDA-approved for the treatment of OCD. The SSRIs are the treatment of choice; their risk–benefit profile is similar to depression treatment, except that, similar to adult treatment, patients may require higher dosing to achieve an effect, and the medications may require a more extended trial to determine their impact. The relevant medications are summarized in Table 21-4.

Medications for Bipolar Disorder. Treating classic mania in children and adolescents is similar to adult treatment. That said, of the medications used in adults, only lithium and several of the antipsychotics are FDA-approved for bipolar disorder in children and adolescents. Divalproex has shown efficacy in randomized studies of bipolar disorder in adolescents. However, it is only

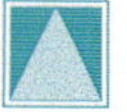

Table 21-4.
Medications FDA-Approved for Obsessive-Compulsive Disorder in Children and Adolescents

Medication	Brand Names	Current Terminology	Mode of Action	Age (yr)	Dosing (mg)[a] Initial Daily Dose	Dosing (mg)[a] Target Daily Dose (Assuming Gradual Increases)
			Serotonin Enhancers			
Fluoxetine	Prozac, Sarafem	SSRI	Reuptake inhibitor (SERT)	>7	10	May increase to 20 after 2 wk Lower weight: 20–30 Adolescents and higher weight: 20–60
Sertraline	Zoloft	SSRI	Reuptake inhibitor (SERT)	6–12 12–17	25 50	Increase by 50/wk. Do not exceed 200.
Fluvoxamine	Luvox	SSRI	Reuptake inhibitor (SERT)	8–17	25	Increase by 25 every 4–7 days. Target 50–200.
			Serotonin–Norepinephrine Enhancers			
Clomipramine	Anafranil	Tricyclic antidepressant	Reuptake inhibitor (SERT and NET)	≥10	25	Titrate to 3 mg/kg/day or 100 mg, whichever is less. May further increase to 3 mg/kg/day or 200 mg whichever is less.

[a]For informational purposes only. Please consult the package insert of a product for specific dosage guidelines.

FDA-approved for epilepsy in children, and using it as a mood stabilizer would be off-label. Quetiapine, which is FDA-approved, shows similar efficacy as divalproex for mania. Carbamazepine and other anticonvulsants are also sometimes used off-label for bipolar disorder in children.

Lithium is FDA-approved for children aged 7 and older with bipolar disorder. Lithium is also used to treat aggression in children. Using lithium requires careful monitoring of blood levels and thyroid function. This requirement, unfortunately, usually means frequent blood draws for a child. Some research suggests that saliva levels may correlate with blood levels, opening the way for a less invasive approach to testing lithium levels.

The mood-stabilizing drugs that are FDA-approved for mania or bipolar disorder are summarized in Table 21-5.

Medications for Anxiety Disorders. SSRI agents are currently the first-line agents in the pharmacologic treatment of anxiety disorders in children and adolescents. The FDA-approved escitalopram in the treatment of GAD in 2023 in youth 7 to 17 years old. The selective serotonin–norepinephrine reuptake inhibitor (SNRI) agent duloxetine is approved in children 7 to 17 years old for the treatment of GAD. Although only escitalopram and duloxetine are FDA-approved for GAD in children and adolescents, a large multisite study, Child/Adolescent Anxiety Multimodal Study (CAMS) provided evidence that sertraline, alone, and especially in combination with cognitive-behavioral therapy (CBT), is efficacious in the treatment of GAD, social anxiety disorder, and separation anxiety disorder in youth 7 to 17 years old. SSRIs that are commonly prescribed clinically, off label, in the treatment of anxiety disorders in children and adolescents include sertraline, fluoxetine, citalopram and escitalopram.

Several benzodiazepines are approved for anxiety disorders in children, and others are used off-label. Although having evidence for their effect on panic disorder and other anxiety disorders, they carry similar risks as for adults of causing sedation, tolerance, and dependence. They should be used carefully, usually short-term, until other psychotherapeutic treatments are effective.

Benzodiazepines are also used for some sleep disorders, including sleep terror disorder and sleepwalking disorder. Again, they should be used only temporarily, as behavioral approaches can affect various sleep disorders. They can also be helpful as a pretreatment for medical procedures.

Buspirone has limited data in pediatric populations but may be used off-label for anxiety disorders. Similarly, venlafaxine has been used off-label for anxiety disorders in pediatric populations.

The medications that are FDA-approved for anxiety disorders in children and adolescents are summarized in Table 21-6. This list should be viewed cautiously as, once the FDA approves a medication for one indication, there is often less incentive for a pharmaceutical company to seek other indications given the time and expense required for FDA approval. Thus, many of the medications currently used for anxiety disorders in children are used off-label. Although not approved, there is at least some data for this practice for various anxiety disorders. Among the approved medications, most are benzodiazepines, which are not considered first-line treatments for many anxiety disorders, at least for long-term treatment. One approved medication, meprobamate, is no longer recommended for any age group.

Summary. The use of psychiatric medications in children and adolescents has dramatically expanded our ability to treat mental health disorders in this vulnerable population.

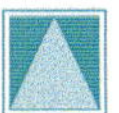

Table 21-5.
Medications FDA-Approved for Bipolar Disorder in Children and Adolescents

Medication	Brand Names	Current Terminology	Mode of Action	Age (yr)	Dosing (mg)[a] Initial Daily Dose	Target Daily Dose (Assuming Gradual Increases)
			Lithium			
Lithium[b]	Eskalith, Lithobid	Mood stabilizer	Enzyme interactions	≥7	<30 kg: 300 BID >30 kg: 300 TID	Titrate to serum trough of 0.8–1.2 mEq/L
			Dopamine–Serotonin Antagonists			
Quetiapine	Seroquel	Atypical antipsychotic (second generation)	Receptor antagonist (D2, 5-HT2) and reuptake inhibitor (NET) (metabolite)	≥10	50	400–600
Olanzapine	Zyprexa	Atypical antipsychotic (second generation)	Receptor antagonist (D2, 5-HT2)	13–17	2.5–5	10, range 2.5–20
			Dopamine–Serotonin–Norepinephrine Antagonists			
Risperidone	Risperdal	Atypical antipsychotic (second generation)	Receptor antagonist (D2, 5-HT2, NE alpha-2)	≥10	0.5	Increase by 0.5–1/day to 2.5 Range: 0.5–6
			Dopamine Partial Agonists			
Aripiprazole	Abilify	Atypical antipsychotic (second generation)	Receptor partial agonist (D2, 5-HT1A) and receptor antagonist (5-HT2A)	10–17	2	Increase to 5 after 2 days, target range 10–30
Valproate[c]	Depakote	Mood stabilizer, anticonvulsant	Yet to be determined	>2	15 mg/kg/day	15–60 mg/kg/day (divided doses)

[a]For informational purposes only. Please consult the package insert of a product for specific dosage guidelines.

[b]Only lithium is approved for bipolar disorder in children. The other medications listed are approved for bipolar mania.

[c]Approved for epilepsy in children. Per FDA guidelines, the safety and tolerability of Valproate in children are comparable to adults (although there is a greater risk of hepatoxicity in children <2 years); however, efficacy for mania has not been established in the studies submitted to the FDA.

While many medications have demonstrated efficacy, concerns remain regarding long-term safety and developmental effects. These concerns are complicated by the fact that most research on the safety of psychiatric drugs in children and adolescents are short-term studies. While these generally are reassuring, limited long-term data exists. We need more research to understand the long-term impacts of these medications on growth, development, and cognitive functioning.

The current research, however, does support the judicious use of psychiatric medications in pediatric populations when clinically indicated. We must carefully consider risk-benefit ratios, including understanding that all the risks may not be known. SSRIs and stimulants have the most robust evidence base, while antipsychotics and mood stabilizers are less well-studied but can play crucial roles in managing more severe conditions.

Future research should focus on long-term safety and efficacy, age-specific dosing guidelines, and the impact of early medication use on neurodevelopment. In addition, more studies are needed on combination treatments and integrating pharmacologic approaches with psychosocial interventions.

As our understanding of child and adolescent psychopharmacology continues to evolve, ongoing vigilance and research are essential to ensure the safe and effective use of psychiatric medications in children and adolescents.

Neurostimulation

Research is ongoing on the use of neurostimulation in children and adolescents for psychiatric disorders. Clinicians should be cautious when considering these treatments, particularly as their effect on the developing brain is inadequately understood. As more data accumulates, some currently only investigational treatments will likely become FDA-approved for use in children. The following is a summary of the current status of some neurostimulation treatments.

Electroconvulsive Therapy (ECT). In 2018, the FDA approved the use of ECT for catatonia or severe major depressive episodes (either from major depressive disorder or bipolar disorder) in patients 13 years and older who are treatment-resistant or who require a rapid response due to the severity of their symptoms.

This ruling was in light of substantial data spanning many decades, indicating that ECT was safe and effective in children. Multiple studies suggest that the response

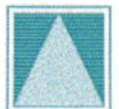

Table 21-6.
Medications FDA-Approved for Anxiety Disorders in Children

					Dosing (mg)[a]	
Medication	**Brand Names**	**Current Terminology**	**Mode of Action**	**Age (yr)**	**Initial Daily Dose**	**Target Daily Dose (Assuming Gradual Increases)**
			Serotonin–Norepinephrine Enhancer			
Duloxetine[b]	Cymbalta	Serotonin norepinephrine reuptake inhibitor	Reuptake inhibitor (SERT and NET)	7–17	30	30–60
Escitalopram[b]	Lexapro	SSRI	Reuptake inhibitor (SERT)	≥7	10	10–20
			GABA Enhancer			
Chlordiazepoxide	Librium	Benzodiazepine anxiolytic	Positive allosteric modulator (GABA-A receptor, benzodiazepine site)	>6 yr	0.5 mg/kg/day divided dose, OR 5 mg PO q6–12hr	5–10 (also approved IV/IM for >12 years, dose range 25–50)
Diazepam	Valium, Diastat	Benzodiazepine anxiolytic	Positive allosteric modulator (GABA-A receptor, benzodiazepine site)	6–12	0.5 mg/kg divided dose	
				>12	0.12–0.8 mg/kg/day divided dose OR 0.04–0.2 mg/kg IV/IM q2–4hr	No more than 0.6 mg/kg within 8 hr
Oxazepam	Serax	Benzodiazepine anxiolytic	Positive allosteric modulator (GABA-A receptor, benzodiazepine site)	>12 yr	Mild/Moderate: 10–15 mg PO q6–8hr PRN; Severe: 15–30 mg PO q6–8hr PRN	Use with caution in 6–12 yr
Meprobamate	Miltown (no longer available in brand form)	Nonbenzodiazepine anxiolytic	GABA-A receptor agonism	Not recommended for use due to risk for toxicity		

[a]For informational purposes only. Please consult the package insert of a product for specific dosage guidelines.
[b]Approved for generalized anxiety disorder.

and remission rate exceed that for either medications or psychotherapy, although there are no head-to-head comparison studies with an adequate design for review.

However, different states require different levels of review before initiating ECT in adolescents. These may include special reviews, such as an assessment from two independent board-certified child and adolescent psychiatrists, at least one with expertise in administering ECT to adolescents. Written consent from the parent and legal guardian is also required; written assent from the patient is often preferred.

Transcranial Magnetic Stimulation (TMS)

The FDA has approved the NeuroStar TMS device as an adjunct for treating major depressive disorder in adolescents aged 15 to 21. This approval was granted in 2018 for the NeuroStar TMS Therapy System, making it the only TMS treatment FDA-cleared for this age group.

This approval was informed by data from data analyzing more than 1,000 NeuroStar patients, of whom about three-quarters showed clinically meaningful improvement in depression severity. The FDA determined from this study and other clinical data that TMS as an adjunct to antidepressants is substantially equivalent in safety to antidepressants alone.

Vagus Nerve Stimulation (VNS)

VNS, previously used for epilepsy in children, was approved by the FDA for patients with epilepsy and depression in patients older than 12. It appears to work by stimulating the ascending pathways of the vagus nerve and altering circuits in the brain stem, midbrain, and cortex. The data was derived from adolescents with epilepsy who, in addition to improvement in their seizures, saw an improvement in their mood when treated with VNS. Further data is needed, particularly in adolescents without epilepsy.

Other Neurostimulation Techniques. Deep brain stimulation and transcranial direct current stimulation (tDCS) are experimental in younger patients. Neither is FDA-approved in children or adolescents.

PSYCHOTHERAPY FOR CHILDREN AND ADOLESCENTS

Psychotherapy is an essential tool in treating various psychological issues in children. Different types of psychotherapies are used depending on the child's needs, developmental stage, and specific psychological problems. We will explore the most common and evidence-based kinds of psychotherapy, their applications, and their efficacy in treating different mental health conditions in children and adolescents.

Psychotherapy with children and adolescents generally begins by establishing rapport through developmentally appropriate psychoeducation regarding the target symptoms and disorders to be addressed. Establishing a therapeutic relationship with a child of any age requires a knowledge of normal development and understanding the context in which the symptoms emerged. Most children do not seek psychiatric treatment; typically, they are brought to a psychotherapist due to symptoms noted by a family member, schoolteacher, or pediatrician. Children often believe that they are being taken for treatment because of their misbehavior or as a punishment for wrongdoing.

As a rule, the younger the child, the more extensively family members participate in the treatment. Even among adolescents, family members are often directly involved in some treatment components to achieve the maximum benefit. In general, successful individual psychotherapeutic interventions with youth also necessitate establishing a therapeutic rapport with parents.

Below, we will consider a variety of psychotherapy techniques. These are not meant to be rigid. They can occur in many settings, such as a private office, clinic, home, or school. Furthermore, many can be done individually, in group settings, or on the internet. They often occur in combination with other treatments, such as with medications, and when multiple clinicians are involved with different aspects of a child's treatment, all must regularly communicate lest treatment become fragmented.

Cognitive-Behavioral Therapy

CBT incorporates principles from behavioral therapy and cognitive psychology. It emphasizes how children may use thinking processes and cognitive modalities to reframe, restructure, and solve problems. A child's distortions are addressed by generating alternative ways of dealing with problematic situations.

CBT is one of the most widely researched and applied psychotherapies for children and adolescents. CBT has shown efficacy in treating depression, anxiety disorders, OCD, ADHD, PTSD, and eating disorders in young populations.

One of the limiting factors in providing CBT to children with OCD, anxiety disorders, and depressive disorders is the lack of sufficient numbers of trained child and adolescent cognitive-behavioral therapists. Internet-based treatments may help fill some of this gap, and studies have shown that internet-based CBT is acceptable to families and patients. Moreover, patients benefit from the treatment, particularly when compared to wait-list subjects.

Justin was a 14-year-old boy from a middle-class family enrolled in the 9th grade at a public school. His parents brought him in for his long-standing history of shyness and anxiety in social situations, which was more evident now that most of his peers were getting together after school, and he was spending his weekends alone. The evaluation revealed social anxiety disorder as the primary disorder. Justin was initially resistant to treatment despite his wish to feel more comfortable with other people and in social situations with peers. After much discussion and some pressure from his parents, Justin began to attend a cognitive-behavioral group treatment for adolescents with social anxiety. Justin became mildly agitated each time he was scheduled for a session; however, once he arrived, he could participate. He began a 16-session course of treatment combining education, cognitive restructuring, behavioral exposure, relapse prevention, and four sessions of parent involvement. As treatment progressed, Justin increased his visibility at school and even attended a school football game with a few peers. Justin told his therapist that he wanted to go to the next school dance but was afraid that he would be embarrassed and have to go home before the dance. The therapists designed several exposures whereby the various things that could happen at a dance were presented to Justin, including being offered alcohol or drugs, having a good time dancing, being left alone or ignored by his friends, or being turned down if he asked a girl to dance with him. As it turned out, Justin's few school acquaintances ignored him and left him at the dance. Justin, prepared for this less-than-desired outcome in his group experience, asked two girls to dance and forced himself to interact with other peers. To his surprise, one girl agreed to dance with him despite his shyness. He considered the evening a success. Justin subsequently went to another social event with a new group of peers who seemed more accepting of him. In Justin's case, practicing responses to potential rejections in the safety of his treatment group was crucial to his success at the dance, and it increased his motivation to continue treatment. Through his treatment, Justin became more and more appropriately prepared, through behavioral exposure and practice, to handle what might previously have been awkward and discouraging situations. (Adapted from Anne Marie Albano, Ph.D.)

Trauma-Focused Cognitive Behavioral Therapy (TF-CBT)

TF-CBT is a specialized form of CBT designed to address the needs of children and adolescents who have experienced trauma. It can help treat PTSD, traumatic grief, and other trauma-related symptoms. It employs techniques such as gradual exposure, cognitive processing of the traumatic event, and enhancing safety skills are vital components. TF-CBT has strong empirical support for reducing PTSD symptoms and improving overall functioning in traumatized youth.

Mindfulness-Based Interventions

Mindfulness techniques have been increasingly incorporated into therapies for children and adolescents. These interventions are used for stress reduction, anxiety, ADHD, and emotion regulation.

Mindfulness techniques include mindfulness meditation, body scan, and mindful breathing. Growing evidence suggests mindfulness-based interventions can improve attention, reduce anxiety, and enhance emotion regulation in young populations. These interventions also have an advantage over some psychotherapies as they do not require as extensive training and are effectively delivered through multimedia or the internet.

Dialectical Behavior Therapy (DBT)

DBT, developed initially for adults with borderline personality disorder, has been adapted for adolescents with emotion regulation difficulties and self-harming behaviors. It employs techniques such as mindfulness, distress tolerance, emotion regulation, and interpersonal effectiveness skills, which are core components. It has been used to treat suicidal ideation, self-harm, eating disorders, and borderline personality traits in adolescents.

Research has demonstrated DBT's significant effect, particularly in reducing self-harm behaviors and improving emotional regulation in adolescents.

Behavioral Therapy

Behavioral therapy modifies observable behaviors through learning theory and operant conditioning principles. Many therapies listed here employ aspects of behavioral therapy, including CBT and DBT. An example of a specific behavioral therapy is Applied Behavioral Analysis (ABA).

Applied Behavior Analysis (ABA). ABA is a therapeutic approach primarily used for children and adolescents with ASDs, though it has also shown efficacy for other developmental disabilities and behavioral disorders. ABA focuses on understanding and changing behavior by systematically applying learning principles.

The primary indication for ABA is ASD, which aims to enhance communication, social skills, learning, and adaptive behaviors while reducing problematic behaviors. The technique involves breaking down complex skills into smaller, manageable steps, and using positive reinforcement to encourage desired behaviors. ABA interventions are highly individualized, with trained therapists conducting detailed assessments to create tailored treatment plans. These plans often involve one-on-one intensive therapy sessions, sometimes up to 40 hours per week for young children with ASD.

The evidence base for ABA is robust, particularly for early intensive behavioral intervention in autism. Numerous studies have demonstrated significant improvements in cognitive functioning, language skills, adaptive behavior, and social skills in children who receive ABA therapy. Long-term studies have shown that many children who receive early intensive ABA interventions achieve higher levels of independence and better outcomes in adulthood. However, it is relevant to note that the intensity and approach of ABA therapy have been subjects of debate within the autism community, with some advocating for more naturalistic and developmental approaches.

Other Behavioral Techniques. Other behavioral approaches used in adults can be helpful for children. For example, exposure and response prevention are used for OCD. It involves practicing confronting the thoughts, images, objects, and situations that provoke obsessions. It uses the behavioral technique of desensitization, in which the patient practices with a manageable but anxiety-producing stimulus until it no longer triggers their ritualistic response. Once mastered, the patient moves to more distressing stimuli until they can master all or many aspects of their OCD.

Jenna was a 13-year-old teen with a family history of anxiety and depression. Her parents brought her to treatment because of recurrent obsessions involving contamination and germs, with corresponding compulsions during which she had convinced her parents to check her food while she washed her hands repeatedly until they became raw and bleeding. The evaluation revealed a fear that the meal would likely be contaminated unless her parents checked her food for bugs or germs. Jenna's parents, attempting to ease her anxiety, would physically pull apart her food and examine it to her satisfaction, often spending upward of 1 hour before each meal. However, this process caused much distress and discord between Jenna and her family. Jenna's hand washing had generalized to almost every daily activity—after opening a door, reading a book, using a pencil, or touching any object she deemed dirty. Jenna's evaluation led to a recommendation of behavioral therapy utilizing exposure and response prevention. This therapy consisted of formulating a hierarchy of her obsessions and compulsions, from the least upsetting (checking food prepared by her mother) to the most disturbing (touching something wet or slimy and then touching her mouth). Systematically, the therapist engaged Jenna first in a series of imaginal exposures to a scene (e.g., "you take a bite of hamburger, and something tastes gritty to you, and you realize that your mom did not check the burger") until her anxiety dropped to an acceptable level. The drop in anxiety typically took approximately 25 minutes. Next, the scene was enacted in vivo, whereby foods were introduced with "contaminants" in them (e.g., putting pieces of uncooked rice into the burger to mimic "grit"), and Jenna ate the food without having her parents check. As treatment progressed, Jenna learned that her chronic fear of becoming sick was not likely to occur.

Similarly, washing rituals were addressed by having her touch items with various substances coating them and then touching her face and mouth. Jenna's treatment entailed a 14-session program during which her parents were taught to assist her with these exposures in the home. Her parents were also instructed to refrain from engaging in her rituals. Relapse prevention plans were added to expand her range of food choices and situational contexts (cafeterias, food stands, restaurants) for exposure. By the end of treatment, Jenna was eating without the need for checking and with minimal anxiety. Moreover, she engaged in many activities without washing after touching each object. (Adapted from Anne Marie Albano, Ph.D.)

Interpersonal Therapy

Originally developed to treat depression in adults, Interpersonal Psychotherapy has been adopted to treat adolescents (Interpersonal Psychotherapy for Adolescents, or IPT-A). IPT-A focuses on improving interpersonal relationships and social functioning. It is mainly used for treating adolescent depression.

IPT-A frames psychological reactions in the context of our relationships with others. It addresses interpersonal challenges such as deficits, role transitions, grief, and interpersonal disputes.

Studies have shown IPT-A to be effective in reducing depressive symptoms and improving social functioning in adolescents.

Family Therapy

Family therapy involves working with the child or adolescent in the context of their family system. Various approaches exist, including structural family therapy, strategic family therapy, and attachment-based family therapy. It is used for a wide range of issues, including behavioral problems, eating disorders, substance abuse, and family conflicts.

As a whole, family therapy has shown positive outcomes in improving family functioning and reducing symptoms in children and adolescents, particularly for externalizing behaviors and substance use disorders.

Conceptual contributions from systems theory, communications theory, object relations theory, social role theory, ethology, and ecology have influenced family therapies. The core premise entails the idea of a family as a self-regulating, open system with a unique history and structure. This structure constantly evolves due to dynamic interaction between the family's mutually interdependent systems and persons who share complementary needs. Increasingly, appreciation of the family system sometimes explains why a minute therapeutic input at a critical junction may result in far-reaching changes.

Play Therapy

Play therapy is primarily used with younger children, allowing them to express and work through their emotions and experiences through play. It is used for trauma, anxiety, depression, and behavioral issues in young children.

Play therapy techniques include both nondirective play and directive play. It offers the benefit of being more engaging and meaningful for a young patient than standard face-to-face therapy. Often, during play, a child will feel more comfortable discussing painful issues with which they are dealing.

Although the choices of play material vary among therapists, the following equipment can constitute a well-balanced playroom or play area: multigenerational families of dolls of various races; dolls representing special roles and feelings, such as police officer, doctor, and soldier; dollhouse furnishings with or without a dollhouse; toy animals; puppets; paper, crayons, paint, and blunt-ended scissors; a sponge-like ball; clay or something comparable; tools such as rubber hammers, rubber knives, and guns; building blocks, cars, trucks, and airplanes; and eating utensils. The toys should enable children to communicate through play. Therapists should avoid fragile objects that can break easily, that can result in physical injury to a child, or that can increase a child's guilt.

Play therapy is supported by considerable research showing that it effectively improves emotional and behavioral problems in young children.

Psychodynamic Therapy

Psychodynamic psychotherapy for children and adolescents is an adaptation of adult psychoanalytic techniques tailored to address the developmental needs and challenges of younger individuals. This approach explores unconscious processes, early life experiences, and relationships to understand and treat emotional and behavioral issues. It is often indicated for children and adolescents experiencing anxiety, depression, trauma, attachment difficulties, and complex family dynamics.

The therapeutic technique differs depending on the child's age and stage of development. With younger children, the therapist may adapt techniques from play therapy, whereas more traditional talk therapy may be more appropriate for older children and adolescents,

While the supporting evidence for psychodynamic therapy in youth populations has historically been limited compared to other modalities, recent research has shown promising results. Several studies have demonstrated its effectiveness in reducing symptoms of anxiety and depression, improving social functioning, and enhancing overall psychological well-being in children and adolescents. However, more rigorous randomized controlled trials are needed to strengthen the evidence base for this approach in youth populations.

Supportive Psychotherapy. Supportive psychotherapy is a type of psychodynamic psychotherapy that tends to be more active and focused on the "here and now" rather than past conflicts. Techniques include psychoeducation for patients and family members, establishing realistic goals, and helping patients improve their adaptive skills by emphasizing healthy defenses against anxiety and stress.

Supportive psychotherapy is beneficial in enabling a well-adjusted youngster to cope with the emotional turmoil engendered by a crisis. It also is used to treat disturbances related to traumatic experiences, losses, mild mood disorders, and mild forms of anxiety.

A 6-year-old boy was brought for treatment because of long-standing severe aggression and destruction of property. In addition to an evaluation for medication, the child was seen in twice-weekly psychoanalytically oriented psychotherapy. The beginning sessions were marked by the repeated need to set limits and contain the child's aggressive behaviors. Two months into treatment, he began to pump himself up, roar, and announce that he was "the Incredible Hulk." He would then stomp around the play therapy room, attempting to destroy the toys. The therapist suggested, "You know you can't really *be* the Hulk. You can *pretend* you are the Hulk, and then maybe we can play this together." After several similar exchanges, the child gradually allowed the therapist to join the game. Over the next 6 months, the boy modulated his behavior to "play the part" of the Hulk without destroying property and limiting himself to less aggressive actions. He understood that he could pretend to be the Hulk without trying to be the Hulk. (Adapted from David L. Kaye, M.D.)

Summary. Psychotherapy offers a range of effective interventions for children and adolescents struggling with mental health issues. While CBT remains one of the most well-researched and widely applied approaches, other therapies such as DBT, family therapy, trauma-focused interventions, and behavioral and psychodynamic interventions have also demonstrated significant efficacy. The treatment choice should be tailored to the child's or adolescent's needs, considering factors such as age, specific diagnosis, and family context. Ongoing research continues to refine these approaches and develop new interventions to serve young populations' mental health needs.

Further Readings

Boaden K, Tomlinson A, Cortese S, Cipriani A. Antidepressants in children and adolescents: meta-review of efficacy, tolerability and suicidality in acute treatment. *Front Psychiatry*. 2020;11:717.

Carr A. Family therapy for adolescents: a research-informed perspective. *Aust N Z J Fam Ther*. 2016;37(4):467–479.

Cohen JA, Mannarino AP, Deblinger E. *Treating Trauma and Traumatic Grief in Children and Adolescents*. 2nd ed. Guilford Press; 2017.

Correll CU, Cortese S, Croatto G, et al. Efficacy and acceptability of pharmacological, psychosocial, and brain stimulation interventions in children and adolescents with mental disorders: an umbrella review. *World Psychiatry*. 2021;20(2):244–275.

Cortese S. Pharmacologic treatment of attention deficit-hyperactivity disorder. *N Engl J Med*. 2020;383(11):1050–1056.

Cortese S, Adamo N, Del Giovane C, et al. Comparative efficacy and tolerability of medications for attention-deficit hyperactivity disorder in children, adolescents, and adults: a systematic review and network meta-analysis. *Lancet Psychiatry*. 2018;5(9):727–738.

Dunning DL, Griffiths K, Kuyken W, et al. Research review: the effects of mindfulness-based interventions on cognition and mental health in children and adolescents—a meta-analysis of randomized controlled trials. *J Child Psychol Psychiatry*. 2019;60(3):244–258.

Fonagy P, Cottrell D, Phillips J, Bevington D, Glaser D, Allison E. *What Works for Whom? A Critical Review of Treatments for Children and Adolescents*. 2nd ed. Guilford Press; 2015.

Koelch M, Fegert JM. Ethics in child and adolescent psychiatric care: an international perspective. *Int Rev Psychiatry*. 2010;22(3):258–266.

Leigh E, Smith P, Milavic G, Stringaris A. Mood regulation in youth: research findings and clinical approaches to irritability and short-lived episodes of mania-like symptoms. *Curr Opin Psychiatry*. 2012; 25(4):271–276.

Lewis YD, Gallop L, Campbell IC, Schmidt U. Effects of non-invasive brain stimulation in children and young people with psychiatric disorders: a protocol for a systematic review. *Syst Rev*. 2021;10(1):76.

Locher C, Koechlin H, Zion SR, et al. Efficacy and safety of selective serotonin reuptake inhibitors, serotonin-norepinephrine reuptake inhibitors, and placebo for common psychiatric disorders among children and adolescents: a systematic review and meta-analysis. *JAMA Psychiatry*. 2017;74(10):1011–1020.

Mehlum L, Ramleth RK, Tørmoen AJ, et al. Long term effectiveness of dialectical behavior therapy versus enhanced usual care for adolescents with self-harming and suicidal behavior. *J Child Psychol Psychiatry*. 2019;60(10):1112–1122.

Oud M, de Winter L, Vermeulen-Smit E, et al. Effectiveness of CBT for children and adolescents with depression: a systematic review and meta-regression analysis. *Eur Psychiatry*. 2019;57:33–45.

Pataki C. Child psychiatry: psychiatric treatment. In: Boland RJ, Verduin ML, eds. *Kaplan & Sadock's Comprehensive Textbook of Psychiatry*. 11th ed. Wolters Kluwer, 2025.

Piacentini J, Bennett S, Compton SN, et al. 24- and 36-week outcomes for the Child/Adolescent Anxiety Multimodal Study (CAMS). *J Am Acad Child Adolesc Psychiatry*. 2014;53(3):297–310.

Pumariega AJ, Rothe E, Mian A, et al; American Academy of Child and Adolescent Psychiatry (AACAP) Committee on Quality Issues (CQI). Practice parameter for cultural competence in child and adolescent psychiatric practice. *J Am Acad Child Adolesc Psychiatry*. 2013;52(10):1101–1115.

Rith-Najarian LR, Mesri B, Park AL, Sun M, Chavira DA, Chorpita BF. Durability of cognitive behavioral therapy effects for youth and adolescents with anxiety, depression, or traumatic stress: a meta-analysis on long-term follow-ups. *Behav Ther*. 2019;50(1):225–240.

Scher S, Kozlowska K. *Rethinking Health Care Ethics*. Springer; 2018.

Solmi M, Fornaro M, Ostinelli EG, et al. Safety of 80 antidepressants, antipsychotics, anti-attention-deficit/hyperactivity medications and mood stabilizers in children and adolescents with psychiatric disorders: a large scale systematic meta-review of 78 adverse effects. *World Psychiatry*. 2020;19(2):214–232.

Strawn JR, Vaughn S, Ramsey LB. Pediatric psychopharmacology for depressive and anxiety disorders. *Focus (Am Psychiatr Publ)*. 2022; 20(2):184–190.

Tan JOA, Passerini GE, Stewart A. Consent and confidentiality in clinical work with young people. *Clin Child Psychol Psychiatry*. 2007;12(2):191–210.

Weersing VR, Jeffreys M, Do MT, Schwartz KTG, Bolano C. Evidence base update of psychosocial treatments for child and adolescent depression. *J Clin Child Adolesc Psychol*. 2017;46(1):11–43.

Weisz JR, Kuppens S, Ng MY, et al. What five decades of research tells us about the effects of youth psychological therapy: a multilevel meta-analysis and implications for science and practice. *Am Psychol*. 2017;72(2):79–117.

22 Special Areas of Interest

PEDIATRIC SLEEP DISORDERS

Sleep Evaluation Methods

One of the primary tools for studying sleep is *polysomnography* (PSG), which incorporates a variety of measures of physiologic changes experienced during sleep. The American Thoracic Society developed a set of recommendations for interpreting pediatric PSG that has become the standard for sleep labs nationally. With the aid of portable technology, PSG is increasingly being performed at home, although the methods and results are not quite as sophisticated as when performed in the lab. While PSG remains the gold standard for sleep studies, other less complicated and less expensive techniques are available for studying various sleep disorders in children and adolescents.

Actigraphy was developed in the early 1970s and has become increasingly used in research studies and clinical practice. Actigraphy allows for studying sleep–wake patterns and circadian rhythms by assessing body movements. The device is typically worn on the wrist and can easily be adapted for home use. With the advent of personal fitness trackers, manufacturers have increasingly been designing better algorithms for gathering data on sleep; however, these devices have shown high variability and many inaccuracies.

SLEEP DISORDERS IN CHILDREN

Approximately 25% of children will suffer from a sleep problem during childhood. The types of problems affecting children vary greatly in their frequency and severity, ranging from the more common bedtime resistance and anxiety to the occasional primary sleep disorders, such as narcolepsy and obstriuctive sleep apneas (OSAS). Regardless of the primary complaint, parents frequently report sleep difficulties among their children, and these reports are remarkably consistent with most researchers identifying up to 50% of preschool children, roughly 30% of school-aged children, and approximately 40% of adolescents as having sleep difficulties. Among a representative US sample of 13- to 16-year-olds, the 30-day prevalence of insomnia was 9.4%, and the lifetime prevalence was 10.7%; further, 88% of the adolescents with a lifetime history of insomnia reported current sleep difficulties, indicating the chronic nature of insomnia among youth. Much higher rates of sleep disorders are generally reported among those with neurodevelopmental and psychiatric disorders. Among children with intellectual disability, for example, 30% to 80% have sleep problems, while 50% to 90% of children with autism spectrum disorders (ASDs) are affected. Despite a high overall prevalence, however, sleep problems are not often discussed during visits with primary care practitioners and are therefore left undiagnosed and untreated.

Classification of Sleep Disorders

The *International Classification of Sleep Disorders*, Third Edition (ICSD-3), the *Diagnostic and Statistical Manual of Mental Disorders*, Fifth Edition (DSM-5), and its text revision (DSM-5-TR) are the primary classification systems for sleep disorders. While the ICSD-3 and the DSM-5-TR cover much of the same ground, the ICSD-3 classification is more comprehensive and precise. The DSM-5-TR specifies 12 main categories of sleep disorders.

Sleep-Disordered Breathing. The term sleep-disordered breathing (SDB) encapsulates a variety of difficulties, including primary snoring, upper airway resistance syndrome (UARS), and OSAS, and it occurs relatively frequently in otherwise healthy children. Although accurate figures are difficult to obtain, perhaps 2% to 5% of all children may be affected by OSAS, and 7% to 12% of children may suffer from primary snoring.

Whereas adults with OSAS most often present with *excessive daytime somnolence* (EDS), children rarely exhibit this symptom and instead tend to present with externalizing behaviors, such as hyperactivity, aggression, social withdrawal, and learning difficulties. In one study, fewer than 15% of children with OSAS exhibited EDS. Diagnosis of OSAS further requires a consistent clinical history and physical examination. Children should also undergo overnight PSG to augment these two diagnostic measures and reveal the extent of the effect on sleep.

Children with OSAS present with loud snoring, sweating, agitated sleep, and various related sleep problems (e.g., persistent enuresis, night terrors, somnambulism, bruxism). EDS, somnambulism, bruxism, and anxiety are also frequently noted in adolescents with OSAS. Physical examination often demonstrates craniofacial abnormalities and adenotonsillar hypertrophy, and PSG indicates frequent apneas/hypopneas and oxygen desaturations. Outcomes of OSAS can include significant health problems, such as failure to thrive, hypertension, pulmonary hypertension with or without cor pulmonale, and mental health problems.

The most common treatment for pediatric SDB is adenotonsillectomy, which cures the problem in approximately 85% of affected children. A continuous positive airway pressure (CPAP) mask is often used for children who fail surgical treatment or for whom surgery is not indicated.

Insomnia. Pediatric insomnia has been much less studied and is more poorly understood than adult insomnia.

The prevalence of pediatric insomnia is estimated at 1% to 6% among general pediatric populations, with a much higher prevalence in children with neurodevelopmental and chronic medical and psychiatric conditions. When including bedtime resistance and disruptive nighttime awakenings, the prevalence of sleep-disrupted behavior approaches 25% to 50% in preschool-aged children. Psychiatric symptoms exist in almost 50% of children with persistent insomnia. Persistent insomnia may also represent an early sign of emotional distress in susceptible children with poorly preserved sleep homeostasis.

The ICSD-3 describes two forms of behavioral insomnia in childhood as unique diagnostic entities to emphasize sleep difficulties that result from inappropriate sleep associations or inadequate parental limit setting. *Limit-setting type* is due to parents having difficulties establishing and enforcing bedtimes. In contrast, the *sleep-onset association type* is characterized by reliance on maladaptive and inappropriate sleep associations such as rocking, watching television, feeding, and falling asleep in the parents' bed. The child usually cannot fall asleep in the absence of these conditions at both bedtime and following nocturnal arousals. Behavioral insomnia generally leads to sleep fragmentation, increased nighttime awakenings, insufficient sleep duration, later bedtimes, and daytime sleepiness.

Good sleep hygiene and behavioral interventions, such as extinction or bedtime fading, are the first recommended treatments for pediatric insomnia. Children who do not respond to behavioral interventions may be considered for the pharmacologic management of their insomnia. There are no US Food and Drug Administration (FDA)–approved medications for treating insomnia in children. Nonetheless, a large study of over 1,000 child and adolescent psychiatrists found that 96% recommended at least one prescription medication, and 88% advised an over-the-counter medication for sleep in a typical month. Despite the lack of FDA approval, however, limited empirical evidence supports the use of melatonin and clonidine for childhood insomnia. Meanwhile, benzodiazepines, guanfacine, pyrimidine derivatives (e.g., zaleplon and zolpidem), sedating antidepressants (e.g., trazodone and mirtazapine), sedating antipsychotics (e.g., quetiapine), and sedating antihistamines (e.g., diphenhydramine, doxylamine, and hydroxyzine) are often employed to improve symptoms of insomnia in children and adolescents but have virtually no solid evidence to support their use.

Coincident with the increasing use of herbal medications and dietary supplements in the United States, several studies have been conducted over the last decade that demonstrate that melatonin is an effective, safe, and well-tolerated agent, especially in cases of sleep-initiation insomnia caused by circadian factors. Several placebo-controlled studies of melatonin in normal, healthy children with idiopathic sleep-initiation insomnia have shown that melatonin administered at bedtime reduces sleep-onset latency time and increases total sleep time (TST).

Little information is available on the use of the nonbenzodiazepine hypnotic agents zaleplon and ramelteon, but studies have found both zolpidem and eszopiclone ineffective for attention-deficit/hyperactivity disorder (ADHD)-related insomnia. In addition, hypnogogic hallucinations and paradoxical agitation may occur when youths receive adult doses of these agents. More safety trials and pharmacokinetic studies are needed prior to recommending these drugs for use in pediatric insomnia.

Cognitive-behavioral therapy for insomnia (CBT-I) is the most effective treatment in adults for decreasing sleep latency and the frequency and duration of nighttime awakenings, improving sleep quality, and increasing TST. CBT-I incorporates several evidence-based psychological and behavioral strategies, including stimulus control (e.g., removing clocks from the bedroom, maintaining a quiet sleep environment), sleep restriction (e.g., limiting the amount of time in bed until the patient is sleeping 90% of the time they are in bed), arousal reduction (e.g., relaxation techniques such as belly breathing and biofeedback), addressing cognitive distortions associated with insomnia (e.g., catastrophizing such as "if I don't fall asleep soon, I'll be a complete wreck tomorrow"), circadian rhythm maintenance (e.g., going to bed and awakening at the same time each day), and sleep education and hygiene. Patients accept CBT-I well; 70% to 80% achieve a therapeutic response, while 40% achieve clinical remission. Numerous randomized studies of adults demonstrate that CBT-I is even more effective for insomnia than sleep medications and that it is equally effective whether delivered one-on-one, in a group setting, or via the internet.

Although most studies of CBT-I have focused on adults, recent research demonstrates its efficacy among pediatric populations as well. Reductions in sleep latency and wake after sleep onset, along with increased sleep efficiency among children and adolescents, have been demonstrated to last at least 6 months posttreatment. In addition, the first randomized controlled trial of CBT-I in adolescents found a medium to large effect size.

While sleep hygiene is typically recommended by practitioners, sleep hygiene alone is not sufficiently effective for treating pediatric sleep difficulties. Discontinuing exposure to blue light via screens for an hour or two before sleep, limiting caffeine, alcohol, and drugs (such as marijuana and nicotine), and creating a comfortable sleep environment with limited light and noise while being judicious about the timing of exercise, are, however, valid sleep hygiene strategies that can augment the utility of CBT-I.

Narcolepsy. Significant strides in the understanding of the etiology of narcolepsy have been taken in recent years as remarkable discoveries have identified a new neuropeptide, hypocretin or orexin, which is linked to animal models of narcolepsy. The exact prevalence of childhood narcolepsy is unknown. The youngest patient on record was age 12 months. In retrospective studies, about one-third of adults with narcolepsy indicate onset prior to 15 years of age and roughly 15% prior to 10 years of age.

Children with narcolepsy are commonly misdiagnosed with other neurologic or psychiatric disorders, such as epilepsy, ADHD, mood disorders, and psychotic disorders. Excessive daytime sleepiness is the most common presentation of narcolepsy in school-aged children, although according to some reports, 50% to 70% of childhood narcolepsy patients present with symptoms of cataplexy. Nighttime sleep is frequently disturbed in patients with narcolepsy, and periodic limb movements during sleep are also common. The diagnosis of narcolepsy requires sleep laboratory assessment, including nocturnal PSG and a multiple sleep latency test.

Effective treatment of narcolepsy in children and adolescents demands establishing a regular sleep schedule, providing extensive education on sleep hygiene, and implementing scheduled daytime naps if possible. Excessive daytime sleepiness in children and adolescents with narcolepsy is commonly treated with psychostimulants such as methylphenidate and dextroamphetamine. Modafinil and armodafinil are alertness-promoting medications that can provide long-lasting benefits and are effective in pediatric patients with narcolepsy.

Tricyclic antidepressants such as clomipramine, protriptyline, and imipramine have long been known to be effective for symptoms of cataplexy. Serotonin-specific reuptake inhibitors and mixed-action antidepressants are used for patients with cataplexy. Sodium oxybate (Xyrem) and calcium, magnesium, potassium, and sodium oxybate in combination (Xywav) have been recently approved by the FDA for pediatric use and are effective for the treatment of excessive daytime sleepiness and cataplexy associated with narcolepsy.

Due to the complexity of narcolepsy symptoms and their effect on child development, a variety of treatment modalities, including individual and family therapy, school advocacy, and academic interventions, should be used to optimize symptom control.

Parasomnias. Parasomnias are disruptive physical acts that occur during specific sleep stages or the transition between sleep stages and include non-REM types (somnambulism and sleep terrors), REM sleep behavior disorder, somniloquy, bruxism, nightmares, and restless leg syndrome (RLS). Although the incidence of general psychopathology in children with non-REM sleep parasomnias is relatively low, the overall prevalence of having at least one parasomnia by age 13 years may be as high as 78%. Although rarely requiring clinical intervention, the events are often very troubling for parents.

SOMNAMBULISM. Somnambulism, or sleepwalking, is relatively common in childhood, with annual prevalence rates approaching 17%. Although somnambulism rarely results in harm to the subject, an episode of somnambulism can become a confusional arousal, in which the likelihood of accidental violence (to oneself or others) is much greater. The prevalence of confusional arousal is less well established, although a 4% incidence was noted in a longitudinal study of 212 children ages 6 to 16 years selected randomly in Stockholm.

SLEEP TERRORS. Sleep terrors are somewhat less common than somnambulism and are challenging to quantify because of the self-report nature of the data and the fact that parents often confuse them with nightmares. Annual incidence rates are as high as 6%, and prevalence rates are as high as 17% among children aged 13 years and younger. Parents of affected children first notice most non-REM parasomnias. However, a large percentage of children have at least one incidence of somnambulism and far fewer present with recurrent and disruptive somnambulism. Sleep terrors follow a similar trend but are less common than sleepwalking. Numerous studies have demonstrated a connection between anxiety levels and parasomnias in children, showing that increased anxiety correlates with an increased prevalence of sleepwalking and sleep terrors.

Although the treatment of non-REM parasomnias has received minimal formal study, numerous measures are effective. In addition to safety measures, the use of scheduled awakenings and naps, and in severe cases, clonazepam or tricyclic antidepressants, may be effective. In addition, a formal sleep study may help reveal SDB as a comorbid disorder for which treatment may reduce the apparent severity of the parasomnia.

SLEEP TALKING. Sleep talking or *somniloquy* is considered the most common parasomnia, with a reported prevalence of greater than 50% in children between the ages of 3 and 13 years. Somniloquy is often comorbid with sleepwalking and sleep terrors, suggesting a common pathophysiology among the three disorders. Nightmares are common among children and adolescents and are only considered abnormal when they are recurrent and cause excessive distress. Although sometimes associated with posttraumatic stress disorder (PTSD), up to 70% of children report that the content of their nightmares is influenced by media seen on television or at the movies. Effective treatment for nightmares generally includes cognitive-behavioral therapy (CBT) and rescripting but can also include hypnotherapy and medication. REM sleep behavior disorder, in which subjects become aroused during REM sleep and "act out" their dreams due to loss of body paralysis, is not generally observed in children and is more closely associated with brain damage and dementia.

RESTLESS LEG SYNDROME (RLS). RLS is an irresistible urge to move the legs, commonly associated with discomfort and pain, partially relieved by movement. In the adult population, RLS has an estimated 10% to 15% prevalence. Periodic limb movement disorder (PLMD), no longer classified by DSM-5-TR, is characterized by episodic limb movements during sleep, generally involving the leg and the ankle and toe extension.

Only recently has the presence of RLS in children and adolescents been elucidated, with studies generally demonstrating a prevalence rate of RLS among the general pediatric population to average around 2%. There is considerable interest in the relationship between RLS, PLMD, and ADHD. The prevalence of RLS in patients with ADHD is estimated to be between 10.5% and 44%, emphasizing the need to consider both diagnoses and the possible interrelationship between them in children and adolescents.

Prior to the diagnosis of RLS, a child often presents with sleep disturbances and daytime impairments, including extreme fatigue, irritability, and hyperactivity, and the discomfort in the extremities that accompanies the disorder is often confused with growing pains. Other qualitative signs suggestive of RLS include an urge to move the legs with a worsening sensation when sitting or lying down, the alleviation of discomfort through movement, and worsening symptoms in the evening. Several studies have demonstrated an autosomal-dominant inheritance for early-onset RLS. Family history, therefore, is a critical indicating factor in diagnosing RLS in children and adolescents.

Most treatments for RLS/PLMD include a pharmacologic component, although proper sleep hygiene is also crucial. Children and adolescents with RLS/PLMD should reduce caffeine intake, eliminate alcohol and tobacco use, avoid stimulating activities prior to bedtime, and minimize sleep deprivation. Low ferritin levels, iron deficiency, and RLS symptoms appear to correlate in both children and adults. Providing ferrous sulfate supplementation for deficient children has been demonstrated to reduce PLMD symptoms. Other medications have also demonstrated efficacy in reducing symptoms. One randomized, double-blind, placebo-controlled study of children with RLS aged 7 to 12 years found a combination of carbidopa/L-DOPA safe and effective. In adults with RLS, dopaminergic medications, including levodopa, pramipexole, and ropinirole, are most often used. Gabapentin may also improve RLS symptoms in children. Although these medications are prescribed to children and can be effective in reducing symptoms, the FDA has not approved these for the treatment of RLS/PLMD in children. As a result, clinicians should administer the medications cautiously and intensively monitor for potential side effects.

CIRCADIAN RHYTHM SLEEP–WAKE DISORDERS. Circadian rhythm sleep–wake disorders occur due to a misalignment between the internal circadian rhythm and the sleep–wake schedule. Over 10% of children are affected by circadian rhythm sleep problems. Delayed sleep phase type occurs in as many as 5% to 10% of adolescents, while advanced sleep phase type is more common in old adults and occasionally in preschool children.

A delay in the normal sleep phase is typical in the peripubertal period, leading to later bedtimes. Extensive homework and extracurricular obligations coupled with early school start times frequently result in excessive daytime sleepiness, academic difficulties, irritability, mood instability, attention and memory impairment, and family conflict. Recognizing the detrimental effects of delayed sleep phase on adolescents, the American Academy of Pediatrics (AAP) has published a policy statement urging a delay in the school start time so that high school students can achieve adequate sleep.

Treatment of delayed sleep phase typically involves sleep education, hygiene, and gradual advancement of the sleep phase. Bright light morning therapy (5,000 to 10,000 lux), along with low-dose melatonin (approximately 500 mcg) about 4 to 5 hours before the desired bedtime, have both been found helpful in advancing the sleep phase after several weeks. Chronotherapy, or the gradual delay in bedtime by 3 hours each night until achieving the desired bedtime, can also be effective, although the schedule is challenging to maintain.

NOCTURNAL ENURESIS. Although no longer classified by DSM-5-TR as a sleep–wake disorder, *nocturnal enuresis* is a frequent occurrence, affecting approximately 30% of 4-year-olds, 10% of 6-year-olds, 5% of 10-year-olds, 3% of 12-year-olds, and 1% of individuals aged 15 years or older. *Primary nocturnal enuresis* (never consistently dry at night) is likely to have a multifactorial etiology and may be due to difficulties with bladder musculature stability, central nervous system arousability, pontine reflex function, internal sphincter tone, functional bladder capacity, nocturnal urine production, and a maturational delay in antidiuretic hormone (ADH) secretion. *Secondary nocturnal enuresis* (previously dry for at least 6 months), by contrast, is typically caused by urinary tract infections, diabetes mellitus, and psychological factors.

Behavioral treatment most commonly involves using an enuretic alarm, which has the highest cure and lowest relapse rates. Other behavioral interventions include bladder training to increase the number of micturitions during the day or to enlarge bladder capacity. The use of reward systems, such as star charts, has also been shown to be helpful. Finally, cognitive therapy (e.g., explaining the enuretic process and maintaining a daily diary), motivational therapy, pelvic floor muscle training, and biofeedback also have some reported utility.

The two medications most commonly accepted as an appropriate pharmacologic treatment for pediatric nocturnal enuresis are desmopressin acetate and imipramine. The use of amitriptyline and anticholinergic agents, such as oxybutynin and tolterodine, however, has also been described.

Sleep Disorders in Children with Psychiatric Disorders

Sleep problems often occur in the context of mental illness, either as primary concerns (e.g., primary insomnia) or secondary concerns (e.g., as a consequence of depression or anxiety). All sleep problems identified early in childhood correlate with anxiety, depression, attentional difficulties, family or parental distress, continued sleep problems, aggression, delinquency, and social problems.

Attention-Deficit/Hyperactivity Disorder. Numerous studies based on parent reports have demonstrated the prevalence of sleep disorders among children with ADHD to be higher than that for healthy controls, controls with other psychiatric illnesses, and healthy sibling controls by up to fivefold. Actigraphy has shown children with ADHD to have greater variation in sleep onset time, wake time, and single-night sleep duration than controls, and in at least one study, there were significantly more bedtime struggles and longer total sleep duration in the ADHD group. Although children with ADHD often have difficulty settling down to sleep and may sleep more total hours than controls, restricting the amount of sleep a child receives in an experimental setting can also result in symptoms of ADHD, including inattention, hyperactivity, impulsivity, and poor cognitive performance.

ADHD is also associated with snoring during sleep. Habitual snoring is three times more common in children with ADHD than in control children drawn from child psychiatry and pediatric clinics. In addition, children with ADHD have a greater frequency of PLMD while maintaining normal sleep architecture. Children with ADHD also suffer from SDB at a greater rate than expected. SDB is associated with poor memory performance on standardized psychometric tests and lower academic achievement in children.

Children with ADHD may also suffer circadian rhythm abnormalities. Among children with ADHD, there is greater inconsistency or instability in time to sleep onset, wake time, and sleep duration than in controls. Furthermore, there is a high prevalence of ADHD among children with chronic sleep-onset insomnia, and sleep-onset insomnia in children with ADHD is associated with later dim-light melatonin release. The use of melatonin near bedtime often improves sleep-onset delay among children with ADHD.

Fragmented or disrupted sleep, rather than lessened TST, may be the culprit behind some children's daytime behavioral changes and disruptions. To that end, recommendations to families with a disruptive or hyperactive child should emphasize basic sleep hygiene. Many children with ADHD take medication regularly, which can further complicate an understanding of their sleep cycle. Much investigation, however, has suggested that children with ADHD still demonstrate more sleep disturbances than controls regardless of medication use, particularly sleep-onset latency, sleep efficiency, and TST.

Opinions vary greatly on how to manage insomnia due to either ADHD or stimulant medications. Typical recommendations include lowering the dose of the stimulant, changing to a shorter-acting preparation, adding a low dose of stimulant (if the insomnia is believed to be secondary to hyperactive "rebound"), or changing to an entirely different stimulant or treatment, such as atomoxetine. If using adjunctive pharmacotherapy, typical medications include melatonin, clonidine, antihistamines (e.g., diphenhydramine, cyproheptadine), and antidepressants (e.g., trazodone, mirtazapine).

Autism Spectrum Disorders. Children with ASDs are also susceptible to sleep difficulties, with prevalence estimates ranging as high as 90%. Younger children and those with more severe cognitive or intellectual disabilities tend to demonstrate increased sleep problems, which often persist over time. The most frequently reported sleep problems among those with ASD include difficulty falling asleep, restless sleep, frequent awakenings with difficulty falling back to sleep, early-morning awakenings, irregular sleep–wake patterns, shortened duration of sleep, dyssomnias, and parasomnias.

Numerous hypotheses exist to explain the reported sleep difficulties among children with ASD, including failure to recognize environmental and social cues, poorly developed circadian rhythms secondary to social deficits, altered melatonin production, and abnormalities in the hypothalamic–pituitary–adrenal axis and serotonin systems. Many treatments have been proposed for children with ASD with comorbid sleep difficulties.

Various behavioral treatments have been used with varying success in the ASD population. Most favorably, the use of proper sleep hygiene techniques, stimulus control, graduated extinction, scheduled awakenings, and daytime nap restriction have all shown utility among children with autism and intellectual disability. Light therapy, in combination with chronotherapy, may also be helpful in children with autism who have circadian rhythm abnormalities. Pharmacologic treatments also have proven to be useful for many, but not all, children with ASD.

Various prescribed medications have reported utility in the treatment of sleep difficulties in the ASD population, including antihistamines, sedating antidepressants, α-2 agonists, benzodiazepines, and antipsychotics. Melatonin has also demonstrated utility in treating children with neurodevelopmental disabilities and autism.

Mood Disorders. Sleep complaints are among the most prevalent symptoms of major depression in children and perhaps the most prevalent symptom among adolescents. Insomnia affects nearly 90% of depressed adolescents, whereas *hypersomnia* affects a considerably smaller proportion, perhaps around 25%. Some adolescents—around 10%—continue to experience insomnia even after the remission of depression. The use of actigraphy in diagnosing sleep problems among depressed children and adolescents highlights the compromised sleep quality and abnormal circadian rhythms these individuals experience while depressed. PSG studies in children with depression often demonstrate decreased REM latencies, increased total REM, and increased sleep-onset time. A recent meta-analysis of PSG characteristics among children and adolescents with major depression demonstrated that increased sleep-onset latency was collectively the strongest PSG marker of depression in youth.

Several large prospective population-based and cross-sectional studies have been conducted in the past decade among adolescents, demonstrating a strong association between sleep problems and suicidality. There is a close relationship between sleep problems and suicide attempts in adolescents who have already engaged in nonsuicidal self-injury. A curvilinear dose–response was observed such that those adolescents with reported TST of 8 to 9 hours per night had the lowest risk for suicidal ideation and attempts. Insufficient sleep duration has emerged as one of the most salient risk factors for suicidality, illustrating the importance of sleep screening as part of a suicide assessment.

Many children who are, or will be, diagnosed with bipolar disorder present with sleep-related symptoms. When depressed, these children may experience exhaustion, distractibility, irritability, and impulsivity at levels significantly greater than at baseline. In contrast, children experiencing mania may have unusual amounts of energy and a decreased need for sleep. Such extremes of sleep behavior warrant clinical assessment.

Seasonal affective disorder (SAD) has a reported prevalence of 3% to 4% in children and adolescents, for whom more than 20% of their parents report that their children are sleepier and generally more tired during the winter months. Studies of children with a diagnosis of SAD have found that they did not differ from controls in the level of nocturnal activity but did experience significantly lower diurnal activity levels and had less robust circadian rhythms, with a reduction in amplitude.

There have been a small number of studies examining the effects of pharmacologic and behavioral interventions in depressed children and adolescents suffering from sleep problems. A combination of improved sleep hygiene and CBT is effective in managing the insomnia and awakenings associated with depression. In those cases that require further treatment, the most effective drug therapy appears to be a combination of an antidepressant with the short-term use of a sedative or hypnotic. As noted previously, however, some children and adolescents experience a paradoxical reaction to these medications, which severely limits their utility.

Anxiety Disorders. Although it is difficult to establish causality between early sleep problems and the later onset of anxiety and depression, it is clear that anxiety and sleep problems are intimately connected in childhood and that the presence of a sleep problem at age 4 years is significantly correlated with the development of depression and anxiety by age 15 years. Fears at nighttime are common among children, with up to 75% of those aged 4 to 12 years reporting such fears, which generally take the form of animals, fictitious characters (e.g., witches, monsters), being kidnapped, or being teased by peers. Although no specific numbers are available, for the majority of children with DSM-5-TR anxiety disorders, sleep problems typically follow. In addition to the aforementioned concerns, anxiety likely predisposes children to parasomnias and nightmares.

The effects of anxiety on sleep are profound, and the clinical presentation depends mainly on the specific disorder. Individuals with *generalized anxiety disorder* (GAD) have a wide range of sleep disturbances, which can include insomnia and hypersomnia. These GAD sleep symptoms may be due to central nervous system hypervigilance and hyperarousal, so the individual cannot relax sufficiently to fall asleep and maintain good sleep quality. Patients with panic disorder tend to present with insomnia, restless and fragmented sleep, and nocturnal panic attacks. These symptoms often result in trouble initiating and maintaining sleep, increased sleep latency, and reduced sleep efficiency.

Posttraumatic Stress Disorder (PTSD). Children and adolescents with PTSD may experience significant sleep difficulties. Individuals with PTSD often have trouble initiating sleep and experience significant nighttime arousals and disruptive nightmares. Because children with PTSD may have flashbacks to their traumatic experiences, bedtime can become a stressful time in which they experience increased anxiety and are unable to relax sufficiently for restful sleep. The accompanying nightmares, which are a characteristic symptom of PTSD, and increased limb movements, which are associated with nightmares, lead to disrupted REM sleep.

Some research suggests that early trauma may exert a sustained impact on sleep persisting into adulthood. Bader and colleagues demonstrated that childhood trauma was the strongest predictor of delayed sleep-onset latency, poor sleep efficiency, and high nocturnal activity during adult years, even after controlling for stress and depression. Similar data has been derived from studying sleep in females who experienced sexual abuse as children, suggesting that traumatic exposures, more so than a diagnosis of PTSD per se, are closely associated with persistent sleep disturbances.

Cognitive and behavioral techniques, systematic desensitization, and imagery rehearsal therapy have demonstrated efficacy in decreasing nightmares and are integral parts of treating the sleep disturbances accompanying obsessive-compulsive disorder (OCD), PTSD, and GAD. CBT, along with systematic desensitization, has been demonstrated to improve the sleep disturbances associated with OCD. In particularly severe cases, serotonin-specific reuptake inhibitors such as fluoxetine, sertraline, and paroxetine further aid in the reduction of symptoms. Children and adolescents with PTSD generally have a complex constellation of symptoms, and the primary psychiatric diagnosis must be treated first before the sleep disturbances will resolve. CBT and play or expressive therapies, in which the children process the traumatic events triggering the PTSD, are very effective, and antidepressants and anxiolytics may hasten the recovery process in combination with other therapies.

CHILD MALTREATMENT

Child maltreatment is pervasive across all socioeconomic classes, races, ethnic groups, and religions. Although the federal government and every state have programs to investigate allegations of abuse, prevent abuse, and educate caregivers, the cases that are reported and substantiated are just the tip of the iceberg of the true prevalence of child maltreatment.

A diverse group of professionals—including child and adolescent psychiatrists, psychologists, social workers, law enforcement, school personnel, pediatricians, dentists, emergency department (ED) workers, and other mental health professionals—are mandated to report suspected child maltreatment.

DEFINITIONS

DSM-5-TR

The somewhat terse classification system provided by the *Diagnostic And Statistical Manual Of Mental Disorders, Fifth Edition, Text Revision* (DSM-5-TR) lists *child physical abuse, child sexual abuse, child neglect, and child psychological abuse*. The four conditions appear in the chapter "Other Conditions That May Be a Focus of Clinical Attention" and in the section "Abuse and Neglect." These categories apply when the focus of clinical attention is the severe mistreatment of one individual by another. Evaluators can distinguish each type of maltreatment: confirmed abuse from suspected abuse; an initial encounter from a subsequent encounter; parental abuse from nonparental abuse; whether the abuse previously occurred during the person's childhood, and whether the mental health services are for the perpetrator of parental or nonparental abuse.

Federal Law

The Child Abuse Prevention and Treatment Act (CAPTA) was passed in 1974 and has been amended several times, most recently in January 2019, by the Victims of Child Abuse Act Reauthorization Act of 2018. In federal law, *child abuse and neglect* mean, as a minimum, any recent act or failure to act on the part of a parent or caretaker that results in death, serious physical or emotional harm, sexual abuse or exploitation, or an act or failure to act which presents an imminent risk of serious harm. In federal law, *sexual abuse* means the employment, use, persuasion, inducement, enticement, or coercion of any child to engage in or to assist any other person to engage in any sexually explicit conduct or simulation of such conduct to produce a visual depiction of such conduct. CAPTA further expands the legal definition of child sexual abuse to include the following terms: rape (and in cases of caretaker or familial relationships, statutory rape), molestation, incest, and prostitution. CAPTA was also most recently amended to include other forms of sexual exploitation of children and victims of sex trafficking.

State Law

A large mass of legal definitions and statutes exist at the state level. The legal definitions of terms related to the maltreatment of children vary from one jurisdiction to another, so clinicians should be aware of their state statutes, with a particular focus on mandatory reporting laws, corporal punishment laws, and the legal age of consent.

Medical Diagnoses

Child maltreatment is a unique area of medicine where the medical diagnosis and legal findings overlap. For this reason, legal definitions and statutes inform the diagnoses. However, the diagnosis of child maltreatment in the clinical setting is independent of the investigative process and is determined based on the medical provider's level of concern for maltreatment. There are also variations in terminology used between the medical and legal fields.

Child Neglect

The most prevalent form of child maltreatment, *child neglect,* is a failure to provide or supervise children and includes acts of commission or omission. Neglect can fall into several categories, including the following:

1. Physical neglect, such as abandonment
2. Nutritional neglect
3. Medical neglect
4. Inadequate supervision
5. Emotional neglect
6. Educational neglect

Neglect may also be chronic, where an individual incident of neglect may not appear harmful, but multiple incidents over time create a negative impact on the child.

Child Physical Abuse

As described above, the minimum definition of *child physical abuse* involves an act on the part of a child's caretaker that results in death, serious physical harm, or imminent risk of serious harm. In the clinical setting, child physical abuse may present with a wide range of symptoms, from subtle bruising on a nonmobile infant to abusive head trauma resulting in long-term disability or death. Determining the level of concern for child physical abuse in the clinical setting depends on several factors, including the constellation of symptoms and injuries, the history provided to explain these injuries, and the developmental capabilities of the child. If there is no history provided to explain the injuries, if the history provided is implausible to explain them, if the child is developmentally incapable of causing the injuries, or if abuse is disclosed, witnessed, or confessed, this warrants a report to the local child protective services and consideration of additional medical evaluation.

Corporal punishment, or physical discipline, includes acts such as spanking or paddling. Each state differs in its laws regarding corporal punishment at home and school. Regardless of state law regarding the use of corporal punishment, if the discipline resulted in serious physical harm or imminent risk of physical harm, it should be considered child physical abuse and reported as such.

Abusive head trauma is a specific type of child physical abuse with potentially long-lasting neurocognitive and mental health impacts related to intracranial injuries and abuse. Medical providers are strongly discouraged from using the term "shaken baby syndrome," as this inappropriately focuses on one specific possible mechanism of injury instead of the abuse itself.

Child Psychological Abuse

Child psychological abuse is a pattern of intentional verbal or behavioral actions or lack of actions that conveys to a child that they are worthless, flawed, unloved, unwanted, or endangered. Child psychological abuse includes the following categories: spurning, rejection or degradation, terrorizing, exploiting or corrupting, denying emotional responsiveness, and isolation. The severity of psychological abuse depends on (1) whether the perpetrator intends to inflict harm on the child and (2) whether the abusive behaviors are likely to cause harm to the child. In contentious divorces, one of the parents may indoctrinate the child to fear or dislike the other parent, thus causing parental alienation between the child and the rejected parent. Depending on the circumstances, one or more of these DSM-5 terms may identify parental alienation: child psychological abuse, parent–child relational problem, or child affected by parental relationship distress.

Child Sexual Abuse

The AAP defines child sexual abuse as occurring when a child is engaged in sexual activities that they cannot comprehend, for which they are developmentally unprepared and cannot give consent, or that violate the law or social taboos of society. Recent definitions and laws have expanded to include children who are victims of human trafficking and internet crimes against children, such as child pornography. State laws vary significantly regarding the age of consent, definitions of terms such as penetration, and timing for evidence collection related to an acute sexual assault. Inappropriate sexual contact with a child can include kissing, fondling, digital–genital, orogenital, genital–genital, and anogenital contact. The vast majority of child sexual abuse is perpetrated in the home by a close household family member.

Children commonly engage in sexualized behaviors with themselves or with other children, described as "sexual play" that is spontaneous, intermittent, mutual, and noncoercive. Normal sexualized behaviors typically include acts such as self-stimulation and voyeurism. It is essential to recognize that these behaviors may be distressing to caregivers but are not an indication that child sexual abuse has occurred. Reassurance and education regarding these behaviors are frequently all that is needed when they present. Sexualized behaviors become problematic when they cross socially unacceptable boundaries, become coercive or aggressive, or represent an early onset of adult sexual activity. When the behaviors become problematic, further interventions to extinguish the behaviors and evaluation for possible child maltreatment may be indicated.

COMPARATIVE NOSOLOGY

The tenth edition of the ICD (ICD-10, Version 2007) has a slightly different way of organizing child maltreatment diagnoses. The ICD-10 has a chapter titled "Injury, Poisoning and Certain Other Consequences of External Causes" and a section titled "Other and Unspecified Effects of External Causes." Within that section is a heading for "Maltreatment Syndrome," which includes the following diagnoses: neglect or abandonment; physical abuse; sexual abuse; psychological abuse; other maltreatment syndromes; and maltreatment syndrome, unspecified. The ICD-10-CM (Clinical Modification) includes codes that enhance the specificity of the abuse or neglect diagnosis. For example, the abuse can be either *suspected* or *confirmed,* and the type of encounter can be either *initial* or *subsequent*.

The 11th edition of the ICD (ICD-11, Version 2019) has a chapter entitled "External Causes of Morbidity or Mortality." Maltreatment is a subsection in this chapter and encompasses physical, sexual, psychological, specified, and unspecified categories. This version of the ICD no longer includes the section "Maltreatment Syndrome." ICD provides extension codes to add details to defined categories. The codes include abandonment and neglect. Under the "Factors Influencing Health Status or Contact With Health Services" chapter, there is coding for personal history of physical, sexual, and psychological abuse and neglect in addition to unspecified and specified history of maltreatment.

EPIDEMIOLOGY

Each year, the Children's Bureau, an agency within the Department of Health and Human Services, collects data on child maltreatment and publishes the results in the document *Child Maltreatment*. The agency estimated that, in 2018, child protective services received approximately 4.3 million reports with concern for abuse or neglect involving 7.8 million children, and 678,000 reports were substantiated. 1.3 million children received postresponse services, and over 200,000 children were placed into foster care. Of the substantiated cases, 61% were for neglect, 11% for physical abuse, 7% for sexual abuse, and 15.5% for multiple types of abuse and neglect. The Children's Bureau estimated that 1,770 children died as a result of maltreatment in 2018, which is more than an 11% increase from the 2014 estimate. Approximately 47% of these deaths were children younger than 1 year of age, and boys (2.87 per 100,000) had a higher fatality rate than girls (2.19 per 100,000).

The data were analyzed for patterns of maltreatment by the sex, age, and race or ethnicity of victims. The age group from 0 to 1 years of age had the highest victimization rate (26.7 per 1,000 children), with the rate of victimization decreasing with increasing age of the victim. The majority of identified child victims were either White (44.5%), Hispanic (22.6%), or African American (20.6%). American Indian or Alaska Native children had the highest rate at 15.2 per 1,000 children, and African American children had the second highest rate at 14.0 per 1,000.

RISK FACTORS

Characteristics of a child that may be risk factors for maltreatment include age less than 4 years old, prematurity, emotional/behavioral difficulties, physical disabilities, and unplanned or unwanted pregnancy. Risk factors associated with caregiver and family characteristics include substance abuse, parental mental illness, lack of understanding of the child's needs or developmental capabilities, caregiver history of child abuse or neglect, and young parental age. Additional family characteristics that are often associated with child maltreatment are low caregiver educational achievement, low caregiver socioeconomic status (SES), single parenthood, a large number of children in the home, nonbiologic caregivers, and domestic violence in the home. Community and societal risk factors include community violence, concentrated neighborhood disadvantages, poverty, and social isolation. These factors may be challenging to identify and assess. It is also essential to be aware of the unconscious bias identification of these risk factors may create, as their presence does not mean abuse or neglect had to have occurred, nor does their absence mean abuse or neglect did not occur. These factors must be considered in the overall context of the individual case. Community and societal factors that may protect a child are a strong extended family and social support system.

DIAGNOSIS AND CLINICAL FEATURES

Physically Abused Children

Abused children display behaviors that should arouse the suspicions of the health professional. For example, these children may be unusually fearful, docile, distrustful, and guarded. However, they may be disruptive and aggressive. They may be wary of physical contact and show no expectation of being comforted by adults, they may be on the alert for danger and continually size up the environment, and they may be afraid to go home.

The literature regarding the psychological consequences of physical abuse and neglect indicates a wide range of effects: affect dysregulation, insecure and atypical attachment patterns, impaired peer relationships involving increased aggression or social withdrawal, and academic underachievement. Physically abused children exhibit a range of psychopathology, including depression, conduct disorder, ADHD, oppositional defiant disorder (ODD), dissociation, and PTSD.

Sexually Abused Children

A variety of symptoms, behavioral changes, and diagnoses sometimes occur in sexually abused children: anxiety symptoms, dissociative reactions and hysterical symptoms, depression, disturbances in sexual behaviors, and somatic complaints.

Anxiety Symptoms. Anxiety symptoms include fearfulness, phobias, insomnia, nightmares that directly portray the abuse, somatic complaints, and PTSD.

Dissociative Reactions. The child may exhibit periods of amnesia, daydreaming, trancelike states, psychogenic nonepileptic seizures, and symptoms of dissociative identity disorder.

Depression. Depression may manifest as low self-esteem and suicidal and self-mutilative behaviors.

Disturbances in Sexual Behaviors. Sexualized behaviors in children toward other children or adults are particularly suggestive of sexual abuse. Behaviors exhibited by young children, such as repeated masturbating, imitating intercourse, or inserting objects into the vagina or anus, are suggestive of sexual abuse. Sexually abused children may display sexually aggressive behavior toward others. Other sexual behaviors are less specific, such as showing genitals to other children. A young child who experienced sexual abuse may manifest age-inappropriate sexual knowledge. In contrast to these overly sexualized behaviors, a child who has been sexually abused may avoid sexual stimuli as they grow and develop.

Somatic Complaints. Somatic signs suggestive of possible sexual abuse include enuresis, encopresis, anal and vaginal itching, and nonspecific somatic complaints such as frequent headaches and stomachaches.

The above symptoms are not pathognomonic of maltreatment. Nonabused children with anxiety disorders and other psychiatric disorders may also exhibit some of the symptoms and behaviors. For example, normal, nonabused children commonly exhibit sexual behaviors such as masturbating, displaying their genitals, and trying to look at people who are undressing.

Approximately one-third of identified sexually abused children may not exhibit observable symptoms. Most adults who were abused as children have no obvious significant abuse-related symptoms. However, the following factors tend to be associated with more severe symptoms in the victims of sexual abuse: greater frequency and duration of abuse, sexual abuse that involves force or penetration, and sexual abuse perpetrated by the child's father or stepfather. Other factors associated with poorer prognosis are the child's perception of being less believed, family dysfunction, and lack of maternal support. In addition, multiple investigatory interviews appear to increase symptoms.

Child Sexual Abuse Perpetrators

A particular pattern or sequence of steps may characterize child sexual abuse that occurs over some time. Victims of sexual abuse recount a gradual progression of boundary violations by the perpetrator, starting with tiny invasions and escalating to serious, overwhelming intrusions. Healthy, self-confident children may rebuff the intrusions directly (via temper tantrums and verbal disagreements), indirectly (through silence and distancing maneuvers), or by adopting a strategy that causes the offender to refrain.

Sexual abuse that occurs over an extended time typically involves close household contacts and may evolve through phases. There may be a period of engagement or "grooming" where the perpetrator gains the child's trust or the trust of their caregivers in order to gain access to the child prior to engaging in inappropriate sexual contact. The sexual contact may be ongoing and escalate over time. Sexual abuse includes any form of inappropriate sexual contact with a child, including but not limited to kissing, digital–genital contact, orogenital contact, anogenital contact, and genital–genital contact. The child may not disclose the abuse for an extended time due to fear, shame, or not feeling like they will be believed or supported, and the perpetrator may engage in threatening ways to keep the inappropriate sexual contact a secret. Sometimes, sexual abuse is discovered accidentally without a disclosure. If the child does not feel safe, supported, or believed, it is not uncommon for the victim to recant, deny, or minimize the abuse.

Long-Term Consequences of Maltreatment

Many adults who were abused as children have no readily identifiable significant abuse-related symptoms. However, epidemiologic studies—such as the Adverse Childhood Experiences (ACE) Study—have shown a link between childhood adversity and adult psychopathology in diverse populations. The physical consequences of maltreatment on the developing brain likely mediate this vulnerability.

EVALUATION PROCESS

The evaluation of a child or an adolescent who may have been physically or sexually abused depends on its circumstances and context. Practitioners must consider whether they are conducting a forensic evaluation, which has legal implications and may ultimately be used in court, or a clinical evaluation done for a therapeutic purpose. A forensic evaluation emphasizes collecting accurate and complete data to determine the level of concern for abuse. The evaluator must preserve the data collected in a forensic evaluation in an audio and video-recorded format and organize the results into a report that attorneys, a judge, and others will read. However, a therapeutic evaluation emphasizes assessing psychological strengths and weaknesses, making a clinical diagnosis, developing a treatment plan, and laying the foundation for continuing psychotherapy. The clinician may also be interested in determining what happened to the child, but it is not so essential to distinguish facts from fantasies. Compared with the forensic evaluation, the psychotherapist does not need to keep such detailed records and ordinarily does not prepare a report for court.

In addition to distinguishing a forensic examination from a therapy meeting, several factors may affect the evaluation of a child who was abused or may have been abused: whether one is a pediatrician in an ED or a child psychiatrist in an office, whether a parent or another person is suspected of the abuse, the severity of the abuse and the victim's relationship to the perpetrator, whether physical signs of abuse are apparent or absent, the age and gender of the child, and the degree of anxiety, defensiveness, anger, or mental disorganization the child exhibits. Often, the examiner must be creative and persistent.

From the psychiatric perspective, the interview is usually the primary source of information, and the physical examination is secondary. In practice, children who present with concerns about child maltreatment typically receive a physical exam proximate to the history being obtained by medical providers or social workers.

Parent Interviews

The evaluator obtains a history from the parents (separately, in most cases) and other pertinent informants, as well as from the child, if verbal. The emphasis of the interview depends on the circumstances.

Suspected Physical Abuse. The examiner should obtain a history from caregivers regarding the cause of the patient's injuries and pertinent past medical history. It is always a consideration that the caregivers are not telling the truth, so it is essential to document the caregivers' history and compare it to the objective clinical findings of the patient to determine a level of concern for maltreatment.

When the child is brought to the emergency room, a detailed and spontaneous account of the injury should be obtained promptly from parents or other caregivers. The interviewer should allow the caregiver to explain, expound, derail, or detour the storyline. Caregivers may provide histories that are implausible for the injuries noted on the child, such as multiple broken bones from rolling off of the couch, or provide no history at all to explain the injuries, such as stating that the patient went to sleep without injuries and woke-up covered in bruises.

Suspected Sexual Abuse. As with physical abuse cases, caregivers involved in child sexual abuse cases may not be telling the truth. This is especially true when there are concerns for child sexual abuse in the home, and the adult caregiver does not believe or support the patient or the caregiver is the possible perpetrator of the abuse. Parents may also fabricate concerns about child sexual abuse during custody disputes. It is important to remember that it is rare for a child to fabricate a report of sexual abuse.

The examiner should determine how the allegation originally arose and what subsequent statements were made; determine the emotional tone of the first disclosure (e.g., whether the disclosure arose in the context of a high level of suspicion of abuse); determine the sequence of previous examinations, the techniques used, and what was reported; try to determine whether the previous interviews were likely to have distorted the child's recollections; review, if possible, transcripts, audiotapes, and videotapes of earlier interviews; seek a history of overstimulation, prior abuse, or other traumas; and consider other stressors that could account for the child's symptoms. The examiner should also ask about exposure to other possible male and female perpetrators.

Psychosocial History Components

1. Symptoms and behavioral changes that sometimes occur in abused children.
2. Confounding variables, such as psychiatric disorders or cognitive impairment, may need to be considered.
3. Family attitude toward discipline, sex, and modesty.
4. Developmental history from birth through periods of possible trauma to the present.
5. Family history, such as earlier abuse by the parents, substance abuse by the parents, spouse abuse, and psychiatric disorders in the parents.
6. Underlying motivation and possible psychopathology of adults involved.

Collateral Information

The evaluator should consider requesting collateral information from the following after obtaining authorizations: protective services, school personnel, other caregivers (e.g., babysitters), other family members (e.g., siblings), the pediatrician, and police reports.

Child Interview

Several structured and semistructured interview protocols exist that maximize accurate information and minimize mistaken or false information provided by children. These approaches include the cognitive interview, which encourages witnesses to search their memories in various ways, such as recalling events forward and backward. The Step-Wise Interview is a funnel approach that starts with open-ended questions and, if necessary, moves to more specific questions. The interview protocol developed at the National Institute of Child Health and Human Development (NICHD) includes a series of phases and uses detailed interview scripts. The Cornerhouse Forensic Interview Protocol is another semistructured, nondirective interview method for alleged victims of child sexual abuse.

Although these protocols may be critical in a forensic context, experienced clinicians endorse flexibility and consistent good-hearted behavior by the interviewer. When seeing any patient, the evaluator must size up the situation and use techniques likely to help the youngster become comfortable and communicative. One victim might need a favorite object (e.g., a teddy bear or a toy truck); another might need a particular person in the interview. Some children are comfortable talking; others prefer to draw pictures. An unrelated joke, a shared cookie, or the picture on the evaluator's wall may lead to a disclosure of abuse. Critical comments might be made while chatting during the break time instead of during the structured interviews.

Interview Process. The interviewer of the child who may have been abused should remember the following principles:

1. Audio and video record the interview.
2. Use a minimum number of interviews (perhaps two or three) because multiple interviews may encourage confabulation.
3. Avoid repetitive questions, either–or questions, and multiple questions, and try to avoid leading and suggestive questions.

4. Use restatement, that is, repeat the child's account back to the child (which allows the interviewer to see whether the child is consistent and ensures that the interviewer understands the child's report).
5. Conduct the examination without the parent present (if the child is young, consider having a family member in the room).
6. Use an appropriate examination technique for the child's age and developmental level.
7. Determine the child's terms for body parts and sexual acts; do not educate or provide/introduce new terms.

Interview Content. The interview should not take the form of an interrogation. The interviewer should note the child's affect while discussing these topics and be tactful in helping the child manage anxiety. Young children may not be able to report all of the relevant information. The examiner should explore the following:

1. Whether the child was told to report or not to report anything.
2. Who was the alleged perpetrator.
3. What the alleged perpetrator did.
4. Location of the incident.
5. When it started and when it ended.
6. Number of times the abuse occurred.
7. How the child was initially engaged and how the abuse progressed over time.
8. How the alleged perpetrator induced the child to maintain secrecy.
9. Whether the child is aware of specific injuries or physical symptoms associated with the abuse.
10. Whether photography or videotaping took place.

The Investigative Interview Protocol

The usual clinical interview may need some modification for evaluating a child who may have been abused. The Investigative Interview Protocol, developed at the NICHD, consists of the following components: introduction, rapport building, training in episodic memory, transition to substantive issues, investigating the incidents, eliciting information that has not been mentioned by the child, collecting information about the disclosure, closing the interview, and concluding with a neutral topic.

Introduction. The interviewer introduces themselves and explains the purpose of the meeting in general terms. The interviewer explains the importance of telling the truth. The child can say, "I don't understand your question" or "I don't know." The child can correct the interviewer if the interviewer makes a mistake.

Rapport Building. The interviewer encourages the child to talk about the child's activities and interests but avoids focusing on television, videos, and fantasy.

Training in Episodic Memory. Asking the child to describe two specific past events assesses the child's memory and models the form of the interview for the child. Using nonleading, open-ended questions, the interviewer asks the child to tell everything that happened on two specific days. The interviewer trains the child to give a free narrative account, the pattern throughout the interview.

Making the Transition to Substantive Issues. The interviewer asks the child to focus on the reason for the interview by making a nonleading statement such as, "I understand that something may have happened to you. Tell me everything that happened from the beginning to the end."

Investigating the Incidents. The interviewer starts with open-ended questions like "Tell me everything about what happened." If the child describes a specific incident, elicit additional information in a nonleading manner by saying, for example, "You mentioned (a particular activity). Tell me everything about that." After posing open-ended questions, the interviewer proceeds with focused questions that relate to the information the child mentioned. For example, "You mentioned a friend was there. What was her name? What was she doing"? This process of investigating the incidents is repeated, which are typically "the last time," "the first time," and "another time that you remember well."

Eliciting Information that the Child Did Not Mention. The interviewer may proceed with direct questions only if they have tried other approaches and forensically important information is missing. For example, "When you told me about the time in the kitchen, you mentioned the man took off his pants. Did something happen to your clothes? Tell me all about that." The interviewer may need to formulate a direct question by using outside information. For example, "I heard you told your mother something happened at school. Tell me everything about that."

Obtaining Information About the Disclosure. The interviewer wants to know how the child came to disclose the alleged abuse. Using nonleading questions, the interviewer may say, "Tell me what happened after (the last incident)" and "Does anybody else know what happened"?

Concluding the Interview. At the end of the interview, the interviewer says, "You have told me lots of things today, and I want to thank you for helping me." The interviewer may also say, "Is there anything else you think I should know?" and "Are there any questions you want to ask me"? The interviewer should not compliment the child with comments such as, "You were very brave to talk about those things that happened." The interviewer may conclude with a discussion of a neutral topic, such as, "What are you going to do today after you leave here"?

Extended Forensic Interview

In typical child abuse investigations, Child Advocacy Centers across the United States widely recommend a single-session forensic interview. Interview protocols, which try to define the ideal single-session interview, assume the child is a willing and able participant who can provide a significant account of the alleged abuse. If the single interview results in an equivocal account of abuse, the interview is flawed, or the details need further clarification, another interview following the same protocol may be required. These single-session interviews may not suffice for children who have difficulty relating to a stranger about emotional, traumatic information. Such children may benefit from a multisession interview process.

The National Child Advocacy Center investigated an extended forensic interview (EFI) model to help determine if such a protocol would be superior to the single-session model for certain children. They investigated its use for children who either (1) did not disclose, but there was other compelling evidence for abuse such as medical findings, (2) the child was unable to provide a full disclosure during the single interview, and (3) the allegations remain unresolved (founded or unfounded) after the single interview. They determined that a six-session EFI was the most efficient model. The results from the field testing showed that the EFI had utility and an equal rate of court outcomes as the single interview model. Thus, for single-session forensic interviews that may have initially been unfounded, the EFI helped to resolve the ambiguity surrounding the allegation in almost two-thirds of cases. Like other interviews, the EFI should be recorded.

PHYSICAL EXAMINATION OF SUSPECTED CHILD MALTREATMENT

A comprehensive medical examination should be performed promptly by a medical professional, preferably one with particular expertise in child abuse. The assessment should include a head-to-toe examination of all body areas, including the anogenital region. Any findings should be objectively documented in the medical record and photo-documented when possible. The medical assessment should also include a comprehensive review of systems, past medical history, birth history, and family history to determine concern for underlying medical or inherited conditions that could contribute to the child's clinical presentation.

Just as there is no single psychological characteristic that is diagnostic of abuse, no single physical injury is diagnostic of abuse when considered in isolation. A medical provider must consider the overall constellation of injuries in the context of the history provided to explain them and the developmental capabilities of the patient. The following is a list of injuries that suggest child physical abuse:

1. Any injury to a preambulatory infant, including bruising, oropharyngeal injuries, fractures, intracranial injuries, and abdominal injuries
2. Multiorgan system injuries
3. Injuries in different stages of healing
4. Patterned injuries
5. Injuries to areas of the body typically protected from accidental injuries, such as the nonbony locations of the torso, ears, face, neck, and upper arms
6. Significant injuries that are unexplained

These injuries may range in severity from minor cutaneous injuries to life-threatening intracranial injuries. The younger the patient, the more at risk they are for severe or fatal injuries. Physical abuse also tends to be repetitive and escalate over time, so it is essential to intervene on behalf of the patient, even when the injuries appear to be minor, to prevent the risk of future harm. These seemingly minor injuries noted on infants are called sentinel injuries, and a thorough medical evaluation is needed promptly to assess for occult injuries or those injuries that are not apparent on physical exam.

Physical Findings of Sexual Abuse

The vast majority of victims of child sexual abuse will have no signs of anogenital injury, especially in the non-acute setting, which represents the largest portion of sexual abuse exams due to the well-known delay in reporting sexual abuse and resiliency of the anogenital region. It is of the utmost importance for medical providers to recognize that an absence of injury does not invalidate the child's report of abuse. Several anogenital exam findings have been described in child abuse literature. Findings strongly suggestive of sexual abuse include certain signs of acute anogenital trauma and residual (healing) injuries. Other signs of sexual abuse include sexually transmitted infections (STIs) (e.g., Neisseria gonorrhea, chlamydia trachomatis, syphilis, human immunodeficiency virus [HIV]), semen identified in forensic specimens from a child's body, and pregnancy.

SPECIAL TESTS AND LABORATORY EXAMINATION

Child Physical Abuse Evaluation

Medical providers must have a standard approach to the evaluation of suspected child physical abuse in order to identify and treat all injuries as promptly as possible and to reduce provider biases regarding which patients should undergo the evaluation. The AAP provides evidence-based recommendations regarding this evaluation based on the patient's age and clinical presentation. All young infants and older patients with concern for neurotrauma should receive a head CT to assess for intracranial injury. For patients whose initial head imaging or exam is concerning for intracranial injury, clinicians should consider advanced neuroimaging via MRI of the brain and spine and dilated fundoscopic exam to assess for retinal hemorrhages. All children under the age of 2 years or young children with developmental disabilities or neurologic compromise should receive a skeletal survey to assess for occult skeletal trauma. All children up to the age of 5 years should have labs obtained to assess for occult abdominal trauma with a follow-up abdominal CT for elevations in these labs or those children with concerns on physical exam for abdominal trauma. A follow-up skeletal survey approximately 2 weeks after the initial study is typically recommended to assess for occult skeletal trauma not identified in the initial study, and siblings of children with concern for child physical abuse should undergo an assessment for injuries due to the inherent risks associated with their sibling's injury.

Child Sexual Abuse Evaluation

State laws vary regarding the timing of evidence collection following acute sexual assault and range from 24 hours to 120 hours, with particular consideration to the age of the victim and their disclosures. The acute sexual assault evaluation should be performed by a trained medical professional, including sexual assault nurse examiners (SANE nurses). The acute sexual assault evaluation includes a thorough head-to-toe examination of the victim and an anogenital exam with photo documentation, typically assisted by medical equipment such as a colposcope. Evidence collection kits vary depending on the state and typically include several swabs designated for specific body areas. The chain of custody must be maintained during and following the evidence-collection process. Depending on the age of the victim and type of contact disclosed by the victim, STI, HIV, and pregnancy testing and prophylaxis may be indicated. In prepubertal patients, the anogenital exam should be external. Anesthesia should only be used if there is concern for internal injuries that cannot be visualized on external exams and may need surgical intervention. If a patient is noncooperative with an exam, the patient should be allowed to refuse the exam with accommodations made to collect as much evidence and information as possible to the extent of the individual patient's comfort level, as the intent is not to retraumatize a victim with the process intended to protect them. When a patient presents with concerns for sexual abuse outside of the acute timeframe established by their state laws, a forensic medical exam should be performed as promptly as possible and includes a head-to-toe exam, including anogenital exam with photo documentation, and any appropriate STI testing indicated by disclosures of sexual contact made by the victim. Most victims will have no findings on the exam. If an injury or STI is identified, a follow-up exam and testing may be indicated to assess for healing and a cure for the disease. Should the patient need HIV postexposure prophylaxis, follow-up with infectious disease experts is commonly indicated, given the prolonged regimen and the need to monitor side effects and compliance.

PSYCHIATRIC CONSIDERATIONS

The psychiatric evaluation of youngsters who may have been abused may involve assessing the patient's credibility. Although children generally tell the truth when they talk about abuse, sometimes, children make false denials (saying that they were not abused when they were) or false allegations (saying they were abused when they were not).

Possible Explanations of Denials of Abuse

A false denial or retraction may occur for several reasons. The perpetrator or family members may have pressured the child to recant the allegation. The pressure may consist of bribery, mockery, or threats of injury. The child may protect a parent or other family member, even without external coercion (i.e., the child takes on this responsibility through role reversal). The child might be frightened or distressed by the investigation and may withdraw participation. For instance, an interviewer could induce a false denial by asking overly challenging questions. A child may be inhibited by shame or guilt; the child may mistakenly assume responsibility for what happened. Finally, the child may have accommodated the abuse, consciously or unconsciously, instead of objecting to it.

Possible Explanations of Allegations of Abuse

A false allegation of abuse, although rare, may occur for several reasons.

Allegations Originating with Adults. Sometimes, a false allegation arises in a parent's or another adult's mind, and the adult imposes this on the child.

PARENTAL MISINTERPRETATION AND SUGGESTION. The parent may have misinterpreted an innocent remark, a neutral piece of behavior, or a benign physical condition as evidence of abuse and may have induced the child to endorse this interpretation. This happens in child custody disputes, as well as in other settings.

PARENTAL DELUSION. The parent and child may share a *folie àdeux*, or the child may give in and agree with a delusional parent.

PARENTAL INDOCTRINATION. A parent may have fabricated the story and induced the child to collude in presenting it to the authorities.

INTERVIEWER SUGGESTION. Previous interviewers may have asked leading or suggestive questions. An interviewer who believes abuse occurred may unwittingly shape a child's responses until the child validates the interviewer's assumptions.

Group Contagion. In epidemic hysteria, people modify what they have heard to meet their emotional needs. Thus, rumors may become more convincing with retelling.

Unconscious or Nonpurposeful Mental Mechanisms in the Child

FANTASY. A younger child may confuse fantasy with reality.

DELUSION. Although rare, older children and adolescents may experience delusions about sexual activities in the context of a psychotic illness.

MISINTERPRETATION. Sometimes, children misunderstand what happened and later report it inaccurately.

MISCOMMUNICATION. The child may misunderstand an adult's question, and the adult may later misinterpret or take the child's statement out of context.

CONFABULATION. Children fill gaps in their memory with whatever information makes sense to them and others at the time.

Conscious or Purposeful Mental Mechanisms in the Child

PATHOLOGIC LYING. Also called *pseudologia fantastica*, this refers to children who tell stories so zealously that they may become convinced of their truth.

INNOCENT LYING. Children may make false statements because that seems to be the best way to handle the situation. Developmentally, this is more likely to happen with younger children.

DELIBERATE LYING. Children may choose to avoid or distort the truth for some personal advantage. This happens more with older children and adolescents.

PERPETRATOR SUBSTITUTION. The child may have been sexually abused and may exhibit symptoms consistent with abuse but may identify the wrong person as the perpetrator, resulting in a false allegation. The child may do this to protect the actual offender, or the child may displace the memories and accompanying emotions onto another individual.

SPECIAL ISSUES

Neonatal Abstinence Syndrome

Neonatal abstinence syndrome (NAS) is another example of the potential maltreatment of a fetus. Newborns exposed to maternal drug use can undergo withdrawal after their birth. This withdrawal can be due to illicit substance use by the mother or iatrogenic addiction (e.g., maternal treatment of a pain condition with opioid medication). The type of substance exposure reflects the newborn's symptoms. Symptoms of NAS encompass high-pitched crying, jitteriness, tremors, convulsions, sweating, fever, mottling, excessive sucking/rooting, poor feeding, vomiting, and diarrhea. A toxicology workup can be done in addition to thorough history taking, although the mother may be reluctant to disclose substance use. About 3% of the 4.1 million women of childbearing age who abuse drugs will continue to use drugs during their pregnancy. From 2000 to 2009, the rate of infants born with NAS rose from 1.2 to 3.4 per 1,000 hospital births per year. Maternal substance use has both medical and developmental concerns for the newborn as well as legal, health, and economic impacts for the mother.

Medical Child Abuse

Medical child abuse, or factitious disorder imposed on another, was formerly known as Munchausen Syndrome by Proxy. This syndrome occurs when a child receives unnecessary and harmful or potentially harmful medical care at the instigation of a caretaker. The perpetrator is usually the mother and often has a narcissistic, histrionic, or borderline personality disorder and thrives on the center-stage position they assume. Medical child abuse is perpetrated by fabrication (falsifying or lying about symptoms) or induction (an act that induces or causes illness, such as poisoning). Frequently, this form of maltreatment has been ongoing for an extended time before medical providers recognize it. In families in which medical child abuse is found, more than one child may be involved consecutively or simultaneously. In extreme cases, children can be killed, seriously injured, terrorized, and experience severe adverse effects from medications or other treatments.

Sex Trafficking

Human sex trafficking is the commercial sexual exploitation of children (CSEC). CSEC includes a large number of crimes against minors, including prostitution, survival sex, internet-based exploitation, and child pornography. While trafficking may involve the physical transfer and movement of the child, these crimes also frequently occur in or close to the home. LGBTQ youth are especially vulnerable to human trafficking related to survival sex. Almost 300,000 American youth are at risk of becoming victims of the commercial sex trade. The average age at which children enter the trade is between 12 and 14 years for girls and 11 and 13 years for boys.

The use of violence, drugs, coercion, and other methods of manipulation are commonplace among the traffickers. If a youth in the sex trade becomes addicted to drugs, the trafficker can use the addiction as a means of control. The National Center for Missing and Exploited Children created the Child Sex Trafficking Team in 2001 due to the need for specialized services in this area. Training of police officers, detectives, and emergency room staff can help to identify youth involved in trafficking.

Teamwork

Child maltreatment cases require a multidisciplinary team (MDT) of medical providers, mental health professionals, law enforcement, and child protective services. Team participation provides consultation, professional support, collaboration, and coordination for continued safety, health, hope, and positive social interactions within the grim realities of case discovery.

In cases of suspected child abuse and neglect, the physician should make an assessment based on a history, a physical examination, and indicated medical studies; should request appropriate surgical, medical, and psychiatric consultations; should diagnose the suspected maltreatment; and should report these concerns promptly to their local child protective services and investigative agencies. Child protective services will determine the safety plan for the patient, which can range from periodic monitoring to out-of-home foster care placement. Members of the MDT may also refer the patient to appropriate mental health services and other needed medical or developmental therapies. These activities, taken together, should be a coordinated team effort.

TREATMENT

Child

The first part of the treatment of child abuse and neglect is ensuring the child's safety and well-being. The child may need to be removed from an abusive or neglectful family to ensure protection but emotionally may feel even more vulnerable in an unfamiliar setting. Because of the high risk of psychiatric symptoms in abused and neglected children, a psychiatric evaluation is in order. Along with providing specific treatments for any mental disorders present, the therapist may have to deal with the immediate situation and the long-term implications of the abuse or neglect. Psychotherapeutic issues include dealing with the child's fears, anxieties, and self-esteem; building a trusting relationship with the therapist in which the child is not exploited or betrayed; and gaining a perspective, over time, of the factors that contributed to the child's victimization. These issues may be addressed in individual or group psychotherapy or both.

The intensity and duration of treatment depend on the severity of the symptoms. If an abused child has no posttrauma symptoms, it is probably adequate to provide a few counseling sessions that include psychoeducation and anticipatory strategies for recognizing problems in the future. For a child who has been minimally assaulted (e.g., a relatively innocuous single episode of fondling by a stranger), it may be adaptive for the child to forget the incident and move on.

Abused children with mild to moderate psychological symptoms have been treated with a form of cognitive-behavioral treatment that has four components: psychoeducation, anxiety management, exposure, and cognitive therapy. *Psychoeducation* includes teaching the child and the caregivers about the nature of maltreatment, offenders, and strategies to avoid future abuse. *Anxiety management* includes teaching children how to use relaxation and other coping strategies to reduce fearful responses to memories and reminders of abuse. *Exposure* refers to talking, drawing, or writing about the abuse experiences. It is usually helpful to have the child share the painful, ugly details of the abusive experiences with the therapist. This may take time and may require therapeutic creativity and flexibility. Although some children may be able to relate the bad things that happened through ordinary conversation, other children may need a variety of play, artistic, or other projective techniques. Some children avoid painful memories through conscious (suppression) and unconscious (repression) mechanisms. *Cognitive therapy* techniques can help the child replace cognitive distortions about the event or negative feelings about themselves.

Abused children and adolescents with very severe symptoms (such as complex PTSD or DESNOS) require extensive treatment. These victims of abuse have been treated with a multimodal approach, including specific psychotherapies such as dialectical-behavioral treatment (DBT), psychotropic medication, and perhaps hospitalization or residential treatment.

Parents

Developing an intervention plan for an abused or neglected child requires assessing the parents' behavior and functioning in several respects. The psychopathology and the prognosis for achieving adequate parenting skills for the abusive parent and the one who allowed the abuse to occur should be assessed. The evaluator should determine whether the parent's dysfunction is confined to this child or involves other children and whether the dysfunction is short-term or long-term (reflecting a lifelong pattern). The evaluator should assess the parent's willingness to participate in the intervention plan and the availability of personnel and physical resources to implement the various intervention strategies. One must consider the risk of additional physical or sexual abuse if the child remains in the home.

Based on the information obtained, several options can be selected to improve the parent's functioning: (1) eliminating or diminishing the social or environmental stresses; (2) lessening the adverse psychological effects of the social factors on the parents; (3) reducing the demands on the parent to a level that is within their capacity through day care utilization or provision of a housekeeper or babysitter; (4) providing emotional support, encouragement, sympathy, stimulation, instruction in parental care, and training in planning for, assessing, and meeting the needs of the child (supportive casework); and (5) resolving or diminishing the parent's inner psychic conflicts (psychotherapy). Some clinics provide group counseling for nonoffending parents.

INTRAFAMILIAL CHILD SEXUAL ABUSE

The first step in the treatment of child sexual abuse perpetrated by a family member is its disclosure, which means overcoming the denial and collusion of the family members and the fear and blame felt by the victim. The perpetrator may leave the home, or protective services may remove the child so the inappropriate sexual contact is not likely to recur. In circumstances where it is possible for the family to reunite or cases where the perpetrator never left the home, family therapy is helpful in re-establishing the group as a functioning unit and developing healthier role definitions for each member. Specific individuals may need therapy regarding unique aspects of their involvement. If the child victim does not feel heard/validated, they can develop a defensive posture and become reclusive, distrusting, and feel unloved, in addition to a host of other adverse psychological sequelae. The nonoffending caregiver may also develop a sense of guilt that erodes their self-confidence and interferes with family relationships. They may feel unworthy of being a parent, resulting in further parenting deficits or overcompensation for perceived faults. When the participants experience severe psychopathology, treatment must focus on the underlying illness. While the perpetrators of abuse are learning to develop internal restraints and appropriate ways to gratify their needs, the external control provided by therapy helps to prevent further abusive behavior. At times, legal agencies are involved to help enforce external controls.

SCHOOL CONSULTATION AND COLLABORATING WITH THE EDUCATIONAL SYSTEM

Schools are second only to homes in influencing child development. They play a crucial role in both academic learning and social–emotional development. The school environment shapes students' cognitive, psychological, social, and behavioral development. Psychiatrists can support students' mental health and well-being by collaborating with educational settings, which can impact both mental health and school performance.

SCHOOL SYSTEMS

Common Terms

Table 22-1 lists the educational terms and acronyms most relevant to the psychiatrist working in the school system; we will discuss some of the most important in the following sections.

Special Education

Special education has six foundational principles: (1) free and appropriate public education (FAPE), (2) appropriate evaluation, (3) Individualized Education Program (IEP), (4) least restrictive environment (LRE), (5) parent and student participation in decision making, and (6) procedural safeguards to ensure that the rights of children with disabilities and their parents are protected and that they have access to the information needed to participate in the process effectively.

The availability of special education and mental health services in schools depends on federal, state, and regional legislation.

Some Key Federal Laws

For most of this country's history, the federal government has generally rejected proposals to fund public education. In the 1960s, however, there was increasing pressure to address educational disparities as part of a more considerable effort to address poverty in America. The US

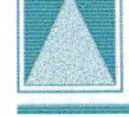

Table 22-1. Common Education Terms

Common Education Terms	Description
LEA: Local Educational Agency	Public authority tasked with administrative control of schools in a region (i.e., county education office, district)
General/Regular Education	Education for typically developing children based on annually reviewed state standards
Special Education	Specially designed instruction under IDEA to meet needs of child with a disability; can include gifted instruction
IDEA: The Individuals with Disabilities Education Act	Federal law: free appropriate public education for children with disabilities, for special education and related services
FAPE: Free and Appropriate Public Education	In IDEA and Section 504, describes education that's at no cost to parents, meets state standards, and meets student's needs
LRE: Least Restrictive Environment	In IDEA, appropriate educational environment, meets special educational needs, and maximizes being with nondisabled peers
IEP: Individualized Education Program	Written statement for each student with a disability that describes how disability affects education, goals, progress, and services
Accommodations	Changes in how student learns material or demonstrates mastery. Does NOT change what is taught or tested
Modifications	Changes to content and performance requirements. DOES include changes to what is taught or tested

Congress passed The Elementary and Secondary Education Act (ESEA) in 1965 as part of President Johnson's "War on Poverty" and aimed to guarantee equal educational opportunity for all students. It authorized funding for various educational programs, professional development, and instructional materials. Since then, Congress has modified and reauthorized the ESEA several times. For example, the Equal Educational Opportunities Act of 1974 prohibits discrimination against students and teachers. The No Child Left Behind Act (NCLBA) introduced standards-based testing, and the Every Student Succeeds Act (2015) modified the NCLBA, shifting accountability to the states and mandating that schools apply the same assessments and standards to students with disabilities as other students.

Perhaps most influential has been the Individuals with Disabilities Education Act (IDEA) (1975, 2004), which mandated FAPE for eligible children with disabilities and set the standards for special education as listed above. It also codifies the rights of parents and guardians in their child's education, including the right to active participation.

DISPARITIES IN THE EDUCATIONAL SYSTEM

Despite these and other laws' attempts to equalize the educational system in the United States, there remain significant disparities that can affect students throughout their lifetime. For example, according to the US Department of Education, Black preschool children experience disproportionate suspensions (more than 2.5 times that of enrolled students), with similar rates continuing in elementary and secondary education. Native American youth are suspended at four times their enrolled population during K-12 schooling and expelled from school at six times their population. Native American and Black youth are also disproportionately referred to and arrested by law enforcement for school-related offenses at least twice the rates of their enrolled populations.

In 2019, the US Commission on Civil Rights reviewed racial and ethnic disproportionality of school discipline for students with disabilities. The report concluded that despite disproportionate discipline for students of color, these students did not commit more disciplinable offenses than their White peers, although they received harsher and longer punishments than did White students. They summarized research showing that out-of-school discipline is associated with poor classroom engagement, more significant school dropout, and juvenile justice involvement. The Commission recommended that federal nondiscrimination laws be enforced, and schools should be provided resources and training for alternatives to out-of-school discipline.

The mental health system can also play an essential role in addressing these disparities by, for example, consulting with educational systems on implementing trauma-informed practices and improving school climate, including student support, engagement, and school connectedness.

COMMON EDUCATIONAL SETTINGS

Psychiatrists may find that their young patients attend various educational settings with varying resources and regulations. They should also consider the strengths and limitations of a school setting in light of the strengths and needs of each child.

Public Schools

Public schools serve 90.5% of the United States students and are funded primarily by state and local governments.

Charter Schools

Charter schools are public schools operating under a legislative contract with a sponsor. These sponsors include state education agencies, special boards, and school districts. Charter schools are given autonomy and flexibility in their curriculum and structure. They must still hold to the same standards as public schools.

Private Schools

Most private schools in the United States are religious (7.6% of all students) or nonsectarian (1.9%). These schools are not under federal jurisdiction unless they receive federal aid. Generally, parents or guardians pay for these schools; however, a school district may choose to pay for a private school if, for example, a student has a disability that the public system would not adequately address.

Homeschooling

About 6% of students K-12 are homeschooled. Regulation of home schools is state-dependent as no federal law governs or mentions homeschooling.

Alternative Programs/Schools. Schools may offer alternative programming for students at risk of dropping out but do not qualify for special education services to serve students at risk of failing academically or dropping out. Examples of students who can benefit from such programming include pregnant or homeless students or victims of domestic violence.

ROLES OF SCHOOL PERSONNEL

Teachers

Teachers are the primary staff involved with students daily. They typically average 23 students per class in elementary school and 20 to 25 in middle and high school.

Special Education Teachers

Special education teachers are credentialed to work with students with learning disabilities or other special needs.

They usually work with small groups of students to provide individualized instruction.

Aides

Aides or paraprofessionals assist teachers or special education teachers. They may be assigned to help a specific student.

School Counselors

School counselors vary depending on their role. Academic or guidance counselors assist in academic or vocational planning. Adjustment counselors or social workers provide psychosocial interventions to students and their families.

School Psychologists

School psychologists conduct educational assessments and help construct individualized educational programs. They may also provide group or individual therapy. They often work for more than one school in a district.

School Administrators

School administrators include principals and vice principals who coordinate services within schools and report to their superintendent. The superintendent is responsible for the educational activities of all district schools and reports to the elected school board (for public schools) or appointed boards (in private schools).

Depending on a student's needs, other professionals include speech-language pathologists, occupational therapists, school nurses, and mental health counselors.

SCHOOL RESOURCES AND PROGRAMMING

In addition to becoming familiar with the types of personnel in a school system, a psychiatrist should also understand the range of resources and programming available at a school.

Multitiered Systems of Support

One overall framework for considering the integration of all supports on a campus is the multitiered systems of support (MTSS), which describes supports generally available to all students on a school campus. Typically, the interventions available are tiered and depend on the target audience and intensity needed. Examples of tiers include:

Tier 1: Universal or primary. This level supports all or most students and includes whole-class approaches and social–emotional learning.

Tier 2: Secondary. Secondary support includes targeted interventions for small groups of students.

Tier 3: Tertiary. Tertiary support involves intensive, individualized support for a few students who do not respond to the less individualized interventions.

Table 22-2 lists example programs in each tier.

In cases where a student needs more formalized support within the general education setting than can be provided within the tiered model, schools may develop 504 plans or an individualized educational program.

504 Plans

504 plans support students needing formal support but not yet requiring an IEP. The name refers to section 504 of The Rehabilitation Act of 1973, which addresses protections for students with disabilities. It applies to students with disabilities affecting major life activities but not requiring special education. 504 plans provide accommodations within general education, such as extended time or preferential seating. The accommodations do not change the content or assessment for a student. Students receiving accommodations are typically subject to the same grading scale as students who are not receiving accommodations. If the student requires more intensive interventions, the plan can include modifications to the content or performance requirements. These accommodations and modifications can follow a person after high school into postsecondary education.

Table 22-3 lists common types of accommodation and modifications.

Individualized Education Program

If a student needs more specialized services and programming than a 504 plan can provide, then a student may be involved in the IEP process. Eligible students qualify for special education services under specific eligibility categories the IEP team sets. IEP assessments include review of records, administration of any indicated testing based on the suspected area(s) of disability, observations of the student, or consulting with outside providers, such as the psychiatrist.

Most initial IEP assessments include formal, standardized tests, especially when the suspected area of disability relates to a student's academic achievement, speech or language functioning, processing, or social, emotional, and behavioral functioning.

If the student meets eligibility criteria (Table 22-4), the IEP team meeting will develop recommendations for the special education programs and services the student needs, known as the team's offer of FAPE. The IEP team can determine (1) goals and objectives based on individual needs, (2) recommended services and programming or placement based on the goals, and (3) accommodations, modifications, or supports based on the recommended placement. The IEP team will also decide on the percentage of time the student receives instruction within and outside the general education setting.

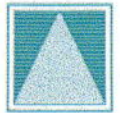

Table 22-2.
Examples of School Social, Emotional, and Behavioral Interventions by Tier of Support

Tier	Target Population	Grade	Intervention	Description	Outcomes
1	Public, Pre-K in historically disinvested, low-income neighborhoods	PS	ParentCorps[a]	Parent and teacher training to create a safe and nurturing environment and improve teacher–parent communication, SEL in the classroom	Improves academics, behaviors
1	Universal	PS, ES	Incredible Years Training for Teachers[b]	Teacher training for positive classroom management	Decreases conduct problems, improves emotion regulation, social skills, and school readiness
1	Universal	ES	Good Behavior Game[b]	Classroom behavior management approach that encourages prosocial behavior through games	Decreases aggressive behavior, substance use, suicide
1	Universal, SEL	ES	Promoting Alternative Thinking Strategies (PATHS)[a]	Teach self-control, feelings and relationships, and social problem-solving	Decreases aggression, disruptive behaviors, delinquency
1	Bullying Prevention	ES	Steps to Respect[b]	Staff training to increase awareness and responsiveness and classroom SEL for bullying	Decreased bullying and bystander behaviors, improved climate
1	SEL, School-Wide Climate Change	ES, MS	Positive Action[a]	Brief classroom lessons from K–8th grade to teach emotions, behaviors, and positive actions	Lower absenteeism, suspensions, grade retention, substance use, violence
1	Substance Use and Violence Prevention	MS	Life Skills Training[a]	Classroom intervention that teaches self-management, social skills, problem-solving, drug resistance	Decreased drug use, violence, delinquency, and risky behaviors
1	Dating Violence Prevention	MS, HS	Safe Dates[b]	10-session dating violence prevention program for MS and HS students	Reduces dating violence, improves communication skills
1–2	Substance Use Prevention	ES, MS	Strengthening Families 10–14[b]	Seven sessions to increase family protective factors and resilience	Decreases substance use, antisocial and aggressive behavior
2	Aggression	ES, MS	Coping Power[b]	5th–6th-grade students receive anger management and social problem-solving, and parents learn parenting skills and family communication (16 months)	Improves academic performance and prosocial behaviors, and decreases substance use and conduct problems
2–3	Traumatic Stress	ES, MS	Cognitive-Behavioral Intervention for Trauma in Schools[b]	CBT-based group intervention for youth exposed to trauma/violence, with optional parent and teacher sessions	Decreases PTSD and depressive symptoms
3	Depression	MS, HS	Interpersonal Psychotherapy Adolescent Skills Training[b]	Short-term intervention focusing on the developmental and interpersonal needs of adolescents and building communication and social problem-solving skills	Improves depression and improves well-being

[a]Blueprints Model Programs.

[b]Promising Programs (https://www.blueprintsprograms.org).

CBT, cognitive-behavioral therapy; ES, elementary school; HS, high school; MS, middle school; PS, preschool; PTSD, posttraumatic stress disorder; SEL, social-emotional learning.

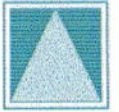

Table 22-3.
Accommodations and Modifications

Categories	Application
Accommodations	
Presentation	• Allow student to audiotape lessons • Allow student to use alternatives to test books (including audio records) • Reduce the amount of work per page • Enlarge print size • Provide adjusted paper for writing and math (e.g., wide-lined notebook paper; enlarged graph paper) • Use multimodal communication, especially for instructions (e.g., pairing auditory and visual information) • Read all instructions aloud to student • Frequent checks for understanding
Response	• Allow alternative response form (i.e., orally vs. in writing) • Only call on student when student raises their hand • Eliminate participation grade/use alternative means for grading participation • Use of a scribe for written responses • Extended time allowances for responses • Opportunities to complete work or take tests in a separate location • Allow student to use a dictionary and/or grade spelling separately. • Do not downgrade for handwriting • Allowances to use a calculator and/or printed math facts sheet (e.g., multiplication table)
Timing/Scheduling	• Extended time allowances for in-class work, homework, projects, and/or tests • Opportunities to take breaks, including movement breaks • Extended time allowances during passing periods • Allowances to take tests over multiple days/periods
Setting	• Allowances to take tests in a separate location (i.e., quieter setting) • Preferential seating to maximize learning (e.g., closest to the source of instruction; at back of room to allow for movement) • Being provided with special lighting or acoustics • Nonpunitive use of sensory tools (e.g., chair band, seat cushion, foot rest)
Modifications	
Assignment	• Spelling tests using alternative words to be tested on • Reduce assignments in amount or modify content significantly • Provide alternative material or assessments that differ from standard grade-level type or amount
Curriculum	• Teach adjusted content and use material that differs from standard level • Adjust grading requirements and standards as expected of same-grade peers • Provide alternative projects with adjusted grade-level materials

Parents and guardians are considered vital members of the IEP team and have the right to participate actively in the IEP meetings and processes.

The recommended IEP services typically include instructional settings such as general education classrooms, Recurrent sleep paralysis (RSP), Special Day Class (SDC), Specially Designed Instruction (SDI), Specialized Academic Instruction (SAI), "push in" (inclusive education with a specialist that assists the student in a general education setting), and "pull out" (student pulled out of the general education class to receive specialized services). The location of services can also vary (on a general education campus or a specialized campus such as a nonpublic school). Additional services may be included depending on specific needs (e.g., speech and language therapy).

Private schools are not required to provide special education services or an IEP. However, they cannot discriminate against a child with a disability for reasons related to that disability. If a private school student qualifies for special education, the services are often through the local public school.

Table 22-5 compares key aspects of 504 plans and IEPs.

ROLES OF PSYCHIATRISTS IN SCHOOL

A psychiatrist in practice may play a collaborative role, working with the school as part of a patient's treatment plan, such as coordinating medication treatment with a school nurse, supporting a teacher with specific behavioral strategies, or as an advocate in supporting a student

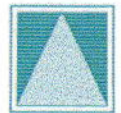

Table 22-4.
IEP Eligibility Categories

Eligible Category	Description	Examples of Disorders/Conditions
Specific Learning Disability (SLD)	Disorder in one or more of the basic psychological processes involved in understanding or in using language (ability to listen, think, speak, read, write, spell, or do mathematical calculations)	• Dyslexia • Dyscalculia • Dysgraphia • Brain injury • Developmental aphasia • Perceptual disabilities
Emotional Disturbance (ED)/Emotional Disability (ED)	One or more of the following characteristics over a long period of time and to a marked degree that adversely affects one's educational performance: A. An inability to learn that cannot be explained by intellectual, sensory, or health factors B. An inability to build or maintain satisfactory interpersonal relationships with peers and teachers C. Inappropriate types of behavior or feelings under normal circumstances D. A general pervasive mood of unhappiness or depression E. A tendency to develop physical symptoms or fears associated with personal or school problems	• Affective/mood disorders • Anxiety disorders • Psychotic disorders • Certain impulse control disorders (including trichotillomania)
Other Health Impairment (OHI)	Having limited strength, vitality, or alertness, including a heightened alertness to environmental stimuli	• Attention-deficit/hyperactivity disorder • Tourette syndrome • Asthma • Diabetes • Epilepsy • Sickle cell anemia
Autism (AUT)	Exhibits diagnostic impairments consistent with the diagnosis of AUT. Educational performance affected by engagement in repetitive activities and stereotyped movements, resistance to environmental change or change in daily routines, and unusual responses to sensory experiences.	• Autism spectrum disorder
Speech/Language Impairment (SLI)	Meets one or more of the following criteria: A. Articulation disorder. B. Abnormal voice C. Fluency disorders D. Language disorder	• Apraxia of speech • Dysarthria • Aphasia • Stuttering • Phonologic disorder • Muteness • Selective mutism
Intellectual Disability (ID)	Subaverage general intellectual functioning, existing concurrently with deficits in adaptive behavior and manifested during the developmental period	Mild, IQ = 50–70 Moderate, IQ = 35–49 Severe, IQ = 20–34 Profound, IQ < 20
Multiple Disabilities	Combination of disorders causing severe educational needs that they cannot be accommodated in special education programs solely for one of the impairments	Combination of conditions
Deaf–Blindness	Requires severe communication and other developmental and educational needs	
Deafness/Hard of Hearing (DHH)	Severe impairment in processing linguistic information through hearing	
Hearing Impairment	Impairment in hearing (permanent or fluctuating) adversely affects educational performance, but that is not included under the definition of deafness	
Orthopedic Impairment (OI)	Severe OIs that include impairments caused by a congenital anomaly and impairments from other causes	• Cerebral palsy • Amputations • Fractures

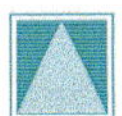

Table 22-4.
IEP Eligibility Categories (Continued)

Eligible Category	Description	Examples of Disorders/Conditions
Traumatic Brain Injury (TBI)	An acquired injury to the brain resulting in total or partial functional disability or psychosocial impairment, or both	
Visual Impairment (VI)	Impairment in vision that, even with correction, adversely affects a child's educational performance	• Partial sight • Blindness

in accessing needed special education services. A school psychiatrist may be an employee of the educational system or an outside organization, such as a community agency or university, who evaluates and treats students referred by the school system, such as through the School-Based Health Centers (SBHCs). A school consultation model involves a psychiatrist who serves as a classroom, school, or district consultant and may provide staff and administrator-level recommendations for system improvement. Finally, a school may ask a psychiatrist to assist the school during a crisis, such as during a disaster or sudden death.

Direct Service Models

Direct service models can involve a psychiatrist providing clinical care for students in the school system or a partnership between community organizations and schools to support an array of mental health services in the school or linked to a community agency. SBHCs and Comprehensive School Mental Health Programs (CSMHPs) are two models that reflect such models of direct service. SBHCs are either in or near a school and integrate health services into schools, improving access for underserved communities. CSMHPs provide tiered mental health services through school–community partnerships. Community mental health staff increasingly partner with school-employed mental health staff and educators to provide this comprehensive, integrated model. Telemental health services are an effective model for remote psychiatric consultation and can improve access in underserved areas.

School Consultation

One role a psychiatrist can have with schools is as a school consultant in response to an identified need or question from the school system.

When consulting with a school, the psychiatrist should consider several key components, including identifying the consultee and establishing confidentiality limits, clarifying the consultation question and expectations, and understanding the biopsychosocial context and how the more extensive system is experiencing the problem. The psychiatrist must also consider legal and ethical factors, such as when parents decline a consult for their child; in this case, the psychiatrist may talk with the school staff but not directly interview or treat the child.

Crisis Response

A school may consult a psychiatrist in cases of student death, preventing violence on campus, or supporting a school during a broader crisis.

Given that death by suicide is a significant cause of death for young people, schools can play a critical role in disseminating universal suicide prevention strategies. One example of an effective intervention is the Signs of Suicide (SOS) program, which teaches students about the warning SOS risk and how to seek assistance from trained school staff. After a death, the psychiatrist can help to prevent a contagion effect.

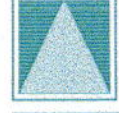

Table 22-5.
Comparison Between 504 Plans and IEPs

Description	504 Plan	IEP
Who qualifies?	1. Has a physical or mental impairment 2. Impairment limits at least one major life activity	1. Meets eligibility criteria for at least one of the Special Education categories 2. Exhibits difficulties that have existed over an extended period of time and, to a marked degree, adversely affect a student's educational functioning
Who typically implements services?	General education staff	Specialized staff (e.g., special education teacher, school psychologist, speech therapist, etc.)
Does school receive funding to implement recommended changes?	No funding	Federal/state/local funding for services
Are protections available postsecondary school?	Yes	No

Although mass shootings are rare, psychiatrists may be called upon to conduct a threat assessment of the potential "risk" that a student may act violently toward others. The psychiatrist should be aware that there are often warning signs of violence, including conversations with other students or threats posted on social media. Structured protocols are available when assessing threats. For example, the Virginia Student Threat Assessment Guidelines to evaluate potential risks.

Psychiatrists may also help a school or a district after a natural or man-made disaster or a catastrophic public health situation, such as the pandemic. Community-wide traumatic events such as these can impact the education, health, and well-being of students but often challenge the school staff and administrators in similar ways. In particular, these types of events can reverberate across multiple social determinants of health, exacerbate existing inequities, and disproportionately affect under-resourced communities of color. Interventions can include creating online training for teachers and other school personnel, supporting students with anxiety, and providing psychological first aid for teachers.

WEB RESOURCES

Table 22-6 provides selected websites describing various school mental health programs.

GAY, BISEXUAL, TRANSGENDER, QUEER/QUESTIONING, INTERSEX, AND ASEXUAL (LGBTQIA) YOUTH

Today's youth are increasingly comfortable with gender and sexuality in the context of greater societal awareness and acceptance of diverse gender identities and sexual orientations. Relatedly, there has been a notable increase in child and adolescent patients seeking gender- and sexuality-related care and support. To provide effective evidence-based care to their gender-diverse and sexual minority patients, psychiatrists can increase their knowledge and comfort with key terminology and concepts and learn to implement trauma-informed LGBTQIA-affirming care models, as discussed in this chapter.

In this chapter, we utilize the term *LGBTQIA*, which stands for Lesbian, Gay, Bisexual, Transgender, Queer/Questioning, Intersex, and Asexual, to refer to gender and sexual minority patients except where data refer to specific subgroups therein. Some of these specific terms represent gender identities, while some represent sexual orientations. It is also worth emphasizing that different LGBTQIA patients use different terms to describe themselves and their identities, and the acronym used by the authors encapsulates a limited number of identities. For example, many youths identify with nonbinary, genderfluid, and/or genderqueer identities. A best practice for the clinician is always to ask the youth what term(s) best describe them and what terms they would like the clinician to use.

SEXUAL ORIENTATION

Many Western cultures take a heteronormative approach to socialization—in other words, many youth are taught that heterosexuality is one's expected sexuality. Parental expectations and assignations of gender begin even before conception and birth and can shape parenting. Hence, LGBTQIA youth often identify a sense of not belonging, a challenge to personal development during adolescence, when norms and fitting in seem to be the social task at hand. As a result, numerous large national studies have found notable mental health disparities between LGB youth and their heterosexual peers, including increased rates of depression, anxiety, suicidality, and substance use. It has also been noted that family support and acceptance are substantial mitigating factors in reducing these risks for LGB youth.

An individual's sexual orientation describes to whom they are physically, romantically, or emotionally attracted (Table 22-7). Sexual orientation is independent of one's sex or one's gender. Sexual orientation has three main components:

1. Identity: how one sees themself
2. Attraction: to what gender(s) is one attracted emotionally, romantically, or physically
3. Behavior: in what acts does one engage and with whom

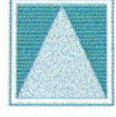

Table 22-6. Website Resources

Category	Description	Site
Blueprints	Registry of evidence-based interventions for healthy youth development	blueprintsprograms.org/
National Center for School Mental Health	National training, practice, research, and policy information	csmh.umaryland.edu
School Threat Assessment	Trainings and resources for threat assessment in schools	schoolta.com/
Social-Emotional Learning	Research, practice, and policy regarding social–emotional learning	casel.org
What Works Clearinghouse	Reviews the existing research on different *programs, products, practices,* and *policies* in education	ies.ed.gov/ncee/wwc/
Wrightslaw	Special education law and advocacy	wrightslaw.com

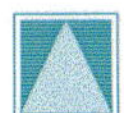

Table 22-7.
Sexual Orientation Terminology

Heterosexual ("Straight")	Attracted to the "Opposite" Sex/Gender
Lesbian	Female-identified attracted to female-identified
Gay	Male-identified attracted to male-identified
Bisexual	Attracted to "both" sexes/genders
Pansexual	Attracted to all sexes/genders
Queer	Denotes identities outside of traditional cisgender heteronormativity. Historically used as a derogatory term but also feels supportive to some.
Allosexual	Having the capacity to be attracted to others in a sexual way
Asexual ("ace")	Not attracted to anyone in a sexual way
Aromantic ("aro")	Not attracted to anyone in an emotional/romantic way

The DSM has a long history of pathologizing LGBTQIA identities, leading to a mistrust of the field of psychiatry and an avoidance of care. Homosexuality was first included in *The Diagnostic and Statistical Manual of Mental Disorders (DSM), First Edition (DSM-I)* (1952), and the original DSM-II (1968) as a "sociopathic personality disturbance." It was later recategorized as a "sexual orientation disturbance" (as opposed to a mental disorder) in a 1974 edition after years of protests. The diagnosis was changed again to "ego-dystonic homosexuality" in the DSM-III (1980) before being revised yet again to remove the word homosexuality (substituted with "sexual disorder not otherwise specified") in the DSM-III-R (1987).

SEX AND GENDER

Although often conflated with each other, sex and gender are distinct concepts. An individual's *sex* is typically *assigned at birth* based on visualized genitalia and, less often, on other physical characteristics and chromosomes. *Sex assigned at birth* is typically described as female, male, or intersex. Of note, intersex is an umbrella term that describes differences in sexual development (DSD) or a range of traits and conditions in which individuals have naturally occurring variations in chromosomes, gonads, or genitals. Differences in sex development are discussed in greater detail later in this chapter.

An individual's *gender* refers to both one's internal identity and the expression of their gender within their social context (Table 22-8).

Nonbinary Identities

Among Western cultures, much of the population is raised using the gender binary as the social norm. Thus, the concept of gender existing on a continuum or a spectrum can be surprising. In fact, many cultures and societies embrace diverse gender identities outside of Western colonization. In the modern day, many children and adolescents embrace nonbinary identities. In other words, many youths express gender identities outside the typical "masculine" or "feminine" descriptors. In the United States, several states legally recognize nonbinary identities.

Gender Dysphoria

Similar to its approach to pathologizing homosexuality, the DSM's approach to transgender identities has been stigmatizing and marginalizing to many. The DSM-III (1980) listed "transsexualism" for the first time. This term was replaced by "gender identity disorder," categorized under Sexual Dysfunctions and Paraphilic Disorders in the DSM-IV (1994). In the DSM-5 (2013), "gender identity disorder" was replaced by "gender dysphoria" (APA, 2023).

The DSM-5-TR (2022) defines gender dysphoria in children as "a marked incongruence between one's experienced/expressed gender and assigned gender, lasting at least 6 months, as manifested by at least six of the following [criteria]." The first criterion, "a strong desire to be of the other gender or an insistence that one is the other gender," is required for the diagnosis. Note that the criteria for gender dysphoria in adults and adolescents varies slightly. Similar to the diagnosis in adolescents and adults, "the condition is associated with clinically significant distress or impairment in social, school, or other important areas of functioning."

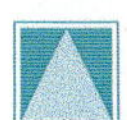

Table 22-8.
Gender Terminology

Gender binary	The division of gender into two separate and "opposite" categories (i.e., male and female)
Gender identity	How one thinks about their own gender (i.e., masculine, feminine, both, neither)
Gender expression	The way one dresses, behaves, and "expresses" oneself
Gender roles	The norms that one's culture creates around male and female identities
Cisgender	One's gender identity coincides with the sex assigned at birth
Transgender	One's gender identity differs from their sex assigned at birth. Umbrella term that can encompass other descriptors such as agender, bigender, gender expansive, gender diverse, gender nonbinary, genderqueer, and genderfluid.
Nonbinary	Describes one's identity as neither fully male nor female.
Transition	The process of changing one's gender expression to match one's gender identity.

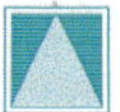

Table 22-9.
Gender Dysphoria in Children/Gender Incongruence of Childhood

	DSM-5-TR	ICD-10	ICD-11
Diagnostic Name	Gender Dysphoria in Children	Gender Identity Disorder of Childhood	Gender Incongruence of Childhood
Duration	≥6 mo		2 yr
Symptoms	Desire to be other gender or insistence one is that gender Preference for cross-dressing in boys, preference for typical masculine, and resistance to typical feminine clothing in girls Preference for cross-gender roles during play Preference for toys/games/activities stereotypically used by another gender Preference for playmates of another gender Rejection of toys/games/activities stereotypically of one's assigned gender Dislike of one's sexual anatomy A desire for sex characteristics of one's experienced gender	Distress about assigned sex	Incongruence between experienced/ expressed gender and assigned sex Strong desire to be a different gender Dislike of their sexual anatomy/ anticipated secondary sex characteristic A desire for secondary sex characteristics to be of a different gender Activities and play typical of the experienced gender
Required number of symptoms	6		
Psychosocial consequences	Distress or psychosocial impairment		
Exclusions		Gender-variant behavior or preferences	Gender-variant behavior or preferences
Symptoms specifiers	With a disorder/difference of sex development (e.g., congenital disorder)		

Tables 22-9 and 22-10 show comparative diagnostic criteria for gender dysphoria between DSM-5-TR, ICD-10, and ICD-11 in children and adolescents, respectively.

Treatment for gender dysphoria consists of gender-affirming care, which may include therapy or psychiatric treatment for gender-linked distress and co-occurring conditions. Youth and adults with gender dysphoria experience higher rates of co-occurring anxiety, depression, suicidality, trauma, and substance use disorders. Research has not shown correlations between gender dysphoria and rates of schizophrenia or bipolar disorder diagnoses. Recent research also points to a strong correlation between ASD incidence among gender dysphoric youth.

Gender Transitions

Gender diversity in children and adolescents has become highly politicized in the United States. Anti-LGBTQIA legislation and lawsuits have focused mainly on bathroom access, youth sports team participation, and access to gender-affirming health care. However, studies show that transgender youth who are supported in their identities experience lower rates of adverse mental health outcomes than those who are not. In the TransYouth Study, investigators found that prepubescent youth who socially transitioned—meaning they lived as their experienced gender, with parental support—demonstrated the same rates of depression as matched cisgender peers. Accordingly, many mainstream medical organizations have published statements and guidelines supporting gender-affirming care, including the American Psychiatric Association (APA), the American Psychological Association, the American Academy of Child and Adolescent Psychiatry (AACAP), the American College of Gynecology, and the Endocrine Society.

Many, and not all, youth with gender dysphoria will wish to transition, which is the process of changing one's gender expression to match one's gender identity. Transitioning *may* include social, legal, and medical changes (Table 22-11).

There is no single protocol for a gender transition; every gender-diverse individual has unique needs and goals. For example, some people opt solely for social or legal transition. Others may wish to engage in any number of medical transition options with their doctors. Of note, many gender-diverse individuals face legal, social, and financial barriers that prevent access to medical-affirming care. Furthermore, the above medical

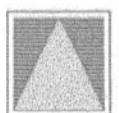

Table 22-10.
Gender Dysphoria in Adolescents and Adults/Gender Incongruence of Adolescence or Adulthood

Disorder	DSM-5-TR	ICD-10	ICD-11
Diagnostic Name	**Gender Dysphoria in Adolescents and Adults**	**Transsexualism**	**Gender Incongruence of Adolescence or Adulthood**
Duration	≥6 mo		
Symptoms	Incongruence between experienced/expressed gender and primary or secondary sex characteristics Desire to be rid of primary/secondary sex characteristics or prevent their development The desire for primary/secondary sex characteristics of another gender Desire to be a different gender Desire to be treated as a different gender A conviction that they feel and react like a different gender	Desire to live and be accepted as a member of the opposite sex Discomfort with one's anatomic sex or sense that it is inappropriate Desire to transition	Incongruence between experienced/expressed gender and assigned sex Desire to transition
Required number of symptoms	2		
Psychosocial consequences	Distress or psychosocial impairment		
Exclusions			Gender-variant behavior or preferences
Symptoms specifiers	With a disorder/difference of sex development (e.g., congenital disorder)		
Course specifiers	Posttransition: living as experienced gender and has undergone ≥1 gender-affirming medical procedure		

procedures have developmental prerequisites and may not be readily accessible to minors. The Standards of Care for the Health of Transgender and Gender Diverse People, Version 8 (SOC8), published by the World Professional Association for Transgender Health (WPATH), provides specific guidance around medical transitions and the treatment of gender dysphoria (see https://www.wpath.org/publications/soc for details).

Mental health clinicians have historically been pushed into a "gatekeeper" role in the medical transition process, as standards of care often require patients to pursue psychological evaluation and obtain surgical readiness evaluation letters from psychiatrists or therapists. Insurance carriers or surgeons mandate these evaluations in some cases. This process can create a complicated relationship between mental health clinicians and their gender-diverse patients. For example, patients may feel pressure to deny mental health symptoms or pursue care to be accepted or "approved" for gender-affirming medical care. Like many individuals who experience social stressors, gender-diverse individuals may benefit from therapeutic or psychiatric treatment. The best clinical practices allow the clinician to support the youth and family before, during, and after the transition process. Clinicians can help youth target mental health symptoms, manage stressors, seek support, and better understand their goals while providing developmental guidance and skills to caregivers to improve youth well-being.

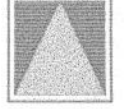

Table 22-11.
Gender Transitions

Social	Changes in name and pronouns, appearance, dress, grooming (e.g., clothes, hair, make-up); nonmedical changes; may include "coming out" to family, school, peers, or others
Legal	Legal name or gender marker change, resulting in the reissuing of government documents (e.g., birth certificate, driver's license, passport)
Medical	Gender-affirming procedures with medical doctors; may include: puberty blockers (i.e., gonadotropin-releasing hormone agonists, like leuprolide), hormone therapies (e.g., estradiol or testosterone), testosterone blockers (e.g., spironolactone), and gender-affirming surgical procedures such as: • For transmasculine/nonbinary patients assigned female at birth: chest masculinization (bilateral mastectomy with chest reconstruction), hysterectomy, phalloplasty, metoidioplasty • For transfeminine/nonbinary patients assigned male at birth: breast augmentation, orchiectomy, vaginoplasty, electrolysis, tracheal shave, facial feminization surgery

Differences of Sex Development (DSD) and Intersex Youth

While the literature on the specific mental health needs of intersex youth remains limited, the first national survey of intersex adults in the United States revealed a high prevalence of lifetime anxiety disorders, PTSD, and depressive disorders. Intersex youth face unique stressors and related mental health symptoms across developmental stages due to the medicalization and pathologization of their bodies from a young age. Some intersex traits present clearly at birth, such as those involving external genitalia, while others manifest during puberty.

Intersex youth experience intense stressors with lifelong consequences, including medically unnecessary surgeries, a lack of support around gender identity development, and the loss of autonomy and agency. Parents, meanwhile, may contend with a sense of urgency around sex assignment, including pressure to consent to genital surgeries without understanding the potential long-term effects on their child and regret irreversible decisions. Often, the justification for an early surgical procedure is to improve long-term mental health by helping the child live a "normal" life—a justification made without evidence and typically by clinicians who do not specialize in mental health. In addition, early medical interventions reinforce sociocultural norms around male and female gender stereotypes, often before the development of the youth's own gender identity.

Overall, there is a great need for increased mental health research, programs, and developmentally appropriate guidelines in caring for youth with DSDs. Mental health professionals can support youth and families in gender identity exploration, navigating challenging health care decisions, and recovery from traumatic stress. In addition, new parents may experience intense and conflicting emotions when deciding on their child's health care plans. Child and adolescent clinicians can also advocate using psychologically sound evidence to determine care for intersex youth at all developmental stages and seek inclusion in pediatric teams who manage DSDs. Finally, they can assist youth and families in identifying community resources and supports that promote mental well-being.

YOUTH TRAUMA AND RESILIENCE

LGBTQIA youth are more likely than cisgender heterosexual youth to experience traumatic stress due to discrimination, harassment, marginalization, and victimization across social systems, including family, school, and health care settings. Examples of common social stressors include family rejection and neglect, harsh discipline and bullying in schools, and anti-LGBTQIA legislation. Youth who experience multiple forms of psychosocial stress are especially susceptible to trauma sequelae across their lifespan. The stage of development during which the stressors occur may also influence their long-term impact. Youth with chronic or pervasive social stressors, particularly unsupportive, rejecting, or dangerous home environments, are at a higher risk for unhealthy behaviors. Consequently, they experience higher rates of the leading causes of morbidity and mortality in adulthood, including ischemic heart disease, cancer, lung disease, and liver disease, than peers without ACE.

Mental Health Inequities Among LGBTQIA Youth

Despite an increase in the number of youths identifying as LGBTQIA, data continue to demonstrate clear inequities in mental health outcomes among LGBTQIA youth compared to their cisgender heterosexual peers. LGBTQIA youth report disproportionate rates of depression, anxiety, suicidal ideation, and suicide attempts. Nearly two-thirds of LGBTQIA youth report symptoms of GAD, and more than half report symptoms of major depressive disorder (MDD). For many LGBTQIA youth, mental health challenges emerge earlier in the life course and persist over time.

Clinicians can understand these disproportionate mental health outcomes by examining the interlocking systems of marginalization and discrimination that compound to produce a variety of unique mental health challenges for LGBTQIA youth living in cis-sexist heterosexist social environments. Intersectional and minority stress approaches, which have strong empirical support in LGBTQIA health disparities research, explain how structural inequities like a lack of access to stable housing and interpersonal anti-LGBTQIA discrimination lead to increased rates of mental health symptoms among LGBTQIA youth. In addition to the adverse outcomes stemming from the external stressors themselves, experiences of anti-LGBTQIA stereotypes and messaging influence internalized psychological processes, such as the perception of the external world as threatening, concealment of identity, and poor self-image. Clinically, providers may observe symptoms related to anxiety, depression, and somatization, in addition to more externalizing symptoms like impulsivity and substance use.

CLINICAL APPROACHES FOR LGBTQIA YOUTH AND THEIR FAMILIES

Intersectional Care for LGBTQIA Youth

To provide effective care, clinicians must thoughtfully explore and assess each youth's unique experiences of stigmatization and support, as LGBTQIA youth do not share a universal experience by any means. For example, asexual adolescents report significantly higher rates of internalized LGBTQIA-phobia than adolescents with other sexual minority identities while experiencing less interpersonal prejudice and engaging in fewer risky behaviors. Notably, LGBTQIA youth of color experience profound inequities across school, juvenile justice, and social welfare settings due to compounding marginalization based on both race/ethnicity *and* gender identity or sexual orientation. Gender-diverse youth of color report more school victimization based on gender identity *and* race/ethnicity than cisgender peers of color, while multiracial Black LGBTQIA students experience more victimization than LGBTQIA students who identify only as Black.

Clinicians must thoughtfully examine connections between observed symptoms and identity-linked social stressors. Like cisgender heterosexual youth, LGBTQIA youth experience an array of mental health challenges, which can be additionally compounded by their experiences of marginalization and social rejection. Existing evidence-based treatments can be tailored to a youth's unique stressors and strengths. For example, CBT can address LGBTQIA identity-related stressors and promote adaptive coping strategies. Modified CBT has been shown to reduce depression symptoms, alcohol use, and HIV risk behaviors among gay and bisexual young men. Trauma-focused cognitive-behavioral therapy (TF-CBT) has been formally adapted to LGBTQIA youth and their families. Additional interventions, such as the Family Acceptance Project, target caregivers' accepting and rejecting behaviors and family caregiver–child communication to improve outcomes among LGBTQIA youth and can be adapted to diverse families.

Addressing Risk Factors and Building Resilience

In addition to experiencing more social stressors, LGBTQIA youth are also less likely than cisgender heterosexual peers to have access to key protective factors that mitigate traumatic stress, including family support, stable housing, and social support networks. In working with LGBTQIA youth, clinicians can focus on family, school, and community support that strongly impact the psychosocial well-being of LGBTQIA youth.

Family support is a critical factor in the mental well-being of LGBTQIA youth, while family rejecting behaviors detrimentally impact youth mental health. Accepting and supportive parental behaviors related to gender identity and sexual orientation reduces the risk of depression and risk behaviors among LGBTQIA youth, buffering the effects of identity-related stressors. Among prepubescent transgender youth, those who socially transition with parental support demonstrate rates of depression and anxiety comparable to cisgender peers. In working with families, the best practice is aligning with caregivers to support their child's well-being rather than challenging deeply held beliefs.

Experiences of acceptance and support in the school setting also significantly impact LGBTQIA youths' mental health, as do bullying and discrimination. School connectedness and safety are associated with better mental health and decreased risk behaviors. Unfortunately, the vast majority of LGBTQIA youth experience verbal harassment and discrimination in school settings. Clinicians can help youth recover from traumatic stress, manage co-occurring conditions, build coping strategies, and locate safe spaces and supports. Caregivers can also advocate in the school setting for inclusion policies, support their youth, and help them connect to affirming community activities.

Trauma-Informed Affirming Care for LGBTQIA Youth

By implementing trauma-informed affirming care, clinicians can play critical roles in recognizing and targeting psychological symptoms that stem from social stressors and marginalization experienced by LGBTQIA youth. Research consistently shows that social support and positive coping strategies can mitigate stress experienced by LGBTQIA youth. Clinicians who practice from a trauma-informed perspective recognize and support the youth's strengths and contextualize symptoms and challenges stemming from lived experiences. In addition, in practicing affirming care, clinicians fundamentally presume that gender and sexual orientation (1) exist on a natural spectrum where no gender identity or expression or sexual orientation is pathologic; (2) can be fixed or fluid and, in regards to gender, binary (male/female) or nonbinary; and (3) may evolve or change over the life course for some individuals. LGBTQIA-affirming care also recognizes that gender and sexual orientation vary across cultures and throughout history. Clinicians can follow specific practices to deliver trauma-informed affirming care to LGBTQIA youth (Table 22-12).

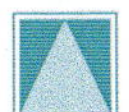

Table 22-12.
Key Trauma-Informed LGBTQIA-Affirming Practices in Clinical Settings

- Collect accurate data on sexual orientation and gender identity, including names and pronouns used
- Use the youth's name and pronouns consistently
- Screen for trauma symptoms and experiences of abuse, discrimination, marginalization, and bullying
- Utilize open-ended questions to discuss sexual orientation and gender identity/expression
- Ensure confidentiality and privacy pertaining to identity
- Engage the youth in collaborative decision-making when feasible
- Avoid gender stereotypes and comments based on appearance
- Make the clinical care space more supportive (e.g., access to gender-inclusive bathrooms, open-ended intake forms)
- Refer to Standards of Care and Continuing Education to stay up-to-date with LGBTQIA care practices

RACISM AND DISCRIMINATION'S IMPACT ON THE HEALTH AND WELL-BEING OF DEVELOPING CHILDREN AND ADOLESCENTS

While several well-known and foundational researchers were investigating the impact of "race" on the health and well-being of children, adolescents, and adults, it was not until 2002 that the Institute of Medicine (IOM)'s Committee on Understanding and Eliminating Racial and Ethnic Disparities in Healthcare produced a seminal document titled "Unequal Treatment: Confronting Racial and Ethnic Disparities in Healthcare." This report demonstrated the impact that historical marginalization and unequal health care access have on the health of Black, Indigenous, and People of Color (BIPOC) in the United States. The report included recommendations for mitigating the injustices in the health care system. However, health care systems have made few changes, and health care disparities remain.

During the midst of the global COVID-19 pandemic and the reactions to the murder of George Floyd, the CDC officially recognized that race and ethnicity remain significant predictors of access, quality, and type of care that patients receive. The CDC director declared that "the pandemic illuminated inequities that have existed for generations and revealed for all of America a known, but often unaddressed, epidemic impacting public health: racism."

In 2019, the AAP published a policy statement that at the time was revolutionary, simply stating, "Racism has a profound impact on the health status of children, adolescents, emerging adults, and their families."

DEFINING TERMINOLOGY

Carl Linnaeus's 1735 taxonomy of humans created the underpinnings of scientific racism that persist to this day, reflecting Eurocentric classifications of groups by the myth of "race." Because of the longstanding use of "race" as a proxy to attribute differences in health and well-being, health disparities have long been framed using race as the construct rather than racism. "Race" has been confounded with social determinants, such that phenotypic appearance has been designated as a key factor in illness and health rather than understanding how the context in which people live, work, and play influences their experiences. "Biologic race" does not determine health and well-being; instead, these are secondary to structural systems and barriers put into place by the social construct of race. More simply, these systems and structures have determined access, quality of care, and, ultimately, the health of people rather than personal choices and decisions.

Throughout this chapter, Black is used to describe African American/African peoples from the African diaspora, Latinx describes Latino/Latina/Latine/Hispanic peoples, Asian American and Pacific Islander (AAPI) describes Asian American/Asian/Native Hawai'ian/Pacific Islanders, and Native American describes Indigenous, First Nations, Alaskan Natives, Native tribes—federally recognized, and not.

Most theorists divide racism into multiple buckets, including larger systems or structures, down to the more nuanced and personalized forms of racism that we see operating between and within individuals (Table 22-13). These differing forms of racism operate constantly, impacting the physical and mental health of individuals, particularly children and youth. When discussing systemic or structural racism, the link to the deliberate construction of neighborhoods, schools, and other foundational systems is critical in understanding how these systems continue to function and negatively impact the lives of BIPOC Americans. While the government purposefully constructed these inequitable systems, other actors maintained and reinforced them. The result has impacted the health of generations of children and families of color. The various deleterious forms of racism, from structural and institutional racism to interpersonal and internalized forms of racism, have multiple impacts depending on the cognitive, regulatory, and emotional development of a child. The experiences of these developing children and adolescents also occur within the larger supports

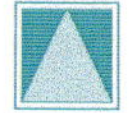

Table 22-13.
Levels of Racism

Levels of Racism	Structural/Institutional Racism	Interpersonal/ Personally Mediated Racism	Internalized Racism	Impact
Definition	• Systematic and historic racial inequities that are embedded into interconnected social, political, cultural, and economic systems such as health care, education, housing, economic, imprisonment • Historically has privileged whiteness and disadvantaged people of color	Face-to-face or covert actions expressing racial prejudice, hate, or bias. These acts can be intentional, unintentional, and include acts of omission and commission	Acceptance by members of the stigmatized races of negative messages and stereotypes affecting self-esteem and self-worth	Psychiatric development morbidity and mortality

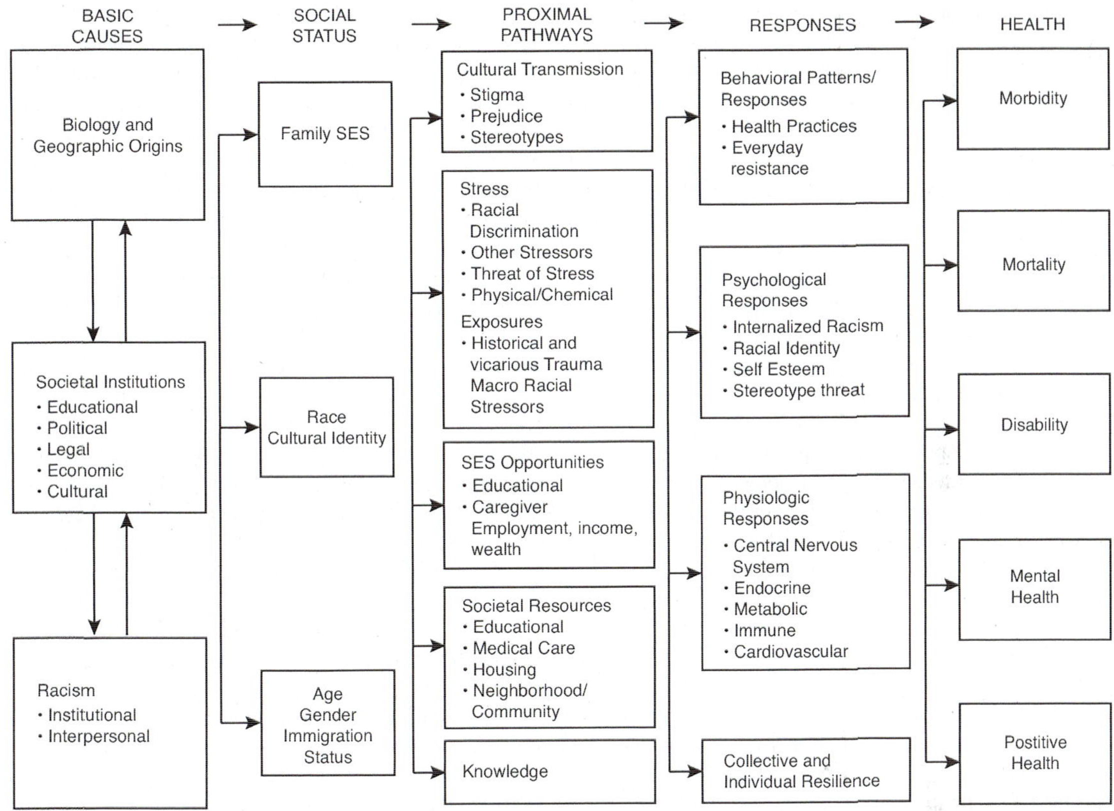

FIGURE 22-1. Pediatric framework for the study of racism and health. (Adapted with permission from Williams DR, Mohammed SA. Racism and health I: pathways and scientific evidence. *Am Behav Sci.* 2013;57(8):1152–1173.)

and systems in which they live, including their parents and primary caregivers, schools and childcare facilities, neighborhoods, and communities (Fig. 22-1).

CONTEXTUALIZING RACE-BASED TRAUMATIC STRESS AS AN ADVERSE CHILDHOOD EXPERIENCE

Racial Stress and Trauma

In 2009, the APA Presidential Task Force on Traumatic Stress Disorder and Trauma in Children and Adolescents first recognized discrimination as a contributing factor to stress in the lives of youth of color. *Racial Trauma* describes "dangerous or frightening race-based events, stressors, or discrimination." Most of the time, racial trauma is not a major, isolated episode but results from an accumulation of sometimes daily, covert acts of racial discrimination. Children and adolescents may experience direct racial trauma through structural inequities (neighborhood environments, lower quality schools, health care, family resources, and the like) or via interpersonal/personally mediated racist experiences. Racism and discrimination are not only social determinants of health but are also increasingly considered ACE and have a direct impact on adult health. Many surveys now acknowledge the impact of racism and discrimination as ACEs, such as the National Survey for Children's Health (NSCH) Philadelphia ACE Survey. For example, due to racism in the adult carceral system, a significant proportion of Black and Latinx youth have incarcerated parents. Youth with incarcerated parents are at increased risk of poverty, criminal activity, drug use, and emotional distress.

In addition, youth of color are also vulnerable to direct, indirect, or vicarious racialized trauma, such as personally experiencing police harassment or witnessing police killings of unarmed Black or Latinx citizens. Resulting symptoms of racial stress and trauma include anxiety, depression, hopelessness, and cognitive distortions about self-esteem and safety. Racial trauma has a detrimental effect on the physiologic, emotional, social, and psychological development of BIPOC children and adolescents. Ongoing racial discrimination and incidents of racial trauma can lead to a range of behavioral health disorders, including post-traumatic symptoms such as hypervigilance and avoidance, PTSD, GAD, or MDD diagnoses.

EMERGING RESEARCH/ NEUROBIOLOGY/NEUROPLASTICITY

The health and development of children and adolescents is shaped by a dynamic process of adaptation (at the molecular, cellular, organ system, and behavioral levels) that begins at conception and extends throughout the life course. The underlying plasticity that influences adaptive capacity (known to decrease with age) can lead to various outcomes influenced by the interactions among individual genetic predispositions and the environments in which pre- and postnatal development unfolds. Crucially, as children's brains develop, the cortical lining thins. Cortical thinning occurs in a typical pattern that begins in the primary sensory cortices, extends to the motor cortices, and ends in the association cortices late in adolescence or early adulthood/transitional age youth. Cortical thinning reflects myelination, and myelination reduces plasticity. Thus, early cortical thinning may shorten the window of developmental plasticity. Cortical thinning is linked to synaptic pruning, potentially limiting the plasticity at later developmental windows. Recent examination of cortical changes throughout development has shown that cortical thickness differences exist between individuals from lower and higher socioeconomic backgrounds across much of the brain in adolescence. When further articulating when these changes first begin, data has shown that in early childhood (ages 4 to 7), the cortex is thinner (reflecting that of an older child) in individuals from lower socioeconomic backgrounds, suggesting that a variety of environmental circumstances may influence cortical thickness differences, and likewise may also be preventable with appropriate evidence-based interventions. The theory that stress accelerates aging is well established, and the theory that early life stress accelerates maturation has been gaining ground.

STRESS, CORTISOL LEVELS, HYPOTHALAMIC–PITUITARY–ADRENAL AXIS

Racial discrimination and the chronic stress associated with racism and poverty have direct effects at the microcellular level and can lead to physiologic dysfunction. Racism increasing cortisol levels reflects the phenomenon of stress neurobiology. With increased stressors, there is a related increase in the sustained release of stress hormones, which is critically important for all adult pregnant women and their developing fetuses. We now know that not only does early exposure to maternal responses to stress shape the developing fetuses' later stress responsivity, but also early postnatal exposure can have similar adverse effects. We are increasingly learning more about the mechanisms involved in these alterations, such that now, an agreement exists, as highlighted in a technical report issued by the AAP, to increase the depth of surveillance. Unceasing stress hormones directly impact cortical structures with neuronal shrinkage of specific areas, including the amygdala, hippocampus, and prefrontal cortex. Reductions in these areas can lead to specific behavioral challenges, including emotional and behavioral dysregulation and later executive function deficits. With the greater elucidation of early neurodevelopmental science, much is now known about how these unrelenting, pervasive stresses with resultant increasing levels of earlier detection of mental health and behavioral challenges lead to increasingly complicated psychiatric presentations later in childhood.

In the past 20 years, this level of sustained exposure to specific stress hormones (cortisol, corticotropin-releasing hormone [CRH], adrenaline, norepinephrine) has often been labeled "toxic stress" secondary to the harm it produces on children's developmental trajectories. This intimate intertwining of systemic racist environments impacting developing brains speaks to the need to not only understand the mechanisms of action involved but also to understand better ways to mitigate these interactions to prevent, intervene, or buttress children of color who are disproportionately bearing the brunt of these disparate endemic conditions. All of this evidence speaks to the importance and understanding that early experiences matter greatly, as these very early experiences can alter neuronal development, leading to lifelong consequences. With growing evidence of the impact that early, repeated, and pervasive stress leads to later physiologic and psychological changes, understanding racism as a modifiable early adversity is critical.

IMPACT OF RACISM AND DISCRIMINATION ON DEVELOPMENT

The health and development of young children are shaped by a process of ongoing, interactive adaptation from the cellular through to cortical systems, beginning at conception and extending throughout the life course. The underlying plasticity that influences adaptive capacity (which decreases with age) can lead to a wide range of positive or negative outcomes influenced by the inextricable interactions among individual genetic/biologic predispositions and the environments in which pre- and postnatal development unfolds. Disparities in physical and mental health impose substantial human and economic costs on societies—and the relation between early adversity and lifelong well-being presents a rich scientific framework for fresh thinking about promoting health and preventing disease broadly, augmented by a deeper focus on how racism exacerbates inequities more specifically.

With increasing longitudinal research, we are beginning to understand the impact that racism and discrimination specifically have on child neurodevelopment at different ages. Secondary to the differing forms of racism as described earlier in the chapter, as well as the differential impacts on developmental stages, this section unpacks how these specific forms of racism and discrimination impact children and adolescents across five developmental stages: infancy and toddlerhood, preschool age, school age, adolescence, and transitional age youth.

Infant and Toddler

There is increasing evidence that environmental exposures including, but not limited to—intrauterine conditions, poverty, ecologic toxicants, psychosocial stressors, maternal ACEs, racism, and traumatic life events—confer significant neurodevelopmental risk prenatally. Furthermore, there is increased evidence that maternal stress-related aberrations in utero are associated with a child's later risk for neuropsychiatric disorders and stress responsivity, as discussed earlier in the chapter. When thinking about the impact of racism on early childhood, it is critically important to understand that pregnant women's experiences of racism and discrimination impact not only their health and well-being but also that of the growing fetus. Crucially, evidence suggests that early environmental influences, including racism, impact children's outcomes, including their behavioral health. Notably, the multiplicity of factors has a worsening impact on early childhood development.

Data reflects that very young children experience both institutional/structural racism, as well as interpersonal or personally mediated racism (indirectly) through their mothers' or primary caregiver's experiences, with evidence identifying that racism created inequities for Black and Brown mothers and children, even before birth. Strikingly, Black babies have the highest incidence of ACEs—more than 1.5 times the national average of two or more. Public health researcher Geronimus developed the analytic framework of weathering, which essentially describes how the health of Black people is harmed by early deterioration secondary to exposure to structural/institutional racism. Her studies have demonstrated that racial discriminatory experiences negatively impact telomeres. The length of telomeres, the end caps of chromosomes that shorten with cellular division, has been used as a marker of epigenetic age. Individuals who have experienced more stress have shorter telomeres. Geronimus has shown that exposure to stressors, such as racism and discrimination, can increase allostatic load, leading to faster aging or "weathering." There is mounting evidence that disparities in the pace of aging begin early in life: children from racially and socioeconomically disadvantaged groups mature faster than their socially advantaged and non-Latinx White peers.

Preschool Age

Recent research has reflected the impact of structural racism and discrimination on early maturation noted by early molar development in preschool-aged children. There is mounting evidence that disparities in the pace of aging begin early in life with children from racially and socioeconomically disadvantaged groups, Black and Latinx children, all maturing faster than their socially advantaged and non-Latinx White peers. Along with these early signs of early maturation as a consequence of racism and discrimination, further evidence reflects that as children age, they become increasingly aware of racism, specifically interpersonal or personally mediated racism, and even begin to struggle with internalized racism. Recent data has shown that Black and non-Latinx White children show pro-White biases by age 4 and that children have preferential play partners, and this can be based on skin color or gender. However, importantly for young children, these biases are based solely on phenotypic differences or skin color, not racist stereotypes. What becomes increasingly clear is that young children have clear in-group preferences. Nevertheless, as these children aged, they focused on individual characteristics, such as shared interests, to determine in-group and out-group membership.

By age 5, Black children attribute social exclusion to their identified race. Less is known about how young children process interpersonal racism and social exclusion or about individual differences in their sensitivity to these experiences. Kenneth and Mamie Clark discussed these issues in the 1940s with the seminal doll study showing the impact of structural racism in the form of school racial segregation and its impact on Black preschoolers in the South. The data showing harm was so compelling that Thurgood Marshall and colleagues used this more than a decade later when arguing the landmark desegregation case of Brown *v* Board of Education.

As described earlier in this chapter, race is a social construct, and very young children initially identify differences in skin color. However, they learn that a value is attached to different skin colors. Theory and research have suggested that implicit intergroup attitudes emerge at comparable levels in adults early in life.

School Age

School-aged children have a different understanding and experience of racial dynamics. Research has demonstrated that non-Latinx White children can exhibit anti-Black bias by the age of 6. Research studies have also shown that non-Latinx White children are more likely to choose other non-Latinx White children as friends over Black, Latinx, Asian, and Native American children. This bias can cause racial bullying at school and the exclusion from academic, school-related (sports, arts, groups), and social activities. This results in racial trauma and negative associations with school, learning, and education for non–White-identifying students.

Moreover, research proves that children who are the only Black children in their class or school are more likely to experience more racist incidents while having less support from teachers, administration, and their peers at school. At 7 years old, most children have developed racial permanency, the understanding that their skin color is unchangeable, and in-group bias. By 9 years old, most children understand their racial or cultural group's status in the broader society.

Children of color are often able to notice when preferential or oppressive racial dynamics play out at school, in their community, and society at large. School-aged children are also able to recognize that racial violence in the form of police killings of citizens, xenophobia against immigrants, and race-based attacks are based on White supremacy. Dr. Alvin Poussaint hypothesized that Black people are not able to express appropriate rage in response to the racial violence that they experience, which results in repressed anger and internalized psychological self-hatred. Elementary school children of color can internalize racism and racial stereotypes, leading them to unconsciously perceive people as having negative or positive characteristics based on race. This can further result in children of color internalizing White supremacy and believing in White superiority. Academic and social rejection by teachers and peers may lead students to avoid school for fear of traumatic school experiences, which then affects students' academic participation and performance in school. In addition, children of color are often aware that their non-Latinx White peers are often given preferential treatment and access to additional resources. Accordingly, despite racial permanency, children of color can unconsciously desire to attain Eurocentric physical features to receive equal treatment at school and in broader society.

10 to 12 Years Old

Research has shown that Black children as young as 10 years old are routinely perceived to be older and less innocent than non-Latinx White children of the same age. This stereotyping leads to differential treatment, with Black children labeled as aggressive, culpable, and needing to be watched and feared. In addition, in Black boys (aged 10 to 15 years), experiences with perceived interpersonal and institutional racism were related to increased internalizing symptoms, such as depression and anxiety, and increased externalizing symptoms, such as anger or aggression. School-aged children of color are also able to identify that racial discrimination threatens safety and security. Direct and indirect experiences of race-based trauma can cause typical trauma symptoms such as fear, helplessness, and worry about the physical safety of children and their family members based on race. Race-based trauma can also affect caregivers' emotional availability, attachment, and ability to help children manage their psychological responses to racial stress and trauma. Racial trauma in school-aged children is associated with distractibility, problems in school, phobias, and other anxiety symptoms.

Dr. Kenneth B. Clark hypothesized that racism creates an unconscious hypervigilance in its victims. Accordingly, as school-aged children age, they can identify differential treatment based on race but may not have the ability to recognize that their problems with mood, behavior, and self-image may be secondary to racism. Consequently, children tend to avoid settings where they feel "othered." A loss of safety and sense of belonging can result in decreased self-esteem and children losing hope, optimism, and belief in a future filled with endless possibilities. Research has shown that by age 12, there is increased pressure for youth to conform to racial in-group beliefs, as evidenced by the tendency to shun nonconforming in-group members.

Early Adolescence

Adolescence is a crucial developmental stage in the life cycle that encompasses numerous physical and psychosocial changes. During this phase, youth become more attuned to their social standing within peer groups and increasingly separate from their family. In addition, adolescents explore their sense of self and personal identity. For minoritized youth, this normative process becomes exceedingly more complex when confronted with increased exposure to institutional, interpersonal, and internalized forms of racism, which threaten central parts of identity and may have deleterious effects on developmental pathways and adolescent mental and physical health.

Several studies have reported higher rates of internalizing disorders among Black, Native American, and Asian American adolescents compared to non-Latinx White adolescents. In a longitudinal, school-based epidemiologic study of adolescent depression encompassing a diverse range of adolescents in grades 7 through 12, minoritized youth were more likely to report higher baseline levels of depression. Secondary analyses identified several factors that predicted a higher risk for the onset of a depressive episode, including Black/Latinx ethnicity, female gender, and low-income SES. Latinx children and adolescents reported the highest levels of depressive symptoms of all ethnic groups across three separate waves of data collection. Asian Americans reported similarly high levels, followed by Black adolescents. Non-Latinx White adolescents had the lowest depressive scores over time, whereas depression scores for all other ethnic groups converged despite initial differences.

Traumatic events (i.e., physical, sexual abuse, witnessing violence) disproportionately impact Black youths. One study demonstrated that 65% of Black youth report traumatic experiences compared to 30% of their peers from other races. In addition, Black youth were more likely to report adverse emotional and behavioral sequelae to trauma exposure, including poor mental health, substance abuse, decreased well-being, and risky sexual behavior. Unique race-based toxic stressors moderate the disproportionate rates of trauma and the associated outcomes observed among African Americans.

Late Adolescence/Transition Age Youth

The transition to adulthood has become a critical window in life, directing some young people on trajectories of increasing advantage and solidification and others on pathways of increasing disadvantage. A seminal study of 422 patients independently observed over 5 years in a psychiatric ED found that after adjusting for psychotic disorders, the severity of disturbance, dangerousness, psychiatric history, use of restraints, time spent in ER, and other factors, Black patients received more antipsychotic doses and less clinical attention than other comparable patients.

RACISM IN SYSTEMS OF CARE

Children and adolescents spend the majority of their time interfacing with different systems of care, including schools, early intervention (EI) programming, child welfare, juvenile justice, and services for those with developmental disorders. However, data reflects structural/institutional racism or interpersonal/personally mediated racism and discrimination impacts these systems. Furthermore, when thinking of barriers or access to care, institutional/structural racism again plays a role in that the creation of redlining or residential segregation in the 1930s in over 200 cities across the United States has left neighborhoods in the 21st century bereft of certain services and infrastructure, thus placing patients farther away from quality care, as well as barriers around the costs of affordable care.

We posit that antiracist, culturally, and trauma-informed approaches that focus on systemic inequities can create more equitable frameworks benefitting the children and adolescents they serve.

Racism in Early Care and Early Intervention

A greater understanding of the mechanisms of early stressors, including racism and discrimination on neurodevelopmental pathways, and how these stressors cause impairment of these critically developing systems has led to more work substantiating the importance and efficacy of early care and EI programming. The EI system was created to ensure that high-quality preventive and EI programming is accessible to very young children to prevent adverse outcomes. Several EI programs have shown efficacy in longitudinal assessments of various health, behavior, development, and educational outcomes. The impact of these programs is notable for children in the first 5 years of life who participate in high-quality programs (e.g., Perry Preschool Program, Carolina Abecedarian Project [BC], Early Headstart, and the like).

As more is known about the criticality of the first 5 years of life and neurodevelopment, understanding the benefits and challenges inherent in early childhood intervention and prevention systems is incredibly important. Evidence shows that implicit racial bias and exclusionary discipline against children begin as early as preschool. Dr. Walter Gilliam's work in preschools highlights how teachers' biases and stigmatized beliefs directly impact young children's (particularly young Black boys with an expulsion rate of 3.6 times more than their non-Latinx White age-matched peers) ability to remain in early educational programming. Understanding how to buttress healthy caregiving to ensure that even when children live in inequitable systems, institutional and federally funded supports exist to level the playing field.

Racism in Educational System

Children of color experience structural/institutional and interpersonal/personally mediated racism daily. Much of a child's time occurs in school, a system purposed to facilitate healthy socioemotional development and equip children with knowledge while serving as a safe, nurturing, and affirming environment. Unfortunately, schools have often served the opposite role for children of color who experience repeated, daily structural and interpersonal racial discrimination in school settings from as early as preschool. Structurally, Black, Latinx, and Native American children are more likely to be educated in school systems with less experienced teachers, less advanced courses, and lower resources than their non-Latinx White peers. Multiple studies have shown that children of color perform better academically in school when they share the same cultural background as their teachers, yet youth of color are less likely to have a teacher, counselor, or principal of the same cultural background compared to their non-Latinx White peers. In addition, due to racial bias, Black and Latinx children score lower on standardized testing than their non-Latinx White peers. Subsequently, these factors impact students' engagement and investment in school, compelling many children of color to mentally and physically "check out" of school early, affecting their educational attainment, income, and status as adults.

In controlled preschool classroom simulations, teachers were more likely to have increased surveillance of Black children and expect misbehavior from them, especially Black boys, even when no behavioral issues were present. Studies have demonstrated that continual correction of students by teachers in front of peers hurts the peers' perceptions of students. Black and Latinx children are viewed as more aggressive than non-Latinx White students. This bias has resulted in Black preschoolers being suspended at a rate of more than three times their White peers. Black girls are six times more likely to be suspended from school than non-Latinx White girls. At school, similar behaviors in Black and White children, such as inattention, talking back to a teacher, or defiance, are often interpreted differently and can result in additional attention and resources for non-Latinx White students versus punishment for Black students.

In addition to disproportionate punishment, academic enrichment, leadership opportunities, and extracurricular opportunities are structured by racism and bias.

Black students are less likely to be recommended for gifted education programs than their non-Latinx White peers because teachers have lower expectations for Black students. Moreover, children of color who are not academically challenged but may experience attentional and behavioral issues in school are more susceptible to racially biased exclusionary disciplinary practices. Multiple studies have shown that Black students are disproportionately punished with suspension and expulsion. Factors influencing suspension include being Black, being male, and being perceived as looking older than their classmates. Black and Latinx youth are also less likely than their non-Latinx White peers to receive a referral by school professionals for an ADHD evaluation.

Exposure to racism in schools can render them unsafe spaces for children of color. This, in addition to other institutional forms of racism (family economics, neighborhood environment, nutrition), contributes to educational inequalities. By high school, Black, Latinx, and Native American youth were more likely to have higher rates of absenteeism and lower graduation rates than their non-Latinx White counterparts. This further exacerbates racial disparities as advanced educational attainment is a significant predictor in life outcomes such as health and economics.

Racism in Special Education

As stated earlier in the chapter, secondary to the impacts of structural racism, youth of color are more likely to have experienced a variety of adverse outcomes, including low birth weight, exposure to lead and environmental pollutants, and living in unsafe neighborhoods, all of these are structural risk factors for developing disabilities. In addition, there is significant bias and structural racism in the rates of disability identification, evaluation, categorization, and access to and utilization of services rendered for Black and Latinx children in the special education system. Children diagnosed with one or more disabilities, such as ASD, emotional disturbance, and hearing impairment, qualify for special education. Black children are more likely to be diagnosed with emotional disturbance or intellectual disabilities; they are underrepresented in ASD and speech and language delay categories. Missed diagnoses mean that instead of receiving accurate diagnoses and appropriate services, Black youth with disabilities are more likely to be suspended than their non-Latinx White peers with disabilities.

Overall, Black and Latinx children are less likely to be enrolled in special education compared to children who are identified as non-Latinx White. However, when placed in special education programs, youth of color are more likely to be placed in the most restrictive educational settings. This means they are more likely to spend 100% of their educational time in segregated, special education settings and are less likely to have access to general education curricula, teaching, and resources. Black and Latinx children in the high school special education system are more likely to be placed in tracks where they earn high school certificates instead of traditional high school diplomas, which prevents them from considering postsecondary education as a possibility. These exclusionary practices for Black and Latinx students in special education have significant repercussions because they restrict Black and Latinx youth to a future of limited job opportunities, income/economics, health, and life trajectories.

Racism in Juvenile Justice System

Importantly, challenges that children of color face in schools are also linked to their involvement in the juvenile justice system, a system that reflects larger societal structural racism. Students who experience exclusionary and punitive disciplinary measures in school are more likely to drop out of school and more likely to become involved in the juvenile justice system. Black, Latinx, and Native American youth are disproportionately represented in the juvenile justice system. According to 2021 data, youths of color comprise 49.8% of the United States population but make up 62% of the youth charged in the juvenile justice system. Racially minoritized teens have higher arrest rates for nonviolent, low-level offenses and noncriminal misbehaviors such as truancy and curfew violations. Research has also shown that race is a strong predictor of youth commitment to facilities where Black youth were more likely to be sent to boot camp or wilderness programs, while their non-Latinx White peers were committed to therapeutic programs such as drug/alcohol diversion programs and mental health facilities. In addition, Black children are five times more likely to be detained in juvenile justice facilities and are more likely to be sent from juvenile to adult court than their non-Latinx White peers.

During incarceration, youth experience solitary confinement, abuse, and possible inadequate access to mental health care or education. Evidence has shown that involvement in the justice system "can lead to lower family functioning, impaired social networks, decreased high school graduation, decreased employment rates, increase in violence and victimization, and poorer mental health outcomes." Subsequently, youth involved in the juvenile justice system are more likely to continue involvement in the justice system throughout adulthood.

Child Welfare

The child welfare system is another system characterized by inequity, racial disparity, and racial disproportionality across multiple levels. Oversurveillance of and overinvestigation of families of color reflect systemic, implicit, and explicit biases that are racialized and extend across every stage of decision-making in the child welfare system, from reporting, investigating, intervention, and the placement process. This includes the types of services to which families are referred, are accessible, the degree of placement instability, and engagement with caseworkers. All of these reflect disparities where Black families have disparate contact and outcomes. Biased decision-making contributes to the fact that caseworkers are more likely to substantiate claims of abuse and neglect for Black and Indigenous families, resulting in disproportionate separation of Black and Indigenous youth from their families. From entry to placement or exit out of the child welfare system, Black children experience more harm, longer lengths of stay, protracted reunification periods, and slower rates of exit compared to other children.

Specifically, the mental health implications of structural racism within child welfare are significant. Researchers have shown how racism impacts mental health access for youth of color in the child welfare system and that despite having similar presentations in symptoms and diagnoses, youth of color have a higher likelihood than non-Latinx White youth to receive psychotropic medication and behavioral health diagnoses. Solutions proposed by researchers, advocates, and policy members include the development of culturally responsive practices, recruiting and retaining foster families of color, and understanding and addressing bias at various decision points.

Developmental Disabilities

Another system in which disparities exist for children of color is within developmental disabilities services. Proper and timely identification, access to treatment, and care are all challenges for BIPOC families. Multiple studies have identified that there are significant racial–ethnic disparities in the identification of ASD. Historically, there were lower rates of identification in Black and Latinx children compared to their peers. Recently, the CDC has shown an improvement in the identification of ASD in Black children. However, lower identification rates for Latinx children persist. Black and Latinx children are still more likely to receive ASD evaluations at later ages and stages of severity than their non-Latinx White peers. Studies indicate that this delay in assessment and diagnosis occurs years after Black parents have voiced concern for their child's development to teachers and pediatricians. Black parents are also more likely to experience difficulties getting ASD evaluations for their children and, on average, visit multiple providers before finally receiving a diagnosis of ASD. This delay in diagnosis denies children of color access to EI (which is related to longitudinal outcomes, including morbidity and mortality), services, and accommodations that are essential in their developmental trajectories and quality of life. Moreover, these children ultimately experience worse health outcomes.

Even when diagnosed with developmental disabilities, children of color are more likely to receive certain diagnoses that reflect racist stereotypes. Black students are twice as likely to be identified as having emotional disturbance and intellectual disabilities as their peers. Native American students are twice as likely to be identified as having specific learning disabilities and four times as likely to be identified as having developmental delays. In addition, children of color with disabilities are more likely to be placed in more restrictive learning environments than their non-Latinx White peers. After diagnosis, research has shown that Black and non-English speaking families receive fewer services for their children with developmental disabilities than non-Latinx White families who have children with developmental disabilities. These differences also occur at the state level, and studies show that regional centers in California that provide services for children with developmental disabilities spend less funding on Black and Asian children than on non-Latinx White children.

RACIAL INEQUITIES IN MENTAL HEALTH TREATMENT AND OUTCOMES

The data reflects how BIPOC patients not only have less access to care, but when they do receive care, it is consistently poorer quality than that obtained by their non-Latinx White peers. Racism and racial bias are woven into the foundation of the American practice of psychiatry, dating back to Rush's 18th-century concept of *negritude* (the belief that having black skin was a disease) and Cartwright's 19th-century invention of *drapetomania* (which believed that enslaved Africans who attempted to escape mental disorder treatable only with physical punishment or amputations). Psychiatric institutions likewise intentionally participated in racial segregation, and even when "integrated," they provided lower standards of care and treatment for Black patients. In the 1960s and 1970s, Black men were disproportionately diagnosed with schizophrenia as the diagnostic criteria included aggression, violence, agitation, and stereotypical terms often attributed to Black men. These disorders were then used to discredit the mental fitness of many Black people who were involved in the Civil Rights Movement. This racialization and criminalization of mental illness also resulted in mental health care and treatment transferring from psychiatric institutions to the carceral system, which disproportionately imprisons BIPOC. To this day, psychiatrists are more likely to diagnose Black patients with schizophrenia and prescribe them higher doses of antipsychotic medications.

Adults of color are also more likely to have worse mental health outcomes than their non-Latinx White counterparts, which is of particular importance when recognizing that the health of the parents or primary caregivers directly influences the healthy development of their child. A child's mental health prognosis depends on the mental wellness of their adult caregivers. In addition, inequities in mental health care extend to children of color. Psychiatrists' racial bias and differences in access to mental health care have resulted in mental health disparities along color lines. Research has shown that implicit and explicit personally mediated racism can affect mental health care delivery and outcomes.

Concerning psychiatric and behavioral health care, recent literature reviews have indicated that ethnic/racial minority children with mental health difficulties are underserved relative to their non-Latinx White counterparts for prevention, access, quality treatments, and outcomes of care. Mental health care systems perpetuate racism and racial bias through the underdiagnosis and misdiagnosis of common pediatric psychiatric disorders and the limited exploration and identification of the manifestations of racial trauma in children. Children and adolescents of color have experienced disparities in mental health care access, diagnostic variability, and treatment availability, resulting in differences in outcomes. Due to structural racism, Black and Latinx youth are more likely to live in areas with a shortage of health providers and, most likely, child psychiatrists. Systemic racism influences treatment seeking and the experience of mental health care for BIPOC children and youth. Studies from the United States cite experiences of racism, discrimination, and culturally incompetent care as barriers to help-seeking behaviors and retention in treatment. Studies in Canada demonstrated that youth are less likely to access outpatient levels of care voluntarily and more likely to initiate treatment in crisis settings or through the criminal justice system. When minoritized youth ultimately access mental health treatment, they are more likely to express dissatisfaction with their care due to experiences of race-based discrimination. In addition, attitudes toward help-seeking are further complicated by cultural background (i.e., first- vs. second-generation immigrants) and views of mental health treatment as a Westernized construct.

According to the 2006 to 2012 Medical Expenditure Panel Surveys, Black and Latinx children had fewer visits to psychiatrists and other mental health professionals and less substance use care than their non-Latinx White peers, even when controlled for mental health impairment, income, and health insurance. This may also show lower identification of mental illness in minority youth and decreased referral rates to psychiatrists from pediatricians and educators. Psychiatric and behavioral problems in youth of color are more likely to result in increased school punishment and incarceration than increased referrals for mental health care. Black adolescents diagnosed with MDD received mental health treatment at a much lower rate than non-Latinx White adolescents. Black and Latinx adolescents, even when severely impaired, were less likely than non-Latinx White adolescents to receive medication or therapy for mood and anxiety disorders. Once care was initiated, youth of color had fewer follow-up mental health appointments than their non-Latinx White peers.

A large portion of all diagnostic processes allows for clinician subjective evaluation, which leaves room for unconscious racial bias. ADHD is prevalent in children of all races and genders. However, non-Latinx White boys are more likely to be diagnosed with ADHD than any other group. By kindergarten, Black children are 70% less likely to receive the diagnosis of ADHD compared to non-Latinx White children, and by high school, non-Latinx White children are almost twice as likely to receive the diagnosis of ADHD as Black children. Further studies have shown that Black and Latinx youth are more likely to receive the diagnosis of ODD and conduct disorder (CD) than the diagnosis of ADHD and are more likely to be diagnosed with ODD and CD than their non-Latinx White peers. These diagnoses make youth more vulnerable to adverse punitive disciplinary action in school, poor school performance, and involvement in the juvenile justice system. Failing to diagnose youth of color with ADHD can significantly alter one's life trajectory; it denies youth essential medications, therapy, and support services, further perpetuating or exacerbating professional and socioeconomic inequalities. Compounding overreporting of ODD and CD and underreporting of depression, anxiety, and ADHD in youth of color is the fact that racial trauma is likely underreported in youth of color due to clinician's lack of awareness, bias, and discomfort surrounding racial topics and the narrow and exclusive scope of the PTSD criteria.

Disparities in mental health diagnosis and treatment have resulted in worsened mental health outcomes for children and adolescents of color. Research from Leventhal et al. showed that self-reported concern about increasing societal discrimination was associated with a higher frequency of substance use, a more significant number of substances used, and higher odds of depression and ADHD symptoms. The suicide rate for Black youth has increased from 2.55 per 100,000 in 2007 to 4.82 per 100,000 in 2017, which is the fastest rate increase for any racial-ethnic group. Compared to their non-Latinx White peers, Black youth under 13 years are twice as likely to die by suicide. Research investigating the impact of perceived racial discrimination among children and adolescents found that exposure to perceived discrimination predicted poorer mental health care outcomes.

THE ROLE OF THE CHILD AND ADOLESCENT PSYCHIATRIST

Child and adolescent psychiatrists are poised to leverage both developmental and structural approaches to understand and respond to structural racism and the resultant adverse mental health outcomes in BIPOC children and youth. By acknowledging the role of racism in child and adolescent mental health, psychiatrists and other mental health professionals can proactively engage in systems-level interventions to identify, mitigate, and prevent the adverse effects that stem from structural, systemic, interpersonal/personally mediated, and internalized racism, thus improving the health and well-being of all children, adolescents, emerging adults, and their families. By using innovative strategies, including having an antiracist approach to clinical practice, engaging not only the family but also community partners, and building resilience through supporting racial–ethnic socialization (R/ES) and racial pride, child and adolescent psychiatrists can improve the equitable care of diverse children.

Intentionally antiracist practices, trauma-informed care, and culturally informed care are essential factors in ensuring the healthy and optimal development of BIPOC children and youth. Psychiatric treatment of minoritized and marginalized youth should fundamentally be strength-based, emphasizing creating safe spaces that foster trust, autonomy, and self-advocacy. Understanding the neighborhoods, schools, and communities where children live and grow is essential to child psychiatric practice. Optimizing clinical care includes understanding the lives and experiences of diverse children, adolescents, and their families, ensuring that prevention and intervention programs interdigitate with real life. Screening for mental health and behavioral issues should always be nuanced and thoughtful, taking into account differential experiences as well as taking into account diverse cultural practices and beliefs.

Building Resilience

Many children and adolescents can thrive even in the face of racist systems and structures that directly impact their lives, neighborhoods, communities, and, ultimately, their development. As important as it is to describe how racism and discrimination can negatively affect developing children, equally important is recognizing that families have support systems that help mitigate the impacts of racism and discrimination.

As has been noted, several studies have identified racism as impacting youths' psychosocial functioning and emotional well-being, particularly around anxiety, depression, and academic functioning. Literature that examines protective and resilience-promoting factors highlights the importance of R/ES and racial pride in decreasing adverse mental health outcomes. As described by Stevenson, Hughes, and colleagues, R/ES represents a diverse set of individual coping skills across various psychosocial domains to mitigate experiences of racial-related tension and stress in interpersonal relationships. R/ES, which includes affirming messages passed on between youth and their caregivers around racial pride and identity, has been particularly important for Black children's academic and socioemotional well-being. Racial–ethnic connectedness is a form of cultural affirmation and pride that can positively impact academic achievement and decrease conduct and emotional problems.

Research and Antiracism

Despite a considerable increase in the number of studies on racism and health in recent years, relatively few have focused on children, adolescents, and transition-age youth. Furthermore, much of the work has focused on the experiences of Black and, to a lesser extent, Latinx children and adolescents, excluding the experiences of Asian Americans, Hawaiian, Pacific Islanders, and Native/Indigenous children and adolescents. The sparse evidence from studies that draw on longitudinal data draws a correlation between racial trauma and poor health but provides few insights about the sensitivity of early exposure, the importance of duration of exposure, precise mechanisms of action, or the latency period between exposure to racism and discrimination and the onset of illness; as a result, we do not fully understand the causal pathways through early childhood and later adolescence. What is known is that the impact of perceived and observed experiences of discrimination and racism on child and family health outcomes can be profound. Future research efforts should (1) focus on nuanced tools to measure perceived racism and its impact on all BIPOC children and adolescents at different developmental ages and (2) explicitly focus on BIPOC youth as they are underrepresented in research, thereby ensuring that prevention and intervention strategies that are created will be as effective in diverse communities.

By ensuring that the research undertaken recruits and includes diverse families and youth, we will ensure more equitable care, treatment access, and holistic preventive strategies. Secondary to the increasing recognition of the dearth of inclusive research on children and youth of color, federal and state agencies are creating legislation to ensure these limitations cease in future funded research mechanisms. Allied organizations are also changing the language they use with youth and their families, enhancing their guidelines to identify and address racism and discrimination and its impact on developing children and youth. Both the AAP and the AACAP have created resources for clinicians, children, and families that highlight the importance of addressing issues of racism and discrimination often and early, recognizing the detriment they have on child and adolescent mental health and well-being.

As this chapter comes to a close, the salient points highlighted throughout the sections include the growing evidence of the significant ways in which multiple forms of racism and discrimination can adversely impact developing children and adolescents. Also highlighted are the burgeoning evidence-based modalities and system changes that, once generalized, will ensure equitable care and treatment for all children. Increasingly, the role of the child and adolescent psychiatrist is to be able to understand emerging principles of neuroscience as they relate to child development and then integrate this understanding with information about the social determinants of mental health. A comprehensive appreciation of child development must include the impacts of racism and discrimination on child health.

This chapter has taken a developmental perspective to articulate how racism and discrimination harm children and youth while ensuring that the science around prevention, intervention, and discussion of systems and practices to prevent, intervene, mitigate, and ultimately treat if necessary are also clearly understood.

INTERNET GAMING DISORDER IN YOUTH

Internet gaming disorder (IGD) was proposed in the United States in 2013 and included in the Diagnostic and Statistical Manual (DSM-5-TR) as a "condition for further study." Clinicians conceptualized it as a potentially impairing psychiatric disorder that might merit inclusion in future revisions of the DSM. At about the same time, the World Health Organization (WHO) considered game addiction a significant public health issue. In 2018, the WHO proposed game addiction as a gaming disorder (GD) and included it in the 11th revision of the International Classification of Diseases (ICD-11).

In the United States, given the paucity of evidence-based clinical studies on GD and the lack of consensus on diagnostic criteria, clinicians and researchers decided to delay its inclusion in the DSM-5-TR, instead including it in their appendix as a condition for further study.

PREVALENCE

Due to variability in screening measures as well as different uses of the diagnostic criteria of IGDs in the ICD-11 and the DSM-5-TR, the prevalence of this disorder in youth and adults remains challenging to determine. Clinicians disagree about how much gaming is too much and what role culture and nationality play.

Prevalence estimates range from 0.7% to perhaps 15% with an average of about 5%. No region or country appears to vary greatly in prevalence (the 15%, however was from a high school in Hong Kong). Although the percentage of persons with internet access has increased with time, the prevalence of IGD has not increased significantly.

DIAGNOSTIC CRITERIA: GAMING DISORDER (ICD-11) AND INTERNET GAMING DISORDER (DSM-5-TR CONDITION FOR FURTHER STUDY)

The DSM-5-TR (Internet Gaming Disorder—condition for further study) and ICD-11 (Gaming Disorder) list similar diagnostic criteria for these disorders. Similarities include repetitive or persistent gaming behavior that impairs functioning in multiple domains (e.g., educational, occupational, interpersonal) for at least 12 months (Table 22-14).

BENEFITS AND RISKS OF ONLINE VIDEO GAME PLAY IN YOUTH

The benefits of internet gaming for youth include promoting problem-solving, cooperation, and connection with peers worldwide. Inherent to all video games is a process of learning rules and objectives. It also teaches

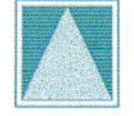

Table 22-14.
Internet Gaming Disorder/Gaming Disorder

	DSM-TR	ICD-11
Diagnostic Name	**Internet Gaming Disorder**	**Gaming Disorder**
Duration	1 yr	Extended period
Symptoms	Preoccupation with online games Withdrawal when games are taken away Tolerance to the activity (needing more time to play) Failed quit attempts Loss of interest in alternative activities Continued use despite insight into gaming as a problem Deceived others about the amount of gaming Use of games to avoid negative moods	Persistent gaming, with: • Loss of control over the behavior • Gaming takes precedence over other activities • Continues/escalates despite negative consequences
Required number of symptoms	≥5	All of the above
Psychosocial consequences	Psychosocial impairment: risked or lost relationships, jobs, or other opportunities due to gaming	Psychosocial or other impairment
Exclusions	Gambling games or pornography sites	Substance or medication-induced, including withdrawal Other mental disorder
Symptoms specifiers		Predominantly online Predominantly offline
Severity specifiers	Mild, moderate, or severe, depending on the number of symptoms and amount of psychosocial consequences	
Comment	Included as a proposed diagnosis under "Conditions for Further Study"	

frustration tolerance, winning and losing gracefully, cooperating with others, and, in some cases, delayed gratification. It can also foster social connection and provide an outlet for otherwise isolated or lonely youths.

However, gaming can also have a negative effect. Children may rely on video gameplay to avoid social and academic challenges. Some gaming environments can also lead to hostility or intimidation of younger children who play with older players or bully less experienced players. Despite many claims, there is no data to support that violent video games lead to violent in-person behaviors in youth, but some games may encourage aggressive or even abusive behavior toward other gamers. In addition, games and the equipment required to play them can be expensive. Games may be free or inexpensive to begin but require increasingly expensive purchases to continue.

BIOLOGIC CORRELATES OF INTERNET GAMING DISORDER

Proposed Neurobiology of Internet Gaming Disorder

IGD shares neurobiologic alterations that are typical for other addictions. Studies have demonstrated the activation of the brain reward regions, which appear similar to substance-related activations. They also show reduced activity in brain areas devoted to executive function and impulse control.

COMORBIDITY

Several comorbid psychiatric disorders are associated with youth who present with problematic or impairing video game use. The strongest associations are with anxiety, depression, ADHD, and anxiety disorders.

Major Depressive Disorder

Depressive symptoms are frequently associated with youth and adults who present with impairment from internet game use. Depressive and IGD symptoms are likely bidirectionally related, consistent with findings in other addictive disorders. The relationship is dynamic, and remission from IGD can improve depressive symptoms.

Attention-Deficit/Hyperactivity Disorder

ADHD may be a mediating factor for IGD. Neurologic reports studies have suggested overlap between the pathways involved in ADHD and IGD. ADHD is also associated with a poor prognosis for recovery and recurrence from IGD.

Anxiety Disorders

IGD is associated with GAD, and social anxiety disorder. When anxiety is present with IGD, the risk of developing depression is increased.

TREATMENT OF INTERNET GAMING DISORDER

There is little evidence for any treatment. There is anecdotal evidence for this, including parent training, motivational interviewing, group therapy, and CBT. Currently, several residential treatment programs for IGD are in operation in the United States and abroad, which offer "digital detox," however, long-term outcomes have yet to be verified.

One case study suggested bupropion as having efficacy, but the evidence is insufficient to recommend a pharmacologic agent apart from those used to treat comorbid disorders.

CLINICAL CONSIDERATIONS

Age-appropriate game choice and boundaries are essential considerations for parents and a skill for clinicians to identify signs of problematic gameplay and provide guidance for parents. Parents' familiarity with and understanding of expectations of schoolwork and other balanced tasks of childhood (exercise, socializing with peers, extracurricular activities, enrichment) at different developmental ages will help them to determine how much gaming and screen time would be appropriate for their child's circumstances. The American Academy of Pediatricians lists recommended time limits based on age (see https://services.aap.org/en/patient-care/media-and-children/).

As the potential for online gaming impairment may rise along with the increased accessibility of gaming devices, screening for IGD is a worthwhile addition to mental health evaluation in youths. Clinicians should begin with open-ended, plain-language questions such as "Tell me about what gaming means to you, "What happens when you find yourself gaming too much"?, and "What does gaming get in the way of for you"?

We do not recommend abstinence since it may promote avoidance of issues rather than help a child learn self-regulation. Gaming is often a coping strategy for many children. In moderation, gaming can represent a beneficial activity, allowing children an opportunity for emotional processing, social play, learning, and a reprieve from life stressors. Clinicians need to understand that although video game use is ubiquitous in today's youth, addiction to video gameplay leading to impairment is rare.

Public Oversight of Online Gaming

Currently, in the United States, the Entertainment Software Ratings Board provides oversight within the video game industry regarding transparency of the content within video games. However, there is no oversight about game content outside of age restrictions on online gambling platforms.

ACKNOWLEDGMENT

The authors would like to acknowledge Dr. Suegee Tamar-Mattis, DO, for graciously offering to consult and review our content related to caring for intersex youth and youth with DSD.

Further Readings

Pediatric Sleep Disorders

American Academy of Pediatrics. School start times for adolescents. *Pediatrics*. 2014;134(3):642–649.

Blake MJ, Sheeber LB, Youssef GJ, Raniti MB, Allen NB. Systematic review and meta-analysis of adolescent cognitive-behavioral sleep interventions. *Clin Child Fam Psychol Rev*. 2017;20(3):227–249.

Buckley AW, Hirtz D, Oskoui M, et al. Practice guideline: treatment for insomnia and disrupted sleep behavior in children and adolescents with autism spectrum disorder: Report of the Guideline Development, Dissemination, and Implementation Subcommittee of the American Academy of Neurology. *Neurology*. 2020;94(9):392–404.

England SJ, Picchietti DL, Couvadelli BV, et al. L-dopa improves restless legs syndrome and periodic limb movements in sleep but not attention-deficit/hyperactivity disorder in a double-blind trial in children. *Sleep Med*. 2011;12(5):471–477.

Gershon A, Singh MK. Sleep in adolescents with bipolar I disorder: stability and relation to symptom change. *J Clin Child Adolesc Psychol*. 2017;46(2):247–257.

Ivanenko A, Crabtree VM, Gozal D. Sleep and depression in children and adolescents. *Sleep Med Rev*. 2005;9:115–129.

Ma ZR, Shi LJ, Deng MH. Efficacy of cognitive behavioral therapy in children and adolescents with insomnia: a systematic review and meta-analysis. *Braz J Med Biol Res*. 2018;51(6):e7070.

Malow B, Adkins KW, McGrew SG, et al. Melatonin for sleep in children with autism: a controlled trial examining dose, tolerability, and outcomes. *J Autism Dev Disord*. 2012;42(8):1729–1737.

Plazzi G, Ruoff C, Lecendreux M, et al. Treatment of paediatric narcolepsy with sodium oxybate: a double-blind, placebo-controlled, randomised-withdrawal multicentre study and open-label investigation. *Lancet Child Adolesc Health*. 2018;2(7):483–494.

Thorpy MJ, Bogan RK. Update on the pharmacologic management of narcolepsy: mechanisms of action and clinical implications. *Sleep Med*. 2020;68:97–109.

Child Maltreatment

Adams JA, Farst KJ, Kellogg ND. Interpretation of medical findings in suspected child sexual abuse: an update for 2018. *J Pediatr Adolesc Gynecol*. 2018;31(3):225–231.

American Professional Society on the Abuse of Children (APSAC). *Forensic Interviewing in Cases of Suspected Child Abuse*. American Professional Society on the Abuse of Children; 2012.

Centers for Disease Control and Prevention, National Center for Injury Prevention and Control, Division of Violence Prevention. Child Abuse and Neglect: Risk and Protective Factors. 2021.

Deblinger E, Mannarino AP, Cohen JA, Steer RA. A follow-up study of a multi-site, randomized, controlled trial for children with sexual abuse-related PTSD symptoms. *J Am Acad Child Adolesc Psychiatry*. 2006;45:1474–1484.

McElvaney R, Greene S, Hogan D. To tell or not to tell? Factors influencing young people's informal disclosures of child sexual abuse. *J Interpers Violence*. 2014;29(5):928–947.

Narang SK, Fingarson A, Lukefahr J; Council on Child Abuse and Neglect. Abusive head trauma in infants and children. *Pediatrics*. 2020;145(4):e20200203.

Nemeroff CB, Seligman F. The pervasive and persistent neurobiological and clinical aftermath of child abuse and neglect. *J Clin Psychiatry*. 2013;74(10):999–1001.

Sege RD, Siegel BS; Council on Child Abuse and Neglect and Committee on Psychological Aspects of Child and Family Health. Effective discipline to raise healthy children. *Pediatrics*. 2018;142(6):e20183112.

Sheets LK, Leach ME, Koszewski IJ, Lessmeier AM, Nugent M, Simpson P. Sentinel injuries in infants evaluated for child physical abuse. *Pediatrics*. 2013;131(4):701–707.

U.S. Department of Health & Human Services, Administration for Children and Families, Children's Bureau. Child Maltreat 2018. 2020.

U.S. Department of Justice, Office of Justice Programs, Office of Juvenile Justice and Delinquency Prevention. Confronting Commercial Sexual Exploitation and Sex Trafficking of Minors in the United States. 2013.

Winters GM, Jeglic EL, Kaylor LE. Validation of the sexual grooming model of child sexual abusers. *J Child Sex Abus*. 2020;29(7):855–875.

School Consultation and Collaborating With the Educational System

Addis S, Greer K, Dunlap L. Effective strategies for alternative school improvement: a practice guide by the national dropout prevention center. *National Dropout Prevention Center*. Successful Practices Network; 2020.

Bostic JQ, Bagnell A. Psychiatric school consultation. An organizing framework and empowering techniques. *Child Adolesc Psychiatr Clin N Am*. 2001;10:1–12.

Cornell D, Maeng JL, Burnette AG, et al. Student threat assessment as a standard school safety practice: results from a statewide implementation study. *Sch Psychol Q*. 2018;33:213–222.

Hoover S, Bostic J. Schools as a vital component of the child and adolescent mental health system. *Psychiatr Serv*. 2021;72:37–48.

Love HE, Schlitt J, Soleimanpour S, Panchal N, Behr C. Twenty years of school-based health care growth and expansion. *Health Aff (Millwood)*. 2019;38:755–764.

Miller DN, Mazza JJ. School-based suicide prevention, intervention, and postvention. In: Flett GL, Saklofske DH, Leschied AW, eds. *Handbook of School-Based Mental Health Promotion: An Evidence-Informed Framework for Implementation*. Springer; 2018:261–277.

Stoiber KC, Gettinger M. Multi-tiered systems of support and evidence-based practices. In: Jimerson SR, Burns MK, VanDerHeyden AM, eds. *Handbook of Response to Intervention: The Science and Practice of Multi-Tiered Systems of Support*. 2nd ed. Springer; 2015:121–141.

US Commission on Civil Rights. *Beyond suspensions: examining school discipline policies and connections to the school-to-prison pipeline for students of color with disabilities*. US Commission on Civil Rights; 2019.

Vona P, Jaycox LH, Kataoka SH, Stein BD, Wong M. Supporting students following school crises: from the acute aftermath through recovery. In: Harrison JR, Schultz BK, Evans SW, eds. *School Mental Health Services for Adolescents*. Oxford University Press; 2017:78–103.

Weisbrot DM. "The need to see and respond": the role of the child and adolescent psychiatrist in school threat assessment. *J Am Acad Child Adolesc Psychiatry*. 2020;59:20–26.

Zirkel PA. Special education law: illustrative basics and nuances of key IDEA components. *Teach Educ Spec Educ*. 2015;38:263–275.

Gay, Bisexual, Transgender, Queer/Questioning, Intersex, and Asexual (LGBTQIA) Youth

American Psychiatric Association. *Diagnostic And Statistical Manual of Mental Disorders*. 5th ed. American Psychiatric Publishing; 2013.

American Psychiatric Association. Gender Dysphoria. 2022. https://www.psychiatry.org/File%20Library/Psychiatrists/Practice/DSM/DSM-5-TR/APA-DSM5TR-GenderDysphoria.pdf

American Psychological Association. Guidelines for psychological practice with transgender and gender nonconforming people. *Am Psychol*. 2015;70(9):832–864.

Becerra-Culqui TA, Liu Y, Nash R, et al. Mental health of transgender and gender nonconforming youth compared with their peers. *Pediatrics*. 2018;141(5):e20173845.

Callens N, Kreukels BPC, van de Grift TC. Young voices: sexual health and transition care needs in adolescents with intersex/differences of sex development—a pilot study. *J Pediatr Adolesc Gynecol*. 2021;34(2):176–189.e2.

Cohen JA, Mannarino AP, Wilson K, et al. *Trauma-Focused Cognitive Behavioral Therapy LGBTQ Implementation Manual*. Allegheny Health Network; 2018.

Coleman E, Radix AE, Bouman WP, et al. Standards of care for the health of transgender diverse people, version 8. *Int J Trangend Health*. 2022;23(Suppl 1):S1–S259.

Drescher J. Out of DSM: depathologizing homosexuality. *Behav Sci (Basel)*. 2015;5(4):565–575.

Eisenberg ME, Resnick MD. Suicidality among gay, lesbian and bisexual youth: the role of protective factors. *J Adolesc Health*. 2006;39(5):662–668.

Keo-Meier C, Ehrensaft D, eds. *The Gender Affirmative Model: An Interdisciplinary Approach to Supporting Transgender and Gender Expansive Children*. American Psychological Association; 2018.

Kidd KM, Sequeira GM, Douglas C, et al. Prevalence of gender-diverse youth in an urban school district. *Pediatrics*. 2021;147(6):e2020049823.

Kosciw JG, Clark CM, Truong NL, et al. *The 2019 National School Climate Survey: The Experiences Of Lesbian, Gay, Bisexual And Transgender Youth In Our Nation's Schools*. GLSEN; 2020.

Ramos N, Barnert E, Bath E. Addressing the mental health needs of LGBTQ youth in the juvenile justice system. *J Am Acad Child Adolesc Psychiatry*. 2021;61(2):115–119.

Ryan C, Diaz R. *Family Acceptance Project: Intervention Guidelines and Strategies*. Family Acceptance Project; 2011.

Strang JF, Meagher H, Kenworthy L, et al. Initial clinical guidelines for co-occurring autism spectrum disorder and gender dysphoria or incongruence in adolescents. *J Clin Child Adolesc Psychol*. 2018;47(1):105–115.

The Trevor Project. National Survey on LGBTQ Youth Mental Health. 2021. https://www.TheTrevorProject.org/survey-2021

Racism and Discrimination's Impact on the Health and Well-Being of Developing Children and Adolescents

Assari S, Moazen-Zadeh E, Caldwell CH, Zimmerman MA. Racial discrimination during adolescence predicts mental health deterioration in adulthood: gender differences among blacks. *Public Health Front*. 2017;5:104.

Berry OO, Londoño Tobón A, Njoroge WFM. Social determinants of health: the impact of racism on early childhood mental health. *Curr Psychiatry Rep*. 2021;23(5):23.

Broder-Fingert S, Mateo CM, Zuckerman KE. Structural racism and autism. *Pediatrics*. 2020;146(3):e2020015420.

Camerota M, Willoughby MT. Prenatal risk predicts preschooler executive function: a cascade model. *Child Dev*. 2020;91(3):e682–e700.

Carter RT, Kirkinis K, Johnson VE. Relationships between trauma symptoms and race-based traumatic stress. *Traumatology*. 2020;26(1):11–18.

Fadus MC, Ginsburg KR, Sobowale K, et al. Unconscious bias and the diagnosis of disruptive behavior disorders and ADHD in African American and Hispanic youth. *Acad Psychiatry*. 2020;44:95–102.

Fadus MC, Valadez EA, Bryant BE, et al. Racial disparities in elementary school disciplinary actions: findings from the ABCD study. *J Am Acad Child Adolesc Psychiatry*. 2021;60(8):998–1009.

Felitti VJ, Anda RF, Nordenberg D, et al. Relationship of childhood abuse and household dysfunction to many of the leading causes of death in adults: the adverse childhood experiences (ACE) study. *Am J Prev Med*. 1998;14(4):245–258.

Graignic-Philippe R, Dayan J, Chokron S, Jacquet AY, Tordjman S. Effects of prenatal stress on fetal and child development: a critical literature review. *Neurosci Biobehav Rev*. 2014;43:137–162.

Jansen MO, Brown TR, Xu KY, Glowinski AL. Using digital technology to overcome racial disparities in child and adolescent psychiatry. *J Am Acad Child Adolesc Psychiatry*. 2022;61(10):1211–1217.

Lindsay S, Li Y, Joneja S, Hsu S. Experiences of racism and racial disparities in health care among children and youth with autism and their caregivers: a systematic review. *Disabil Rehabil*. 2025;47(5):1061–1080.

Love B, Hayes-Greene D. *The groundwater approach: building a practical understanding of structural racism*. Racial Equity Institute; 2018.

MacKinnon N, Kingsbury M, Mahedy L, Jonathan E, Ian C. The association between prenatal stress and externalizing symptoms in childhood: evidence from the Avon longitudinal study of parents and children. *Biol Psychiatry*. 2018;83(2):100–108.

Marrast L, Himmelstein DU, Woolhandler S. Racial and ethnic disparities in mental health care for children and young adults: a national study. *Int J Health Serv*. 2016;46(4):810–824.

Masten AS. Resilience theory and research on children and families: past, present, and promise. *J Fam Theory Rev*. 2018;10(1):12–31.

McDermott CL, Hilton K, Park AT, et al. Early life stress is associated with earlier emergence of permanent molars. *Proc Natl Acad Sci U S A*. 2021;118(24):e2105304118.

McDonald SW, Madigan S, Racine N, Benzies K, Tomfohr L, Tough S. Maternal adverse childhood experiences, mental health, and child behavior at age 3: the all our families community cohort study. *Prev Med*. 2019;118:286–294.

Mendez DD, Scott J, Adodoadji L, Toval C, McNeil M, Sindhu M. Racism as public health crisis: assessment and review of municipal declarations and resolutions across the United States. *Front Public Health*. 2021;9:686807.

Paradies Y, Truong M, Priest N. A systematic review of the extent and measurement of healthcare provider racism. *J Gen Intern Med*. 2014;29(2):364–387.

Priest N, Doery K, Truong M, et al. Updated systematic review and meta-analysis of studies examining the relationship between reported racism and health and well-being for children and youth: a protocol. *BMJ Open*. 2021;11(6):e043722.

Saleem FT, Anderson RE, Williams M. Addressing the "myth" of racial trauma: developmental and ecological considerations for youth of color. *Clin Child Fam Psychol Rev*. 2020;23:1–14.

Sevon MA, Levi-Nielson S, Tobin RM. Addressing racism and implicit bias part 1: a response to the framework for effective discipline. *Communique*. 2021;49(5):10–12.

Trent M, Dooley DG, Dougé J; Section on Adolescent Health, Council on Community Pediatrics, Committee on Adolescence. The impact of racism on child and adolescent health. *Pediatrics*. 2019;144(2):e20191765.

Van den Bergh BRH, van den Heuvel MI, Lahti M, et al. Prenatal developmental origins of behavior and mental health: The influence of maternal stress in pregnancy. *Neurosci Biobehav Rev*. 2020;117:26–64.

Wilkinsom A, Laurore J, Maxfield E, et al. Zero to three: the state of babies yearbook. *Policy Brief*. 2021.

Williams DR, Lawrence JA, Davis BA. Racism and health: evidence and needed research. *Annu Rev Public Health*. 2019;40:105–125.

Internet Gaming Disorder in Youth

Feng W, Ramo DE, Chan SR, Bourgeois JA. Internet gaming disorder: trends in prevalence 1998–2016. *Addict Behav*. 2017;75:17–24.

Gentile DA, Bailey K, Bavelier D, et al. Internet gaming disorder in children and adolescents. *Pediatrics*. 2017;140(Suppl 2):S81–S85.

Kim NR, Hwang SS, Choi J, et al. Characteristics and psychiatric symptoms of internet gaming disorder among adults using self-reported DSM-5 criteria. *Psychiatry Investig*. 2016;13(1):58.

King DL, Chamberlain SR, Carragher N, et al. Screening and assessment tools for gaming disorder: a comprehensive systematic review. *Clin Psychol Rev*. 2020;77:101831.

Liu Lu, Yao YW, Li CR, et al. The comorbidity between internet gaming disorder and depression: interrelationship and neural mechanisms. *Front Psychiatry*. 2018;9:154.

Pataki C, Bostic JG, Tabor-Furmark KS, et al. Functional assessment of social media in child and adolescent psychiatry. In: Beresin EV, Olsen CK, eds. *Child and Adolescent Psychiatry and the Media*. Elsevier; 2019:93.

Razjouyan K, Khademi M, Dorandish ZY, Davari-Ashtiani R. An investigation into the frequency of addiction to video games in children with attention-deficit hyperactivity disorder. *J Family Med Prim Care*. 2020;9(2):669–672.

Rumpf HJ, Achab S, Billieux J, et al. Including gaming disorder in the ICD-11: the need to do so from a clinical and public health perspective. *J Behav Addict*. 2018;7(3):556–561.

Wang CY, Wu YC, Su CH, Lin PC, Ko CH, Yen JY. Association between internet gaming disorder and generalized anxiety disorder. *J Behav Addict*. 2017;6(4):564–571.

Weinstein A, Leroux M. Neurobiological mechanisms underlying internet gaming disorder. *Dialogues Clin Neurosci*. 2020;22(2):113–126.

Zajac K, Ginley MK, Chang R. Treatments of internet gaming disorder: a systematic review of the evidence. *Expert Rev Neurother*. 2020;20(1):85–93.

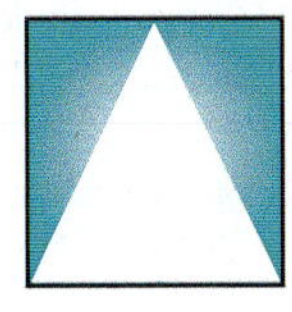

Index

Page numbers followed by *f* indicate figures and page numbers followed by *t* indicate tables.